Lecture Notes
in Business Information Processing

247

More information about this series at http://www.springer.com/series/7911

Theodor Borangiu · Monica Drăgoicea
Henriqueta Nóvoa (Eds.)

Exploring
Services Science

7th International Conference, IESS 2016
Bucharest, Romania, May 25–27, 2016
Proceedings

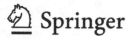
Springer

Editors
Theodor Borangiu
Faculty of Automatic Control
and Computers
University Politehnica of Bucharest
Bucharest
Romania

Monica Drăgoicea
Faculty of Automatic Control
and Computers
University Politehnica of Bucharest
Bucharest
Romania

Henriqueta Nóvoa
Faculty of Engineering - FEUP
University of Porto
Porto
Portugal

ISSN 1865-1348 ISSN 1865-1356 (electronic)
Lecture Notes in Business Information Processing
ISBN 978-3-319-32688-7 ISBN 978-3-319-32689-4 (eBook)
DOI 10.1007/978-3-319-32689-4

Library of Congress Control Number: 2016935960

Printed on acid-free paper

This Springer imprint is published by Springer Nature
The registered company is Springer International Publishing AG Switzerland

Foreword

Service Science was launched by IBM as an open code initiative more than ten years ago in an attempt to integrate different knowledge domains contributing to the study and better understanding of service systems. Since the preliminary proposals, it was clear that the organization, functioning, and development of service systems had to be based on a new conceptualization of services, on relationship governance, and on a new qualification of value generation, as service research has pointed out all along the last decades of scientific production.

In order to address and cope with such demanding theoretical issues in the search for a better understanding of service systems, the service community was inspired by a multicultural approach capable of catalysing into Service Science the scientific contributions proposed by researchers coming not only from IBM, but also from academia and experts in IT, management, and consumer behaviour, sociology, computer science, engineering, and many other disciplines.

Service scientists have accordingly approached the Service Science research path with an open mind and aggregating attitude, inherently and strongly based on T-shaped programs on a global basis, in an attempt to capture intriguing suggestions from different research streams, all interested in advancing knowledge on service systems as well as their modelling and operative traits.

Since 2004 a relevant worldwide community has grown, a community still engaged in this long-lasting process of defining the research boundaries and scientific goals of this inclusive Service Science discipline; however, not all cultural domains have accomplished rewarding results and, moreover, further effort ought to be placed in the integration of various cultural domains.

Within this cross-cultural research setting comes the 7th International Conference on Exploring Service Science, IESS 1.6, an event gathering scholars and researchers from all over the world balancing different categories of scientists and different lines of research — from different perspectives:

- Business oriented vs. technology oriented
- Fundamental vs. applied
- System science foundation vs. computer science support

To approach Service Science, management, and engineering subjects from these multiple innovation perspectives, and to guarantee a cross-cultural approach to Service Science main issues and focus, a number of topics of interest were defined, including: service exploration processes; business transformation through service science; new service business models; modelling of the service consumer needs; service design methodologies and patterns; IT-based service engineering; service orientation in the digital enterprise; modelling and design of IT-enabled service systems; product-service systems; service innovation strategies and solutions; service sustainability; governance of service systems; service system networks; education and skills for service design and management.

The numerous papers received and presented in this volume were grouped into 13 sessions, covering the aforementioned topics. The technological perspective adopted by many scholars balances the managerial point of view of others, once more demonstrating the strong interest of Service Science in an open-minded and interdisciplinary community.

The IESS 1.6 conference met its main goals: to gather scientists working in the Service Science domain, to find out about their most recent research work trying to orient R&D in Service Science toward fundamental contributions leading to this new science, and to encourage new types of service innovation based on this research.

Despite the encouraging results accomplished by the Service Science research context over the last decade, a long research path still has to be pursued in search of even more challenging advances. An overview of the scientific production of our community, in fact, shows that scholars ought to look for more integration among various cultural domains, in order to give rise to this new science and to demolish the cultural boundaries that still appear in the shades of this scientific production.

Service scientists in the future could aim for the production of more interdisciplinary papers, written by scholars coming from different research contexts, and increase the cross-cultural references within each scientific production.

This challenging advance calls for an open-minded attitude brought on by curious researchers willing to study and deepen models and theories according to their specific field of interest, and of course it needs a production systems (journals, book series, reviewers) in line with this approach. The Service Science community is ready for this; hence, let us play a key role in advancing Service Science research in this direction!

February 2016   Francesco Polese

Preface

This volume gathers the peer-reviewed papers that were presented at the 7th International Workshop on Exploring Service Science, IESS 1.6, organized during May 25–27, 2016, by the CIMR Research Centre of the Faculty of Automatic Control and Computer Science, University Politehnica of Bucharest, Romania.

The workshop gathered academic scientists and practitioners from the service industry and their worldwide partners in a collegial and stimulating environment. According to its tradition, IESS 1.6 covered major research and development areas related to Service Science foundations, service engineering and management, service innovation, service orientation of processes, applications in service sectors and ICT support for services.

Services comprise about 75 % of mature economies today, being also a fast-growing sector in emerging economies. This motivates an intense preoccupation to establish the philosophy of a new management and marketing, which highlights a paradigm shift away from the goods-dominant (G–D) logic. This paradigm is the theoretical concept of service-dominant (S–D) logic, fundamental for the service system developments reported in IESS1.6 papers; services are seen as the real protagonists of interactions and transactions.

A broader perspective shows that service systems evolve within dynamic environments and interact, in a network, with other service systems. Also, they may have other interconnected service sub-systems, and thus service systems may have to face external disturbances from the environment, but also internal disturbances generated by one of their sub-systems. Thus, a main challenge in the development of a service system is to design it in a way that ensures the flexibility and adaptability crucial for its survival, or, in other terms, for its viability. From this perspective, the Viable System Model (VSM) is an initial point of such a development strategy, as pointed out by some authors.

The IESS1.6 event includes papers that extend the view on different concepts related to the development of the Service Science domain of study, applying them to frameworks, advanced technologies, and tools for the design of ICT-based service systems.

The perspective introduced by this approach connects Service Science fundamental concepts to business-related concepts. In the Service Science approach, service organizations are studied as service systems evolving in their environment (service system ecology), in the pursuit of their business goal, according to a service business model. Service business models reflect the features of the service sector to which the organization belongs and describe activities for services as business processes. Successful service business models are crucial for the service system viability and they are related to service innovation.

As IESS 1.6 papers describe, specific items of service business models such as target markets and customers, product offerings or value propositions, distribution channels (activities for services), and constraints and profits, together with the description of case studies and business solutions in various service sectors, are analysed and debated.

The book is structured in 13 parts, each one grouping a number of chapters describing research in current domains of service science, from fundamentals, theories, and concepts to models, frameworks, and implementing solutions for societal services (health care, education, administration) and the service industry.

From service theory to solutions, these book sections are: Part 1 – Service Exploration Theories and Processes; Part 2 – Modelling Service Requirements and Management of Business Processes; Part 3 – Value Co-creation Through Knowledge Management and User-Centric Services; Part 4 – Service Design Methodologies and Patterns; Part 5 – Service Innovation and Strategy; Part 6 – IT-Based Service Engineering; Part 7 – Servitization in Sustainable Manufacturing: Models and Information Technologies; Part 8 – Product-Service Systems; Part 9 – Business Software Services and Data-Driven Service Design; Part 10 – Web Service Design and Service-Oriented Agents; Part 11 – IoT and Mobile Apps for Public Transport Service Management; Part 12 – e-Health Services and Medical Data Interoperability; Part 13 – Service and IT-Oriented Learning and Education Systems.

The book offers a new vision on complexity, big data, and context-awareness in data-driven services for the contextual businesses, Service-oriented enterprise architectures, and service-oriented agents in Web and cloud services, by combining emergent ICT, control with distributed intelligence, and multi-agent frameworks for complex, networked service design and management.

The scientific work reported in the workshop technical sessions foster service innovation by allowing different stakeholders to arrive at a consensus in terms of service science fundamentals and build together the future knowledge base in the field of service science.

All these aspects are covered in the present book, which we hope you will find useful reading.

February 2016   Theodor Borangiu
                                                                                             Monica Drăgoicea
                                                                                             Henriqueta Nóvoa

Organization

IESS 1.6 was organized by the CIMR Research Centre of the Faculty of Automatic Control and Computer Science, University Politehnica of Bucharest, Romania, during May 25–27, 2016.

Steering Committee

Michel Léonard	University of Geneva, Switzerland
João Falcão e Cunha	University of Porto, Portugal
Eric Dubois	Luxembourg Institute of Science and Technology, Luxembourg
Theodor Borangiu	University Politehnica of Bucharest, Romania
Monica Drăgoicea	University Politehnica of Bucharest, Romania
Marco de Marco	Università Cattolica del Sacro Cuore, Italy
Henriqueta Nóvoa	University of Porto, Portugal
Gerhard Satzger	Karlsruhe Service Research Institute, Germany
Mehdi Snene	University of Geneva, Switzerland

Conference Chair

Theodor Borangiu	University Politehnica of Bucharest, Romania

Program Chairs

Monica Drăgoicea	University Politehnica of Bucharest, Romania
Henriqueta Nóvoa	University of Porto, Portugal

Sponsoring Institutions

International Society of Service Innovation Professionals, ISSIP
Luxembourg Institute of Science and Technology, Luxembourg
Romanian Academy of Sciences
IBM Romania

International Program Committee

Sabrina Bonomi	University of Verona, Italy
António Brito	University of Porto, Portugal
Bettina Campedelli	University of Verona, Italy
Jorge Cardoso	University of Coimbra, Portugal
María Valeria de Castro	Universidad Rey Juan Carlos, Spain
Sergio Cavalieri	University of Bergamo, Italy

Contents

IT-Based Service Engineering

**Servitization in Sustainable Manufacturing: Models and Information
Technologies**

Product-Service Systems

Business Software Services and Data-Driven Service Design

Service and IT-Oriented Learning and Education Systems

Service Exploration Theories
and Processes

Decision-Making in Smart Service Systems: A Viable Systems Approach Contribution to Service Science Advances

Francesco Polese[✉], Aurelio Tommasetti, Massimiliano Vesci,
Luca Carrubbo, and Orlando Troisi

Department of Business Sciences - Management and Innovation Systems,
University of Salerno, Via Giovanni Paolo II 132,
84084 Fisciano SA, Italy
{fpolese,tommasetti,mvesci,
lcarrubbo,otroisi}@unisa.it

Abstract. In contemporary dynamic markets, approaches to management based on systems theory have assumed increasing relevance, leading firms to valorise a holistic optic to challenge environmental changes. In particular, Viable Systems Approach (vSA) symbolizes the aforementioned holistic view of enterprises, introducing some innovative concepts that renovate traditional managerial paradigms in terms of decision-making. Simultaneously, in the field of service research, Service Science can be interpreted as an all-encompassing framework investigating the efficiency of firms, which are in turn intended as service systems; there are numerous points of convergence between Service Science research stream and the vSA. Therefore, this paper aims to combine the two, highlighting the common features, in order to propose insights for an integrated and shared macro level conceptualization of service systems and smart service systems. The main goal is to demonstrate the opportunities for capturing emerging contributes to Service Science advances. This can be achieved by fostering different views and paradigms, such as the vSA, thus avoiding a possible "missed call" from the existing worldwide Service Science research community.

Keywords: Viable Systems Approach · Viable systems · Service Science · Smart service systems · Decision-making

1 Introduction

The paper aims to analyse the potential contribution of Viable Systems Approach (vSA) to advance Service Science (SS), with a specific focus on decision-making in Smart Service Systems (SSS). Systems Theories as vSA are a useful lens for better understanding complex phenomena and help us to manage and plan modern dynamics in any kind of organization in terms of resource integration, system interaction and viable behaviours. SS studies of service systems and particularly the advances about SSS in any field of interest foster the ground upon which scholars and practitioners try to deepen new ways of decision-making in order to reduce surrounding complexity.

© Springer International Publishing Switzerland 2016
T. Borangiu et al. (Eds.): IESS 2016, LNBIP 247, pp. 3–14, 2016.
DOI: 10.1007/978-3-319-32689-4_1

The decision maker, by adopting a systems framework, better valorises the continuous information exchange and increases comprehension of the context in which he/she operates, by being able to valorise the multiple contributions of Actors within the process of value generation. In this mainframe, SSS are a new generation of service systems that are particularly interesting due to their scalable, adaptable and reactive traits. *vSA* seems to be the right meta-model to better understand SSS dynamics. In fact, its assumptions appear to magnify learning processes, adaptive configurations, systems balance and resonant interactions, all of which appear to be among the key features of SSS.

The main goal of this manuscript is to demonstrate the opportunity for capturing emerging contributes to Service Science advances by fostering different views and paradigms, such as the *vSA*, avoiding a possible "missed call" from the existing worldwide Service Science research community.

The first part of this work focuses on *VSA* insights, highlighting its origins and its application for complexity and decision-making; next, an analysis of systems dynamics (regarding value co-creation, quality of performances, competitiveness) under the *vSA* lens is conducted.

The paper's findings are directed to the decision-making in SSS analysis, looking for a sustainable management of contextual emergence of complex environment in which organizations operate today. In this way, some of the foundational concepts of *vSA* (FCs) are used to highlight several insights useful for SS.

Within the paper, several "boxes" are shown; in these how *vSA* mainstream helps decision-making process in service systems are detailed.

Further a combined SS-*vSA* interpretative model for decision-making is proposed to give a new possible framework for the understanding of complex phenomena.

Finally, the possible contribution of *vSA* in the evolving general definition of SSS is presented as a synthesis of all arguments here afforded.

2   *vSA* as a Lens for Understanding Complex Phenomena

2.1   Systems View

Today business scenarios are characterized by globalization, social and political evolutions, technological innovation and other factors that determine a rising hyper-competition. This, in turn, leads to complexity. This phenomenon, examined by many disciplines, refers to the inability of organizations to act in an unstable context, in which rules are not 'a priori' defined and the risk is high. To tackle this uncertainty, firms should broaden their boundaries and establish relationships with other entities operating in the same environment (i.e., other public or private companies, institutions and all the stakeholders involved in their conduct; we can refer to these as Actors).

This fundamental assumption has gradually led to the foundation of the general system thinking as a sort of a mindset representing an underlying common thread of current managerial models [1]. This paradigm, based on a logical-formal approach to the observation of every system in nature, society and scientific domains, evolved during the last century into the so-called systems theories [2–6]. Using this lens, observers (i.e., scholars, practitioners, managers, and others) can fully understand a phenomenon. They do this not only by breaking it up into elementary parts and then reforming it (as reductionism does); that is considered as a necessary but not sufficient condition for a total comprehensive vision [7]. Systemic views help, in fact, in taking into account any situation that can occur, intending any phenomena as a whole, as the right *continuum* between holism and reductionism.

In line with this shift from "the part to the whole" [8], various theoretical frameworks with different focuses were elaborated [9–11]. Between them, the *Viable Systems Approach - vSA* [12, 13], rooted in systems thinking and based on the *Viable System Model - VSM* [14], stands out from other systemic theories for its capacity to define complexity and to introduce adequate tools to solve it.

Systems theories understand *organizations* as a set of logical components generating a higher-level system that is different from the sum of the single elements producing mutual benefits for each member. To survive in a complex environment, *organizations* (like firms or companies) should relate to other systems in the environment.

In any context, there are many aspects which each organization has to focus on. Linear relationships, the quantity of actors involved in the same context and specifically related to each other, the evolution in demand, the constant *indeterminacy* of the future, the difficulty of making correct decisions and to survive in the long run are some of the main features increasing the level of complexity to be managed and reduced [15]. From a systems theories point of view, complexity is a subjective concept, not interpretable in absolute terms, that can be studied only through the understanding a specific context by a government of an organization seeking to make a wise decision [16]. In fact, in addressing complex situations, we should take into account that the level of complexity is perceived differently by observers (cfr. *variety*), or by the same observer in different moments (cfr. *variability*).

vSA has 10 foundational concepts (FCs) to focus on in order to synthesize properly its main assumptions [17]; most of them appear to be helpful ways to describe the topic we want to deepen. The dynamic point of view, instead, promotes the transition from an objective to a subjective manifestation of complexity, considering that the definition of the context made by decision makers is influenced by their own particular perception of the context. «The interpretation of complex phenomena requires interdisciplinary approaches, and should synthesize both a reductionist view analyzing specific constituents and parts (and their relations) and a holistic view capable of observing the whole» (*vSA* - FC3). Indeed, in the passages from the whole to the parts (and vice versa) the contribution of relations (static, structural) and interactions (dynamic, systemic) is fundamental to their role in the observed phenomenon (reality).

2.2   Dealing with Service Research

The systems vision, completely embraced by *vSA*, is also espoused by theories pertaining to different areas, such as service research, which in turn has been characterized in recent decades by a shift towards a holistic conception of consumption as an interactive, multi-subject, comprehensive process, being at the same time beneficial (or Actors) to all the parties involved [18].

Among the numerous service theories proposed, *Service science, management, engineering and design* (known as SS, SSMED, or Service Science) [19] is certainly one of the most appreciated worldwide. Introduced to better understand the role of service in today's society and to start a long-term open source project, this framework aims at unifying the thinking of scholars, academic institutions, and professionals in a general perspective focused on service. Such a discipline emerged to address the lack of an integrated and multidisciplinary framework for studying the design, the delivery and the evaluation of services [20]. In this sense, the contribution deriving from different domains can help to improve and foster advances in knowledge, surpassing what is on the edge. Starting from SS studies, it is especially interesting to verify in which ways *vSa* supports the design and functioning of service systems, and, particularly, their decision-making process.

The units of analysis of SS are service systems, conceptualized as a «dynamic value co-creation configuration of resources, including people, organizations, shared information (language, laws, measures, methods), and technology, all connected internally and externally to other service systems by value propositions» [21, p. 5]. These open systems are: (1) capable of improving the state of another system through sharing or applying its resource and (2) capable of improving their own state by acquiring external resources [21].

Furthermore, to take into account the proactive adaptation of organizations to the variable contextual conditions as a key factor for competitiveness and survival in the long run, the notion of SSS [22] was formulated. The mechanism of learning is central to these systems, since these entities are capable of self-reconfiguring themselves in order to perform enduring behavior among engaged actors [23]. SSS are thus based upon interactions among actors, and dynamically perform through reactive and pro-active behavior within their wider relational context [24].

Under a systems view, «Systems are open for their connection with many other systems exchanging resources. A system's boundary realizes a filter with regard to the external complexity. It is changing and comprises all their activities and resources needed within the system evolutionary dynamic» (*vSa*– FC4). This concept represents evidence of the common thread between *vSa* and SS itself [25]. In detail, as discussed in following paragraphs, SS can benefit from the *vSa*'s assumptions, both from a theoretical point of view, thanks to concepts such as complexity and viability addressing organizations to better manage uncertainty, and from a practical standpoint, directing management to the implementation of more competitive and sustainable actions.

3   *vSa* as a Model for Decision-Making of Smart Service Systems

Based on the difference between holistic and reductionist view, *vSa* re-defines traditional managerial theories by adapting old conceptualizations to today's economic and social background. The new main framework affects insights for decision- making, particularly through the introductions of two aspects: (1) the transition from environment to context through the identification of external systems; (2) the distinction between consonance and resonance and between structure and system;

First, *vSA* considers organizations (including firms and enterprises) as viable systems (VS) whose final goals is survival over time; then, relationships with stakeholders are essential in the first place to comprehend the context in which we operate and, secondly, to use this knowledge to tackle variety and variability.

The various and homogeneous groups of potential stakeholders can be identified as supra-systems or sub-systems [12]. Sub-systems (employees, property, finance, etc.) are internal to the system and ought to be directed by managers in order to contribute to the system's finality [26]. Supra-systems are external and overruled by the system, and are hierarchically ordered based on critical resources they possess and of their influence on the system (supplying, distribution, consumers, public administration, media, etc.).

The selection of supra and sub-systems leads firms to the passage from a macro level, the environment comprising all the potential stakeholders, to a meso-level, the effective context in which all the stakeholders are selected to gain an organization's specific objectives.

BOX 1 - *How vSA helps decision-making in service systems:*
Managers that govern business plans, strategies and operations should possess the ability to organize relationships, transforming survival impulses into decisions contributing to the establishment of both internal and external equilibrium while simultaneously achieving efficiency.

Another implication for decision-making is related to the structure–system dichotomy, coinciding with the opposition between consonance and resonance. The structure refers to the set of correlated physical elements of organizations (human resources, equipment), defining what is proper to the structure and what is extraneous to it [27]. It includes components, to which a manager attributes a specific function, and a set of stable links between the components.

On the contrary, the system perspective overcomes organizational boundaries concerning the concrete relationships between components emerging during the ongoing interactions, leading to the emergence of a potential system from the structure.

Further, the *vSA* concepts of consonance and resonance connect to the concepts of structure and system. Consonance is the structural compatibility between the actors of a system representing the potential relations among them (static vision), while resonance is the actual harmonic interactions (dynamic vision) concretely occurring [12]. The physical components of structure may relate potentially in many different ways: from a structure, in fact, many systems may arise, depending on the peculiarity of the specific decision-making process.

The key role of *vSA*'s assumptions in supporting decision-making assumes particular relevance for business, especially when considering that firms can be viewed, in a service science optic, as service systems [28].

BOX 2 - How vSA helps decision-making in service systems:
Maximizing all the contributions shared by a single company and its stakeholders'
top management should renew the internal resources possessed by the firm, giving
rise to more specific skills that enable creation of inimitable added value.

Both SS and vSA see modern organizations as systems, challenging traditional management canons and theoretical models [29]. Therefore, this integration consists in the new interpretation of service systems in the light of vSA's principles that can strengthen the notion, broadening the perspective of this study.

The starting point of these two frameworks is the identification of networks of relationships in the contemporary economic environment; this reticular configuration leads in both cases to the transition from a reductionist and short-term vision to a holistic and long-term viewpoint. VS in the first case and service systems in the second one are intended as an integrated whole of interacting connections.

Another fundamental thing is the acknowledged importance of the exchange of intangible resources, which produce new knowledge, consequently creating new rules for the understanding of complexity determining survival conditions. In fact, one of the key concepts of SS, as shown by the definition of service system itself, valorizes the role of knowledge and information.

In parallel with service systems' pursuit of a common goal, vSA introduces the notion of equifinality, based on the achievement of different but mutual goals for each subject, determined by a synergy of objectives produced by resources exchange [17].

Starting from these sequential theoretical intersections, highlighting the similarities between the two frameworks, VSA can offer many practical implications, concretely identifying the conduct decision makers should implement to survive in the context and to gain sustainable advantages.

BOX 3 - How vSA helps decision-making in service systems:
In order to obtain new knowledge, managers should have a proactive behavior and to make it sustainable really, they ought to actively react to environmental transformations, predicting the possible alterations of context, interpreting the changes, and accepting all the risks connected with this conduct.

In summary, even if SS and vSA simultaneously affirm the predominance of collective interests over individual ones, the innovative feature of vSA can be individuated in the transition from a traditional competitive view to a more sustainable resonant (win–win) logic. This optic based on the establishment of dynamic interactions with contextual entities in order to adopt an adaptive and proactive behavior, is necessary to survive in an increasingly complex environment. This leads to a re-thinking of the value generation process, first in terms of multi-part contributions at all levels of co-creation phases [30].

4   *VSA* as a Support for the Definition of Smart Service Systems: New Proposal for a Combined *VSA*-SS Interpretative Model

The principles of *VSA* are essentially convergent with SS's assumptions; in particular, *VSA* contributes to better define and clarify the essence and the functioning of service systems, especially considering that the conceptual nature of SSS has not yet been defined sufficiently.

Indeed, viable systems might conceptually "include" SSS, since the aspect of smartness does not conceptually contain all the features of viability [17]. As discussed before, viability implies a long-range vision concerning the enduring characteristics that enable a service system to survive over time through consonance and resonance, while smartness is not adequately analysed, since its relation to the attainment of a sustainable advantage deserves further attention. It follows that viability represents an essential and necessary prerequisite to operate in the contemporary context, and smartness is a trait of proactive behaviour: if a viable system is always a, smart system, not all smart systems are viable systems.

In other words, service systems are smart if they react to circumstances and make a rational and efficient use of resources, a concept that is not different from *VSA*'s suggestions on the role of consonance and resonance to acquire enduring viability. In addition, all the sub-systems of a viable system share a common goal, a determined finality pursued by the whole system, similar to the way in which smart service systems are oriented towards enduring performance and towards satisfaction of all the involved actors.

The governance of viable/smart service systems (VS/SSS) should direct the system towards a final goal, transforming static structural relationships into dynamic interactions with other entities [31]. Therefore, an efficient government should have the ability to organize relationships, thus contributing to the equilibrium of the system and to the satisfaction of supra-systems.

BOX 4 - How VSA helps decision-making in service systems:
To implement SS's sustainable vision, managers need key knowledge about internal factors (distinctive elements, know-how, skills, expertise, capacity, technology, etc.) and should take into account threats and opportunities arising from the context. The consideration of the needs of other entities can significantly limit in such a case the autonomy of decision-making and the flexibility of the system.

This endogenous limitation could make it difficult to coordinate service system's entities due to the intrinsic independence of the top management of each system in determining and pursuing its own mission. To bridge this gap, service system's managers should try to enhance interests' convergence, addressing the policies of each entity towards shared activities [32].

However, in balancing exogenous needs, it may be difficult to identify an adequate relational asset within a group of aggregative but heterogeneous elements. Hence, effective governance is fundamental in order to reinforce relationships' resonance.

The integration between the two frameworks can be accomplished through the adoption of a methodology taking advantage of the above-examined conceptual relations from both a design and a managerial point of view.

BOX 5 - How vSA helps decision-making in service systems:
Managers should elaborate specific strategies intended to harmonize and valorise the structural diversity and the contrasting interests of various entities, fostering the emergence of a circular process of value co-creation generating an overall synergy of knowledge, superior to the simple sum of the singular contributions of each actor involved.

The implications for decision-making entailed by vSA allow to combine the concept of viable systems (VS) with the notion of SSS, matching the aforementioned four basic characteristics of the latter (people, organizations, technology, shared information) with the various components of the network systems postulated in vSA. In vSA, the dimension of *people* could be related to all the members involved in the service delivery process, then both sub-systems (including employees and the human factor within the operating structure- OS) and supra- systems, comprising suppliers, consumers and co-makers in general. In fact, the challenge of SS lies not only in the formal construction of technology or organizational interactions, but also in the formation of people and in the configuration of their role as workers for the knowledge of the system [33]. *Organizations*, as mentioned, are not physically accessible resources, equipped with the ability to establish formal and informal relationships with other stakeholders. In this context, organizations are supra-systems (governmental political supra-system, labour supra-system, etc.) designed to encourage each member to participate in the service while establishing constraints and legislative and institutional rules to regulate the conduct of companies. Through the *sharing of information* (and of immaterial resources in general) then, according to vSA through the establishment of trust-based relationships permitting a circular exchange of knowledge among all the actors involved, consumers/ citizens can participate in the life of an enterprise, expressing their needs, and also providing their opinions about the service and offering possible solutions. In short, they can be considered as real 'experts' who collaborate in the design of the offer.

As shown in Fig. 1, thanks to the systemic vision shared by the two research streams, decision-makers (DM) studying the context and starting from a macro-environment can select meta- and meso-environments. In this way, complexity is gradually reduced moving to complication and identifying the key partners with whom establishing consonance and then resonance, according to win-win logic. In an integrated viewpoint combining SS with vSA, DM can enjoy a careful choice of stakeholders. Then, thanks to an appropriate training of human capital, they can create, through the sharing of information, a circular path of knowledge exchange generating co-learning, and thus innovation and sustainable advantage in the long run [34].

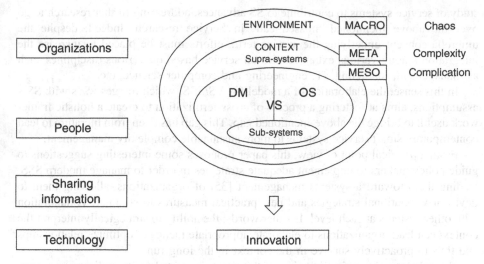

Fig. 1. An integrated model for decision- making combining *vSA* and SS: toward VS/SSS (**Source**: Authors' elaboration.).

5   Discussions, Implications and Future Research to Avoid a Potential "Missed Call"

In the light of the common holistic view embraced by both the examined theories, the present paper undertakes a discussion aimed at individuating the similarities between *vSA* and SS, highlighting the practical implications entailed by *vSA* that permit to pinpoint the concrete consequences that the conceptualization of this framework involves in terms of suggestions for decision-making.

Summarizing the debate's results, the points of contact between *vSA* and SS concern in particular three features: the key role of relationships to challenge environmental instability; the new collaborative logic contrasting with the old competitive vision; and the necessity of adopting a systems management of contemporary enterprises. Even if these similarities stress an underlying and shared all-inclusive mentality, *vSA*, by detaching from the sole theoretical level, appears to provide some concrete proposals that challenge the issue of current hyper-competition. As a result, since *vSA*'s assumptions can be situated at the bottom of organizational strategies, it can be sustained that the implications of the application of this theory to SS, and particularly to service systems, are both theoretical and managerial.

From a conceptual perspective, the study could help researchers and academics to understand the functioning and the relational dynamics of organizations, providing them with insights useful to address them to a systematization of the notion of SSS, which proposes an all-encompassing optic, which can be easily espoused by other theories.

Moreover, by taking advantage of *vSA*, which combines biology, social science, physics and tektology (the last is a discipline synthesizing the previous branches), the current work shows the benefits deriving from the adoption of several domains in the study of service systems to contribute to SS advances, addressing further research to go over the above mentioned 'missed call' in Service research. Indeed, despite the umbrella concept underlying the service term, efforts must be placed to increase the integration among various extant studies on service based on various disciplines such as management, marketing, IT, engineering and computer science, etc.

In this sense, the elaboration of a model for VS/SSS, which merges *vSA*'s with SS's assumptions, aims at fostering a process of cross-fertilization to create a holistic framework useful to bridge the above-mentioned gap. This gap has risen from literature to lead contemporary smart service systems to more sustainable complexity management.

From a practical point of view, this paper proposes some interesting suggestions to guide policy makers to implement adequate strategies in order to manage modern SSS, leading them toward a systems management [35] of organizations, allowing them to devise new relational strategies and new practical measures to stimulate collaboration with other systems at each level. In other words, the ability to strategically interpret the context can lead organizations to elaborate appropriate tactics to optimize relationships and thus to proactively survive in the context in the long run.

Nevertheless, the main limitation of this work is related to its preliminary nature, representing only a starting point for directing future research in this area. Actually, the assumptions introduced here require further empirical studies designed to investigate the relationship between the level of collaboration of a service system and its governance effectiveness, as well as the relationship between the systems management of service systems and the generation of innovation and satisfaction for each actor.

In this sense, the present paper only sets the foundations for concretely validating the implementation of smart service systems across different kinds of services, especially considering that these systems are capable of improving the quality of service [17] and hoping for the creation of a general unifying vision connecting various managerial and service theories.

References

1. Barile, S., Polese, F., Pels, J., Saviano, M.: An introduction to the viable systems approach and its contribution to marketing. In: Barile, S. (ed.) Contribution to Theoretical and Practical Advances in Management, vol. 2, pp. 1–37. Aracne, Roma (2013)
2. Bogdanov, A.: Tektologiya: Vseobschaya Organizatsionnaya Nauka. Berlin and Petrograd, Moscow (1922)
3. Bogdanov, A.: Essays in Tektology: The General Science of Organization. Intersystems Publications, Seaside (1980). Trans. By George Gorelik
4. Von Bertalanffy, L.: General System theory: Foundations, Development, Applications. George Braziller, New York (1968)
5. Laszlo, E.: The Systems View of the World: A Holistic Vision for Our Time. Hampton Press, New Jersey (1996)
6. Meadows, D.H.: Thinking in Systems: A Primer. Chelsea Green Publishing, Chelsea (2008)
7. Barile, S., Saviano, M., Polese, F., Di Nauta, P.: Reflections on service systems boundaries: a viable systems perspective. The case of the London borough of sutton. Eur. Manag. J. **30**, 451–465 (2012)

8. Capra, F.: The web of life. Doubleday-Anchor Book, New York (1997)
9. Boulding, K.: General systems theory - the skeleton of science. Manage. Sci. **2**(3), 197–208 (1956)
10. Maturana, H.R., Varela, F.J.: Autopoietic systems. BLC Report 9, University of Illinois (1975)
11. Senge, P.M.: The Fifth Discipline, The Art and Practice of the Learning Organization. Doubleyday Currency, New York (1990)
12. Golinelli, G.M.: L'approccio sistemico al governo dell'impresa. L'impresa sistema vitale. CEDAM, Padova (2000)
13. Barile, S.: L'impresa come sistema. Contributi sull'Approccio Sistemico Vitale. Giappichelli, Torino (2006)
14. Beer, S.: The viable system model: its provenance, development, methodology and pathology. J. Oper. Res. Soc. **35**(1), 7–25 (1984)
15. Ng, I., Badinelli, R., Polese, F., Di Nauta, P., Löbler, H., Halliday, S.: S-D logic research directions and opportunities: the perspective of systems, complexity and engineering. Mark. Theory **12**(2), 213–217 (2012)
16. Barile, S., Carrubbo, L., Iandolo, F., Caputo, F.: From 'EGO' to 'ECO' in B2B relationships. J. Bus. Market Manag. **6**(4), 228–253 (2013)
17. Barile, S., Polese, F.: Smart service systems and viable service systems. Serv. Sci. **2**(1/2), 21–40 (2010)
18. Barile, S., Saviano, M., Pels, J., Polese, F., Carrubbo, L.: The contribution of VSA and SDl. Perspectives to strategic thinking in emerging economies. Manag. Serv. Qual. **24**(6), 565–591 (2014)
19. Maglio, P.P., Spohrer, J.: Fundamentals of service science. J. Acad. Mark. Sci. **36**(1), 18–20 (2008)
20. Spohrer, J., Maglio, P.P., Bailey, J., Gruhl, D.: Steps toward a science of service systems. IEEE Comput. **40**(1), 71–77 (2007)
21. Spohrer, J., Vargo, S.L., Maglio, P.P, Caswell, N.: The service system is the basic abstraction of service science. In: Proceedings of the 41st Annual Hawaii International Conference on System Sciences, pp. 104–104. IEEE Press, Honolulu (2008)
22. Demirkan, H., Spohrer, J., Krishna, V.: Service Systems Implementation. Springer, New York (2011)
23. Mele, C., Pels, J., Polese, F.: A brief review of systems theories and their managerial applications. Serv. Sci. **2**(1/2), 126–135 (2010)
24. Carrubbo, L.: La Co-creazione di valore nelle destinazioni turistiche. RIREA, Roma (2013)
25. Mele, C., Polese, F.: Key dimensions of service systems in value-creating networks. In: Demirkan, H., Spohrer, J., Krishna, V. (eds.) The Science of Service Systems, pp. 37–59. Springer, New York (2011)
26. Barile, S.: L'impresa come sistema. Contributi sull'approccio sistemico vitale. Giappichelli, Torino (2008)
27. Laumann, E.O., Marsden, P.V., Prensky, D.: The boundary specification problem in network analysis. In: Freeman, L.C., White, D.R., Romney, A.K. (eds.) Research Methods in Social Network Analysis, pp. 61–89. Transaction Publishers, New Brunswick (1992)
28. Bartlett, C.A., Ghoshal, S.: The multinational corporation as an interorganizational network. Acad. Manag. Rev. **15**(4), 603–625 (1990)
29. Barile, S., Spohrer, J., Polese, F.: System thinking for service research advances. Serv. Sci. **2**(1/2), i–iii (2010)
30. Wieland, H., Polese, F., Vargo, S., Lusch, R.: Toward a service (Eco) systems perspective on value creation. Int. J. Serv. Sci. Manag. Eng. Technol. **3**(3), 12–25 (2012)

14   F. Polese et al.

31. Pels, J., Barile, S., Saviano, M., Polese, F.: VSA and SDL contribution to strategic thinking in emerging economies. In: Gummesson, E., Mele, C., Polese, F. (eds.) Service-Dominant Logic, Network & Systems Theory and Service Science: Integrating Three Perspectives for a New Service Agenda, p. 100. Giannini Editore, Napoli (2013)
32. Polese, F., Di Nauta, P.: A viable systems approach to relationship management in S-D logic and service science. Bus. Adm. Rev. Schäffer-Poeschel **73**(2), 113–129 (2013)
33. Tommasetti, A., Vesci, M., Troisi, O.: The internet of things and value co-creation in a service dominant logic perspective. In: Colace, F., De Santo, M., Moscato, V., Picariello, A., Schreiber, F.A., Tanca, L. (eds.) Data Management in Pervasive Systems, pp. 3–18. Springer, Berlin (2015)
34. Barile, S., Polese, F., Calabrese, M., Iandolo, F., Carrubbo, L.: A theoretical framework for measuring value creation based upon Viable Systems Approach. In: Barile, S. (ed.) Contributions to Theoretical and Practical Evidences in Management. A Viable Systems Approach (VSA), vol. 2, pp. 61–94. Aracne, Roma (2013)
35. Barile, S.: Management Sistemico Vitale. Giappichelli, Torino (2009)

On a Qualitative Game Theoretic Approach of Teacher-Student Interaction in a Public Higher Education Service System

Virginia Ecaterina Oltean[✉], Theodor Borangiu, and Monica Drăgoicea

Faculty of Automatic Control and Computers, Politehnica University of Bucharest,
Splaiul Independenței 313A, 77206 Bucharest, Romania
ecaterina_oltean@yahoo.com, borangiu@cimr.pub.ro,
monica.dragoicea@acse.pub.ro

Abstract. Public higher education services receive nowadays intense attention from the society from at least two perspectives: the high level professional performances requested by companies and public administration as final customers of the educational service system, on one side, and the problem encountered by the authorities in deciding how to dedicate the financial support for universities from the public budget, taking into account also the present state of the labour market and its trend, on another side. Starting from empirical considerations, this paper proposes an ontology model of a generic public higher education service system and several scenarios regarding a qualitative game modelling approach of a Teacher-Student interaction when this service system is placed in an emerging economy and, comparatively, in a mature free market economy.

Keywords: Bimatrix game · Dominant strategy · Decision system · Evolutionary game · Strategic game · Extensive form game · Value co-creation · Service system ontology

1 Introduction and Motivation

Higher education services receive nowadays intense attention from the society from at least two perspectives: on one side, there is an increasing need, among the final beneficiaries - companies and public administration - of the higher education service system for human resource capable of high level professional performances, according to the complex tasks and duties arising in a global and interconnected world, so everyone, including the students, ask for quality in the educational process; on another side, public education is in general entirely sustained from the public budget, so the government, as central authority, has to choose criteria to dedicate the financial support for universities, including the introduction of a hierarchy among these public institutions, taking into account also the present state of the labour market and its trend.

The formal approach in describing the service interactions in public education systems is not straightforward, firstly because, when talking about decision systems and

© Springer International Publishing Switzerland 2016
T. Borangiu et al. (Eds.): IESS 2016, LNBIP 247, pp. 15–29, 2016.
DOI: 10.1007/978-3-319-32689-4_2

games, the strategies as well as the associated gains for each rational agent are rather complicated to be defined, as they concern human behaviour. Moreover, regarded as service systems [1], public education systems are strongly interconnected with the economic environment and with the cultural tradition, among others, so a formal model of the decisions and options in the educational service process [2] has to emphasize also the influences of other systems in the service system ecology.

There are multiple viewpoints in the literature from which the decisions and options in educational systems are analyzed and tackled as decisions systems and games. An important common feature of these studies is that the dynamic 'economic theory of education' [3] is employed as a modelling basis for decisions and interactions in educational systems. Also, the student's achievements are considered to have a public good nature and the actors involved are considered as rational agents [4]. The key challenge is that individuals and governments often face hard choices because of the scarce resources they possess, on one side, and the fact that education is a process with long term effects, on the other side, so a potential "mistake" in decision making cannot be quickly "corrected".

Despite the huge diversity of studies available, depending on the economic environments of the service systems one can distinguish three main classes of viewpoints and subjects in the analysis of public higher education service systems.

In case of emerging economies in democratic countries, the public financial resources are rather scarce, and the problem is the policy of government subsidization for education in presence of the constitutional right to education. An analysis on this subject, discussing also specific costs and key performance indexes is given in [5].

In high-competitive economies, the focus is on the battle for advanced technologies, requiring top human knowledge and competence. Fukiharu [6] discusses the problem of reforming public universities in Japan, to promote higher technologies in presence of global competition, with focus on maximization of universities' prestige as a function of quality of teaching and research. From the perspective of educational costs, Şahin [7] uses a game-theoretic model to analyze the relation between tuition subsidies and the student's motivation for professional effort.

Enlarging the perspective, some studies consider the national public education systems only as subsystems of a global, interconnected system. When students can choose between several universities, passing from one country to another, not only competition, but also other effects may appear. From this viewpoint, Franck and Owen [8] propose a two-country game-theoretic framework focused on the nexus between human capital formation and international migration, in a framework where students can choose, balancing between costs and quality, to study home or abroad, with distinctive brain drain and/or gain effects that can arise.

Starting from authors' educational and research experience, from informal discussions between academia and business and also from concrete educational policies in some of Eastern-European democracies, with specific budget allocation mechanisms for low salaries in education, this paper proposes an integrative, empirically-based perspective on higher education service systems from three view points: the ontological structure, the value co-creation paradigm and the teacher-student interaction model as a qualitative bimatrix game.

The quest for an integrated view is motivated by the need of constructing generic, unified qualitative models of higher education service systems, as a prerequisite for understanding the internal and external systemic interactions on one side, and for developing quantitative research frames and building key performance indexes for higher education quality.

Based on authors' previous work [2] and on the foundational concepts of Service Science [1], an ontology structure of a public higher education service system and a description of a two-stage value co-creation process are introduced in Sect. 2. Section 3 proposes several qualitative game-theoretic models of the Teacher-Student interaction in an emerging economy and, comparatively, in a mature free market economy. Concluding remarks are finally formulated.

2 Specific Aspects in a Public Higher Education Service System Ontology

2.1 Entities, Stakeholders, Activities and Interactions in a Public Higher Education Service System

Recall that Service Science (SS) is based on ten foundational concepts: *resources, entities, access rights, value co-creation interaction, governance interaction, outcomes, stakeholders, measures, networks* and *ecology* [1], which can be configured, around the *service system, service* and *value proposition* concepts, as a conceptual description or SS worldview [2, 9].

One can consider higher education services as information services, but in a more complex and broader sense than the one specified in [10], where "information processing services deal with the collection, manipulation, interpretation, and transmission of data to create value for the client."

Starting from the generic model discussed in [2], an ontology structure of a higher education service system is proposed in Fig. 1. The main stakeholders are: the Teacher, as initiator of the educational service, based on creation of educational value propositions, the Student, as beneficiary and participant to the educational service and potential Graduate, the Employer, as observer, potential sponsor and principal beneficiary of the educational service, and the public Authority, as decision maker in what concerns the educational policy and financing.

A key feature of a higher education service system is that the Student, as stakeholder, is not customer in the usual sense, because the final beneficiary of the educated human resource, as main service outcome, is the Employer and, in a broader sense, the society, i.e. the ecology of the educational service system.

Strictly speaking, the Employer is part of the ecology of the public educational service system, but he may be involved in the configuring and sponsoring of specific educational programs, influencing the value propositions, on one side, and as consumer of the human resource, by jobs offerings, on the other side.

A second important feature of the public higher education service system is, as already emphasized in Sect. 1, the fact that it provides not only immediate, short term outcomes, but also long term outcomes, for at least one generation.

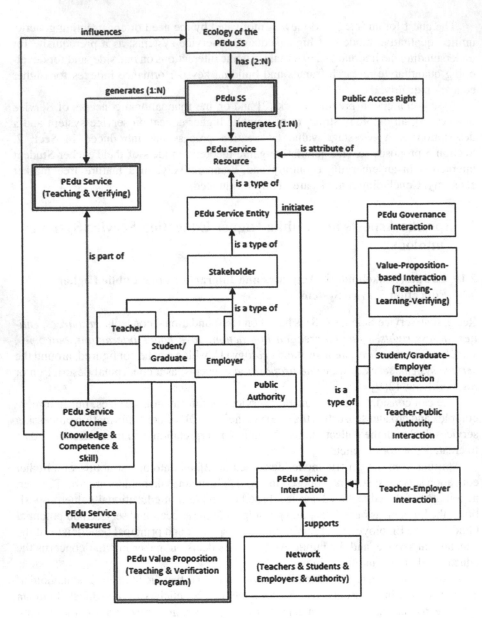

Fig. 1. A Public Educational Service System (PEdu SS) ontology – an instance of the general ontology proposed in [2].

The relations between the Employer, the public higher education system, requiring financial support and the Authority as decision maker are influenced by the economic environment (Fig. 2).

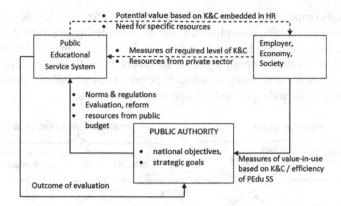

Fig. 2. The relations between the Public Educational Service System (PEdu SS), the socio-economic environment (employer, economy, society) as final beneficiary of the educational service and the authority, as provider of the main financial support for public education; the PEdu SS offers value based on knowledge and competence (K&C) embedded in the educated human resource (HR); in emerging economies, the dashed links are weaker or absent.

A third important feature of the public educational service system is the difficulty to elaborate key performance indexes and service measures. Finally, the question that remains is how valuable is the educated human mind, compared to the less educated one. The quest for a quantification of education value drives to a discussion concerning the value co-creation and the utility function.

2.2 Value Co-creation in a Public Higher Education Service

The general value co-creation perspective proposed in [11] concerns the two main stakeholders of a service, the customer as value creator and co-producer and the service provider, as value facilitator and co-creator, so the corresponding joint utility function of a service is constructed by adding the value-in-use, important for the customer to the total firm's profit [12].

Based on the ontological structure (Fig. 1) and on the specific features of the public education service system, the view of the educational value co-creation process has to be adapted into a two-stage paradigm, in which the former student, as beneficiary in the teaching-learning-verifying service interaction becomes facilitator of value based on knowledge and competence as employee, while the employer and the society are the final beneficiaries of the educational service (Fig. 3).

At a first stage, the utility value concerns acquiring knowledge, competence and also ability for further learning by the Student, and the service consists of teaching and verifying: the Teacher proposes a teaching and verifying program and the Student studies and gets knowledge and competence; in this interaction, both Teacher and Student may adapt their methods and expectations after first evaluations, in the ongoing learning process. The Student may also quit, and then value is not co-created.

After the Student graduates, he becomes human resource in economy and society and interacts, in the labour market, with the Employer: the Graduate makes an offer of knowledge and competence, the Employer makes a job offer, and they negotiate. If the former Student, as Graduate, is employed, value is co-created as he gets a salary payment and generates future value in the working process. This value generated in the second-stage is as higher as the company's goal is to produce goods and services with high added value, implicitly containing the already acquired knowledge and competence of the former Student, including his ability as creative problem solver.

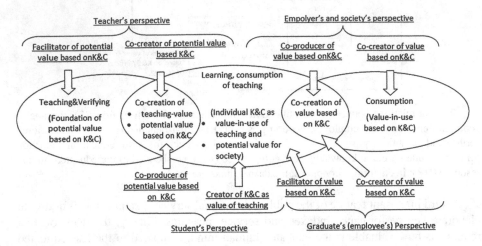

Fig. 3. Co-creation of potential value, based on knowledge and competence (K&C) acquired through education is a prerequisite for co-creation of value based on K&C in society.

The quantification of the value embedded in the goods and services is only partly reflected by the company's results, as the human resource carries also the germs of future development, through innovation and creativity. In emerging economies, the creativity and innovation of human workforce do not get, in general, a central role in the labour market, as the companies cannot compete for new innovative products and services, implying, in general, high initial costs and technologies. These aspects influence not only the relations between the employers and the employees, but also the expectations of the Student, when deciding to participate to a higher education program, and also the teaching and verification program offered by the Teacher. Consequently, the final value generated by a public higher education service system is in general lower in emerging economies, even if the human potential of learning, innovating and creation is high.

3 Decisions and Game Models in Public Higher Education Services

In the sequel, in terms of evolutionary games, Teacher and Student signify a large population of - more or less - identical teachers and students, respectively, as players in the educational game model. Their actions and the corresponding game outcome result from a dynamic process, rather than of rational analysis. The authority decides upon the financial support for the educational system and the corresponding norms, policies and regulations, at a tactic level. The proposed qualitative scenarios are empirically deduced by extrapolating qualitative observations on socio-political, economic and educational realities in Eastern-Europe countries to a generic emerging economy environment. A comparison with a qualitative scenario placed in a generic mature free market economy, deduced on similar empirical considerations regarding advanced European countries, is finally discussed.

3.1 The Public Authority's Decisions in a Generic Emerging Economy Environment

The description of the economic and social environment is synthesized by the following aspects, composing the basic assumption for the decisions that the public authority will make.

Assumption 1. (1) The economy is in transition, so the local and external markets are changing, not always in favour of existent local economic traditions and heritage. (2) The national companies have not yet the capacity to produce goods and services with high and very high added value. (3) The foreign companies are not yet interested to develop local design and research centres, but are mainly focussed on execution of their own projects with cheaper local workforce. (4) Part of the local companies has financial difficulties, so the authority expects to face also a certain rate of unemployment or, at best, to face a low level of salaries.

   Public authority's strategic objective is to maintain *global social peace* and to ensure an (even unstable) social equilibrium by democratic actions. As economic performance and welfare cannot reach the level of national expectations, the public authority has to ensure *the survival* of the two main (populations of) entities acting and interacting in the public higher education service system: Student and Teacher.

   The situation described in Assumption 1 has several consequences for the public educational system, which the public authority must face in its attempt to maintain the social peace.

Consequence 1: *there is no supplementary financial support for education and no direct relation or cooperation between the universities and the final beneficiary of the educational service.* The authority cannot propose and impose laws and regulations aimed to improve the financial support for the higher education public sector from private sources. In theory, the desired supplementary financial support is supposed to consist of dedicated contributions of the companies interested in those sectors for which public faculties ensure specific *knowledge and competence* (K&C), attested by licence's and master's degrees. Hence: (1) the only financial resources for public higher education are the public central and local budgets, both under pressure and (2) the companies (national or foreign) are not motivated and interested to get their human resources in partnership with the public universities, as they can get "cheap" workforce without need of significant recruitment effort.

Consequence 2: *there is no Student's motivation for research and top knowledge, the Student has simultaneously a full time job to survive, so he is also employee.* Due to consequence 1, in context of assumption 1, the authority cannot ensure the financial support of the Student at a corresponding level. In his effort to survive, the Student has also a job. This affects negatively (1) his presence and participation at the classroom activities and also (2) his interest for research and top knowledge, as he compares his actual duties as employee to the educational program, and finds the educational offering of the public universities disconnected from reality. At a psychological level, the Student perceives that there will be no social and financial reward, in the future, from getting high level professional knowledge, and, moreover, the effort implied by the study is in general incompatible with practicing his current job.

The public authority is well informed about the consequences 1 and 2, so it has to make some decisions to encourage the Student to remain in contact with the university, but with the price of some compromise.

Public authority's decision 1: *not to ask too much professional effort or rigorous classroom presence from the students.* In view of its main objective (global social peace), the public authority decides not to eliminate from educational programs those students who will not systematically participate to the classroom activities, and to (tacitly) allow them to pass their examinations in a large time interval after the teaching program was over.

Assumption 1 and consequence 1 imply also the next consequence.

Consequence 3: *the Teacher will have a very low salary level.* As the budget allocated for higher education is relatively small, the authority cannot ensure a corresponding level of the Teacher's salary.

Confronted with consequence 1 and having as priority the maintenance of its *strategic objective* (also for political, electoral reasons), the public authority makes a second compromise, this time in a way that mimics the interest for a competition between teachers and universities.

Public authority's decision 2: *the money is allocated to support the Student, not the Teacher's salary directly, but the Teacher has an employment contract of indefinite duration.* The financial mechanism for supporting the public higher education system implies money allocation for the Student, not for the Teacher, so if the students' number decreases, there will be a lower salary level for the educational staff of the public universities. In parallel, in order to ensure social peace, the educational staff has employment contract with indefinite duration, provided that it makes effort to attract and maintain a relatively high number of students in the universities.

The possible implications of these decisions, in context of an emerging economy, depend on one side, objectively, on the fact that it is more difficult for the Teacher to manage the didactic activity with a high number of students and a relatively low level of the educational budget, and on the other side, subjectively, on the ethics and psychological profile of the main agents interacting in the public higher education service system: Teacher and Student.

3.2   Strategies and Gains in Teacher-Student Interaction

Recall that in the sequel one considers that all high school teachers and all students constitute large populations of (more or less) identical and rational players, respectively called Teacher and Student. Depending on the basic feature of the psychological profile of Teacher and Student, several bi-matrix game models are proposed next. The common elements of these models are the set of payoff values and the corresponding set of strategies.

For both players the proposed qualitative payoff values are very high (H), high (h), low (l) and very low (L), with $P = \{H, h, l, L\}$ and

$$H > h > l > L. \tag{1}$$

The strategies of both players reflect their radical options regarding their professional attitude. In accomplishing his professional duties, the Teacher can play *Verify* or *Don't Verify*. *Verify* implies teaching at a corresponding level of competence and also verifying the level of knowledge of the Student through rigorous examination. However, examining with rigour might eliminate part of the students and diminish the population of students accordingly. *Don't Verify* implies teaching at a corresponding level of competence but without, or followed only by a superficial examination, thus ensuring a conservation of the population of students, and also a conservation (or increase) of the level of financial support received by the university. Denote the set of strategies of the player I by $I = \{Verify, Don't\ Verify\}$.

When choosing his strategy, the Teacher is supposed to make a decision based on three non-convergent criteria: *professional effort*, *risk to lose money* and *professional prestige*; the Teacher establishes a hierarchy among these criteria and, in a simplified behavioural model, he allocates a qualitative level, *high* ($\uparrow$) or *low* ($\downarrow$), to each criterion. So, for example, if the Teacher cares mostly about his professional prestige, despite the low salary level then he wants *professional prestige*$\uparrow$ with highest priority, and the level of the other criteria is less important. In this case, he will choose the strategy *Verify*. On the contrary, if the minimization of the financial risk is dominant, then the Teacher will consider *risk to lose money*$\downarrow$ with highest priority and he will choose the strategy *Don't Verify*, as in this case there is no risk to lose students.

The Student may choose between *Study* and *Don't Study*. *Study* implies the interest for K&C, in view of a better competitiveness in the global market of human resource, that is the Student is determined to study and to pass rigorously all the examinations. *Don't Study* means the that the Student is focussed mainly on its current job and, eventually, on obtaining, without significant effort, a licence or master degree, so he will study very little or not at all and will consider himself in general advantaged if the Teacher chooses *Don't Verify*. Denote the set of strategies of the player II by $II = \{Study, Don't\ Study\}$.

When choosing his strategy, the Student will make a decision based on three criteria, which, as in the case of player I, are not all convergent: *knowledge*, *risk to lose the degree* and *professional effort*; the Student establishes a hierarchy among the criteria and, similarly to the simplified behavioural model of the Teacher, he allocates a qualitative level *high* ($\uparrow$) or *low* ($\downarrow$), to each criterion. So, for example, if he wants *knowledge*$\uparrow$, then he chooses the strategy *Study* which implies also *risk losing the degree*↓, accepting also *professional effort*↑.

3.3   Scenarios and Game Models of Teacher-Student Interaction in a Generic Emerging Economy Environment

In all scenarios, the Teacher's objective *risk to lose money*↓ has highest priority and will imply that the strategy *Don't Verify* is dominant, thus ensuring his survival. Hence all scenarios are bad from this viewpoint.

The first scenario: the Student and the Teacher want both to perform, but only if their economic survival is ensured. The game model is depicted in Fig. 4a, b. The Teacher wants *risk to lose money*↓ with highest priority, and with lower priority *professional prestige*↑, so *Don't Verify* is a dominant strategy and the game becomes a decision problem for the Student. The Student considers *knowledge*↑ with highest priority, so the strategy *Study* is dominant and the outcome is (h, h) for the strategies $(Don't\ Verify, Study)$: the Teacher survives but worries about having a lower prestige and the Student studies but he is not tested properly for his knowledge.

The second scenario: the Teacher wants only to survive, without care for losing prestige but the Student wants to acquire knowledge. The game model is depicted in Fig. 4c, d. The Teacher's strategy *Don't Verify* is dominant and the game becomes again a decision problem for the Student. The Student wants *knowledge*↑ and also *risk losing the degree*↓, so he plays *Study* and the outcome is (H, h) for the strategies $(Don't\ Verify, Study)$: the Teacher survives without caring for losing his prestige and the Student studies but he is not tested properly for his knowledge.

The third scenario: the Teacher wants only to survive and the Student is not interested in knowledge, but only in acquiring the degree without much effort. The game model is depicted in Fig. 4e, f. The Teacher's strategy *Don't Verify* is dominant, the Student knows this and he wants *risk losing the degree*↓ but also *professional effort*↓, so he plays *Don't Study*. The outcome is (H, h) for the strategies $(Don't\ Verify, Don't\ Study)$.

The fourth scenario: the Teacher wants only to survive, without care for losing his professional prestige and the Student is interested neither in knowledge, nor in acquiring the degree, but, eventually, only in his job. The game model is depicted in Fig. 5a, b. The Teacher wants *risk to lose money*↓ with highest priority, so *Don't Verify* is a dominant strategy and the game becomes a decision problem for the Student. The Student considers *professional effort*↓ with highest priority, so he will choose to play *Don't Study*. The outcome is (H, H) for the strategies $(Don't\ Verify, Don't\ Study)$. The game is symmetric and this scenario is the worst.

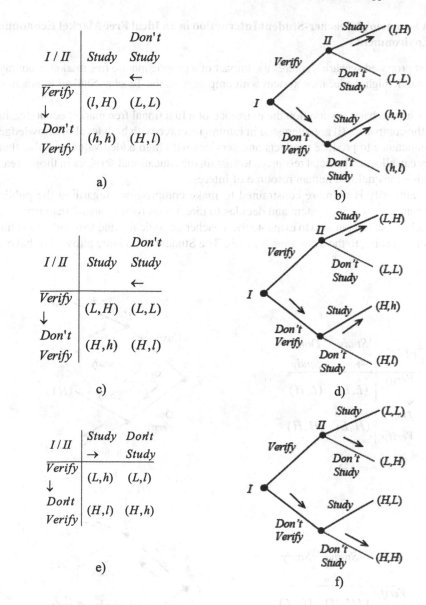

Fig. 4. The game between Teacher (player *I*) and Student (player *II*) in an emerging economy, in strategic and extensive form: the first scenario (a) and (b), the second scenario (c) and (d) and the third scenario (e) and (f); the qualitative gains are very high (*H*), high (*h*), low (*l*) and very low (*L*).

3.4   A Scenario of Teacher-Student Interaction in an Ideal Free Market Economic Environment

The next proposed scenario captures the impact of a generic mature free market economy on the public higher education system with emphasis on the Teacher-Student interaction model.

Consider as basic assumption the existence of a functional free market economy, in which the companies (i) are interested in human resource with high level of knowledge and competence to produce products and services with high added value and also that (ii) they can allocate financial resources to sustain the educational services in those areas generating the qualified human resource of interest.

The authority is no more constrained to make compromises regarding the public higher education service system and decides to direct important financial resources for the Teacher's salary but also to evaluate the Teacher periodically and to decide upon his contract according to the evaluation's result. The Student is no more allowed to have a

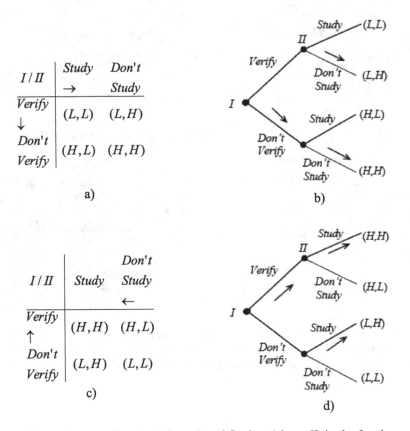

Fig. 5. The game between Teacher (player *I*) and Student (player *II*) in the fourth scenario, representing the worst case, placed in an emerging economy (a) and (b) and in the fifth scenario, placed in a functional free market economy (c) and (d).

job during his semester. The number of students in a classroom is diminished in order to raise the quality level of the educational service.

The fifth scenario: the Teacher and the Student want both to perform. The game model is depicted in Fig. 5c, d. The Teacher wants *professional prestige*↑ with highest priority, so *Verify* is a dominant strategy and the game becomes a decision problem for the Student. The Student considers *knowledge*↑ with highest priority, so he will choose to play *Study*. The outcome is (H, H) for the strategies (*Verify*, *Study*).

The game is also symmetric and is the opposite of the game in the fourth scenario.

4 Concluding Remarks

The increasing interest in modelling and analyses of higher education service systems is motivated both by the problem of costs and by the need for higher levels of knowledge and competence, in a competitive, global economic environment.

The variety of viewpoints reported in the literature reflects the diversity of issues regarding public higher education, but also a lack of integrative models, aimed to provide general frameworks for discussions and solutions.

This contribution proposes a step in this direction, and starting from strictly empirical and qualitative considerations, introduces general modelling frameworks of public higher education services from two perspectives.

Firstly, the ontological specificity of a public higher education system is discussed in Sect. 2, having as starting point the ontology of a generic service system introduced in [2]. In the framework of Service Science, the most relevant particular feature of a higher education service system is that the Student is not a client but, together with the Teacher, it is one of the two main stakeholders, while the final beneficiary is the Employer and the society, not only in present, but also in the future time interval of a generation. This aspect is reflected also in the chained structure of the value co-creation process: initially the knowledge and competence is acquired in the Teacher-Student interaction, and afterwards, the Student becoming a Graduate is employed and co-creates value for the companies and for the society in general.

Secondly, a qualitative bimatrix game model is introduced in Sect. 3, for the analysis of the Teacher-Student interaction conditioned by economic and political decisions, norms and regulations, on one side, and by personal options and motivations of the actors, on the other side.

The scenarios proposed in case of an emerging economy show that, in context of scarce public resources, an educational policy based on a strategic objective called, in brief "social peace", drives systematically to a low quality of the educational process.

More specifically, if the Teacher's salary is low and conditioned by the number of students and if the private companies are not contributors to the financial support of higher education, then whatever the personal options of the involved actors are, the need for survival is dominant for both of them.

In contrast, in an ideal mature free market economy, the direct and feedback relations between universities and private companies decrease the pressure on the public educational budget and stimulate both Teacher and Student to co-create value.

The proposed qualitative approaches are thought as starting points for developing future research frames dedicated to higher education quality, integrating specific instruments such as interviews and statistical data processing. The problem of constructing reliable key performance indexes for evaluation of educational services, as well as the quest for alternative efficient higher education paradigms in emerging economies remains subject of debate; for example, in Eastern European countries one can argue about the possibility to balance between the basic economic and standardization principles of the Bologna Process [13] and a reconsideration of older valuable viewpoints regarding organization of education and research, like the contribution in this area of the Nobel Prize winner P.L. Kapitsa [14].

References

1. Spohrer, J., Anderson, L., Pass, N., Ager, T.: Service science and service-dominant logic. Paper no: 2, Otago Forum 2, Academic Papers (2008). www.business.otago.ac.nz
2. Borangiu, Th, Oltean, V.E., Drăgoicea, M., Falcão e Cunha, J., Iacob, I.: Some aspects concerning a generic service process model building. In: Snene, M., Leonard, M. (eds.) IESS 2014. LNBIP, vol. 169, pp. 1–16. Springer, Heidelberg (2014)
3. Hezel, F.X.: Recent Theories of the Relationship between Education and Development (1974). http://micsem.org/pubs/articles/education/frames/rectheorfr.htm
4. Correa, H., Gruver, G.W.: Teacher-student interaction: a game theoretic extension of the economic theory of education. Math. Soc. Sci. **13**(1), 19–47 (1987)
5. Selim, T.H.: The education market in Egypt: a game theory approach. Economic Research Forum, Working paper Series, Working Paper 442 (2008). https://ideas.repec.org/p/erg/wpaper/422.html
6. Fukiharu, T.: The reform of higher education in Japan: a game-theoretic analysis of intensified competition. In: MODSIM 2005 the International Congress on Modelling and Simulation, Modelling and Simulation Society of Australia and New Zealand, pp. 1007–1013, December 2005. http://www.mssanz.org.au/modsim05/papers/fukahiru.pdf
7. Şahin, A.: The Incentive Effects of Higher Education Subsidies on Student Effort. Federal Reserve Bank of New York Staff Reports, no. 192 (2004). https://www.newyorkfed.org/medialibrary/media/research/staff_reports/sr192.pdf
8. Franck, B., Owen, R.F.: International migration of brains, educational competition and national interests: a two-country, game-theoretic approach. In: ETSG 2014 the 16th Annual Conference of the European Trade and Study Group, LMU Munich and Ifo Institute, September 2014. http://www.etsg.org/ETSG2014/Papers/352.pdf
9. Lemey, E., Poels, G.: Towards a service system ontology for service science. In: Kappel, G., Maamar, Z., Motahari-Nezhad, H.R. (eds.) ICSOC 2011. LNCS, vol. 7084, pp. 250–264. Springer, Heidelberg (2011)
10. Katzan Jr., H.: Foundations of service science: concepts and facilities. Journal of Service Science **1**, 1–22 (2008) (Third Quarter 2008) The Clute Institute (2008). http://www.cluteinstitute.com/ojs/index.php/JSS/issue/view/468
11. Grönross, C., Voima, P.: Making Sense of Value and Value Co-Creation in Service Logic. Hanken School of Economics, Helsinki (2011)
12. Tringh, T.H., Liem, N.Th., Kachitvichyanukul, V.: A game theory approach for value co-creation systems. Prod. Manuf. Res. An Open Access J. **2**(1), 253–265. http://dx.doi.org/10.1080/21693277.2014.913124

13. Bologna Process. https://en.wikipedia.org/wiki/Bologna_Process
14. Kapitsa, P.L.: Basic factors in the organization of science, and how they are handled in the U.S.S.R. (originally published in *Daedalus*, J. Amer. Acad. Arts and Sciences, 102, 167—176 (1973)) In: Experiment, Theory and Practice, Articles and Addresses, 183–197, D. Reidel Publ. Co., Dodrecht, Holland (1980)

Service-Dominant Strategic Sourcing: Value Creation Versus Cost Saving

Laleh Rafati[(⊠)] and Geert Poels

Faculty of Economics and Business Administration, Center for Service Intelligence, Ghent University, Tweekerkenstraat 2, 9000 Ghent, Belgium
{laleh.rafati,geert.poels}@UGent.be

Abstract. The concept of strategic sourcing recognizes that procurement is not just a cost function, but supports the firm's effort to achieve its long-term objectives. Organizations more and more expect from their chief procurement officer (CPO) to develop long-term and short-term plans in procurement. Typically, however, procurement is driven by a *tactical spend management* sourcing process aimed at cost saving targets, which is not able to support organizations in achieving strategic objectives like innovation, value creation, sustainable competitive advantage and long-term partnerships. A paradigm shift from a tactical way of thinking about sourcing to a more strategic way of thinking is needed by focusing on value-driven targets. To help realize the new paradigm of value-driven management in sourcing, we designed a systemic view on strategic sourcing based on Service-Dominant Logic and (service) systems thinking. We used this systemic view to develop the conceptual basis of a new modeling and analysis language that helps organizations in exploring sourcing alternatives according to value-driven management.

Keywords: Strategic sourcing · Value-driven management · Service-Dominant Logic · Capability sourcing

1 Introduction

The growing importance of supply chain management has led to an increasing recognition of the strategic role of procurement [1]. Procurement has evolved from mere buying [2] and has recently been recognized as a critical driving force in the strategic management of supply chains [3]. Procurement is not just a cost function, but supports the firm's effort to achieve its long-term objectives [4]. Organizations more and more expect from their chief procurement officer (CPO) to develop long-term and short-term plans in procurement. Generating and measuring savings, safeguarding quality, ensuring delivery availability, enhancing value creation, fostering partnerships and innovation will remain the top priorities of CPOs in supply chain management for the next coming years [5]. Procurement is, however, driven by a *tactical spend management* process aimed at cost saving targets, which is not able to support organizations in achieving strategic objectives like innovation, value creation and long-term partnerships [6]. A paradigm shift from a tactical way of thinking about sourcing to a more strategic way of thinking is needed by focusing on value-driven targets. Cox [7, 8] introduced a

© Springer International Publishing Switzerland 2016
T. Borangiu et al. (Eds.): IESS 2016, LNBIP 247, pp. 30–44, 2016.
DOI: 10.1007/978-3-319-32689-4_3

strategic view on sourcing as value-driven management in which sourcing is a cross-functional process that is based on a deep understanding of an organization's value creation processes and what is needed for performing these processes. To help realize value-driven management, we designed a systemic view on strategic sourcing based on Service-Dominant Logic and (service) systems thinking. We used this systemic view to develop the conceptual basis of a new modeling and analysis language that helps organizations in exploring sourcing alternatives according to the new paradigm of value-driven management. Our research methodology was Design Science Research [9], which is the standard research methodology used in the Information Systems discipline for designing new artifacts that solve unsolved problems or improve upon existing solutions.

Section 2 defines strategic sourcing as a sub-process of procurement and analyzes current techniques of strategic sourcing, which focus strongly on cost saving targets. Section 3 characterizes strategic sourcing as value-driven management and subsequently elaborates on our research objectives. Section 4 introduces our systemic view of strategic sourcing by taking a service ecosystem perspective of an organization that is focused on value creation instead of cost savings. Section 5 defines a strategic sourcing conceptualization as the conceptual basis of a new modeling language that helps implementing strategic sourcing as value-driven management. Section 6 presents a proof of concept evaluation that demonstrates by means of a case study of IT outsourcing in a large university hospital how a model-driven strategic sourcing approach based on our envisioned modeling language helps exploring strategic sourcing alternatives from a value-driven management perspective. Finally, Sect. 7 concludes and outlines future research.

2   Strategic Sourcing as Tactical Spend Management

Strategic sourcing is traditionally seen as a sub-process of procurement as described in [4, 10] (Fig. 1). The procurement process starts with spend analysis and ends with payment and is composed of two distinct phases: sourcing and purchasing. The sourcing phase encompasses the source-to-contract (S2C) sub-process of procurement with three executive steps: (1) spend analysis to collect and analyze spend data and then identify potential opportunities for cost reduction; (2) strategic sourcing to select the most appropriate go-to market sourcing strategies and then selection and evaluation of suppliers in alignment with the strategic goals of the firm; and (3) contract management for controlling and tracking the formal and legal agreements with suppliers to fully exploit the value of the contract arrangements. The purchasing phase encompasses the purchase-to-pay (P2C) sub-process procurement with three executive steps: (1) the purchase requisition; (2) the purchase order and order confirmation; (3) the delivery notification and invoice payment.

The current techniques for strategic sourcing such as the Purchasing Category Portfolio of Kraljic [11] the Cox Power Portfolio model [12] and the purchasing chessboard approach [13] focus strongly on cost savings targets through applying spend analysis, supply market analyses and positioning techniques. They have been criticized for approaching strategic sourcing as a tactical spend management process

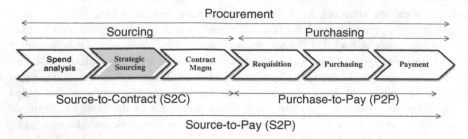

Fig. 1. Procurement process

rather than as a process of strategic importance to the organization [6, 14, 15]. Furthermore, the analyses do not consider all of the variables, which are required for assessing and evaluating the complexity of the supply market, the value of purchasing categories, the power of suppliers against buyers, and strategic sourcing alternatives [7, 14, 15]. In the next section, we present a new (strategic) way of thinking for strategic sourcing that caters for this shortcoming.

3   Strategic Sourcing as Value-Driven Management

According to the strategic thinking promoted by Cox [8], sourcing is a cross-functional process that focuses on "leverage value for money trade-offs", not just "tactical cost savings". For value-driven management, the CPO should consider both the demand and supply bases for value creation to support the firm to achieve its strategic goals such as sustainable competitive advantage, enhancing value creation, increasing quality, mitigating risk, driving innovation and fostering long-term partnerships. Therefore, the CPO needs to manage the interactions between the organization's buyers, its suppliers and its internal and external customers by considering the resources, competencies and capabilities and relationships (e.g. customer-provider and buyer-supplier) of both the supply and demand side. Hence, requirements to realize-value driven management are a holistic view on the value chain and a more rigorous analysis of category value by considering both cost-down KPIs and value-driven KPIs. According to these requirements, we define our research objectives as **Objective (1)** Design a systemic view on strategic sourcing with emphasis on value creation to realize strategic sourcing as value-driven management. **Objective (2)** Develop a conceptual modeling language for the systemic exploration of strategic sourcing alternatives towards both cost saving and value creation targets. In the following section, we introduce our systemic view of strategic sourcing to realize value-driven management.

4   Service-Dominant Strategic Sourcing

We believe that a systemic view on strategic sourcing that emphasizes the value creation by an organization will help realizing value-driven management. It is our position that the interpretation of complex emerging phenomena like value creation is greatly facilitated by a systems view that synthesizes both a reductionist perspective (i.e., analyzing elements and their relations) and a holistic perspective (i.e., being capable of observing the whole) [16]. We therefore propose a service ecosystem perspective for strategic sourcing as a systemic view that is based on the Viable Systems Approach (vSa) [17, 18] and Service-Dominant Logic (S-D Logic) [19]. The vSa is a systems theory that is increasingly getting attention in service research due to its contribution to understanding complex phenomena such as value co-creation. S-D Logic provides a framework for thinking more clearly about the service system and its role in competition [20] and survivability [19], which are two main objectives of strategic sourcing.

A viable system is defined as a system that survives, is both internally and externally balanced, and has mechanisms and opportunities to develop and adapt, and hence to become more and more efficient within its environment [21, 22]. A service ecosystem is then defined as a viable system of service systems connected (internally and externally) by mutual value creation interactions realized through service exchanges [23]. This ecosystem view is founded on S-D Logic, which is an important theoretical framework for the study of service systems [24, 25]. The S-D Logic views a service system as a dynamic value co-creation configuration of resources that is connected internally and externally to other service systems by value propositions through service exchanges [26]. While the traditional view on (tactical) sourcing is more a 'goods-dominant' worldview of suppliers and buyers as senders and receivers of goods (hence procurement's focus on realizing cost savings), the value-driven management view on (strategic) sourcing matches better the value co-creation interpretation of provider-customer relationships as in S-D Logic [20]. Therefore, a service ecosystem perspective for strategic sourcing introduces a way of thinking about strategic sourcing in terms of S-D Logic. We observe a clear similarity between S-D Logic concepts and strategic sourcing concepts (as value-driven management), as defined below in Table 1.

Table 1. S-D logic and strategic sourcing mapping of concepts

S-D Logic concepts	Strategic sourcing concepts
Operand Resources as usually tangible, static and passive resources that must be acted on to be beneficial, e.g., natural resources, goods, and money [26, 27].	**Resources** as the firm's assets that require action to make them valuable and beneficial for the firm to sustain competitive advantage. Strategic resources enable organizations to sustain competitive advantage, if the resources are Valuable, Rare, Inimitable, and Non-substitutable (VRIN) [28, 29].
Operant Resources as usually intangible, dynamic and active resources that act upon other resources to create benefits, e.g., knowledge, skills [26, 27]. They are the essential component of differentiation and the fundamental source of competitive advantage [30].	**Competencies** are the firm's specific strengths that allow a company to gain competitive advantage [31].

(Continued)

Table 1. (*Continued*)

S-D Logic concepts	Strategic sourcing concepts
Service System as a configuration of resources (at least one operant resource) that is capable of providing benefit to other service systems and itself [26].	**Capability** is a configuration of the firm's resources and competencies that makes the firm able to achieve and sustain competitive advantage. *Dynamic capabilities* are the firm's capacities and abilities to reconfigure its resource base internally and externally to achieve the sustainable competitive advantage [32]. Dynamic capabilities act on operational capabilities [33, 34].
Service is the application of operant resources for the benefit of another party [26]. Service is the fundamental basis of value creation through economic exchange. *Competitive advantage* is a function of how one firm exchanges its services to meet the needs of the customer relative to how another firm exchanges its services [30]. *Surviving* is a function of how the firm exchanges its services to be able to survive and thrive in its surrounding environment [35]. Service is the primary source of competitive advantage and survivability. However, "the only true source of sustainable competitive advantage and survivability is the operant resources that make the service possible" [29].	**Service** is the application of competencies to achieve competitive advantage or survivability. *Competitive advantage* is the ability to create more economic value than competitors. It is a firm's profitability that is greater than the average profitability for all firms in its industry. Furthermore, *sustained competitive advantage* is a firm maintaining above average and superior profitability for a number of years [31]. The primary objective of strategic sourcing is to achieve a sustained competitive advantage (in a commercial domain) or survivability (in a non-commercial domain), which in turn results in superior profit or long-term viability.
Actors are engaged in the service exchanges as value co-creators through *actor-to-actor (A2A) relations* [31] at the micro, meso, and macro level [36, 37]. They are essentially doing the same thing: creating value for themselves and others through resource integration [38]. An actor can only offer a value proposition concerning some services and cannot solely create value for the beneficiary actor [37, 39].	**Actors** as buyers, suppliers, internal customers and external customers are able to create value through participation in a value network with various relationships like supplier-buyer relationship and customer-provider relationship in both the demand and supply sides of the value chain [20].
Value is an increase in the viability (survivability, well-being) of the system. Value comes from the ability to act in a manner that is beneficial to a party [40]. A *value proposition* establishes connections and relationships among actors [37, 39]. The process of co-creating value is driven by *value-in-use* (value actualization), but mediated and monitored by *value-in-exchange* (value capturing) [35].	**Perceived value** is defined by customers, based on their perceptions of the usefulness of the product on offer. **Exchange value** is realized when the product is sold. It is the amount paid by the buyer to the producer for the perceived value [41]. Strategic sourcing derives from value co-creation, which in the provider role serves as value proposition to customers, in the supplier role serves as value facilitation to customers, and in the customer role serves as value actualization [20].

Given these similarities, we define strategic sourcing as *a strategic process for organizing and fine-tuning the focal firm's resources, competencies and capabilities internally and externally through A2A interactions with suppliers, buyers, internal and external customers, in order to achieve (sustainable) competitive advantage or survivability, which in turn results in value as superior profitability or long-term viability.* In the next section, we use this systemic view of strategic sourcing to design a conceptualization as the foundation of a modeling language that can be used for the systemic exploration of strategic sourcing alternatives, in line with value-driven management.

5 C.A.R.S – A Conceptual Modeling Language for the Systemic Exploration of Strategic Sourcing Alternatives

Conceptual modeling is our proposed approach for exploring strategic sourcing alternatives and options from a service ecosystem perspective as described in the previous section. To create conceptual models that describe sourcing alternatives, a domain-specific modeling language [42] for strategic sourcing is needed. Such language is defined by a conceptualization of strategic sourcing. We introduce the C.A.R.S (Capability – Actor – Resource – Service) conceptualization as a new language for strategic sourcing modeling (Fig. 2). There is a clear mapping between the C.A.R.S concepts and the core concepts of S-D Logic as we apply them based on Table 1 to design a systemic view on strategic sourcing. The C.A.R.S concepts are defined as follows:

- **Capability** is 'What the actor Can do' for competitiveness and survivability. Capability as a configuration of C.A.R.S resources is the capacity and ability of an actor to create value through service exchange. The capability of an actor represents its potential long-term effects on the achievement of sourcing strategic objectives. Therefore, we define value-driven KPIs of strategic sourcing based on the capabilities of actors in the demand and supply side of the value chain.
- **Actor** is 'Who is the Resource Integrator' that provides service, proposes value, creates value and captures value. According to common sourcing relationships, suppliers offer value propositions to the focal firm; the focal firm (as a buyer) purchases service from suppliers; the focal firm (as a provider) delivers service to the customers; customers perceive and use value; and finally the focal firm captures value from both the demand and supply sides. All actors involved are co-creators of value in the value chain.
- The **Resource** base is 'What the actor Has' that provides the capability to create value. The resource base notion includes tangible and static resources (e.g., goods), as well as intangible and dynamic resources (e.g., competencies and skills). As in Table 1 we distinguish between assets (i.e., operand resources in S-D Logic) and competencies (i.e., operant resources in S-D Logic). Resources are distributed across the market and can be configured to create capabilities.
- **Service** is 'What the actor Does' that is exchanged with other actors for competitiveness and survivability. Service is the application of resources to create value. We use this notion to illustrate the performance dimension of actors to achieve

sourcing operational objectives (bottom-line results). Therefore, we define cost-down KPIs of strategic sourcing based on the performance of an actor like cost, quality, and delivery time.

The next section presents a proof of concept evaluation of C.AR.S as the conceptual foundation of a modeling and analysis language for exploring strategic sourcing alternatives in line with value-driven management. We demonstrate the use of our model-driven strategic sourcing approach using an IT outsourcing case-study in the university hospital UZ Gent.

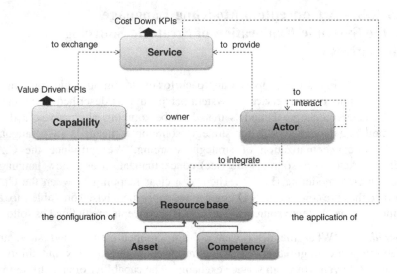

Fig. 2. C.A.R.S conceptualization and viewpoints

6 A Case-Study of Model-Driven Strategic Sourcing

The focus of model-driven strategic sourcing using C.A.R.S is on capability sourcing for value creation instead of identifying cost saving strategies for purchasing categories. Capabilities are the key to alignment and successful strategy execution. Capabilities exist across the value chain and in order to achieve profitability an organization must learn to manage capabilities that other parties in the value chain possess [43–45]. Firms must learn to govern a network of capabilities. Right sourcing allows having a sharper focus on the differentiating capabilities. On the other hand, incorrect sourcing decisions limit agility and increase costs [46].

We take an IT (out)sourcing case in the healthcare domain for demonstrating our model-based exploration of strategic sourcing alternatives and options. We describe this IT (out)sourcing scenario based on existing business/working papers about the healthcare IT contracts and agreements of UZ Gent [47]. Furthermore, we did a reality check with the chief information officer (CIO) of UZ Gent for a proof of concept evaluation of the proposed model-driven approach. In the following, we illustrate how a strategic sourcing decision maker like the CIO can apply our proposed model-driven method to explore strategies and recommendations for sourcing IT capabilities in the hospital. Model-driven strategic sourcing with C.A.R.S entails performing the three activities of strategic sourcing using techniques for capability sourcing, as explained below:

Step 1: Determine capability positioning: This step aims at positioning C.A.R.S capabilities by considering both the demand and supply side of the value chain to find opportunities for cost saving and value creation. Inspired by Cox's criticality analysis [12], we introduce capability criticality analysis based on two dimensions of capabilities: the competitive advantage potential (i.e., commercial criticality) to create more economic value that results in superior profitability and the resource base availability (i.e., operational criticality) to achieve superior performance. The first dimension determines the competition degree of capabilities for sustainability and profitability such as sustainable competitive advantage (SCA), competitive advantage (CA), temporary competitive advantage (TCA) and parity competition (PC). The second dimension determines the criticality degree of the resource base configured by the analyzed capabilities, to achieve superior performance such as valuable resource base (V), rare resource base (R), inimitable resource base (I) and non-substitutable resource base (N). The result of the capability criticality analysis is a 2 × 2 capability portfolio model with four categories: critical-strategic capability, strategic capability, critical-tactical capability and tactical capability.

Figure 3 is a C.A.R.S model of UZ Gent that shows the exchange of two services for the benefit of internal and external customers of UZ Gent. These services are healthcare core services including clinical services and care services and healthcare supporting services including business administration services and ICT communication services. For UZ Gent, the value is the differentiation of healthcare core services and the low costs of healthcare supporting services. For exchanging these two services, UZ Gent requires four IT capabilities: healthcare core management (HCM), healthcare information management (HIM), hospital infrastructure management (HIN) and hospital business management (HBM). These hospital IT capabilities are based on various healthcare IT resources that provide the capacity to act, such as skills (e.g., clinical skills, business skills, ICT skills, technical skills, organizational skills), technologies (e.g., displays, monitors, workstations, projectors, video walls), software (e.g., image processing software and ERP software), systems (e.g., HIS, CIS, RIS, LIS, PACS, reporting system, decision support system and hospital-wide management information systems) and standards (e.g., Health Level-7 and DICOM).

Referring to the supply side of the value chain, Cerner, Xperthis, Agfa Healthcare, Barco, Infohos, Carestream Healthcare, GE Healthcare and Nexuz Healthcare are potential suppliers to provide healthcare core services. On the other hand, SAP, Oracle, Microsoft, EMC, Dimension Data, Realdolmen, HP, PHILIPS, Fujifilm, Dell and Siemens are potential suppliers to provide the healthcare supporting services. According to the hospital spend analysis, 40 percent of total cost (IT spending) has being spent on core services and 25 % of total cost has being spent on supporting services.

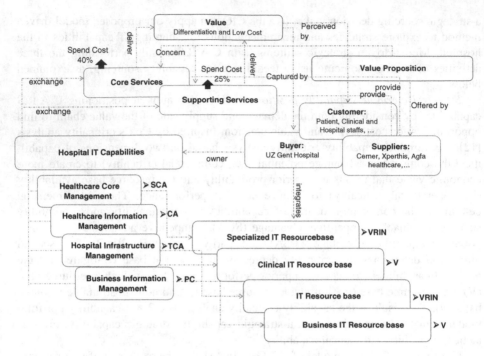

Fig. 3. C.A.R.S model of UZ Gent IT capabilities

The results of the capability criticality analysis have been added to Fig. 4.

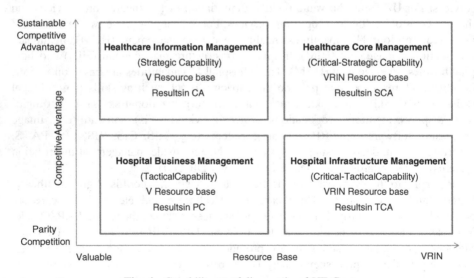

Fig. 4. Capability portfolio matrix of UZ Gent

Step 2: Determine (Buyer-Supplier) Dependency Positioning: This step aims at positioning the dependencies between buyers and suppliers for setting relationship strategies in the supply market. Our proposed approach classifies a buyer-supplier dependency into four categories (buyer dominance, supplier dominance, interdependence and independence) based on two dimensions, supplier power and buyer power, which are measured by (1) the *essentiality* and *substitutability* of the exchanged service [48] between buyer and supplier and (2) the *capabilities, resources and competencies* of both buyer and supplier to exchange service. Figure 5 shows a C.A.R.S model that zooms in the HIS/RIS/PACS service that is provided by one of UZ Gent's suppliers, Agfa Healthcare, which is a specialized healthcare IT solution provider. This service is part of the healthcare core services that are exchanged by the HIM capability of UZ Gent.

The buyer-supplier dependency analysis showed that the HIS/RIS/PACS service is a common healthcare information system for UZ Gent with low-level criticality and low-level financial impact. On the other hand, this service is a core service of Agfa Healthcare with high-level criticality and high-level financial impact. There are more than five alternative suppliers (i.e., Xperthis, Barco, Infohos, Carestream Healthcare, GE Healthcare, Nexuz Healthcare and IBM Healthcare) to provide this exchanged service in the supply market with low-level switching costs. Moreover, there are less than three alternative buyers (i.e., one university hospital and two general hospitals) to request this exchanged service in the demand market resulting in a high-level searching cost. Therefore, the relationship between UZ Gent and Agfa Healthcare is positioned as a *"buyer dominance"* relationship.

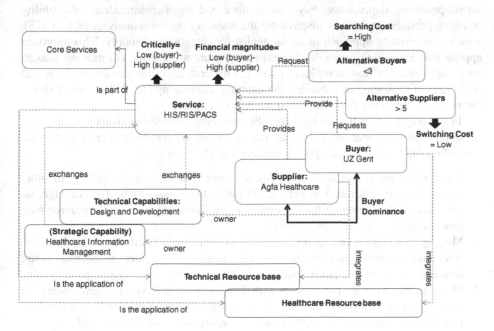

Fig. 5. C.A.R.S dependency model between UZ Gent and Agfa Healthcare

Figure 6 shows the results of dependency analyses other UZ Gent suppliers.

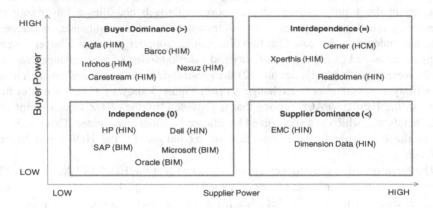

Fig. 6. UZ Gent - Suppliers dependency matrix

Step 3: Identify capability sourcing strategies: This last step aims at developing a portfolio for classifying capability sourcing and setting sourcing strategies. The technique proposed as Capability Sourcing Portfolio Analysis classifies capability sourcing into 16 categories based on the outcomes of the previous steps: the capability positioning (i.e., tactical capability, tactical-critical capability, strategic capability and strategic-critical capability) and (2) the buyer-supplier dependency positioning (i.e., interdependence, dependence, buyer dominance and supplier dominance). Capability sourcing portfolio analysis is inspired by the sourcing portfolio analysis of Cox [28], which is an existing approach to set strategies for categories of supply. This approach applies two leveraging principles for exploring sourcing options: (1) moving into an easy supply market (low complexity) and (2) understanding the current position and seek ways of exploiting or balancing the existing relationship [12, 31]. Figure 7 shows the results of applying this analysis to the UZ Gent case.

For example, according to the capability sourcing portfolio analysis and its leveraging principles, for sourcing healthcare core management (HCM) as a critical-strategic capability, the strategies and options available to UZ Gent are:

1. Develop an integrated health system in-house (insourcing) for selling to other hospitals (new customers) in the market (advantage: innovation; disadvantage: no cost saving) by improving the internal IT capabilities and internal IT resource base *(according to leveraging principle1)*;
2. Moving into Market and Leverage positions (outsourcing) for cost reduction (disadvantage: no value creation), however, if there are no suppliers in the market and leverage positions, this is not viable option *(according to leveraging principle1)*;
3. Maintain the strategic partnership with Cerner through long-term agreements for value creation such as differentiation (disadvantage: lock-in partnership) and reduce risk through master data management *(according to leveraging principle2).*

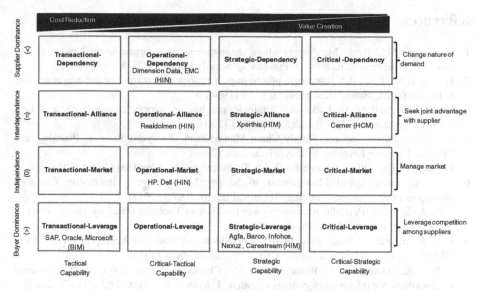

Fig. 7. UZ Gent capability sourcing portfolio

7 Discussion and Future Research

The CIO of UZ Gent believes that the current focus of strategic sourcing is on cost saving metrics (e.g., total cost of ownership, quality, and delivery time) rather than value creation factors (e.g., capabilities, competencies and resources). He realizes that the hospital really needs to create value by participation of its suppliers, internal and external customers to achieve sustainable competitive advantage. The model-driven strategic sourcing approach presented in this paper can support strategic sourcing decision makers like the CIO to achieve value creation targets (e.g., innovation and long-term partnerships) through providing a (IT) capability portfolio (extended by considering both the demand and supply sides) and a dependency portfolio (extended by considering all potential suppliers in the market) for strategic sourcing decision-making. We proposed a modeling and analysis language (C.A.R.S) for exploring strategic sourcing alternatives to support firms to achieve their strategic goals such as innovation (through finding new customers, services, products and partners), sustainable competitive advantage and long-term partnerships. Our future research includes (1) formalizing the C.A.R.S conceptualization and viewpoints as a capability–oriented enterprise modeling language; (2) proposing a concrete syntax for the C.A.R.S meta-model; (3) providing modeling guidelines as way of working; and (4) analyzing the possible construction of KPIs by considering various techniques such as AHP, linear programming and fuzzy set theory for supporting strategic sourcing decision-making.

References

1. Anderson, P.H., Rask, M.: Supply chain management: new organizational practices for changing procurement realities. J. Purchasing Supply Manag. **9**(2), 83–95 (2003)
2. Ellram, L.M., Carr, A.S.: Strategic purchasing: a history and review of the literature. Int. J. Phys. Distrib. Mater. Manag. **30**(1), 9–19 (1994)
3. Chen, I.J., Paulraj, A., Lado, A.: Strategic purchasing, supply management and firm performance. J. Oper. Manag. **22**(5), 505–523 (2004)
4. Weele, A.: Purchasing and Supply Chain Management. Analysis, Strategy, Planning and Practise, Cengage Learning EMEA, Hampshire (2010)
5. Berger, R.: The CPO's Agenda for 2014. Technical report, Aberdeen Group (2014)
6. Cox, A.: From Spend Management to Supply Management - Improving Category Management & Strategic Sourcing. Technical report, IIAPS (2015)
7. Cox, A.: Sourcing Portfolio Analysis: Power Positioning Tools for Category Management & Strategic Sourcing. Earlsgate Press (2014)
8. Cox, A., Ireland, P.: Value Flow Management: How to Create and Appropriate Value from KPI-Driven Companies and Supply Chains. Earlsgate Press (2015)
9. Peffers, K., Tuunanen, T., Rothenberger, M., Chatterjee, S.: A design science research methodology for information systems research. J. Manag. Inf. Syst. **24**(3), 45–77 (2007)
10. Cox, A.: Sourcing portfolio analysis and power positioning: towards a "paradigm shift" in category management and strategic sourcing. Supply Chain Manag. Int. J. **20**(6), 717–736 (2015)
11. Kraljic, P.: Purchasing must become supply management. Harvard Bus. Rev. **61**(5), 109–117 (1983)
12. Cox, A.: Understanding buyer and supplier power: a framework for procurement and supply competence. J. Supply Chain Manag. **37**(1), 8–15 (2001)
13. Schuh, C., Kromoser, R., Strohmer, M.F., Pérez, R.R., Triplat, A.: The Purchasing Chessboard™, pp. 55–207. Springer, Heidelberg (2009)
14. Cox, A.: Improving Procurement Competence. Technical report, IIAPS (2014)
15. Cox, A.: Power Positioning & Sourcing Portfolio Analysis. Technical report, IIAPS (2015)
16. Von Bertalanffy, L.: The meaning of general system theory. General system theory: foundations, development, applications, pp. 30–53 (1972)
17. Ng, I., Parry, G., Maull, R., McFarlane, D.: Complex engineering service systems: a grand challenge. In: Ng, I., Parry, G., Wild, P., McFarlane, D., Tasker, P. (eds.) Complex engineering service systems, pp. 439–454. Springer, London (2011)
18. Barile, S., Polese, F.: Smart service systems and viable service systems. Serv. Sci. **2**(1–2), 21–40 (2010)
19. Vargo, S.L., Maglio, P.P., Akaka, M.A.: On value and value co-creation: a service systems and service logic perspective. Eur. Manag. J. **26**(3), 145–152 (2008)
20. Eltantawy, R., Giunipero, L., Handfield, R.: Strategic sourcing management's mindset: strategic sourcing orientation and its implications. Int. J. Phys. Distrib. Logistics Manag. **44**(10), 768–795 (2014)
21. Beer, S.: Brain of the Firm. The Penguin Press, London (1972)
22. Beer, S.: The viable system model: its provenance, development, methodology and pathology. J. Oper. Res. Soc. **35**(1), 7–25 (1984)
23. Vargo, S.L., Lusch, R.F.: From repeat patronage to value co-creation in service ecosystems: a transcending conceptualization of relationship. J. Bus. Market Manag. **4**(4), 169–179 (2010)

24. Maglio, P., Spohrer, J.: Fundamentals of service science. J. Acad. Mark. Sci. **36**(1), 18–20 (2008)
25. Vargo, S.L., Lusch, R.F., Akaka, M.A.: Advancing service science with service-dominant logic: Clarifications and conceptual development. In: Handbook of Service Science, pp. 133–156. Springer, New York (2010)
26. Vargo, S.L., Akaka, M.A.: Service-dominant logic as a foundation for service science: clarifications. Serv. Sci. **1**(1), 32–41 (2009)
27. Poels, G.: The resource-service-system model for service science. In: Trujillo, J., Dobbie, G., Kangassalo, H., Hartmann, S., Kirchberg, M., Rossi, M., Reinhartz-Berger, I., Zimányi, E., Frasincar, F. (eds.) ER 2010. LNCS, vol. 6413, pp. 117–126. Springer, Heidelberg (2010)
28. Barney, J.B.: Firm resources and sustained competitive advantage. J. Manag. **17**(1), 99–120 (1991)
29. Barney, J.B.: Gaining and Sustaining Competitive Advantage, 2nd edn. Prentice Hall, Upper Saddle River (2002)
30. Lusch, R.F., Stephen, L., Vargo, S.L., Matthew, O.: Competing through service: Insights from service-dominant logic. J. Retail. **83**(1), 2–18 (2007)
31. Hill, C., Jones, G.: Strategic Management: An Integrated Approach, 10th edn., Cengage Learning (2012)
32. Helfat, C., Finkelstein, S., Mitchell, W., Peteraf, M., Singh, H., Teece, D., Winter, S.: Dynamic Capabilities: Understanding Strategic Change in Organizations. Wiley, New York (2009)
33. Zollo, M., Winter, S.G.: Deliberate learning and the evolution of dynamic capabilities. Organ. Sci. **13**(3), 339–351 (2002)
34. Teece, D.: A dynamic capabilities-based entrepreneurial theory of the multinational enterprise. J. Int. Bus. Stud. **45**(1), 8–37 (2014)
35. Vargo, S.L., Maglio, P.P., Akaka, M.A.: On value and value co-creation: a service systems and service logic perspective. Eur. Manag. J. **26**(3), 145–152 (2008)
36. Akaka, M.A., Vargo, S.L., Lusch, R.F.: An exploration of networks in value cocreation: a service-ecosystems view. Rev. Market. Res. **9**, 13–50 (2012)
37. Vargo, S.L., Akaka, M.A.: Value co-creation and service systems (Re)formation: a service ecosystems view. Serv. Sci. **4**(3), 207–217 (2012)
38. Wieland, H., Polese, F., Vargo, S.L., Lusch, R.F.: Toward a service (eco) systems perspective on value creation, pp. 12–24 (2012)
39. Cardoso, J., Lopes, R., Poels, G.: Service systems: concepts, modeling, and programming, pp. 1–91. Springer (2014)
40. Vargo, S.L., Lusch, R.F.: Service-dominant logic: looking ahead. Presentation at the Naples Forum on Service, pp. 14–17 (2011)
41. Bowman, C., Ambrosini, V.: Value creation versus value capture: towards a coherent definition of value in strategy. Br. J. Manag. **11**, 1–15 (2000)
42. Thalheim, B.: The science and art of conceptual modelling. In: Hameurlain, A., Küng, J., Wagner, R., Liddle, S.W., Schewe, K.-D., Zhou, X. (eds.) Transactions on Large-Scale Data- and Knowledge-Centered Systems VI. LNCS, vol. 7600, pp. 76–105. Springer, Heidelberg (2012)
43. Rafati, L.: Capability sourcing: a service-dominant logic view. In: Proceedings of the 8th Mediterranean Conference on Information Systems, p. 8 (2014)
44. Rafati, L., Poels, G.: Introducing service-oriented organizational structure for capability sourcing. In: Leonard, M., Snene, M. (eds.) IESS 2014. LNBIP, vol. 169, pp. 82–91. Springer, Heidelberg (2014)

45. Rafati, L., Poels, G.: Capability sourcing modeling: a high-level conceptualization based on service-dominant logic. In: Iliadis, L., Papazoglou, M., Pohl, K. (eds.) CAiSE Workshops 2014. LNBIP, vol. 178, pp. 77–87. Springer, Heidelberg (2014)
46. Loftin, R., Lync, R., Calhoun, J.: The Sourcing Canvas: A Strategic Approach to Sourcing Decisions. Technical report, Accelare (2011)
47. Sijnave, B.: The care information system of the future is VIRTUAL. Technical report in Presentation at 18de Colloquium Automatisering en zorgverlening, Affligem, Belgium (2014)
48. Jacobs, J.: Dependency and vulnerability: an exchange approach to the control of organizations. Adm. Sci. Q. **19**(1), 45–59 (1974)

New Service's Expectation Positioning
by Applying Cumulative Prospect Theory

Soe-Tsyr Daphne Yuan[✉] and Hsi-Yun Wang

Service Science Research Center, National Chengchi University, Taipei, Taiwan
{yuans,101356024}@nccu.edu.tw

Abstract. In the context of service innovation, the question of when to assess a new service by customer and how to achieve personalized assessment are yet to be explored. This is especially true under the situations of uncertainty when it comes to bringing the effectiveness of new service's promotion and decision making, i.e., for service provider to attain service competitiveness and for potential service customer to decide whether to try the new service. Accordingly, an appropriate expectation positioning method proposed in this study aims to collect and analyze psychological information from potential service customer in order to make service promotion decisions capable of achieving service provider's purpose as well as satisfying service customer, utilizing Cumulative Prospect Theory.

Keywords: New service expectation positioning · Cumulative prospect theory · Customer expectation · Behavior economics · Behavior change · Psychological value

1 Introduction

The service business environment nowadays faces challenges as the quantity of new services keeps rising. In Service Profit Chain, if service providers want to let customer satisfy, they should have attractive service designed and delivered to meet targeted customers' needs [1]. There are some critical questions to which service businesses should respond. First, it is to let potential customers or target market know the new service can increase their utility value that they really concern. Second, it is imperative to find a more effective way to assist potential customers who need to decide whether or not to try the new service. From the view of customers, when individuals make decision whether to try a new service after receiving the new service's information, it will trigger a cycle of stages of change addressed in the transtheoretical model [2]. This model proposes changing behavior as a process of five stages. The five stages include pre-contemplation (no desire to change behavior and ignoring problem), contemplation (conscious of problem but not yet to change behavior), preparation (ready and committed to change behavior), action (changing behavior) and maintenance (maintaining the change).

On the way from the second step to the third step of the behavioral change cycle, it is contemplation step to preparation step; by analogy, it is customer's new service decision making that takes place during the time before they have the willingness to try

© Springer International Publishing Switzerland 2016
T. Borangiu et al. (Eds.): IESS 2016, LNBIP 247, pp. 45–59, 2016.
DOI: 10.1007/978-3-319-32689-4_4

a new service and intend to take action in the immediate future. At this period of time, individuals must be aware of the pros of changing but also can identify the cons. The stage with longest time (as possibly long as six months) is the contemplation stage [3, 4]. This study aims to improve the effectiveness of individuals decision evaluation at this stage.

Another factor to inference individuals' decision making and assess the trying of a new service is "unfit expectation" that attributes to they not feeling worth trying the new service. We argue that individuals can have a more appropriate expectation by deducting some bias when considering the potential benefits and the possibly increased utility of using the new service.

In addition, individuals make decisions relying on their psychological activities, system 1 or system 2, i.e., thinking fast or slow [5]. This can also be applied to the situation of making the decision of positioning expectation of using a new service. We apply existing knowledge of psychological activities to design an IT artifact to cope with individual's possible thinking bias, illusion, *etc.* and achieve new service's proper expectation positioning. This study focuses on how to attain an appropriate expectation through individuals' system 2 psychological activities (consideration, analysis and comparison) on judging whether new service could bring in increased utility value.

To this end, our study presents a method of new service expectation positioning that applies Cumulative Prospect Theory (CPT) [6] of which the underlying philosophy is to help individuals make decision toward their maximum utility. CPT computes the utility value of decisions according to personal perception (psychological value and probability weight). According to an individual's perception, it is able to figure out what the individual really concerns and what phenomena would possibly occur. The method can then find a more appropriate expectation, suggest the individual to re-position the expectation, let the individual feel gaining more benefits and be willing to try the new service.

The paper is organized as follows. Section 2 presents the basic concepts of our method. Section 3 describes the method's IT artifact, its component modules and an illustrating scenario. Section 4 provides some preliminary evaluations, followed by the discussion. Finally, the conclusion is provided in Sect. 5.

2 Basic Concepts

In Cumulative Prospect Theory (CPT), an individual has a reference point which is influenced by the individual's expectation, environment and society and so on [7]. It is used synonymously with the term "current reference point" to mean reference point that is generated by the individual's intuition. Taking the current reference point as the balance point, it is able to compute the gain and loss for a decision. But, current reference point usually is not appropriate enough to represent a decision maker's status quo. When individuals face an uncertainty event, fast thinking (system 1) usually leads individuals to jump to a conclusion and affect their decision [8]. There exist thinking bias that makes individuals be not able to properly assess the utility value. The examples include the focusing effect as the tendency to place too much importance on one attribute and the impact bias as the tendency to overestimate the length or the intensity of the impact of future feeling status, and so on. Because of thinking bias, decision makers usually overestimate or underestimate the expectation of decision outcome.

As depicted in Fig. 1, CPT has two functions (value function and weight function) that are generated from interacting with an individual, and the two functions represent the psychological value and the attitude of probability weight of the individual [6]. The psychological value refers to the subjective value of each attribute for each individual. The attitude of probability weight refers to the subjective cumulative probabilities about how people tend to overweight extreme/unlikely events but underweight average/common events. Therefore, these two functions (value function and weight function) solve the weakness of expected utility theory. In addition, the functions can manifest the personal perception of the individual.

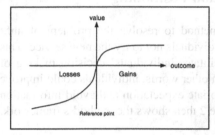 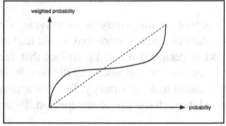

Fig. 1. Value function and weighted cumulative probabilities function in CPT (Source: [6])

Our method aims to pick up the high-weight attributes through a series of steps in order to find out a more proper reference point with system 2. This new reference point is generated based on the decision maker's psychological value, psychological behavior and the other issues the decision maker concerns. We anticipate it can reflect the individual's real situation, and it can help the decision maker position a suitable expectation. Letting decision making under a suitable expectation will bring decision maker more utility value.

On the other hand, there are lots of attributes that should be considered in the moment at which individuals are making decisions upon uncertainty event, such as the amount of monetary, the cost of wasting time, material, self-principles or regulations and the others dependent on the encountered events. Most weight, priority and level of loss aversion are changing and affect individuals' value and behavior over time. Individuals usually care different things, someone care money more than time, or vice versa. Individuals may focus on different aspects (attributes) on the same event, thence they have different levels of loss aversion on different attributes. In addition, the attributes that an individual concerns depend on the event. How to generate the right value function for the right attribute to the right person in order to properly assess the utility value is a critical issue.

This study aims at assisting service providers (businesses) to promote their new service and help service receivers (individual customers) to improve their assessment. It not only helps businesses deliver advantages of their services to potential customers, but also helps potential customers have an appropriate and fit expectation on the uncertainty event. This study assumes the category of "new service" to be the services classified as major innovation, start-up business and new services for the market presently (ones regarded as radical innovation as addressed in Johnson et al. (2000)'s work [9]).

In short, according to the Transtheoretical (stages of behavior change) Model [2], individuals usually spend a lot of time on assessing whether the pro's utility value being more than that of the con's utility value. Our method intends to make individuals have a more effective changing cycle and make them create more utility value from the changing cycle. After getting the positive consequence from the assessment, individuals would be able to move to the next step of behavior change.

3 Method of New Service Expectation Positioning

The purpose of this study is to provide a method to resolve the problem of unfit expectation of a new service that would lead individuals not to try the new service. This method is designed as an IT artifact that facilitates individuals' decision making of trying new service and assessing the benefit. In other words, individuals could improve their decision making strategy, find the appropriate expectation and avoid information distorted through the use of our method. Figure 2 then shows the method's framework.

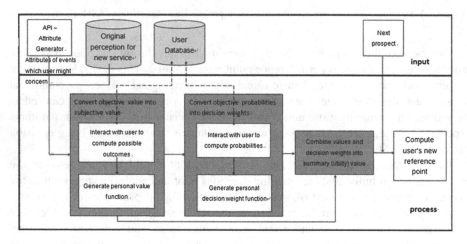

Fig. 2. Framework for the method of new service expectation positioning

An individual action of deciding whether to try a new service is regarded as an event. The method will start from the insight of an event at the API-Attribute Generator in the beginning. The insight of the event refers to the descriptions of the core features of a new service. The method will also attain additional feature information that the individual might concern by mining some on-line resources via the Attribute Generator API. The method also receives next prospect of service provider, in order to compare with the final utility to guarantee the effectiveness of our method. This study regards each attribute being associated with its value function and decision weight function.

After receiving specific attribute and an individual's original reference point, the method starts to interact with the individual to collect data (original expectation of new service, attitudes of risk aversion) from User Database. The method will convert the objective value into subjective value, and convert objective probabilities into decision weights, and then generate the value function and the decision weight function respectively. Combining the value function and the weight function, the method will then compute the utility value for the new service. After computing the utility value that the individual concerns, a new reference point will be passed down to the individual in order to provide a better expectation positioning of the new service. Finally, it would compare the utility value and the next prospect, in order to guarantee that the utility value corresponds to the next prospect.

3.1   Generate Personal Value Function Module

In order to evaluate the psychological value from user who desires to make decision of trying a new service, this module is for converting objective value into subjective value in order to generate the personal value function. The procedure of this module is as follows:

(1) **Receive the Information:** including attribute information which an individual might concern, original reference point, attitudes of risk aversion, from the original perception of a new service. The definition of receiving information are as follows:

- Attribute information that an individual might concern: the new service has its own attributes related to the core features. Some of these attributes are signification to the individual. The method would focus on these attributes to generate the value function, such as the attribute of success match ratio for an online dating service.
- Original reference point: The expectation of the new service when the individual receives the information of new service at the first time, such as the success match ratio being 75 % of an online dating service.
- Attitudes of risk aversion (λ): The attitude of facing an uncertainty or risky decision such as the individual whose attitude of risk aversion is 0.88.

(2) **Interact with the individual:** In order to acquire several outcomes of the new service from the individual, apply the original reference point (original expectation of new service) to design customized questions to interact with the individual. The method will automatically generate binary questions according to the individual's original reference point. The method applies the approach of Certainty Equivalent (CE) to elicit possible outcomes [10]. With the chaining CE approach, it can pick probabilities p_i first and elicit the outcomes of certainty equivalent [11]. The midpoint chaining is a special case of the chaining CE approach, when only one probability $p_1 = 0.5$ is used [12]. The following example takes the monetary attribute as an exemplar question.

> Q: You have an opportunity of gaining 100 dollars with 50%. Are you willing to exchange with a gain of 75 dollars for certainty?

If the individual answers "yes", the method will modify $75 to become lower (i.e., $37.5, the medium point within the range which is lower than 75: $0 \sim 75$). It is represented at the left side of Fig. 3. On the contrary, if the individual answers "no", the method will modify $75 to become higher (i.e., $87.5, the medium point within the range which is higher than 75: $75 \sim 100$). It represents at the right side of Fig. 3. After the method progresses five rounds of interactions and gets the sixth outcome, it achieves convergence (e.g., Fig. 4) and stop the interactions, moving to next procedure.

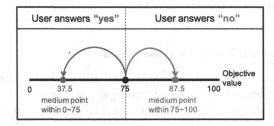

Fig. 3. Rule of interacting.

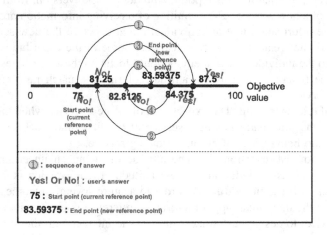

Fig. 4. Exemplar process diagram of step-by-step operations

(3) Demonstrate the new reference point: With the outcomes of the previous step, the method demonstrates the new reference point, which is generated in the last round of the previous step. The last outcome undergoes the most operations of system 2, and the method interprets it as the most appropriate new reference point. Regarding the new reference point as the origin, the remaining outcomes are then converted relative to the origin.

(4) Generate the value function: Substitute the variables (including x, λ that are illustrated as the followings) to the value function of Formula (1), and then compute the utility of the new service.

The equation and definition of variables as following.

$$v(x) = \begin{cases} x^\alpha & \text{if } x \geq 0 \\ -\lambda(-x)^\beta & \text{if } x < 0 \end{cases} \tag{1}$$

v(x): Personal value function of new service for the individual (decision maker) and referring to the psychological value of the outcome *x* that is a possible outcome of an uncertainty decision.

α **and** *β*: Power for gains/losses. Both approximately equal to 0.88.

λ: The attitude of facing an uncertainty decision.

(5) Pass down the outcomes: pass down the outcomes to next module (Generate Personal Decision Weight Function Module).

3.2 Generate Personal Decision Weight Function Module

In view of CPT, researches proposed that the weak point of Prospect Theory can be resolved by cumulative functional [13]. It means to cumulate probability, instead of using pure probability to assign weight to outcomes. This module generates the entire cumulative distribution function, instead of each probability separately. The purpose of this module is also converting objective probabilities to decision weights to generate the decision weight function. The procedure of this module is as follows:

(1) **Receive the information:** receive the outcomes value from previous module (Generate Personal Value Function Module).

(2) **Interact with the individual:** assign the probability to each outcome by interacting with the individual. The method applies different levels of probabilities to design the question, in order to recognize the risk attitude of each outcome. Different levels of probabilities will be illustrated and exemplified below.

The method will automatically generate a question according to the standard sequence of outcomes from Generate Personal Value Function Module. Each outcome should be assigned a probability weight; therefore, this module will progress a number of times (the number is equal to the number of outcomes). In every round the method will ask the individual a question and get a response.

> Q: Imagine you own a gamble which either pays \$100 or \$0. Someone offers you a sure payment of \$75 in exchange for this gamble. Would you accept the sure payment if the chance of winning the gamble were _____% (Hershey, 1985)?
>   ☐ 10% ☐ 50% ☐ 90%

Three options are offered to choose by the individual, 10 %, 50 % and 90 %, represent small-probability, indifferent and large-probability, respectively. This is because the existing researches address that individuals have distorted perception about extreme probability (extremely small or extremely large) [14].

(3) **Generate weight function:** substitute the variables (including p, γ, δ, that are illustrated as follows) to the weight function, and then compute the probability weight of the outcome. The method applies the Formula (2) to compute the probability weight of the outcomes including gains and losses (e.g., 75, 87.5, 81.25, 84.375). The output of this module is the probability weights of outcomes.

The equation and definition of variables as following.

$$W^+(p) = \frac{p^\gamma}{(p^\gamma + (1-p)^\gamma)^{1/\gamma}}, \quad W^-(p) = \frac{p^\delta}{\left(p^\delta(1-p)^\delta\right)^{1/\delta}} \tag{2}$$

w(p): Personal decision weight function of a new service for an individual (decision maker) and referring to the decision weight of the probability of outcome *p* of an uncertainty decision.
γ **and** δ: Probability weighting parameter for gains/losses. Typically, the value of γ is 0.61 and δ is 0.69 [6].

3.3   Compute Utility Value Module

Before individuals are willing to try the new service, they usually have "expectation" in their mind. Then, the individuals usually compare their "expectation" with the value of the new service which they really receive. The method applies the CPT to assess the expectation of the new service for an individual. This method can achieve personal psychological value and personal probability weight. Therefore, the method takes the format of CPT to demonstrate the expectation (it is also called utility value) of new service for user. In order to combine the psychological value and probability weight to let individual try the new service, the method computes the expectation (utility value) through Formula (3) of utility value. Based on the core concept to compute the utility value for a decision, the equation assumes for the assessment phase in simplest form and definition of variables are shown below [15].

$$U = \sum_{i=1}^{n} w(p_i)v(x_i). \tag{3}$$

U: Utility value of new service.

i: All of possible outcomes of the new service for an individual.

$w(p_i)$: This value is from Generate Personal Decision Weight Function Module and is the Personal decision weight function of new service for the individual (decision maker). refers to the decision weight of the probability of outcome i.

$v(x_i)$: This value is from Generate Personal Value Function Module and refers to the Personal value function of new service for the individual (decision maker). $v(x_i)$ is the psychological value of the outcome x_i.

To multiply each outcome value of new service and weight of outcome of new service, it is to summarize all results. The final value is the utility value (expectation) of current attribute for current decision. The method will use this result (expectation) to compare with the Next Prospect and recommend to try or not to try the new service. The aforementioned is using one specific attribute of new service to describe the operation of the method.

Assuming there are more than one attributes of new service which the individual concerns, the method will repeat above process several rounds. The method will get specific utility value (expectation) from different attributes of new service in every round. Thus, the method will use these utility values (expectation) to compute the weighted means. The final weighted means is regarded as the utility value (expectation) of new service in the current decision.

3.4   An Application Scenario

Taking a new service of online dating service i-Part as an example, i-Part was established in 2003, and it is the biggest online dating platform in Taiwan. In the online dating service industry, i-Part was known as a radical innovation service for it proposing a virtual way of making friends with high success match ratio. Although i-Part is already the industry leader, they must think about how to sustain their competitive advantage in light of the other competitors such as iMatchBox and DateMe-Now, and how to make more potential customers change their behavior by having the willingness of trying their service. Our method hopes to help those potential customers to cognize the really expected service and help service provider to deliver the features of new service that the potential customers really concern.

For example, single Johnny receives an advertisement banner of i-Part showing the success match ratio of 70 %. However, Johnny thinks that i-Part should have a success match of 90 % (i.e., current expectation). The method will apply the current mental state (current expectation) to find out his other psychological state (psychological value, probability weigh) through interacting with Johnny. The method will compute the new expectation (assumed as 75 %) and then compare with next prospect (i.e., the expected utility value assumed by i-Part that declares having the 70 % success match ratio).

In above situation, our method hopes to adjust Johnny's expectation via the interactions with his mental system (system 1 and system 2). Our method is to provide him with an appropriate expectation of i-Part with the graph of value function which can let him understand his real psychological value. This can also make Johnny more understand the maximum benefit of i-Part based on Johnny's true psychological state.

4   Evaluation

In this study, we implemented our method into a service system and used a set of experiments to evaluate whether our method proposed in Sect. 3 can make individuals proceed the behavioral change cycle (i.e., willingness of trying new service) and gain more utility from a new service. In addition, the method intends to help new service providers do service promotion. The underlying assumption is that those potential customers are in their contemplation stage of behavior change. That is, they are aware that their problems and would like to verify if their needs can be achieved and create more utility through using a new service. There are 30 experiment subjects; 11 of them are graduate students and 19 of them are founders of service providers, experimenting with two scenarios of encountering new services (Online Shopping Service and Music Streaming Services). Figure 5 depict the experiment process journey.

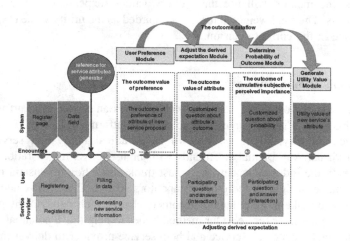

Fig. 5. The subject's journey of the experiment process

The propositions that are to be investigated include:

- **Proposition 1:** Provide a derived expectation of new service (by adjusting individuals' expectation positioning) based on real-time interactions could be used to change individuals' behavior intention.
- **Proposition 2:** People who are in the contemplation step of behavior change cycle can gain more utility through our method than those who are in the pre-contemplation step (i.e., they are yet to be aware of their problems).

Based on Cumulative Prospect Theory, our method adjusts an subject's reference point of an attribute of new service with the interacting questions and answers, using the 30 experiment subjects to do the preliminary test. Subjects can choose if they are to willing to exchange or not based on the options prompted by our system by "Yes" or "No" button and all the interactions will be recorded. The starting value is a subject's current reference point about an attribute of the service. If the subject moves on the next section, the value will be adjusted by the subject's answer. (it will progress 5 times to record 6 outcome values and the value will range in 0 ~ 100).

After adjusting the subject's expectation, the system will compute the utility value of willingness to try the new service. We observe the results of utility values of each new service's attribute, in order to verify if the utility is increased by the adjusting of our system.

We will describe the evaluation results in following two subsections in details. In Sect. 4.1, we explain the utility value which is computed by our system for each experimental subject. In Sect. 4.2, we focus on the URICA score and experimental subjects' behavior change. In addition, we will interpret the results and give some managerial discussion.

URICA questionnaire [16] is a scorecard to distinguish the stage of behavioral change cycle which an individual is situated in.

4.1   Proposition 1 - Utility Value

When individuals perceive that utility is increased, it will prompt individuals to move to the next step of behavioral change. We analyze the utility of new service's attribute. In order to verify the utility is a certainty increase after interacting with our system. The results show this modification is effective, and there are about 66.67 % subjects will gain more utility and have the willingness to try new service (see the Utility (modified) bar of Fig. 6). That is, we can say that the adjusting by interacting and generating a derived expectation of new service in terms of calculating the utility of new service could be used to change the individuals' behavior intention.

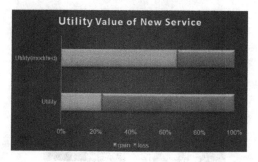

Fig. 6. Proportion of utility value (gain or loss) of new service

In addition, we collected the data about the perception and the confidence of adjusting, and there are five levels. To verify whether the adjusting of derived expectation is perceived (and whether there is confidence about the derived expectation of attribute provided by the system) after interacting with the system five-round respectively, we asked subjects to choose the level of perceived adjusting. The score 1 and 2 point mean negative consciousness of adjusting (and negative confidence of adjusting), score 3 point means they don't have specific consciousness (and confidence) about adjusting, score 4 and 5 point mean positive consciousness (and confidence) of adjusting. Therefore, we want to justify that the subjects' consciousness is larger than score 3 point, and it means our system can result in positive consciousness of adjusting. On the other words, the score larger than 3 point means our system can successfully adjust subjects' derived expectations with their cognitive perception. We used One-Sample T test with 95 % confidence interval and verified that mean of conscious (and confidence) of adjusting is significant larger than score 3 point.

Meanwhile, individuals' ability to make decisions by mental activity can be categorized into two types. To verify whether these two types (system 1, system 2) would alternately operate to assess decisions, we asked the subjects to assign the proportion of their decision ways after they interact with our system. We found that subjects use both system 1 and system 2 (mental activity) to make decision (answer the customized questions provided by our system). We also found subjects who use system 2 no less than (equal or more than) system 1 would be more effectively to have their expectation adjusted.

4.2   Proposition 2 - URICA Score

The Proposition 2 investigates the effect of the interaction way to progress behavioral change. We calculated the 30 experiment subjects' URICA score, including before and after interacting with our system. We classify subjects' evolution of URICA scores (behavioral change state) into two categories (See Fig. 7), including precontemplation stage and contemplation stage, and then we interpret their reasons as follows. The result of descriptive statistic shows that among the 30 subjects, 11 of them are in precontemplation stage and 19 of them are in contemplation stage.

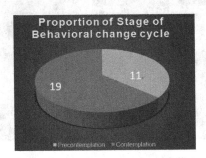

Fig. 7. Proportion of behavioral change cycle

We break down both of the two categories in order to observe which situated stage of subjects can make URICA score increase. Figure 8 shows the evolution of URICA score of each stage category.

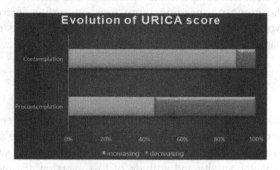

Fig. 8. Evolution of URICA score

The result of descriptive statistic shows that in precontemplation stage there are 11 experimental subjects and there are 5 subjects' URICA score being increased. The proportion of increased URICA score population is about 45.45 %. In contemplation stage, there are 19 experimental subjects and there are 17 experimental subjects' URICA score being increased. The proportion of increased URICA score population is about 89.47 %. Based on the statistic results we found that subjects in contemplation stage interacting with our system is more effective to change their behavior intention than subjects in precontemplation stage.

4.3 Discussion

The purpose of our method is to incite some intrinsic motivation of individuals and let them have the willingness to try a new service (i.e., a behavioral change). After adjusting the derived expectation and receiving the increased utility, the subjects might express that they have willingness to try new service. It brings sufficient intention to stimulate them to do behavioral change. At least from the psychological aspect, they want to do behavioral change and it's a good beginning.

It is a novel way to promote a new service for new service provider. It is very different from existing marketing approaches for this way of utilizing the psychological data to promote the new service. Through figuring out the subjects' preferences and provide proper derived expectations of the new service to make them have the willingness to try new service. In addition, the detailed mental activity (the sequence, proportion and so on) can also bring some aspirations to service provider. This is an occasion to take advantage of the adjusting that can encourage the subjects to think what they really need and concern to stimulate their willingness of trying the new service.

Since our method can help the subjects to adjust their unfit expectation with their mental activities, the analysis data and performance of our system can help new service provider to redesign their new service and marketing plan so as to make individuals have the willingness to try their new service. Our method can also make most subjects have the consciousness and the confidence on the adjusting and stimulate them to do behavioral change. In addition, subjects who spend more time on surfing internet are easier to use our system and complete the operations and have the willingness to try new service. In the group of spending more time on surfing internet such as the founders and co-workers of service providers much appreciate this research's originality and performance.

5 Conclusion

In this paper, we address the problem how to motivate to progress behavioral change (during contemplation stage and preparation stage) for new service's promotion and decision making in terms of the psychological method of adjusting unfit expectation. By leveraging the mental activity and attitude of loss aversion, the method assembles them within the structure of Cumulative Prospect theory, and construct the utility function to achieve the motivation purpose. Through this method, individuals can be stimulated to have the willingness to try a new service, and providers are able to get some inspiration about adjusting their service and marketing promotion.

However, we also note several limitations in our study besides using a limited number of experiment subjects. First, the limited scope of "new service" of radical innovation are more appropriate to apply our method. This is because individuals usually make progress on the procedure of behavioral change when they assess whether or not to adopt a discontinuous technological change (radical innovations). Second, the numerical presentation of derived expectation could be re-designed to become more intuitive and clear to individuals. In this study, we regard the utility value as the role of a KPI for whether customers being willing to try a new service. The future work can extend the role of such a KPI in a broader context of firm's strategy; for example, when there are several alternative new service candidates to be selected, or when there are differences between segments of customers and some new services may be more adequate to a certain segment than others. In addition, the method could further incorporate additional information (e.g., cultural traditions and other aspects) to characterize customer's behavior.

References

1. Heskett, J.L., Schlesinger, L.A.: Putting the service-profit chain to work. Harv. Bus. Rev. **72**, 164–174 (1994)
2. Prochaska, J.O. Johnson, S., Lee, P: The transtheoretical model of behavior change. In: The Handbook of Health Behavior Change (Second Edition), vol. 12, pp. 38–48 (1998)
3. Patten, S., Vollman, A., Thurston, W.: The utility of the transtheoretical model of behavior change for HIV risk reduction in injection drug users. J. Assoc. Nurses AIDS Care **11**(1), 57–66 (2000)
4. Prochaska, J., DiClemente, C., Norcross, J.: In search of how people change: applications to addictive behaviors. J. Addict. Nurs. **47**(9), 1002–1114 (1992)

5. Stanovich, K.E., West, R.F.: Individual differences in reasoning: implications for the rationality debate? Behav. Brain Sci. **23**, 645–665 (2000)
6. Tversky, A., Kahneman, D.: Advances in prospect theory: cumulative representation of uncertainty. J. Risk Uncertain. **5**, 297–323 (1992)
7. Bandura, A., McClelland, D.C.: Social Learning Theory. Prentice-Hall, Englewood Cliffs (1977)
8. Kahneman, D.: Thinking, Fast and Slow. Farrar, Straus and Giroux, New York (2011)
9. Johnson, S.P., Menor, L.J., Roth, A.V., Chase, R.B.: A critical evaluation of the new service development process: integrating service innovation and service design. In: Fitzsimmons, J.A., Fitzsimmons, M.J. (eds.) New Service Development Creating Memorable Experiences, pp. 1–32. Sage Publications, Thousand Oaks (2000)
10. Farquhar, P.: Utility assessment methods. Manage. Sci. **30**, 1283–1300 (1984)
11. Keeney, R., Raiffa, H.: Decisions with Multiple Objectives: Preferences and Value Tradeoffs. Wiley, New York (1976)
12. Krzysztofowicz, R., Duckstein, L.: Assessment errors in multiattribute utility functions. Organ. Behav. Individ. Perform. **26**(3), 326–348 (1980)
13. Quiggin, J.: Subjective utility, anticipated utility, and the allais paradox. Organ. Behav. Individ. Decis. Process. **35**(1), 94–101 (1985)
14. Gonzalez, R., Wu, G.: On the shape of the probability weighting function. Cogn. Psychol. **38**, 129–166 (1999). organizational behavior and individuals decision processes
15. Kahneman, D., Tversky, A.: Prospect theory: an analysis of decision under risk. J. Econometric Soc. **47**, 263–291 (1979)
16. DiClemente, C.C., Prochaska, J.O.: Toward a comprehensive, transtheoretical model of change: stages of change and addictive behaviors. Plenum Press (1998)

Enabling Service Business Models Through Service Processes

Nikhil Zope[1(✉)], Anand Kumar[2], and Doji Lokku[3]

[1] Tata Consultancy Services, Mumbai, India
nikhil.zope@tcs.com
[2] Tata Consultancy Services, Pune, India
anand.ar@tcs.com
[3] Tata Consultancy Services, Hyderabad, India
doji.lokku@tcs.com

Abstract. With increasing importance of business models in modern businesses and continuous business models innovations, it is becoming important to know whether the current processes support proposed business model or can be modified to support the proposed business model. This aspect of Business model innovation is known as business model implementation and it has received little attention in business model related research. In this paper, we explore the relationship between various business model elements with service processes, so that one can systematically assess process readiness for a business model in the future. Focus of this paper is on implementation of new or modified business model in an existing organization already delivering offerings.

Keywords: Business model · Business model elements · Service process · Process characteristics

1 Introduction

Process literature is spread across various topics like business process modelling, business process reengineering, process modelling, process reasoning, service processes, services blueprinting and so on. These topics address concerns like rethinking the way business works, delivering committed quality, recognizing how people contribute, coordinating work and operational know-how.

Business excellence and performance management models like Balanced Scorecard, discuss how strategy can be trickled down to operations. However, these process research threads, do not address how business models are implemented or understood at an operational level.

Business Model has been referred to as the entity that aids in extracting out the inherent value from an offering of a business. It consists of the value proposition, market segment, value chain element, competitive strategy and the like [1].

In present times, economy is dominated by services and becoming increasingly dependent on digital technologies, and innovation. Services innovation is considered essential for any business, which is looking to compete and survive in the long run.

© Springer International Publishing Switzerland 2016
T. Borangiu et al. (Eds.): IESS 2016, LNBIP 247, pp. 60–71, 2016.
DOI: 10.1007/978-3-319-32689-4_5

Business model is one of the key elements in service innovation, as it defines how value is exchanged between the participants in a business transaction (traditionally, provider and customer).

Business model innovation affects the entire organization [2, 3]. It involves designing new business models towards intended innovation and then implementing it, to achieve the innovation results. Experimentation to arrive at the finalized business model to be implemented, is also considered as the vital part of business model innovation. Chesbrough [4] discusses the need for organizational processes and authority for managers to experiment with business models and to take decisions based on the results, of these experiments. In the 4I framework proposed by Frankenberger et al. [5], four stages in business model innovation has been described: initiation, ideation, integration and implementation. Business model implementation however is a widely neglected issue [6]. The scope of this paper includes processes related to integration and implementation stages. These stages include integration of business model with existing infrastructure and organizational processes as well as new practices which are to be incorporated. We consider business model experimentation to be outside the scope of this paper.

Enabling the business models is not just limited to creating required infrastructure (e.g. for web based sales, creating website and payment gateways) but also making sure that the service processes involved in delivering the service offering are aligned to the business models. Alignment of a service process to proposed business model is a research question that has not been addressed till now. In this paper, we aim to take the first step by exploring the relationship between elements of a business model and service processes.

2 Business Model & Gaps in Business Model Implementation

Business Model as a concept started getting popular in late 90's. It started with discussions surrounding internet business and the concept subsequently matured as one of the fundamental ways to look at businesses. A business model is the organization's 'core logic' for creating value for its customers and stakeholders [7]. Osterwalder et al. [6], define a business model as a conceptual tool that contains a set of elements and their relationships and allows for expressing the business logic of a specific organization. They [6] further consider business model as description of the value an organization offers to one or several segments of customers, and of the architecture of the organization and its network of partners for creating, marketing, and delivering this value and relationship capital, to generate profitable and sustainable revenue streams.

Various researchers have defined business model in terms of the elements that it constitutes. Gassman et al. [8], propose four questions, which when answered explicated can be used to make business models tangible. The four questions are: (1) Who is the target customer, (2) What is the value proposition towards the customer, (3) What is the value chain behind the creation of this value, and (4) What is the revenue model that captures the value.

Joan Magretta [10] asserts that a good business model remains essential to every successful organization, whether it's a new venture or an established player.

Business model gives holistic picture of a business, depicting how all elements in the system (factors inside and outside of the organization) work together [10–12]. Chesbrough [9] highlights the importance of business models by stating, that a mediocre technology pursued within a great business model may be more valuable than a great technology exploited via a mediocre business model. Various researchers view business model as planning, managing and analyzing tool for an organization. Demil and Lecoque [13], state that business model lens can help in analyzing the functioning and architecture of a specific organization. Explicitly recognizing business model for an organization can help an organization, respond faster to changes in the business environment [6]. Business Models can also help an organization to improve upon alignment of strategy, business organization and technology [6].

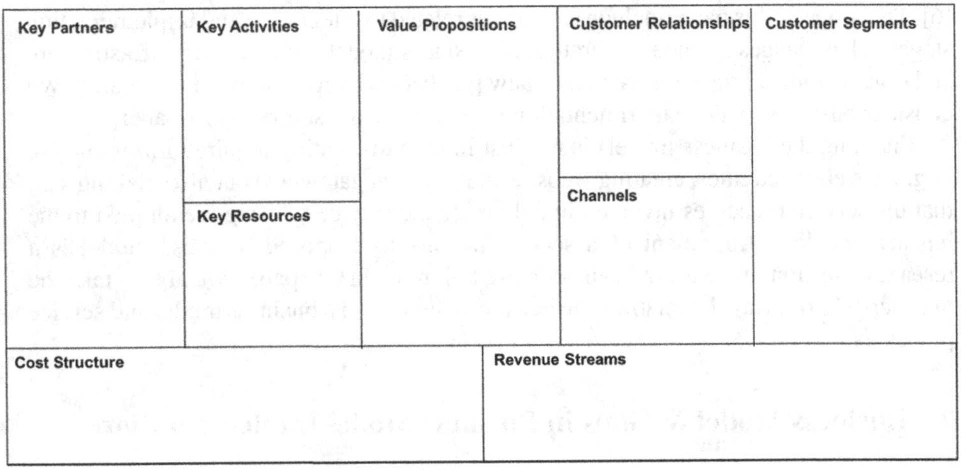

Key Partners	Key Activities	Value Propositions	Customer Relationships	Customer Segments
	Key Resources		Channels	
Cost Structure			Revenue Streams	

Fig. 1. The business model canvas [15]

Business Models can be the way an organization operates to ensure its sustainability [13]. Such sustainability can be achieved by innovating and evolving business models to address possible future for business organizations.

Osterwalder [14] proposed nine building blocks that can be used to describe a business model completely. The nine building blocks are: Value Proposition, Target Customer, Distribution Channel, Relationship, Value Configuration, Core Competency, Partner Network, Cost Structure, and Revenue Model [14].

Osterwalder and Pigneur [15] further worked on these nine building blocks and created business model canvas, as shown in Fig. 1, which can be used to design a new business model as well as describe existing business models for any organization. This business model canvas has become a standard that has been adopted across industry and by academics. We also choose to use the business model canvas as a reference for establishing relationship between business model and service processes. We explore each business model element in the next section.

Business Model implementation and management include the "translation" of the business model as a plan into more concrete elements, such as a business structure (e.g. departments, units, human resources), business processes (e.g. workflows, responsibilities) and infrastructure and systems [6]. Mark Johnson [16], defines business model implementation as an effort largely focused on testing and validating assumptions, while integrating key resources and processes required to deliver on the customer value proposition and profit formula. The current literature on business model implementation is more focused on overcoming the people resistance and resistance due to organization's dominant logic. It does not systematically address how proposed business model manifests as structure and process. Good business model design and implementation, coupled with careful strategic analysis, are necessary for technological innovation to succeed commercially [11]. Wirtz [17], discusses business model implementation similar to implementation of a plan without dwelling on the impact on processes. In direct reference to processes, Zott and Amit [18], suggest two set of parameters that activity systems designers needs to consider with respect to business model. The two set of parameters are: design elements (content, structure and governance) that describe an activity system's architecture, and design themes (novelty, lock-in, complementarities and efficiency) that describe sources of its value creation. Zott and Amit [18], define an activity system as a set of interdependent organizational activities centered on focal firm, including those conducted by the focal firm, its partners or customers etc. Zott and Amit [18], discuss this view from the perspective of creating new organization, however these identified set of parameters are also valid for existing organizations that are looking to implement new business models. Zott and Amit [18], although successfully view business model from the perspective of processes, they lose connection of important business model abstractions in this view.

3 Elements of Business Models and Service Processes

As discussed in previous section, we take nine business model building blocks proposed by Osterwalder and Pigneur [15] as basis for the study. Keeping with the generic terminology, we refer each of these building blocks as an element of business model. In this section, we take each of these business model elements and explore their relationship with service processes.

3.1 Customer Segments

It defines the different groups of people or organizations an enterprise aims to reach and serve [15]. Organizations may group customers into distinct segments based on common needs, common behaviors, or other attributes. Osterwlader and Pigneur [15], also specify the conditions in which different customer segments may be defined:

Customer groups represent separate segments if:

- Their needs require and justify a distinct order
- They are reached through different Distribution Channels
- They require different types of relationships
- They have substantially different profitability
- They are willing to pay for different aspects of the order

Based on these variations in customer needs that define customer segments, the following questions can help understand how well service processes support customer segments:

- How much customization/personalization do service processes support?
- What and how many customer segments are we targeting for the service? Answer to this question dictates –
  - Expected variability and dynamism to be designed in service processes
  - Priority of service quality attributes with respect to each customer segment

3.2   Value Propositions

It describes the bundle of products and services that create value for a specific customer segment [15]. Value proposition is what an organization proposes to benefit the customer through its offerings. Value proposition may define not just benefits from the offering but also what additional or different value, an organization proposes to provide, to differentiate itself from competition.

Value propositions may be tricky to relate directly to service processes, as they get designed in the offerings. However when a characteristics like customer experience is part of value proposition, it should be addressed with due consideration to service processes. Also manifestation of all the design, with respect to value proposition, must be clear in the interactions with the customer. Related process steps in service processes must be designed such that organization can clearly communicate the value proposition at the appropriate steps.

Following questions help in assessing the impact of value propositions on service processes:

- What are the tangible and intangible parts/characteristics of processes, delivering the value proposition?
- What performance parameters must process satisfy, to deliver the value proposition?
- What needs do we satisfy with our service? How do we satisfy them?
- How do we assert our differentiator with respect to competitors?
- What characteristics of service processes represent our value proposition (needs satisfaction+ differentiator)?
- What is the invariable part of processes – the one that defines the service offering by the provider?

3.3   Channels

It describes how an organization communicates with and reaches its customer segments to deliver a value proposition [15]. Channels are customer touch points that play an important role in the customer experience [15]. Channels is thus one of the ways through which value proposition would impact/determine the service process. We find following questions relevant with respect to exploring relationship between channels and service processes:

- How communication channels are utilized in entire service value chain (right from advertising service offering to end of its delivery)?
- What is the waiting time added/reduced due to channels?
- How the process is different due to real time communication/feedback?
- What is the overall communication strategy in service processes?

3.4 Customer Relationships

It describes the types of relationships an organization establishes with specific customer segments [15]. Osterwalder and Pigneur [15] further argue that an organization should clarify the type of relationship it wants to establish with each customer segment. Relationships can range from personal to automated. What kind of customer relationship an organization wants, is a conscious decision that must be supported through the service processes, while delivering the service offerings. In typical services business, customer relationships cover the following functions: delivering the service offering and supporting it; to help customer realize the benefits of the service offering; and help customer in getting right things which are related to delivered service offering but not directly part of it.

Following concerns can be used to understand the influence of customer relationships on service processes:

- What qualities/characteristics must process satisfy, to achieve desired kind of customer relationships?
- Strategy with respect to customer relationships
- Touch points with customer in processes
- Communication channels used, their influence and constraints on processes and dynamics of processes
- Types of interactions with customers

3.5 Revenue Streams

Revenue Streams is the cash an organization generates from each customer segment (costs must be subtracted from revenues to create earnings) [15]. Successfully answering the question, "For what value, is each customer segment really willing to pay?" allows the organization to generate one or more revenue streams from each customer segment [15]. Each revenue stream may have different pricing mechanisms, such as fixed list prices, bargaining, auctioning, market dependent, volume dependent, or yield management [15].

A business model can involve two different types of revenue streams [15]:

- Transaction revenues resulting from one-time customer payments
- Recurring revenues resulting from ongoing payments to either deliver a value proposition to customers or provide post-purchase customer support

Following questions can highlight the relevance with respect to service processes:

- Are the activities segregated/separated appropriately to support measurement on which price is paid by customer (e.g. if customer pays based on number of transactions, are the processes organized so that number of transactions can be measured)?
- What flexibility do service processes offer to customers for paying? How revenue is distributed in service processes, is it lump sum or is it at various milestones? On what basis are the milestones decided?

3.6   Key Resources

It describes the most important assets required to make a business model work [15]. These resources allow an enterprise to create and order a value proposition, reach markets, maintain relationships with customer segments, and earn revenues [15]. Different key resources are needed, depending on the type of business model [15]. Key resources can be physical, financial, intellectual, or human. Key resources can be owned or leased by the organization or acquired from key partners [15].

Following questions can help establish relationship between key resources and service processes:

- What dependencies across activities are induced by these key resources? Scheduling, ordering of activities, etc.
- How are the key resources acquired in service processes?
- In what form are the key resources?
- How are the key resources shared across service processes? And different instances of same service process (one instance for each service transaction)?

3.7   Key Activities

It describes the most important things an organization must do to make its business model work [15]. Every business model calls for a number of key activities. These are the most important actions an organization must take to operate successfully [15]. Like key resources, they are required to create and order a value proposition, reach markets, maintain customer relationships, and earn revenues [15]. And like key resources, key activities differ depending on business model type [15].

This element of business model is directly part of service processes:

- What is the core service and activities representing them?

3.8   Key Partners

Key partnerships are the network of suppliers and partners that make the business model work [15]. Organizations forge partnerships for many reasons, and partnerships are becoming a cornerstone of many business models. Organizations create alliances to optimize their business models, reduce risk, or acquire resources [15].

We can distinguish between four different types of partnerships [15]:

- Strategic alliances between non-competitors
- Coopetition: strategic partnerships between competitors
- Joint ventures to develop new businesses
- Buyer-supplier relationships to assure reliable supplies

From the service processes perspective, it is important to know how interactions with these key partners and dependencies on them affect the processes. Following questions can help in establishing the relationship:

- What dependencies does key partners induce in service processes?
  - Resources required during performing activities
  - Activities performed by partners themselves
- Do we have contract such that waiting time is zero or minimal for acquiring resource or activity to be performed by key partner?

3.9   Cost Structure

It describes all costs incurred to operate a business model. Creating and delivering value, maintaining customer relationships, and generating revenue, all incur costs [15]. Such costs can be calculated relatively easily after defining key resources, key activities, and key partnerships [15].

Following questions can help in exploring how cost structure affects service processes:

- What are the financial constraints process must adhere to?
- What is the allowed flexibility in terms of financials?
- What mechanisms are built into the processes to handle financial constraints?
- What is the flexibility allowed for people in processes, to take decisions involving costs, in order to respond to dynamic needs, in service processes?

4   Analyzing the Influence on Service Processes

In previous sections we have briefly discussed different business model elements and questions that can help in establishing the relationship of these elements with service processes. In order to further understand how service processes support business model, we look at different elements in a process and analyze how each business model element influences process elements. In our previous work [19], we have used various process modeling approaches and languages to arrive at a process meta-model. Details of these process modeling approaches and languages can be found in our previous work [19]. Process elements identified in this meta-model [19] have been utilized to analyze influence of business model elements on service processes. Figure 2 shows the process meta-model.

We briefly summarize some elements of the process meta-model relevant to the scope of this paper. The meta-model represents different elements of a process and

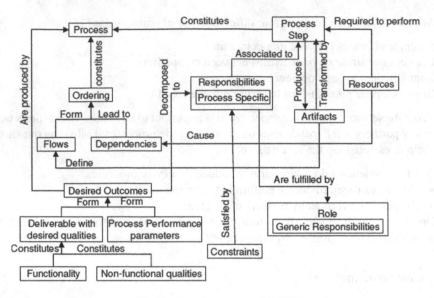

Fig. 2. Process meta-model [19]

relationships between those elements. A process exists for a certain purpose, which could be a service or a product. This service or product is considered as deliverable of the process. This deliverable has certain qualities that it must meet according to certain specification. Along with the deliverable, the process itself has some expected performance parameters like cost, time and flexibility. A deliverable with desired qualities, along with process performance parameters, form the desired outcomes of the process. A process has process steps organized in particular arrangement that makes the set of process steps into a process. Each step requires certain resources to be used in order to carry out the process. Performing each process step results in artefact/s that lead towards the deliverable. Each process step also represents a responsibility that an actor must fulfill, while playing the relevant role. A responsibility signifies meeting the artefact specification and correct execution of the relevant process step. A role signifies the required competence and knowledge to fulfil a set of responsibilities.

We extract the following elements from this process meta-model: activities (process steps), resources, process performance parameters, process constraints, and process flow. To address the specific influence, we take process flexibility and process performance parameter (time) as different elements, which are part of process characteristics. We define process flexibility as the degree to which process can be changed dynamically, in terms of variation of process steps, allocation of resources, etc. Variation of process steps may result from change in parameters for desired outcomes or alternate techniques to achieve some objective or to cope with additional cost/time constraints. Similarly allocation of resources may require change due to alternate techniques or additional cost/time constraints. With this information, we discuss how each business model element influences different process elements, based on the questions we discussed in the previous section.

- Customer segments primarily determine variations that service processes must support. Appropriate process flexibility must be designed in to processes, in order to serve varying needs of targeted customer segments and variations of service characteristics for them.
- Value propositions define what value an organization proposes to provide to targeted customer segments. Apart from the variations that must be designed to serve different segments, value propositions will influence different characteristics that processes must possess.
- Channels which determine the way organization communicates with its partners and customers, can manifest into activities related to channels in the communication and can affect significantly in terms of time taken to perform certain activities, by providing instantaneous information available for carrying out the activities.
- Customer relationships put requirements like speed required from processes, type of authority people require to manage the relationships. We consider these requirements as part of process characteristics. In further study, we can isolate the specific characteristics that customer relationships determine.
- Revenue streams apart from choosing how to get paid and related measurements, do not affect service processes. Both the requirements can get manifested in terms of related activities in service processes.
- Key resources are part of resources to be managed within processes affecting the process flow and dependencies within the process activities.
- Key activities can be directly considered as part of activities in the processes.
- Key partnerships dictate how resources are acquired and also the activities dependent on them. Cost structure determines the financial constraints under which processes must operate.

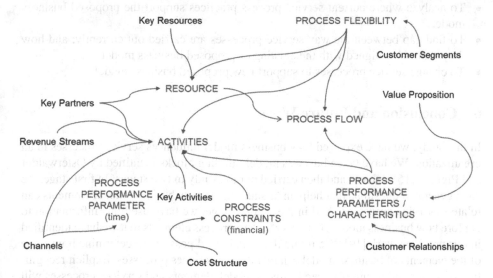

Fig. 3. Influence of business model elements on service process elements

Figure 3 summarizes our analysis with respect to influence of business model elements on aspects of service processes, pictorially.

5 Discussion

Business model innovation cannot be complete without the implementation of designed or changed business model(s) in the business organization. Implementing the business model requires it to be operationalized in terms of existing service processes within the organization. The limited study we have performed, states the relationship of each business model element with elements of service processes. It also presents questions in relation to each of the business model element to determine how it will affect organizational service processes. The relationship with business models can be seen in terms of activities within the process; the sequence of those activities (process itself); and process characteristics like process flexibility, time, resource utilization, etc. Such outcomes can help management in making appropriate changes to organizational processes to enable a newly designed business model. Such outcomes can also be used to determine gaps by noticing the influences and questions that were ignored while creating the business model implementation plan. Customer segments, key partners, key resources, key activities, value proposition, and the other business model elements provide all the necessary inputs required to design new service processes, in the case of a new service offering with a new business model, as it is being added to the organization.

In summary, relationship between business model elements with service processes and its elements can help with the following:

- As input for design of service processes for a service
- To analyze where current service process practices support the proposed business model
- To find gap between the way service processes are carried out currently, and how they should be aligned with the existing or proposed business model
- To change service processes to support new proposed business model

6 Conclusion and Future Work

In this study, we have explored how business model influences service processes in an organization. We have taken business model building blocks identified by Osterwalder and Pigneur [15] as basis and then carried out the study in two stages. In first stage, we have generated questions that help understanding on how business model elements can relate to service processes. And in the second stage, we have used this information to explore how business model elements relate to process elements that we have identified in our previous work [19]. We found that it is indeed possible to determine how some of the elements of business model can manifest in services processes. Explicit recognition of such relationship between business model elements and services processes will ensure successful implementation of a business model, by bringing out clearly how it can be operationalized.

As future work, we plan to explore the proposed questions in Sect. 3 in detail by studying a few real life cases, to arrive at a specific way a business model manifests in service processes. Further details added through case study can be used to prepare a framework that can guide how business models can be operationalized in an organization.

References

1. Lokku, D., Zope, N., Kumar, A.: Role of business models in realizing value: a perspective through 'value framework' and 'open innovation'. In: Tactics Conference (2012)
2. Amit, R., Zott, C.: Value creation in e-business. Strateg. Manage. J. **22**, 493–520 (2001)
3. Nair, S., Paulose, H., Palacios, M., Tafur, J.: Service orientation: effectuating business model innovation. Serv. Ind. J. **33**(9–10), 958–975 (2013)
4. Chesbrough, H.: Business model innovation: opportunities and barriers. Long Range Plan. **43**, 354–363 (2010)
5. Frankenberger, K., Weiblen, T., Csik, M., Gassmann, O.: The 4I-framework of business model innovation: a structured view on process phases and challenges. Int. J. Prod. Dev. **18**(3–4), 249–273 (2013)
6. Osterwalder, A., Pigneur, Y., Tucci, C.L.: Clarifying business models: origins, present, and future of the concept. Commun. Assoc. Inf. Syst. **16**(1), 1–25 (2005)
7. Linder, J.C., Cantrell, S.: Changing Business Models: Surveying the Landscape. Accenture Institute for Strategic Change, Cambridge (2000)
8. Gassmann, O., Frankenberger, K., Csik, M.: The St. Gallen Business Model Navigator. Working Paper, University of St. Gallen, St. Gallen (2013)
9. Chesbrough, H.: Open Innovation: The New Imperative for Creating and Profiting from Technology. Harvard Business School Press, Cambridge (2003)
10. Magretta, J.: Why business models matter. Harv. Bus. Rev. **80**, 86–92 (2002)
11. Teece, D.J.: Business models, business strategy and innovation. Long Range Plan. **43**(2), 172–194 (2010)
12. Zott, C., Amit, R., Massa, L.: The business model: recent developments and future research. J. Manage. **37**(4), 1019–1042 (2011)
13. Demil, B., Lecocq, X.: Business model evolution in search of dynamic consistency. Long Range Plan. **43**, 227–246 (2010)
14. Osterwalder, A.: The Business Model Ontology: A Proposition in a Design Science Approach. Doctoral Thesis at University of Lausanne. (2004). http://www.uniempre.org.br/user-files/files/TheBusiness-Model-Ontology.pdf
15. Osterwalder, A., Pigneur, Y.: Business Model Generation: A Handbook for Visionaries, Game Changers, and Challengers. Wiley, New York (2010)
16. Johnson, M.W.: Seizing the White Space: Business Model Innovation for Growth and Renewal. Harvard Business Press, Boston (2010)
17. Wirtz, B.W.: Business Model Management. Gabler, Wiesbaden (2010)
18. Zott, C., Amit, R.: Business model design: an activity system perspective. Long Range Plan. **43**(2), 216–226 (2010)
19. Zope, N., Nori, K.: Process Meta-modeling: A Design Perspective, Technical Report at Tata Consultancy Services, Hyderabad (2008)

Modelling Service Requirements
and Management of Business Processes

Experience from a Modelling and Simulation Perspective in Smart Transport Information Service Design

Monica Drăgoicea[1]([⊠]), Denisa Constantinescu[2], and João Falcão e Cunha[3]

[1] Faculty of Automatic Control and Computers, University Politehnica of Bucharest, 313 Splaiul Independentei, 060042 Bucharest, Romania
monica.dragoicea@acse.pub.ro

[2] Higher Technical School of Computer Engineering, University of Málaga, Bulevar Louis Pasteur, 35, 29071 Málaga, Spain
denisa.constantinescu@uma.es

[3] Faculty of Engineering - FEUP, University of Porto, Rua Dr. Roberto Frias, 4200-465 Porto, Portugal
jfcunha@fe.up.pt

Abstract. This paper presents experience obtained in modelling and simulation of stakeholder-driven interactions for improved transport service design. The presented results describe value-aware, service model driven design artefacts supporting smart transport service development. The Socio-Technical System Engineering process is used in order to generate modelling and simulation artefacts, based on an executable representation of requirements. As a case study, the paper presents an improved design approach for a city transport information service to support travellers with valuable information regarding planning a trip in a city. This attempt to integrate agent-based modelling and simulation experience into the development of smart transport services emphasises the role of the development platform that provides tools for model analysis, validation, simulation, and real-time animation. The development platform's role in transposing the above mentioned aspects in practice is emphasized and integration guidelines of the STSE process steps with the IBM Rational Rhapsody®development platform are described.

Keywords: Service systems engineering · Modelling and simulation · Service engineering process · Smart transport

1 Introduction

Developing complex service systems requires today the application of different perspectives of related research and practice. They originate from several areas such as service science, service management, operations research, and service design and engineering. Service Systems Engineering is a commonly used term today to define a specific development approach that accounts for systematically

© Springer International Publishing Switzerland 2016
T. Borangiu et al. (Eds.): IESS 2016, LNBIP 247, pp. 75–88, 2016.
DOI: 10.1007/978-3-319-32689-4_6

and quantifiable design, development, operation, and maintenance of service systems [1–4]. In the Service System Engineering approach, a good service outcome and a good process of service delivery are expected to be produced, such as the service will be well perceived by the customers [5]. In this perspective, a service is seen as the outcome generated in a service system that has to fulfil customer expectations [6,7].

Supporting improved service delivery systems involving value-based collaboration between service actors requires a new generation of IT-enabled service systems driven by customer requirements and collaboration between actors in order to co-create value through continuous interaction and service system reconfiguring [8–10].

Modelling, definition, and design of the service organization, processes and data structures are required in the service development process [3]. However, traditional Systems Engineering tools have to be properly integrated in order to be effectively used in the Service Systems Engineering perspective [11,12].

Recent research literature on service, service systems and service innovation highlights the role of modelling approaches in structuring the development opportunities generated in close encounters of service and technology [13–16]. At the same time, actual service systems can be described as complex socio-technical systems, integrating business functions, technology and human resources, whose aim is the creation of value and benefit through the generated services [17–20].

Recent advances in digital technologies, combined with a traditional Model Driven Engineering (MDE) approach, foster greater flexibility in developing complex models not only as documentation artefacts in service design, but also as central artefacts in more structured service engineering activities.

In this respect, this paper describes the application of the *Socio-Technical Systems Engineering* (STSE) process introduced in [17] for smart transport service design and development. The STSE process is defined as a Modelling and Simulation Based Systems Engineering (M&SBSE) process used to guide improved design aiming to capture value co-creation service interactions embedding customer experience in service design and delivery activities.

Section 2 presents related work in service modelling and aligns the steps in the STSE process with modelling and design activities in Rational Rhapsody®, a system development platform in which models can be directly interpreted and executed. The case study presented in Sect. 3 approaches the development of a real time service able to provide integrated information on planning a trip by bus or alternatively by taxi. The working solution proposed here raised different questions regarding real world implementation of such services [17]. This attempt to integrate agent-based modelling and simulation experience into the development of smart transport services emphasises the role of the development platform that provide tools for model analysis, validation, simulation, and real-time animation. As a consequence, the developed models can be defined consistently with user needs. Section 4 concludes the paper.

2   Related Work

In service and service system modelling several techniques and tools are used today, originating both from management practice and engineering and scientific expertise [7]. Recent references present work in progress in this respect, and four different points of view on service systems modelling can be highlighted [17]: (a) activity modelling; (b) resource allocation modelling; (c) service networking modelling; and (d) value co-creation interaction modelling. Considering the modelling of services, a family of languages named *-USDL (the Unified Service Description Language) was proposed to provide computer-understandable descriptions for business services [21,22]. However, all these attempts of modelling service systems from different perspectives are still in early stages of development.

Different aspects of service modelling are presented in [23], taking into consideration a component model, a resource model, and a process model. The Service Systems Engineering methodology is used in [2] to describe an intelligent transportation system and a dynamic Smart Grid service system. The modelling framework SEAM is investigated in [24] to be applied to the design and analysis of viability in service systems.

Several other works try to align value modelling with a more systematic development process such as the model driven approach in the system engineering perspective [25–28]. The role of modelling and simulation for service systems development is also emphasized [10,17,29,30].

The STSE process introduced in [17] defines the required steps to generate modelling and simulation artefacts to formally visualize service entities interactions, as UML and agent based executable models, using a socio-technical description in service systems. Table 1 presents the defined steps aiming to create specific outputs in terms of *model artefacts* to be used later for implementation and bottom-up integration to support new service development.

The final output of the top-down design perspective is the *agent based implementation model* that is used to evaluate the emergent properties through collaboration among interacting entities. The four steps in the organization view account for the creation and reuse of the *requirements based scenarios* that will later assist the subsequent bottom-up integration activities.

In the subsequent sections the role of the development platform in transposing the above mentioned aspects in practice is emphasized and integration guide-

Table 1. Steps in the STSE process, according to [17]

	Step 1	Step 2	Step 3	Step 4
STSE: socio-technical engineering	Social needs identification	Scenario definition	Formal model design	Agent based operational modelling
Inputs	Stakeholders' needs	System requirements	Use cases	Agent based architectural model
Outputs	System requirements	Use cases	Agent based architectural model	Agent based implementation model (executable)

Table 2. Mapping of analysis, modelling and implementation activities from the STSE process with Rational Rhapsody

Rational Rhapsody	Modelling and design activities with Rhapsody	STSE Process
Analysis model perspective	Requirements modelling	Step 1
	Use case modelling	Step 2
	Agents' interaction modelling	Step 3
State model perspective	State diagram modelling	Step 3
Object model perspective	Modelare diagrame de pachete	Step 4
	Modelare diagrame de clase	Step 4
Implementation model perspective	Java/Ada/C++/etc. code	Step 4
Animation perspective	Animated sequence diagrams (simulation)	Verification and testing
	Animated state diagrams (simulation)	

lines of the STSE process steps with the IBM Rational Rhapsody®development platform are described. This visual development environment for embedded, real time or technical application software development based on the UML and SysML modelling standards offers support for *high-level modelling* [31]. Model execution is possible through *simulation* and *real-time animation*.

Table 2 presents the correspondence between the modelling and design activities in Rational Rhapsody and the design steps defined by the STSE process [17].

Step 1. Social needs identification. Identification of stakeholders needs; definition of value co-creation interactions. A requirements document is created to define overall system functionalities and performance criteria for system validation is defined.

Step 2. Scenario definition. Definition of value propositions; development of a use case model; composition of a business scenario. Accordingly, the agent based simulation scenarios are defined in an environment that allows validating different aspects of social interaction between the service consumer and the service provider.

Step 3. Formal model design. Development of a formal model of the proposed working scenario. The proposed architecture of the agent based model should meet the service delivery requirements extracted from the user needs. It should integrate value propositions defined by the service provider.

Step 4. Agent based operational modelling. Transformation of the functional requirements into a coherent description of the service functionalities through model execution. This value-proposition-based interactions phase has to express negotiations between the customer and provider involving specified value propositions.

3   Modelling of Smart Transport Services

In this section a double perspective of service provider and service customer in a case of smart transport service development is presented. It follows the working scenario depicted in [17] for a city transport information service to support travellers with valuable information regarding planning a trip in a city. Smart decisions involve evaluation of new public transport routes availability, extension of available routes, improvement of working shifts, acquisition of supplementary vehicles and improvement of existing business plans. Through their interaction with registered service customers, service providers may gather information about utilization degrees of travel routes in the city, utilization degrees of transport vehicles, evaluation of peak hours, or seasonal trends.

- *Service customer.* An user (tourist) uses a smartphone mobile service application in order to plan his trip in a new city. He intends to access current information through the mobile device, trying to make smart decisions on daily travelling while interacting on-line with different transport service providers, taking into consideration personal preferences (budget, as time and money);
- *Service provider perspective.* Through his mobile device, a service customer can access the mobile information service available in an *open virtual service enterprise environment* to which several service providers can adhere. Service providers may formulate smart decisions that involves new value propositions.

Figure 1 presents the components of the design and analysis model that is used to validate the application of the STSE process to the particular case of smart transport services.

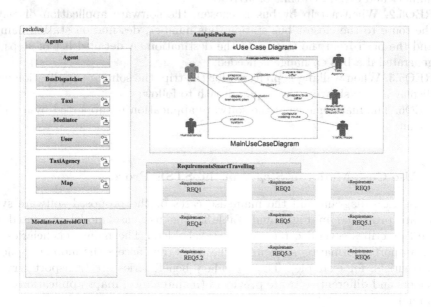

Fig. 1. Package diagram (Rational Rhapsody®)

3.1   Requirements Modelling in *Step 1* of the STSE Process

The analysis of the above mentioned working scenario in the STSE process perspective leads to the definition of the following functional requirements of software application that implements the proposed information service:

- REQ1. The information service should be able to generate possible routes for three modes of transport in a city, bus, taxi, and walking. Therefore, the software application has several *interactions* with bus and taxi dispatchers. It has to compute the walking route through interactions with a map application;
- REQ2. The software application allows to generate a list of transport offers according to the user's preferences and restrictions (destination, time, cost, transport modes);
- REQ3. Transport offers will be listed orderly according to the user's preferences. They will be prioritized according to the price of the trip (p) and the duration of the trip (d);
- REQ4. The user may opt to choose one travel route or to cancel the service;
- REQ5. Each generated transport offer has to include a description containing the transport mode, duration and cost. The following *service interactions* are defined:
- REQ5.1. When a trip by taxi is chosen, the software application solicits the corresponding taxi dispatcher, then informs the taxi service user (taxi ID number and estimated time of arrival);
- REQ5.2. When a trip by bus is chosen, the software application displays the route to the closest bus station, bus number, destination station name, and the path from the station to the destination. A detailed list of steps is generated if a bus exchange is needed;
- REQ5.3. When walking is preferred for the trip, the software application will display a map showing the required path to follow;
- REQ6. The maintenance of the software application is supported by a technician.

3.2   Use Case Model in *Step 2* of the STSE Process

The use case diagram and the main use cases of the proposed software systems are presented in Fig. 1 and Table 3. The use case model presented in Table 3 describes several categories of stakeholders. The main beneficiaries of the transport information system are the users that access the mobile application (tourists, for example). The secondary beneficiaries are transport service providers and different software providers (maintenance, maps applications, for example).

Table 4 lists the actors that interact with the software application implementing the transport information system. The correspondence with agents integrated in the agents based architectural model in *Step 3* in Sect. 3.3 is also specified.

Table 3. Use case model

Use case	Description	Actors	Type	Cross-Ref
Prepare transport plan	User agent request transport. Mediator agent interacts with Taxi Dispatcher, Bus Dispatcher, and Traffic Maps agents to prepare travel offer with user preferences. This use case includes Prepare taxi offer, Prepare bus offer, and Compute walking route use cases.	User	main	REQ1 REQ2
Display transport plan	Transport application returns to the user transport choices or details about transport mode. According to user choice, Mediator sends to user instructions to reach the destination (taxi - taxi ID, estimated arrival time); bus - route to the closest bus station, bus number, destination station name, path to final destination; walking - route to destination on map).	User	main	REQ1 REQ2 REQ4 REQ5 REQ5.1 REQ5.2 REQ5.2 REQ5.3
Prepare taxi offer	Transport application interacts with Taxi Agencies to prepare taxi transport offers, and to plan taxi trips on user request	Taxi Agency	secondary	REQ5.1
Prepare bus offer	Transport application interacts with Bus Dispatcher agents to prepare bus transport offers	Bus Dispatcher	secondary	REQ5.2
Compute walking route	Mediator interacts with maps application to prepare walking routes on user request	Traffic Maps	secondary	REQ5.3
Maintain system	Technician performs maintenance operations on system	Maintenance	secondary	REQ6

3.3   Agents' Interaction Model in *Step 3* of the STSE Process

Agents' interaction modelling (based on UML sequence diagrams - *analysis model perspective* in Rational Rhapsody) and agents' behavioural modelling (based on UML state diagrams - *state model perspective* in Rational Rhapsody) are integrated in the *Step 3* of the STSE process. The behaviours of the *User* (service customer) and *Mediator* (transport information system) agents are depicted in Figs. 2 and 3.

State diagram in Fig. 2 models internal behaviour of *User* agent. The following states are defined according to its behaviour and possible interactions with other agents: InitiatingTransportSession, FillingTransportForm, Waiting, FollowingWalkingInstructions, FollowingBusInstructions, and FollowingTaxiInstructions.

State diagram in Fig. 3 presents the reactive evolution of the *Mediator* agent interacting with a *User* type agent.

The output of *Step 3* in STSE process (*Formal model design*) is the proposed architecture of the agent based model, consisting of a set of agents, the environment in which they operate, agent communication protocol, and the set of general rules according to which they execute their actions and access resources [17].

According to this specification, in Table 5 the agent interaction protocol for resource allocation in the particular case of smart transport services design is presented. It is used to further validate the application of the STSE process in this case study through model execution (simulation and real-time animation).

Table 4. Agent types

Use case diagram elements	Agent Type	Aim	Interacts with
User	**User**	Request transport with personal preferences	Mediator Taxi Bus
Transport System	**Mediator**	Mediates interactions between users and other actors	User Bus dispatcher Taxi Dispatcher Maps
Bus dispatcher	**Bus Dispatcher**	Coordinates Bus Dispatcher agents activity	Mediator Bus
Taxi agency	**Taxi Dispather**	Coordinates Taxi Dispatcher agents activity	Mediator Taxi
–	**Taxi**	Transport by taxi	Taxi Dispatcher User
–	**Bus**	Transport by bus	Bus dispatcher User
Maintenance	**Maintenance**	Software application maintenance	Mediator
Traffic Maps	**Maps**	Traffic information (walking route maps)	Mediator

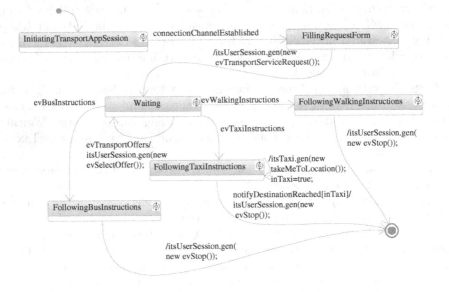

Fig. 2. State diagram - *User* agent

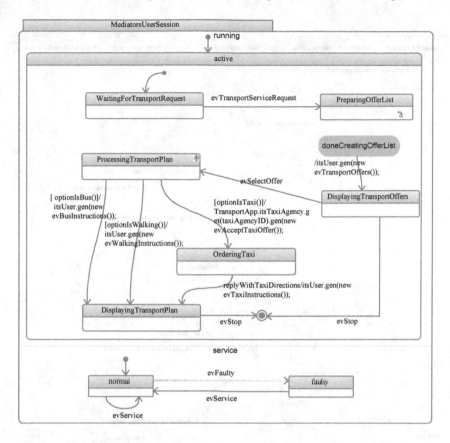

Fig. 3. State diagram - *Mediator* agent

3.4   Value-Proposition-Based Interaction Evaluation in *Step 4* of the STSE Process

In **Step 4** (*Agent based operational modelling*) the functional requirements defined in the previous stages are transformed into a coherent description of the service functionalities through model execution. From a service engineering perspective, the outcomes of the STSE process, artefacts created to automatically support consistency among design steps and effective integration of customer experience and stakeholder requirements through iterative cycles related to service design, are validated through simulation.

Figure 4 presents an animated sequence diagram describing the interaction among agent entities to fulfil a taxi order request. This is a model artefact related to the execution of the UML model describing the service interactions.

Listing 1 presents an excerpt of the execution logs in Rational Rhapsody describing the self-organizing properties of the proposed multiagent model.

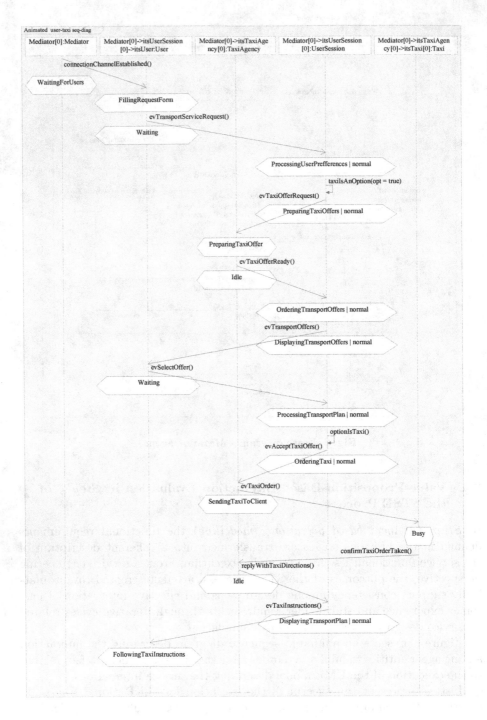

Fig. 4. Animated sequence diagram - Taxi request interaction

Table 5. Agent interaction protocol for allocation of transport resources

Agent	State	Next state	Trigger	Actions
	InitiatigTransportSession	FillingRequestForm	connectionChannelEstablished	-evTransportServiceRequest
	FillingTransportForm	Waiting	-	-
	Waiting	FollowingBusInstructions	evBusInstructions	-
	Waiting	FollowingTaxiInstructions	evTaxiInstructions	-
User	Waiting	FollowingWalkingInstructions	evWalkingInstructions	-
	Waiting	Waiting	evTransportOffers	evSelectOffer
	FollowingWalkingInstructions	FIN	-	evStop
	FollowingBusInstructions	FIN	-	evStop
	FollowingTaxiInstructions	FollowingTaxiInstructions	-	takeMeToLocation
	FollowingTaxiInstructions	FIN	-	evStop
Taxi	Idle	Idle	notifyTaskCompleted	-
Agency	PreparingTaxiOffer	PreparingTaxiOffer	evTaxiOfferRequest ev AccceptTaxiOffer	evTaxiOrder
	PreparingTaxiOffer	SendigTaxiToClient	-	evTaxiOrderReady
	SendingTaxiToClient	Idle	confirmTaxiOrderTaken	replyWithtaxiDirections
Bus	Idle	PreparingtransportPlan	evBusOfferRequest	evBusOfferReady
Dispatcher	PreparingTransportPlan	Idle	-	-
	WaitingForUsers	SettingUpNewUserSession	requestUserConnection	-
	SettingUpNewUserSession	WaitingForUsers	-	-
	running :	active	-	-
	WaitingForTransportRequest	PreparingOfferList:	-	-
	PreparingOfferList:	ProcessingUserPrefferences	-	-
	ProcessingUserPreferences	PreparingTaxiOffers	-	evTaxiOfferRequest
		PreparingWalkingOffer	-	evWalkingOfferRequest
		PreparingBusOffer	-	-
	PreparingTaxiOffers	SortingTransportOffers	evTaxiOfferReady	-
	PreparingWalkingOffer	SortingTransportOffers	evWalkingOfferReady	-
	PreparingBusOffer	SortingTransportOffers	evBusOfferReady	-
	SortingTransportOffers	DisplayingTransportOffers	-	evTransportOffers
	DisplayingTransportOffers	ProcessingTransportPlan	-	-
Mediator		FIN	evSelectOffer	-
		DisplayingTransportPlan	evStop	-
	ProcessingTransportPlan	DisplayingTransportPlan	evBusInstructions	-
		OrderingTaxi	evWalkingInstructions	-
	OrderingTaxi	DisplayingTransportPlan	replyWithTaxiDirections	evAcceptTaxiOrder
	DisplayingTransportPlan.	FIN	evStop	evTaxiInstructions
	normal	faulty	evFaulty	-
	normal	normal	evService	-
	faulty	normal	evService	-
Taxi	WaitingForOrder	Busy	evTaxiOrder	confirmTaxiOrderTaken
	Busy	WaitingForOrder	takeMeToLocation	notiFyDestinationReached
		Busy	-	destACK=true;
Traffic	Idle	PrepareWalkinOffer	evWalkingRequest	-
Maps	PreparingWalkingOffer	ComputingRoute	confirmWalkigRequest	-
	ComputingRoute	Idle	-	evWalkingOfferReady
		Idle	replyWithWalkingDirections	-

Listing 1: Taxi Request Interaction - execution log

```
>>User: STATE InitiatingTransportAppSession
>>Mediator: Connection established. New user session created.
>>Mediator::UserSession: default transition to initial state
>>Mediator::UserSession::Active: STATE WaitingForTransportRequest
>>Mediator::UserSession::Active: evTransportServiceRequest event
  ---> transition to PreparingOfferList STATE
....
>>Mediator: STATE WaitingForUsers
>>User: connectionChannelEstablished event ---> transition to
  FillingRequestForm STATE
>>User: STATE FillingTransportRequestForm
...
>>Mediator::UserSession::Active: evTransportServiceRequest event --->
  transition to PreparingOffersList STATE
>>Mediator::UserSession::Active: STATE PreparingOffersList
>>Mediator::UserSession::Active::PreparingOfferList default transition
  to ProcessingUserPrefferences STATE
>>Mediator::UserSession::Active: STATE ProcessingUserPrefferences
>>Mediator::UserSession::Active::PreparingOfferList: evTaxiOfferRequest
event ---> transition to PreparingTaxiOffers STATE
>>TaxiAgency: evTaxiOrderRequest event ---> transition to
  PreparingTaxiOffer STATE
>>TaxiAgency: STATE PreparingTaxiOffer
>>TaxiAgency: evTaxiOfferReady event ---> transition to Idle STATE
...
>>Mediator::UserSession::Active::PreparingOfferList:
  evTransportantionOffersReady event ---> transition to
  OrderingTransportationOffers STATE
>>Mediator::UserSession::Active::PreparingOfferList: STATE
  OrderingTransportationOffers
>>Mediator::UserSession::Active: evTransportOffers event --->
  transition to DisplayingTransportOffers STATE
...
>>Mediator::UserSession::Active: STATE OrderingTaxi
>>TaxiAgency: evTaxiOrder event ---> transition
  to SendingTaxiToClient STATE
>>TaxiAgency: STATE SendingTaxiToClient
>>Taxi: STATE Busy
>>Taxi: notifyDestinationReached event --->
  transition to WaitingForOrder STATE
>>TaxiAgency: replyWithTaxiDirections event
  ---> transition to Idle STATE
>>Mediator::UserSession::Active: evTransportationInstructions
  event --->  transition to DisplayingTransportPlan STATE
...
```

As a further development perspective, it is worth to evaluate if such an information system architecture can be used in combination with other traveller information services, such as hotel information service or a city attraction information service. In addition, the system can be also embedded with extra information services, such as weather or air pollution data.

4   Conclusions

This article discusses the possibility of integrating agent-based modelling and simulation experience into the development of improved services. It suggests formalizing service design endeavours towards the integration of customer experience, validated through service interaction modelling. The procedure proposed to be followed in order to obtain modelling artefacts supporting the creation of improved services uses a high-level visual modelling approach. The role of the development platform in transposing the above mentioned steps in the STSE process in practice is emphasized and integration guidelines of this M&SBSE process with the IBM Rational Rhapsody®development platform are described. The agent based implementation model for service prototyping is created in Rational Rhapsody. The obtained agent based executable model is suitable for obtaining qualitative simulation results and performing quantitative evaluations on operational aspects in transport service delivery. Rational Rhapsody supports model-to-text transformations from which software artefacts can be generated, such as source code in different programming languages.

References

1. Tien, J.M., Berg, D.: A case for service systems engineering. J. Syst. Sci. Syst. Eng. **12**(1), 13–38 (2003)
2. Lopes, A.J., Pineda, R.: Service systems engineering applications. Procedia Comput. Sci. **16**, 678–687 (2013)
3. Pineda, R., Lopes, A., Tseng, B., Salcedo, O.H.: Service systems engineering: emerging skills and tools. Procedia Comput. Sci. **8**, 420–427 (2012)
4. Sum, J.: Service Systems Engineering: Framework and Systems Modelling. Institute of Technology Management, National Chung Hsing University, Taichung 40227, Taiwan ROC, January 2014
5. Dabholkar, P.A., Overby, J.W.: Linking process and outcome to service quality and customer satisfaction evaluations: an investigation of real estate agent service. Int. J. Serv. Ind. Manag. **16**(1), 10–27 (2005)
6. Slack, N., Chambers, S., Johnston, R.: Operations Management. Hall Financial Times, Prentice Hall (2010)
7. Borangiu, T., Dragoicea, M., Oltean, V.E., Iacob, I.: A generic service system activity model with event-driven operation reconfiguring capability. In: Borangiu, T., Trentesaux, D., Thomas, A. (eds.) Service Orientation in Holonic and Multiagent Manufacturing. SCI, vol. 544, pp. 159–175. Springer, Heidelberg (2014)
8. Breidbach, C.F., Maglio, P.P.: A Service Science Perspective on the Role of ICT in Service Innovation. In: ECIS 2015 Proceedings at AIS Electronic Library (AISeL), 23rd European Conference on Information Systems, Münster, Germany, Research-in-Progress Papers, Paper 33 (2015)
9. Ponsignon, F., Smart, A., Maull, R.: Service delivery systems: a business process perspective. POMS College of Service Operations 2007 Meeting. London Business School, London (2007)
10. Peng, Y.: Modelling and Designing IT-enabled Service Systems Driven by Requirements and Collaboration. Ph.D thesis, Linstitut national des sciences appliques de Lyon (2012)
11. Guide to the Systems Engineering Body of Knowledge (SEBoK) v.1.4. http://sebokwiki.org/
12. INCOSE Systems Engineering Handbook: A Guide for System Life Cycle Processes and Activities, 4th edn. Wiley (2015)
13. Ostrom, A.L., Parasuraman, A., Bowen, D., Patricio, L., Voss, C.: Service research priorities in a rapidly changing context. J. Serv. Res. **18**(2), 127–159 (2015)
14. Bowen, D.E., Schneider, B.: A service climate synthesis and future research agenda. J. Serv. Res. **17**(1), 5–22 (2014)
15. Sanchis, A., Julián, V., Corchado, J.M., Billhardt, H., Carrascosa, C.: Improving human-agent immersion using natural interfaces and CBR. Int. J. Artif. Intell. **13**(1), 81–93 (2015)
16. Billhardt, H., Julián, V., Corchado, J.M., Fernández, A.: Human-agent societies: challenges and issues. Int. J. Artifi. Intell. **13**(1), 28–44 (2015)
17. Drăgoicea, M., Cunha, J.F., Pătraşcu, M.: Self-organising socio-technical description in service systems for supporting smart user decisions in public transport. Expert Syst. Appl. **42**(17–18), 6329–6341 (2015)

18. Beaumont, L.C., Bolton, L.E., McKay, A., Hughes, H.P.N.: Rethinking service design: a socio-technical approach to the development of business models. In: Schaefer, D. (ed.) Product Development in the Socio-sphere, pp. 121–141. Springer International Publishing, Switzerland (2014)

19. Carroll, N.: Service science: an empirical study on the socio-technical dynamics of public sector service network innovation (Doctoral Dissertation, University of Limerick) (2012). http://www.academia.edu/

20. Edvardsson, B., Tronvoll, B., Gruber, T.: Expanding understanding of service exchange and value co-creation: a social construction approach. J. Acad. Mark. Sci. **39**(2), 327–339 (2011)

21. Barros, A., Oberle, D.: Handbook of Service Description: USDL and Its Methods. Springer Science+Business Media, New York (2012)

22. Cardoso, J., Pedrinaci, C.: Evolution and overview of linked USDL. In: Nóvoa, H., Drăgoicea, M. (eds.) IESS 2015. LNBIP, vol. 201, pp. 50–64. Springer, Heidelberg (2015)

23. Böttcher, M., Fhnrich, K.P.: Service systems modeling: concepts, formalized meta-model and technical concretion. In: Demirkan, H., Spohrer, J.C., Krishna, V. (eds.) The Science of Service Systems. Service Science: Research and Innovations in the Service Economy, pp. 131–149. Springer Science+Business Media, LLC, New York (2011)

24. Golnam, A., Regev, G., Wegmann, A.: On viable service systems: developing a modeling framework for analysis of viability in service systems. In: Snene, M., Ralyté, J., Morin, J.-H. (eds.) IESS 2011. LNBIP, vol. 82, pp. 30–41. Springer, Heidelberg (2011)

25. Wang, Z., Ducq, Y.: Value-Driven Business Service Modelling. NICST2013, New and smart Information Communication Science and Technology to support Sustainable Development, Clermont Ferrand, France, September 2013. http://edss.isima.fr/workshop/

26. Xu, X., Wang, Z.: Value-aware service model driven architecture and methodology. In: Mazzeo, A., Bellini, R., Motta, G. (eds.) E-Government ICt Professionalism and Competences Service Science. IFIP International Federation for Information Processing, vol. 280, pp. 277–286. Springer Science+Business Media, LLC, New York (2008)

27. MSEE Manufacturing SErvices Ecosystem: D11.2 Service concepts, models and method: Model Driven Service Engineering. http://cordis.europa.eu/

28. Chen, D., Ducq, Y., Doumeingts, G., Zacharewicz, G., Alix, T.: A model driven approach for the modelling of services in a virtual enterprise. In: Zelm, M., Sanchis, R., Poler, R., Doumeingts, G. (eds.) Enterprise Interoperability: I-ESA'12 Proceedings, pp. 181–187. Wiley, New Jersey (2012)

29. Alix, T., Zacharewicz, G., Vallespir, B.: Service systems modelling and simulation: the sergent distributed approach. In: Mertins, K., Bénaben, F., Poler, R., Bourrières, J.P. (eds.) Enterprise Interoperability VI, pp. 357–367. Springer International Publishing, Switzerland (2014)

30. Yih, Y., Chaturvedi, A.: Service enterprise modelling. In: Salvendy, G., Karwowski, W. (eds.) Introduction to Service Engineering, pp. 135–158. Wiley, New Jersey (2010)

31. The Rational Rhapsody family from IBM. Collaborative systems engineering and embedded software development. http://www.ibm.com/

Process Modeling as Key Technique for Embedding the Practices of Business Process Management in Organization

Elena Fleacă[✉], Bogdan Fleacă, and Sanda Maiduc

Faculty of Entrepreneurship, Business Engineering and Management,
University Politehnica of Bucharest, Spaiul Independentei 313, 060042 Bucharest, Romania
{elena.fleaca,bogdan.fleaca,sanda.maiduc}@upb.ro

Abstract. The growing competition asks for high efficiency in business with the aid of Business Process Management (BPM). This article proposes a practical initiative to incorporate and leverage the BPM into organization. The research commences with the overview on the proliferation of BPM in academic community and industry. The authors modeled the appropriate processes to provide the frame for understanding and applying the BPM methodology within any organization. The obtained result, Supplier – Input – Process – Output – Customer (SIPOC) diagram maps out flow and process relationships that help document and communicate stakeholders how BPM processes should be performed.

Keywords: Business process management · Process modelling · Innovation

1 Introduction

During the last decades, the major concern on delivering business improvements has emerged in a strategic initiative with the aid of optimizing work and the relationships between organization's stakeholders such as employees, suppliers, and customers. This emerging capability of organizations to deliver rapid business change is known as Business Process Management (BPM), and it represents a revolution in running business operations.

The effectiveness and efficiency of any organization are shed to light on the new paradigm based on looking at the management processes and the role of automation of work within and across the organization, enabling thus a rapid and iterative change of business processes.

The evolving nature of Business Process Management (BPM) and the growing needs of BPM expertize have determined plenty of researches in the attempt of defining and integrating all dimensions, methods, and views of the phenomenon.

Based on these circumstances, the paper aims to investigate different views of business process management concepts from the scientific literature and to review key underpinnings, as widely accepted standard in BPM industry. The authors adopted a managerial perspective of BPM and modeled the related processes using the SIPOC

© Springer International Publishing Switzerland 2016
T. Borangiu et al. (Eds.): IESS 2016, LNBIP 247, pp. 89–99, 2016.
DOI: 10.1007/978-3-319-32689-4_7

diagram (Supplier – Input – Process – Output – Customer). The results depict a high level processes needed for adopting and leveraging BPM in organization, and also help facilitate process understanding being a bridge document between business users and IT specialists or business analysts.

2   Research Framework

In order to fulfill the paper objectives, the research was conducted based on the following qualitative research methods: (i) exploratory research on recent studies from the industry best practices and academia to analyze key attempts within BPM approaches; (ii) qualitative analysis of the three references best practices from dedicated industry: ABPMP (Association of Business Process Management Professionals), IIBA (International Institute of Business Analysis), and APQC (American Productivity and Quality Center); and (iii) modeling the processes required for adopting and leveraging BPM in organization.

According to scholars, there are at least two BPM mainstreams within academic environment: a wider approach based on a managerial perspective of BPM in organization, and a narrow approach focused on the IT tools using BPM platforms and suites [1].

The managerial perspective of BPM has its roots early in 1990 s with the reconceptualization of the entire organization by thinking in terms of comprehensive processes, followed by Total Quality Management and Six Sigma with a focus on statistical quality control techniques to continuously improve the organization processes [2].

As organizations were becoming more process oriented, the unit of analysis consisted of the concept of process has attracted a plenty of studies. The researchers have agreed on embedding the process analysis under the business process management area. In this regard, BPM has been defined as a key part of management by which it enables understanding, documenting, modeling, simulating, and executing end-to-end processes toward an ongoing improvement of organizational performance [3, 4].

During last decades, the advent of IT and the highly-changing marketplace demands have determined enterprises to change their business model by defining new strategically directions to offer added value to all key stakeholders [5]. The process modeling based on Enterprise Resource Planning (ERP) and work flow management helped organizations to automate a lot of work operations. The Enterprise Resource Planning (ERP) was designed to facilitate the flow of information within the boundaries of organization and manage the connections to all stakeholders [6].

In other attempt to automate the work processes, IT specialists from BPM domain have established a common modeling language, Unified Modeling Language (UML) that provides a standard way to visualize, specify, construct, and document the artifacts of a software-intensive system. As useful communication tool, the UML facilitates interactions and reduces confusion among BPM stakeholders by defining the vocabulary of any object-oriented system and by providing the rules for a graphical representation of the system modeled [7].

To further investigate the attempts to create a bridge that link the managerial and IT approaches in BPM field, the scholars tackled the organization from the socio-technical view and understood its processes with the aid of system analysis. They have proposed a metamodel for understanding, analyzing and designing socio-technical systems. Consequently, the organization was perceived as a socio-technical system comprised of work systems in which people and equipment interact using information, technology, and other resources to produce products/services used by internal or external customers. The metamodel comprised of a coherent subsets of the ten groups of items: work system, organization, enterprise; work system, process, and activity; activity, product/service, and customer; customer and participant; information; technology; inputs and resources used by an activity; infrastructure; environment; strategy. By defining the groups of items and by clarifying their relationships and functioning, it is aimed to improve the understanding and collaboration between business professionals and IT specialists [8, 9].

The industry and academia collaborated and created a worldwide knowledge database to response to the growing need for a deeper understanding of business process management. The Association of Business Process Management Professionals (ABPMP) has articulated the knowledge within the BPM profession with the aid of several knowledge areas accepted as best practices [10].

Released in 2013, BPM CBOK version 3.0 is providing a comprehensive overview of the issues, best practices and lessons learned by coherently integrating key concepts, methods and tools into a wide range of common activities and associated tasks within the following knowledge areas: process modeling, process analysis, process design, process change and transformation, process performance measurement, and process performance improvements.

Another key intake nurtured from the evolution of business process management is referring to the widely accepted standard Business Analysis Body of Knowledge (BABOK Guide) developed by the International Institute of Business Analysis (IIBA). It has proposed a systematic vehicle for creating, monitoring and sharing new knowledge in business processes area with the aid of the current generally accepted practices in terms of process owner, process analyst or process architect roles [11].

The seven knowledge areas, focused exclusively on the business need and adding business value, describe appropriate processes required to complete the business effort; to identify and understand the stakeholders' needs and concerns; to manage issues and changes to the business solution scope; to identify, refine and clarify the business need; to prioritize and progressively elaborate business solution requirements; and finally to assess, identify gaps in solution, and determine necessary workarounds of change to the solution [11].

Another purposeful arrangement of business processes was brought to light by the well-known framework developed by the American Productivity and Quality Center. Through an out of box thinking, the Process Classification Framework proposed different process models that help practitioners to reduce ambiguity and to organize enterprises processes into two groups with a twelve enterprise-level categories [12].

The operating processes group consists of five operating processes such as: develop vision and strategy; develop and manage products and services; market and sell products and services; deliver products and services; and manage customer service. The aim of this group is to set, create and fulfill the stakeholders demand, being tightly connected to the enterprise value chain.

The management processes group helps to ensure a coherent functioning of the enterprise by setting the goals and by enabling to achieve these with the aid of capable resources. This group consists of seven specific processes such as: develop and manage human capital; manage information technology; manage financial resources; acquire, construct, and manage assets; manage enterprise risk, compliance, and resiliency; manage external relationships; develop and manage business capabilities [12].

3   Results and Discussions

Applying process modelling principles for embedding business process management within organizational settlements requires a thoroughly understanding of the phases related to designing, launching, and implementing the process-centric work.

As scholars highlighted, the critical success phases for commencing the business process management endeavor are consisting of analyzing the organization strategy and business model, developing the processes architecture, running the processes architecture, and monitoring and controlling the execution of processes [13].

The authors have taken advantage of one of the basic quality tools, and modeled the related processes within each phase with the aid of SIPOC diagram (Supplier-Input-Process-Output-Customer). The SIPOC technique has enabled authors to display the sequence of steps and related activities, decision points, and the overall order of processing by mapping the operational details which exist within the horizontal value chain of the model [14].

The steps embedded in each phase mainstream the best practices and lessons learned from dedicated literature and organize the logical flow from the inception to the completion point of the planning endeavor [13, 14].

Phase 1 Analyze the Organization Strategy and Business Model. This phase is intended to depict and understand the means of achieving the business mission. As Fig. 1 suggested, the correctness of the process is required to define and articulate the business model and value proposition by carefully take into consideration main inputs such as: organizational process assets, knowledge data base, and environmental factors.

The organizational process assets are consisted of the mission, vision and core values, product portfolio mixt, internal processes and procedures, lessons learned from previous experiences, historical information, and other artifact or practice from the organization involved, that can be used to perform the analysis of the organization. The knowledge data base is comprised of commercial databases, market place conditions, and human resources availability [14].

Another key input for the planning effort is referring to the organizational environmental factors which may enhance or constrain the planning and analyzing options such the organizational culture, structure and charts, industry standards, geographic distribution of resources and facilities [14].

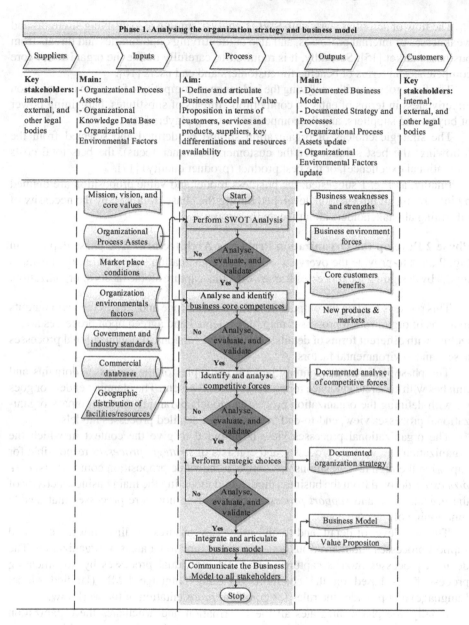

Phase 1. Analysing the organization strategy and business model				
Suppliers	Inputs	Process	Outputs	Customers
Key stakeholders: internal, external, and other legal bodies	Main: - Organizational Process Assets - Organizational Knowledge Data Base - Organizational Environmental Factors	Aim: - Define and articulate Business Model and Value Proposition in terms of customers, services and products, suppliers, key differentiations and resources availability	Main: - Documented Business Model - Documented Strategy and Processes - Organizational Process Assets update - Organizational Environmental Factors update	Key stakeholders: internal, external, and other legal bodies

Fig. 1. Analyzing the organization strategy and business model phase.

The prerequisite is referring to taking into consideration all these inputs in performing the related activities during this phase so that the expected outputs, documented business model and appropriate strategy and processes, should work throughout the entire organization.

The flow of activities starts with SWOT analysis aiming at identifying strengths and weaknesses of internal processes, and also at identifying opportunities and threats from business market [15]. Secondly, it is required to carefully define the organization core competences in terms of benefits for customers and end users [16].

The flow goes on with analyzing the influence of competitive forces on organization effectiveness in terms of entry of competitors, threats of substitutes, bargaining power of buyers and suppliers, and the competition among players [16].

The strategic choices of organization should be defined and selected from the following: the best solution for the customer (customer focus), the bets total costs (operational excellence), or the best product (product quality) [17].

Finally, as Fig. 1 suggested, the business model and value proposition are defined by integrating all information developed during the phase, followed by the necessity of informing all stakeholders about the main outputs.

Phase 2 Develop the Organization Processes Architecture. The phase depicted in Fig. 2 aims to provide the overview of the current situation derived from the business model by designing the processes frameworks that capture all the facets of organization.

This phase is feed on the outputs from the previous one and creates the main outputs in terms of organization processes map, documented and agreed upon processes architecture with different forms of details, and updated versions of organizational processes assets and environmental factors.

The phase begins with defining general principles of the processes domains and finishes with concrete guidance for processes development. The planning endeavor goes on with defining the organization processes models pyramids that encompass organizational processes view, end-to-end processes and detailed processes models.

The organizational processes view is intended to give the context in which the organization can view its processes and consists of *strategic processes* responsible for capturing the high level relationships between the value proposition components, *core processes,* derived from the business model, and modeling the main business activity of the organization, and *support processes* representing non-core processes that enable functioning of the core ones.

The next level of detail, end-to-end processes, ensures the link between core and support processes and the various activities from functional areas of organization. The detailed processes models capture and model individual processes by documenting process flows based on the common modeling language UML (Unified Model Language) that provides the rules for graphical representation of the workflow.

Finally, the phase integrates all the information and articulates the organization processes architecture by organizing the processes in a hierarchy expressing the *core processes* responsible for delivering value to the customers and the *support processes* responsible for managing the value chain, effectively and efficiently.

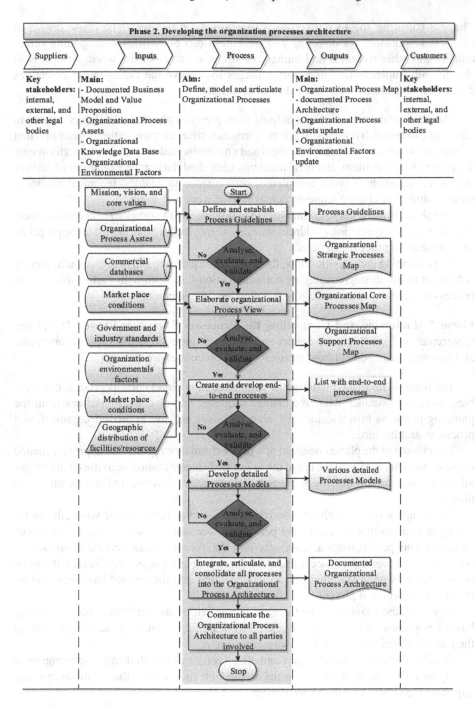

Fig. 2. Developing the organization processes architecture phase.

Phase 3 Running the Organization Processes Architecture. The phase drown in Fig. 3 is responsible for directing and managing process work by integrating stakeholders and other technical and human resources to carry out the work. Also, it is in charge with implementing necessary changes to achieve the organization objectives captured by business model and value proposition.

The phase mainstreams all the outputs from previous phases and delivers outputs in terms of process deliverables, work performance data, change requests, and updated versions of organizational process assets and environmental factors. Work performance data are raw observations and measurements identified during the execution of end-to-end processes such as work completed, performance indicators, technical measurements, number of change requests, actual cost of work and so on.

The phase is intended to communicate and work with various stakeholders to meet their needs and expectations, addresses issues as they occur, and facilitates appropriate engagements in process activities.

By performing the activities flow, the approved organizational processes architecture is brought to life through managing communication flow within all parties involved in process work and also on managing stakeholders' engagements.

Phase 4 Monitoring and Controlling the Processes Execution Phase. The phase, represented in Fig. 4, aims to collect and distribute process performance information, and assesses measurements and trends to effect process improvements.

The phase is nourished with inputs from execution phase such as process deliverables, work performance data, and change requests, and also with baselines from the planning phase as business model, value propositions, and approved organizational processes architecture.

The outputs of the phase consisted of work performance reports and approved change requests are delivered with the aid of the integrated change control activities that analyze all change requests to determine preventive, corrective actions, and follow up action plans.

The complexity of this phase is derived from the two dimensions in which the monitoring and controlling processes are performed: *the static focus,* related to the inputs and/or outputs performance assessments, and *the dynamic focus,* related to the way of performing the work, the process itself. By approving or by rejecting changes, it will be assure that only approved changes are incorporated into the revised baselines, and go through the execution phase.

However, the monitoring and controlling activities are performed on an ongoing bases being inserted in each phase related to designing, launching, and implementing the process-centric work within the organization.

Finally, to increase the efficiency and effectiveness of stakeholders' engagements, it is required to control their commitment through monitoring the relationships and adjusting the strategies for engaging them.

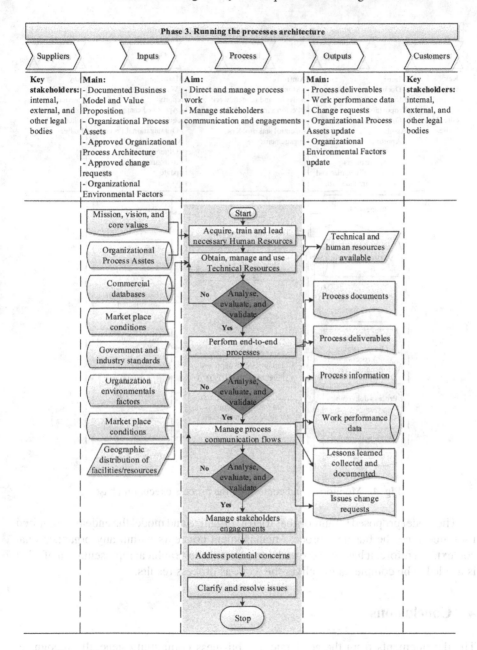

Fig. 3. Running the organization processes architecture phase.

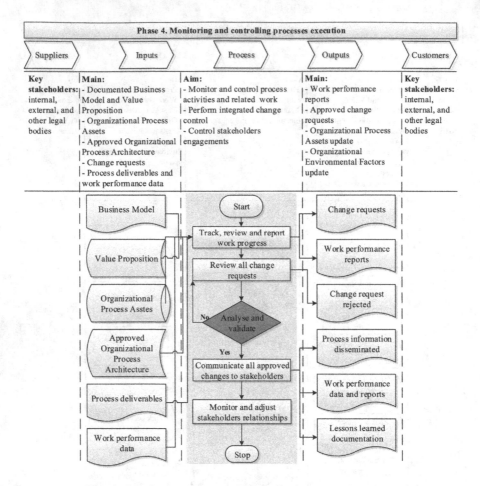

Fig. 4. Monitoring and controlling the process execution phase.

The model proposed by authors has tried to organize and model the endeavor required for embedding the business process management concepts within any organizational context. Therefore, it has been created a conceptual and graphical representation of what is needed to be completed to deliver the work as process results.

4   Conclusions

The developments from the academic and business community generally recognize, accept and promote the process-managed organization's thinking. As the processes are not an end in themselves but rather a vehicle toward fulfilling the organization objectives based on capturing the needs and expectations of customers, an important cross-cutting issue is referring to the conceptual endeavor that integrates all the work needed for a process-centric approach.

Having a broad scope, the proposed methodology maps out inputs, outputs, sequencing activities, and the relationships with different processes' stakeholders and is relying on the knowledge generally recognized as good practices in various industries and business sectors.

To further develop the model, it is envisaged to test the steps within each flowchart in different organizational settings, and to collect necessary feedbacks for adjusting the inputs, outputs, and related activities.

In this way, the paper tried to emphasis the benefits of using a structured approach in the organization, to facilitate the understanding of business process management endeavor, and also to coherently communicate with all stakeholders.

References

1. Bandara, W., Chand, D.R., Chircu, A.M., Hintringer, S., Karagiannis, D., Recker, F., van Rensburg, A., Usoff, C., Welke, R.: Business process management education in academia: status, challenges, and recommendations. Commun. Assoc. Inf. Syst. **27**, 744–776 (2010). AIS Electronic Library.
2. Hammer, M., Champy, J.: Reengineering the Corporation: a Manifesto for Business Revolution. Harper Collins, New York (1993)
3. Jaston, G., Nelis, G.: Business Process Management: Practical Guidelines to Successful Implementation. Elsevier Ltd., Burlington (2006)
4. Fleaca, B., Fleaca, E.: An Exploratory Study on Organization Processes Taxonomy. Bull. USAMV Horticulture. **70**, 310–318 (2013)
5. Harmon, P.: The Scope and Evolution of Business Process Management. Springer, Heidelberg (2010)
6. Bidgoli, H.: The Internet Encyclopedia. Wiley, New Jersey (2004)
7. Booch, G., Rumbaugh, J., Jacobson, I.: Unified Modelling Language User Guide. Addison Wesley Professional, Indianapolis (2005)
8. Alter, S.: The Work System Method for Understanding Information Systems and Information System Research. Commun. Assoc. Inf. Syst. **1**, 90–104 (2002). AIS Electronic Library
9. Association for Information Systems. http://aisel.aisnet.org
10. Guide to Business Process Management Common Body ok Knowledge. Association of Business Process Management Professionals. http://www.abpmp.org/
11. International Institute of Business Analysis: Guide to the Business Analysis Body of Knowledge. International Institute of Business Analysis, Toronto (2009)
12. Process Classification Framework version 6.0.0., American Productivity and Quality Center, http://www.apqc.org/knowledge-base/documents/apqc-process-classification-framework-pcf-cross-industry-pdf-version-600
13. Jaston, G., Nelis, G.: Business Process Management: Practical Guidelines to Successful Implementation, 2nd edn. Elsevier Ltd., Burlington (2008)
14. A Guide to the Project Management Body of Knowledge. Fifth Edition. Project Management Institute Inc, Pennsylvania (2013)
15. Porter, M.: Competitive Strategy: Techniques for Analyzing Industries and Competitors. Free Press, New York (1980)
16. Hamel, G., Prahalad, C.K.: Competing for the Future. Harvard Business School Press, Boston (1994)
17. Treacy, M., Wiersma, F.: The Discipline of Market Leaders. Harper Collins, New York (1997)

Towards a Flexible Solution
in Knowledge-Based Service Organizations:
Capability as a Service

Hasan Koç[(⊠)], Kurt Sandkuhl, and Michael Fellmann

Chair of Business Information Systems, Institute of Computer Science,
University of Rostock, Albert-Einstein-Str. 22, 18059 Rostock, Germany
{hasan.koc,kurt.sandkuhl,
michael.fellmann}@uni-rostock.de

Abstract. To improve their chances of survival, enterprises need to cope with the challenges caused by today's dynamic markets, regulations, customer demands, novel technologies, etc. The shift towards a service-oriented economy as underlined by the concept of Service-Dominant (S-D) Logic is gaining traction within the Service Science community and industry. This shift towards service-dominated business models makes it even more important for enterprises to be agile to meet the rapidly changing customer demands. This demand for agility is reinforced in the context of knowledge-based service organizations (KBSOs), for which flexible service provision is a fundamental requirement. Against this background, we argue that the capability-driven design may provide the KBSOs the required degree of flexibility. Towards this goal, we present an approach for the capability-driven design of enterprises. More precisely, our contributions are (i) the introduction of a capability-based paradigm that contributes to the design of flexible services in KBSOs, (ii) an architecture of our service design and deployment environment and (iii) a demonstration of using our approach based on a real-world use case from an organization in the utilities industry. Our results and insights are based on our work in the EU-FP7 project "Capability as a Service in Digital Enterprises" (CaaS).

Keywords: Capability modelling · Service science · Context-aware services · Knowledge-based services · Context modelling · Capability as a service

1 Introduction

Service is a broadly applied term in Economics and Computer Science. The roots of service lie in division of labor and development of capabilities by various entities that compete and cooperate [1]. The Service Science field is a relatively young discipline investigating different facets of services. Service-Dominant (S-D) Logic focuses on the shift from the exchange of tangible goods toward the exchange of intangibles, specialized skills and knowledge, and processes and reflects the rise of the Service Economy [3]. Knowledge is an operant resource and it is the foundation of competitive advantage. Enterprises operating in this economy have to adapt their services frequently due to increased competition, changes in the market and technology. Capabilities are

© Springer International Publishing Switzerland 2016
T. Borangiu et al. (Eds.): IESS 2016, LNBIP 247, pp. 100–111, 2016.
DOI: 10.1007/978-3-319-32689-4_8

enablers of competitive advantage, they help companies to continuously deliver a certain business value in dynamically changing circumstances [4], which allows adaptation and dynamic design of services.

An important aspect in the Service Science research is the knowledge-based service organization (KBSO). Despite being defined in different ways, KBSOs are characterized with the need of higher flexibility in the service provision, i.e. the *ability to cope with specific needs, expectations and preferences of the clients* [5]. Vargo and Lusch define services as *the application of specialized competences (knowledge and skills) through deeds, processes, and performances for the benefit of another entity or the entity itself* [3] and Alter argues that capabilities reside in the "competences" part [6]. Based on these interpretations, the work focuses on how KBSOs can exploit their capabilities to deliver flexible services by applying the Capability-driven Development (CDD) method, which is being developed in an EU FP-7 research project "Capability as a Service" (CaaS).

The main contributions of the paper are (i) the introduction of a capability-based paradigm that contributes to the flexible service design in KBSOs, (ii) the architecture of service design and deployment environment and (iii) showcasing the approach in a use case from an organization in utilities industry.

The remainder of the paper is structured as follows. In Sect. 2, we analyze the literature in order to state the problem, report on research streams suggesting solutions towards flexible service provision and finally derive requirements for a possible solution. Against this background, in Sect. 3, the CaaS paradigm as well as its methodology, capability-driven development (CDD), are introduced. Following that, Sect. 4 presents a real-world use case in a KBSO to showcase our approach. Finally, Sect. 5 concludes the work and discusses our findings.

2 Problem Relevance and Related Work

Two of five foundations of service systems as studied by Spohrer et al. include an adaptive internal organization responding to the dynamic external environment and a dynamic configuration of resources [1]. This view is supported by Tohidi [7], which emphasizes the role of flexibility in today's enterprises offering services. Flexibility in this case means having a higher degree of adaptability in responding to new demands of the market. Furthermore, Hachani, Gzara and Verjus [8] emphasize that enterprises operate in a changing environment, both the external and internal constraints have an influence on service delivery and remaining competitive is even a harder challenge.

Different research streams relate to the design of flexible services. Among these, Business Process Management (BPM) in general and context-aware business processes and application of business rules in particular are considered most relevant. BPM is increasingly used in cross-boundary organizational processes including unstructured components [9]. In order to reach a higher degree of flexibility, the first possible solution could be adding functionality to BPM languages and making them context-aware, as suggested in [10, 11]. The second possible solution could be extending the boundaries of business process modelling languages, such as using approaches for modelling process variants [12] and relating them to the business rules, for instance by using DROOLS [13].

Furthermore, declarative approaches for business process modeling could also be considered (e.g. [25, 26]). However, declarative process specifications are hard to create and read in contrast to imperative approaches, especially for non-modelling experts.

We have identified a number of publications that list the shortcomings of such solutions in KBSO such as [5, 9] and enriched them based on our experiences in the CaaS project [14, 15]. First of all, it is a challenging task to capture all relevant knowledge in a formal business process model since (i) the processes are complex and have many variants and (ii) organizations and their processes are evolving to adapt to the changes. Second, it is hard to focus on the flexible parts of the services in enterprise models that capture all possible variations. Third, in a KBSO, knowledge workers experience and tacit knowledge is vital for service provision and it is hard to capture this knowledge with business process models. Fourth and last, the solution approaches cannot close the gap between business requirements and technical implementations. This necessarily has a negative influence on the communication between the stakeholders on various levels, such as business analysts, solution engineers and operators.

The Computer Science literature adopts the black box view of services. Proposals in this field seem to focus on aspects related to data and control flow [16, 17]. Thus, the definitions put emphasis on technical services, such as web services and IT-infrastructures needed to realize them. They neglect internal details and how service is performed, which obviously is relevant from the business point of view [18]. We regard services as a socio-technical aspect of organizations rather than a purely technical aspect. Based on this view and the identified problems above, two main requirements that the solution should fulfill have been derived:

- REQ 1: Business services should be designed in an understandable way for the stakeholders, who do not necessarily have a deep IT knowledge. To facilitate understanding, the solution should benefit from enterprise modelling approaches and should not only cover the technical aspects of service delivery.
- REQ 2: To support different roles participating to service design and delivery, a method should be engineered that addresses the modelling of business services depending on the application context, enterprise goals and operational standards.

3   Capability as a Service: A Novel Paradigm

This section introduces an approach that contributes to the flexible design of IT-based business services by explicitly taking into account business goals and delivery contexts, which is being developed in the CaaS project.

The main objective of CaaS-project is the creation of an integrated approach consisting of a *method*, *tools* and *best practices* that enable enterprises to sense and take advantage of changes in business context. The CaaS method for capability-driven development (CDD) consists of various components addressing different modelling aspects, such as context modelling, business process modelling and pattern modelling. The method is supported by the CDD environment, i.e. the *Capability Design Tool* (CDT), the *Capability Context Platform* (CCP) and the *Capability Delivery Navigation Application* (CNA) (cf. Section 3.2). Three industrial cases from e-government, finance and business process outsourcing (BPO) serve as basis for developing and validating the CDD approach. Section 3.1 focuses on the methodological and design aspects of CDD whereas Sect. 3.2 presents the architecture of the environment.

3.1 Context-Aware Design of Services

The CDD follows a component-oriented method conceptualization, each addressing different modeling aspects (REQ 2). The *enterprise modeling* component captures strategic objectives related to the service in a transparent and measurable way. The component specifies the business services by using a model-based approach and represents them with a visual modeling language to support understandability (REQ 1). The *Context modeling* method component identifies potential application context(s) where the business service is supposed to be deployed. Finally, the *Pattern elicitation* component investigates reusable design-time or run-time elements. The method components are based on the CaaS meta-model [2], which is illustrated in Fig. 1 and described below.

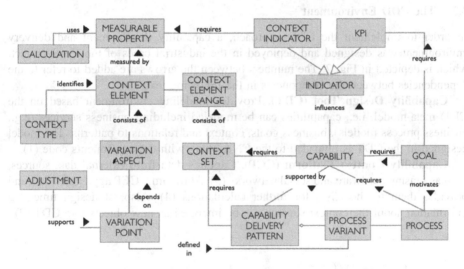

Fig. 1. Refined CDD meta-model based on [2]

Capability is defined as an ability to continuously deliver business value in dynamically changing circumstances (cf. [19]). In the literature, capabilities are perceived as fundamental abstraction instruments in business service design and they are related to the organizational strategies [4]. Vargo and Lusch [3] define services as *the application of specialized competences (knowledge and skills) through deeds, processes, and performances for the benefit of another entity or the entity itself*. Based on this definition, Alter [6] argues that capabilities reside in the "competences" part. Due to its root in strategic management, the notion of capability is a less technical-oriented concept and takes a business point of view. On the other side, services usually take a technical point of view and are concerned about the implementation aspects (cf. Sect. 2 and [17]). Unlike services, capabilities are perceived to be easier to link to the drivers and goals of the business and they are becoming a useful concept to business stakeholders [20]. This relates to the fact that it is still not clear how Service Science should address the managerial aspects of service-oriented technologies whereas capabilities provide an abstraction for business stakeholders on technical and IT-Services perspectives [21].

In terms of service design, capabilities enable flexible utilization of resources in various contexts and aim to support a model-based configuration of services. This part is represented in CDD meta-model with the concepts of *Context element* (the contextual factor), *Context element range* (configurable and relevant value ranges of a context element for the service at hand), *Context set* (a set of relevant ranges, which are monitored during runtime), *Measurable property* (attributes used to calculate the context value), *Variation point* (gateways that require contextual knowledge at runtime to be resolved) and *Adjustment* (adaptation of the service to the new situation by selecting an appropriate process variant). The detailed explanation of the CDD meta-model concepts can be found in [19].

3.2   The CDD Environment

In order to implement the CDD approach, a capability development and delivery environment was designed and deployed in the industrial cases of the CaaS project, which is depicted in Fig. 2. The numbers between the arrows are added to refer to the dependencies between the components in the following text.

Capability Design Tool (CDT). Provides modeling environment based on the CDD meta-model, i.e., capabilities can be modeled including business services (e.g., business process models), business goals, context and relations to patterns. The model designed in the CDT is uploaded to the CNA along with the adjustments code (1).

Capability Context Platform (CCP). Captures data from external data sources, such as sensing hardware and social networks (5). At runtime, CCP aggregates data and provides them to the CNA for further calculations (4). Also, at design time, the information about the context sources can be imported as new objects into CDT (2).

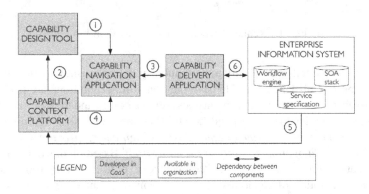

Fig. 2. The Architecture of the CDD Environment

Capability Navigation Application (CNA). Includes a module for monitoring context and KPIs. Moreover, the capability delivery adjustment algorithms are built-in here. The algorithms continuously evaluate necessary adjustments and pass capability delivery adjustment commands to the CDA for adapting the service to its application context (3).

Capability Delivery Application (CDA). An interface between the CNA and the Enterprise Information System of the organization in order to receive capability delivery adjustment commands from the CNA (3) and to provide the adjustment commands in line with the actual service application context (6).

4   Application of the CDD in a KBSO

4.1   BPO Use Case from Utilities Industry

This section reports from the application of the CDD method in SIV group, a vertically integrated enterprise from Rostock, Germany. The group specifically serves the utility industry and acts in the market mainly in two different roles. As an *ISV*, the group has a long-standing market presence in developing and selling the industry-specific ERP platform kVASy®, a software product that provides support functions specifically for the utility services industry.

As a *BSP*, the group uses the kVASy platform to offer digital services to utility companies. Within the European Union, the commodity markets are strictly regulated. Given the strict regulation and growing complexity, public utilities increasingly consider outsourcing of their business processes to external service providers. In this respect, the subsidiary of the SIV group, SIV Utility Services GmbH, is a KBSO and offers digital services to the players (market roles) of the energy sector running kVASy®.

The purpose of the use case is the transmission of energy consumption data from one market role to another. Energy data is exchanged in MSCONS format, which is a member of the EDIFACT specification family. Messages received by a market role are validated against an underlying informal data model and then the transmitted values are imported into kVASy®. Basically, this process includes a file-level check, a validation step and the processing of the individual meter readings. The exceptions in the former two steps can be remedied automatically by the ERP system.

However, the problems in the processing of the meter readings cannot be resolved without a manual intervention. For any exception, the BSP acts as a clearing center, i.e. having a direct access to the client's environment, a knowledge worker regularly checks the client's Business Activity Monitor (BAM) for failed MSCONS import processes. This causes organizational efforts, such as the arrangement of BSP's human resources schedule. Then, based on the contractual agreement between the BSP and the client, the responsible party clears the exceptional message. This decision depends on various factors such as the backlog size of the customer, message type that has thrown an exception or the type of the commodity, which are captured in the contractual agreement. The agreement as such cannot respond to customer demands, particularly when certain deadlines must apply to the message that are specified by the regulatory authority. The organization aims to design a flexible solution related to the routing of the exceptional cases. The envisioned solution introduced in the next section has to support a dynamic behavior in order to decide whether or not an individual clearing case has to be cleared by the client or by the BSP.

4.2 Dynamic and Flexible Clearing Services

SIV group has established business process models underlying the offered services, hence for the capability-based design of the clearing services, a slightly updated version of the process-first capability design method is applied [22]. The method consists of four components, each addressing important concepts (cf. Section 3.1), the notation to represent them as well as the sequence of activities (procedures) to be followed. The method components as well as their application in the use case are explained in the following.

Component 1– Define Scope. In order to design the capabilities, the method user first selects the service and sets the scope of the capability design. The selection can depend on various factors, such as optimizing the services with high process costs or managing services that are affected from the changes. The scope of the capability delivery is set to increase the throughput of MSCONS messages as well as the rate of automation by adjusting the service to the application context. To select the related services, the method proposes the approach introduced in [23], which basically classifies the services in a matrix based on four enhancers, "quality, time, flexibility, and cost".

After consultation with domain experts and business service managers, the "exception clearing in market communication" service is selected, which should deliver "dynamic BSP clearing" as a capability. This capability envisions offering context-aware services to support flexible exchange of messages, where faulty processes must be cleared.

Component 2– Develop or Update Enterprise Models. This method component ensures that selected business process models are up-to-date and applies changes if required. Moreover, to check if business goals are satisfied during the capability delivery, KPIs are developed. If no goals model is available, they are developed based on the guidelines proposed in [24]. Since an alignment of the goals is required on the business service level, method user should rather model the capability related goals and not the enterprise objectives on a general basis. Finally, goals, business process models, KPIs and capabilities are related, which is used as input in the next method component. This method component uses BPMN 2.0 and 4EM Notation [24] to represent the important concepts, such as goals, processes and KPIs.

Clearing of the faulty cases is a knowledge-centric task, hence the BSP's domain experts are predominantly *knowledge workers*. Nevertheless, we observed during the method application that the knowledge workers follow predefined *case handling instructions*, when clearing the messages. The handling instructions include service specifications and best-practices in service delivery in a textual form. This caused ambiguous definitions of the solution implementation as well as low degree of formality, hindering the envisioned flexible service provision. Using the guidelines provided by the method component, we created business process models of case handling instructions. Moreover, we developed the goals model by involving the domain experts in the modelling sessions. In the last step, we related goals, business process models and the "dynamic BSP clearing" capability, which should help in understanding the influence of the contextual factors to the processes.

Component 3 – Context Modelling. This method component models the context of the capability delivery, which is the potential application context of the deployed service. For this purpose, the designer executes three activities subsequently, "find variations, capture context element" and "design context", which are defined in the following.

Find Variations. Identifies the variability in the business process models and focuses on the reasons causing such variations. By further analyzing variability in the subsequent activity, the method user aims to elicit a context element. The activity also provides the method user with the guidelines on what constitutes a process variant and how to distinguish variability from standard decision points.

For the SIV use case, the variations in the business process models were analyzed. To do so, we used the guidelines provided by the method, (e.g. *"different than a decision point, a process variant is always relevant for capability delivery. For each decision point, evaluate the condition expression at the gateway and determine how the decision is met, i.e. data-based, event-based or context-based"*). As a result, 15 process variants were identified, which are being executed by the knowledge worker at BSP when clearing a message.

Capture Context Element. We argue that contextual information can stem from the factors of change, since they mainly cause variations in the service provision. Thus a substantial analysis of process variants underlying the service is required to capture a context element. The method proposes three guidelines for this activity, namely (i) to be classified as a context element, the change factor must be measurable, i.e. its value must be retrieved from an information system, (ii) context element is an external influence on the process, which should not exist as a process instance or data in the system and (iii) context elements are decisive for the resolution of variation points.

In the SIV use case, we investigated the factors influencing the case clearing of a knowledge worker. Alongside with the schedule of the knowledge workers in BSP, the clearing policy establishes the main factor for resolving the variation point, which is a gateway that is resolved in accordance with the service context. A clearing policy typically includes specifications about the message types, market roles, exception clearing type and critical backlog. Each time a knowledge worker clears the case, (s)he compares the actual values of these parameters with the values from the clearing policy. As such, these are external to the processes and thus selected as context elements, which are decisive for capability delivery (cf. Fig. 3).

Design Context. The activity defines ways to measure the context elements and to identify their relevant ranges, which are then put in a container (context set). The context set is linked to the goals and business process models, which is the capability

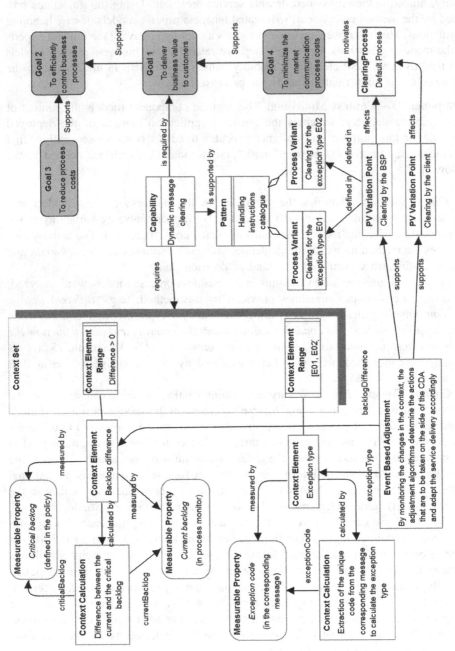

Fig. 3. Context-aware Business Service in a Capability Model

model of the selected service. In SIV use case, we conducted workshops and expert interviews to define the context element ranges. As the context elements have a common degree of similarity in each of the clients, we benefited from defining context elements only once and updating their valid ranges for different clients (cf. Fig. 3).

Component 4– Adjustments Modelling. Specifies the calculations of context values. Based on such calculations, the CNA adjusts the capability delivery in line with the service application context (cf. **Fig. 2**). After completing this method component, the capability model is now ready to be implemented, monitored and adjusted at runtime.

The developed capability model within the Capability Design Tool (CDT) is simplified and illustrated in Fig. 3. The right side of the model captures the organizational goals. The middle part represents the required business processes, reusable solutions and their specifications. Last but not least, left side of the model includes context modelling and adjustment modelling parts, i.e. which configurations and rules are necessary to adapt the service delivery to its application context and which processes are influenced by the changes.

5 Discussion and Outlook

Enterprises operate in changing environments and the shift towards a service-oriented economy based on S-D logic makes it even more important for enterprises to be agile. As stated in the 4th foundational premise of S-D logic, *knowledge is an operant resource* and *it is the foundation of competitive advantage* [3]. In this work, we focused on KBSOs as they require higher flexibility in the provision of services.

In terms of services notion, Computer Science literature adopts a rather technical view and neglects business needs. Necessarily, a solely technical view hinders reaching a common understanding in an enterprise, which is a prerequisite for offering flexible services. To close this gap, we used the notion of *capabilities*, which has its roots in strategic management and adopt a business perspective. Hence, this work contributes to context-aware business service modelling with a recent approach developed in an EU FP-7 research project "Capability as a Service" (CaaS).

The engineering of the CDD method was necessarily an iterative process and the method has undergone several versions, each of which has been evaluated by using different approaches. Currently, the industrial project partners prepare for a successful implementation of CaaS results, including the runtime environment as described in Sect. 3.2. During the application of the CDD method, we have observed that the capability-driven design may provide the KBSOs the required degree of flexibility in the following ways:

- By relating the business services to the application contexts and the goals of the enterprise to be reached, the notion of capability provides an abstraction from technical concepts of services.
- By reducing the gap between various stakeholders due to leveraging a model-based approach, i.e. the business analysts, solution engineers and knowledge workers understand what part of the service provision is flexible (context model), how they

are configured (adjustment model) and how it all contributes to the enterprise strategy (goals model). Moreover, due to the methodological support, the modelling endeavors can be documented systematically and made transparent for all stakeholder types.

- By representing the knowledge workers' tacit knowledge to a great extent in the capability models. Still, a complete automatization of the clearing procedures is not possible, which is a limitation of the approach.
- By not requiring changes in service provision to trace back the influenced business processes and updating them. Instead, the context model and the adjustments model are updated and the capability model is redeployed to the CNA (cf. arrow 1 in Fig. 2.). Hence, the number of process variants as well as the complexity of business process models are expected to diminish.

These merits of our approach should be validated by analyzing qualitative and quantitative data available when the CaaS results are implemented. Therefore, we are currently working on a final evaluation of the artefact. Another limitation is the modelling of the reusable solutions part, i.e. patterns modelling. In SIV use case, the case handling instructions deliver best-practices applicable to the clearing services offered to the clients. Although such instructions might include initial pattern candidates, we think that further analysis is required concerning this part of the method which will be part of our future work.

References

1. Spohrer, J., Golinelli, G.M., Piciocchi, P., et al.: An integrated SS-VSA analysis of changing job roles. Serv. Sci. **2**(1–2), 1–20 (2010)
2. Zdravkovic, J., Stirna, J., Henkel, M., Grabis, J.: Modeling business capabilities and context dependent delivery by cloud services. In: Salinesi, C., Norrie, M.C., Pastor, O. (eds.) CAiSE 2013. LNCS, vol. 7908, pp. 369–383. Springer, Heidelberg (2013)
3. Vargo, S.L., Lusch, R.F.: Evolving to a new dominant logic for marketing. J. Mark. **68**(1), 1–17 (2004)
4. Cutter Consortium. http://www.cutter.com/content-and-analysis/resource-centers/enterprise-architecture/sample-our-research/ea110504.html
5. Faria, J.A., Nóvoa, H.: An agile BPM system for knowledge-based service organizations. In: Nóvoa, H., Drăgoicea, M. (eds.) Exploring Services Science. LNBIP, vol. 201, pp. 65–79. Springer International Publishing, Cham (2015)
6. Alter, S.: Making a science of service systems practical: seeking usefulness and understandability while avoiding unnecessary assumptions and restrictions. In: Demirkan, H., Spohrer, J.C., Krishna, V. (eds.) The Science of Service Systems, pp. 61–72. Springer, Boston (2011)
7. Tohidi, H.: Modelling of business services in service oriented enterprises., Procedia Comput. Sci. **3**, 1147–1156 (2011). World Conference on Information Technology
8. Hachani, S., Gzara, L., Verjus, H.: Business process flexibility in service composition: experiment using a PLM-based scenario. In: van der Aalst, W.M.P., Mylopoulos, J., Rosemann, M., et al. (eds.) Exploring Services Science. LNBIP, vol. **82**, pp. 158–172. Springer, Berlin Heidelberg (2011)

9. Stavenko, Y., Kazantsev, N., Gromoff, A.: Business process model reasoning: from workflow to case management. In: CENTERIS 2013 - International Conference on Health and Social Care Information Systems and Technologies, Procedia Technology, vol. 9, pp. 806–811 (2013)
10. Rosemann, M., Recker, J., Flender, C.: Contextualisation of business processes. Int. J. Bus. Process Integr. Manage. 3(1), 47–60 (2008)
11. van der Aalst, W.M.P.: Business process configuration in the cloud: how to support and analyze multi-tenant processes. In: 2011 IEEE 9th European Conference on Web Services (ECOWS), pp. 3–10. IEEE Computer Society Press, New York (2011)
12. Hallerbach, A., Bauer, T., Reichert, M.: Context-based configuration of process variants. In: 3rd International Workshop on Technologies for Context-Aware Business Process Management (TCoB 2008), pp. 31–40 (2008)
13. Browne, P.: JBoss Drools Business Rules: Capture, Automate, and Reuse Your Business Processes in a Clear English Language That Your Computer Can Understand. From Technologies to Solutions. Packt Pub, Birmingham (2009)
14. Bravos, G., Grabis, J., Henkel, M., Jokste, L., Kampars, J.: Supporting evolving organizations: IS development methodology goals. In: Johansson, B., Andersson, B., Holmberg, N. (eds.) BIR 2014. LNBIP, vol. 194, pp. 158–171. Springer, Heidelberg (2014)
15. Koç, Hasan, Sandkuhl, Kurt: A business process based method for capability modelling. In: Matulevičius, Raimundas, Dumas, Marlon (eds.) BIR 2015. LNBIP, vol. 229, pp. 257–264. Springer, Heidelberg (2015)
16. Ferrario, R., Guarino, N.: Towards an ontological foundation for services science. In: Domingue, J., Fensel, D., Traverso, P. (eds.) Future Internet - FIS 2008: First Future Internet Symposium, FIS 2008, pp. 152–169. Springer, Berlin (2009)
17. Polyvyanyy, A., Weske, M.: Flexible service systems. In: Demirkan, H., Spohrer, J.C., Krishna, V. (eds.) The Science of Service Systems, pp. 73–90. Springer, Boston (2011)
18. Ferrario, R., Guarino, N.: Commitment-based modeling of service systems. In: Snene, M. (ed.) Exploring Services Science. LNBIP, vol. 103, pp. 170–185. Springer, Heidelberg (2012)
19. Bērziša, S., Bravos, G., Gonzalez, T.C., et al.: Capability driven development: an approach to designing digital enterprises. Bus Inf Syst Eng. 57(1), 15–25 (2015)
20. Antunes, G., Borbinha, J.: Capabilities in systems engineering: an overview. In: Cunha, J.F., Snene, M., Nóvoa, H. (eds.) Exploring Services Science. LNBIP, vol. 143, pp. 29–42. Springer, Berlin Heidelberg (2013)
21. Mikalef, P.: Developing IT-enabled dynamic capabilities: a service science approach. In: Johansson, B., Andersson, B., Holmberg, N. (eds.) BIR 2014. LNBIP, vol. 194, pp. 87–100. Springer, Heidelberg (2014)
22. España, S., Grabis, J., Henkel, M., Koç, H., Sandkuhl, K., Stirna, J., Zdravkovic, J.: Strategies for capability modelling: analysis based on initial experiences. In: Persson, A., Stirna, J. (eds.) CAiSE. LNBIP, vol. 215, pp. 40–52. Springer, Heidelberg (2015)
23. Andersson, B., Johannesson, P., Zdravkovic, J.: Aligning goals and services through goal and business modelling. Inf. Syst. E-Bus. Manage. 7(2), 143–169 (2009)
24. Sandkuhl, K., Stirna, J., Persson, A.: Enterprise Modeling: Tackling Business Challenges with the 4EM Method. The Enterprise Engineering Series. Springer, Heidelberg (2014)
25. van der Aalst, W.M.P., Pesic, M.: A declarative approach for flexible business processes management. In: Eder, J., Dustdar, S. (eds.) BPM 2006 Workshops. LNCS, vol. 4103, pp. 169–180. Springer, Berlin Heidelberg (2006)
26. van der Aalst, W.M.P., Pesic, M.: DecSerFlow: towards a truly declarative service flow language. In: Bravetti, M., Nunez, M., Zavattaro, G. (eds.) Web Services and Formal Methods. LNCS, vol. 4148, pp. 1–23. Springer, Heidelberg (2006)

A Three-Dimensional Approach for a Quality-Based Alignment Between Requirements and Architecture

Carlos E. Salgado[1(✉)], Ricardo J. Machado[1], and Rita S.P. Maciel[2]

[1] Centro ALGORITMI, Universidade do Minho, Guimarães, Portugal
carlos.salgado@algoritmi.uminho.pt, rmac@dsi.uminho.pt
[2] Dep. de Ciência da Computação, Universidade Federal da Bahia, Salvador, Brazil
ritasuzana@dcc.ufba.br

Abstract. The relation between requirements and architecture is a crucial part of an information system, standing as one of the main challenges for its successful development, with traditional projects focused on the connection of functional requirements with architecture components having a tendency to ignore quality concerns. As the quality attributes of a system support its architecture high level structure and behavior, also being highly related to its early nonfunctional requirements, there is a pressing need to align these two realities. Following our solution for aligning business requirements with services quality characteristics by derivation of a logical architecture, we now propose the specification of a metamodel and method supporting a three-dimensional approach for handling the alignment of quality issues between requirements and architecture. Taking advantage of a cube structure and method definition within a SPEM approach, which is adaptable to model variations, our proposal contributes to an improved aligned and traceable solution.

Keywords: Quality · Architecture · Requirements · Alignment · Three-dimensional · Modeling

1 Introduction

The transition from and consequent alignment between requirements and architectures has consistently been one of the main challenges during information system development, namely in the development of software solutions [1]. One of its key focuses is on creating architectures that satisfy requirements and their underlying intent, while addressing software quality attributes and supporting traceability management. Also, as human intervention is indispensable due to the complexity of the tasks involved, a certain level of automated support in the form of a tool is essential [2]. Dependencies that exist between requirements and architectures have been referred to as the twin peaks of requirements and architecture, where one of its challenges is preventing the vulnerabilities of traditional projects that focus mainly on functionality while ignoring quality concern [3].

Quality issues are ever present in the development and evolvability of an architecture, where the connection to the nonfunctional side of requirements raises a number of

© Springer International Publishing Switzerland 2016
T. Borangiu et al. (Eds.): IESS 2016, LNBIP 247, pp. 112–125, 2016.
DOI: 10.1007/978-3-319-32689-4_9

questions [4]. These answer problems as the management of requirements whilst simultaneously stressing the automation benefit of its transformation to architectures, or the need for more efforts to explicitly deal with requirements traceability while providing better tool support. One solution is using models in the requirements phase, serving as input for model-driven transformations and making further use of them in an automatic manner. This profits from the use of model-based techniques in the improvement of productivity, efficiency, and software development process quality and effectiveness [5]. It also strengthens the foundation of the software system and its architecture, connecting its high level structure and behavior to the quality attributes.

Our recent work on deriving a service-oriented architecture from business requirements tries to answer some of these issues [6], nevertheless it is not easily operationalized by users due to the diversity of concepts involved and representations of the different perspectives. This led us to propose an approach regarding the alignment between the quality attributes of service/request pairs in a service-oriented architecture and the functional and nonfunctional side of its originated business requirements [14]. There, the quality architecture attributes choice and representation is defined in line with the CISQ Software Quality Characteristics [10], the service/request pairs in the form of SoaML participants [6], and the functional and nonfunctional requirements based on the PGR approach [11].

Accordingly, the relation between functional and nonfunctional requirements (PGR), and from these to architectural services/requests can be viewed as a three-dimensional reality, lifting views from the plain one-dimensional prescriptions [7] while added to the comfort perceptions presented to users by cube-like structures ([8, 9]). So, recurring to the 4SRS-SoaML logical architecture derivation method, in a SOA environment, from PGR-based requirements [6], the derived service/request pairs stand as a third dimension, which can then be extended with a CISQ mapping. This due, we propose a solution for the representation of the three related perspectives in a cube like structure, following those three axis, the PGR-SOA Cube.

The main objective for this cube is that it can be understood and handled by different users, for diverse visualization and processing purposes. Also, as the entire method follows a model-based approach, its operationalization can be traced back and forth through the different perspectives, allowing for complete traceability and an aligned solution, while facilitating future tool development. To further support this solution, it has associated a specification of its method in the Software and Systems Process Engineering Metamodel (SPEM) [12], where, due to the its features, the method is tailored according to the project needs.

This document follows in Sect. 2 with background research information on topics supporting this work. Then, Sect. 3 presents our proposal for the PGR-SOA metamodel representation of its associated cube structure and respective tailorable method to handle their visualization and processing. Next, this proposal is demonstrated in Sect. 4, and in Sect. 5 it is discussed and framed inside the related work in the area, analyzing contributions, current research status and future work ahead. Finally, some conclusions are drawn for this paper.

2   Background

This section presents some background research on the topics supporting this work, namely functional and nonfunctional requirements elicitation, service-oriented logical architecture derivation and software quality characteristics. Regarding functional and nonfunctional requirements elicitation, we center our attention on the PGR metamodel and its associated method for eliciting and relating process, goals and rules requirements. Next we take a glance at the V-Model and its integrating 4SRS-SoaML method for the derivation of a logical architecture in SOA environments, from the previously elicited business requirements. The section closes with a synthesis on the software quality characteristics topic, where it focuses on the CISQ standard referential.

2.1   Functional and Nonfunctional Requirements

Use cases are one of the most popular techniques for eliciting functional requirements in the design of information systems (IS/IT), whether it involves the development of a new system or the reengineering of business processes. Also, nonfunctional decisions about what goals to pursue and on selecting the appropriate strategies to achieve them are always vital. Notwithstanding other elicitation methods and techniques for eliciting goals and rules associated to i* or KAOS [13], our choice for PGR [11] is due to its more complete and business oriented side, which help in defining the business requirements specification for business modeling, and promote the alignment questions between business and IS/IT comprised in process-oriented approaches.

The PGR metamodel and its accompanying method support and guide the elicitation of business goals and rules from process-level use cases, to ensure a better and more comprehensive elicitation of business requirements, functional and nonfunctional. This could allow for better and continuous alignment between business and IS/IT, with improved traceability, building a strong focus on the business model strategy. Its top-down approach initiates on top-level use cases, with elicitation of the respective goals and rules, then drilling down to leaf-level use cases by refinement of goals, including objectives, and rules, with its associated strategies, tactics and policies.

2.2   Service-Oriented Logical Architecture Derivation

Derivation of a candidate logical architecture is seen as a path for achieving the intended logical design for an information system. Integrated in a V-Model approach where the leaf-level use cases serve as its input, the Four-Step-Rule-Set-SoaML (4SRS-SoaML) method iterates and derives a logical architecture, built on SoaML participants, of the future system-to-be (i.e., the base for the information system logical architecture) [6]. The referred process-level V-Model is framed inside the analysis phase of software development, creating context for product design. In its vertex, the process-level 4SRS-SoaML method execution assures transition from the problem to the solution domain, by transforming process-level use cases into service-level architectural participants, which results in the creation of a validated architectural model and allows for architecture componentization and service-oriented development.

Besides providing a business and strategic view of the system, by taking into account the associated business-side information, it strengthens the future validation and certification of the solution architecture. Also, it answers to the increased complexity and challenges posed by new realities, and the emergence of more robust, cross-domain, solutions, by taking advantage of the SoaML concepts, in order to build a stronger alignment between business and IS/IT solutions. SoaML participants are derived, as well as their respective requests, services, and properties, in so defining the service providers and consumers in a system, where they may play the role of service provider, consumer or both. After deriving the participants, the service/request channels between aggregated participants are also identified and integrated in a higher-level super-participant.

2.3 Software Quality Characteristics

ISO 25010 defines the Quality Characteristics (QC) for Software Systems, with QC being composed by several quality sub-characteristics, each consisting of a collection of quality attributes that can be quantified as Quality Measure Elements (QME). These QME can either be counts of structural components or violations of rules of good architectural or coding practice. Four main QC were selected as the most important targets for automation, namely: Reliability, Security, Maintainability, and Performance Efficiency.

Each QC is decomposed into a set of issues, each issue is decomposed into a set of rules and each rule is translated into a violation. All these measures can be used in evaluating and managing IT business applications, providing international standard definitions against which organizations, service providers and software vendors can implement automated measurement of the structural quality of software. Accordingly, the Consortium for IT Software Quality (CISQ) recently released the Specifications for Automated Quality Characteristic Measures [10], a specification for automating the measurement of those four Software QC.

3   The PGR-SOA Cube

Our proposal for a three-dimensional approach for a quality-based alignment between requirements and architecture is grounded in the early derivation of a service-oriented logical architecture, via SoaML participants, from the functional side of the elicited business requirements for an information system [14]. Furthermore, there is the implicit relation and alignment of their, respectively associated, services' quality characteristics of logical architecture components, with the nonfunctional side of business requirements. These are supported by the Service-oriented Architecture (SOA) paradigm and the consortium for IT software quality (CISQ) metrics [10], and by a functional and nonfunctional requirements base assembled within a process, goal, rule (PGR) trio [11].

This approach, from now on designated as the PGR-SOA Cube, is twofold. On one side, there is a metamodel for representation of the functional processes (in the form of use cases), the nonfunctional (with its goals and rules details), the services (in the form of SoaML participants); and the measures of the CISQ (related to software quality characteristics). Complementarily, we detail a method to handle the generated cube-structure, with its constituent activity and associated tasks, work products and roles. This method is first specified, and then further tailored and organized, using the SPEM specification [12] for soundness and clarity reasons.

3.1   PGR-SOA Cube Metamodel

The PGR-SOA Cube follows on our previous work in deriving a services' logical architecture from process use cases, widely accepted on the functional side of requirements elicitation. These last combine with business goals and rules as one prominent solution on the nonfunctional counterpart, in a previously proposed PGR metamodel [11]. Complementarily, the services in the logical architecture have associated CISQ issues, which can then align with the referred goals and rules, concluding the metamodel constituents (Fig. 1).

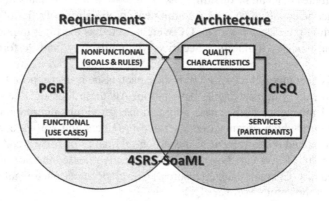

Fig. 1.   PGR-CISQ's requirements-architecture alignment

Following this work on relating processes (represented by use cases), goals and rules (PGR) in the problem domain, we now aim to align and represent this business information in the architecture product related view. As previously referred, the CISQ quality characteristics measures [10] present themselves as an important contribute for this issue. In order to support this alignment between business requirements, in the problem domain, and architectural product characteristics, in the solution domain, a new metamodel for relating PGR, SoaML and the CISQ software quality characteristics was proposed [14].

Processes, goals and rules maintain their relation, with processes connecting to participants via the previously referred 4SRS-SoaML derivation. Each participant counts with its respective services and requests, with services counting with related CISQ Software Characteristics. As each request pairs up with a service, it automatically counts with the same quality characteristics. Moreover, the goals and rules information connects directly to the SoaML BMM container, associated to a Service Interface. This strengthens the linkage between the two worlds, one more business-like and the other more technology-associated. This way, a service can easily reference its business origins as well as its technological quality characteristics.

This relation has been previously explored in a method for generating the services' quality characteristics in a logical architecture from business requirements via SoaML participants [14]. There the CISQ elements associated to each of the detailed individual elements of the nonfunctional part of the PGR requirements. According to our latest 4SRS-SoaML method [6], each leaf-level use case requirement aligns directly with one or more candidate SoaML participants (Fig. 1) in the architecture.

According to the PGR-SOA Cube simplified metamodel in Fig. 1, the service elements present themselves as a third standpoint connecting to the already existing two-dimensional realities of use cases, and goals and rules. On the relation between these three perspectives, an associated cube-like structure is built along three axis: use cases, goals and rules, and services (Fig. 2). Then, a set of CISQ measures connect directly with this triple in a cubie element.

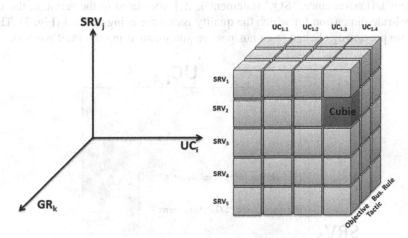

Fig. 2. (UC$_i$; SRV$_j$; GR$_k$) axis and associated cube-structure

The length of the process perspective is variable and depends on the number of leaf-level use cases of the elicited information system structure (four in this example: UC$_{1.1}$, UC$_{1.2}$, UC$_{1.3}$ and UC$_{1.4}$). Regarding the services perspective, it is linked to the number of participants that were derived from the initial set of leaf-level use cases (five in this example: SRV$_1$, SRV$_2$, SRV$_3$, SRV$_4$ and SRV$_5$). For the goals and rules perspective, its length is related to the three low-level constituents inherited from the BMM representation, namely:

- Objective, associated to Goal;
- Tactic, associated to Strategy;
- Business Rule, associated to Policy.

Although this last perspective follows a more fixed length status, additional goals and rules measures can be added to the PGR-SOA Cube as needed, all depending on the intended level of detail or project specificity.

The intersection of elements from those three perspectives represents a cubie element, as the $(UC_{1.4}, SRV_2, Objective)$ example in Fig. 2. Inside each cubie, there is room for the information regarding the system/software quality characteristic issues, in the form of statements associated with CISQ measures. To define issues for each CISQ measure, we define tuples with system/software quality characteristics (SQC) measures and statements (SQC, 'Statement'). These tuples follow on the main four CISQ measure dimensions:

- Reliability;
- Performance;
- Security;
- Maintainability.

As an example, a cubie could be made out of a set of tuples {(Reliability, 'SQC statement'), (Performance, 'SQC statement'), ...} associated to the services, use case and goal-rule dimension for which the quality issues are being defined (Fig. 3). These tuples are previously elicited from business requirements using the PGR method.

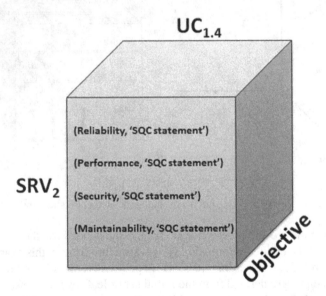

Fig. 3. Example of a PGR-CISQ cubie, with $((O_i; T_j, BR_k), SQC)$ tuples

This metamodel allows for the representation of information relating to the three perspectives and the detailed tuples of SQC measures and statements. Also, recurring to the associated cube-structure, it is possible to adapt its visualization according to the different intentions of its diverse users (business-process analyst, systems analyst, software architect, etc.).

3.2 PGR-SOA Cube Method

The PGR-SOA alignment method can only be applied after performing the use case diagram elicitation, including the deduction of the goals and rules down to the leaf-level use cases with the PGR method, and also the execution of the 4SRS-SoaML method, which generates the candidate logical architecture composed of participants interconnected by services and requests.

In order to handle the information in the metamodel and the associated cube-structure, we propose the design of a generic activity (using SPEM specification), with its required detailed tasks, work products and roles. The activity is comprised of five tasks, four work products and a software architect user role (Fig. 4), which allow to complete the alignment between the nonfunctional PGR requirements of the leaf-level use cases with the quality characteristics of the architectural participants.

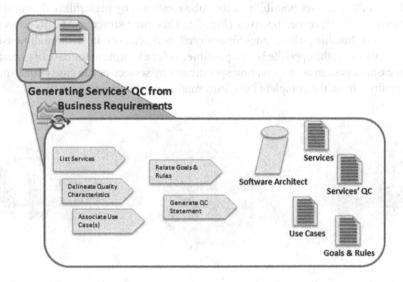

Fig. 4. Proposed activity with its tasks, work products and roles

Regarding the tasks, three are associated with handling of each cube perspective and two are associated to the alignment of the services quality characteristics with SQC measures and the consequent action to perform in each cube element (cubie). Concerning the work products, three are associated to each cube perspective and one is associated to the SQC measures to align with (composing the set of cubies).

So, the first three tasks involve the handling of the use cases, the goals and rules, and the services. These are the work products that form the structure of the PGR-SOA cube, while the fourth and fifth involve the processing of the SQC measures inside each cubie, as well as the definition of the SQC statements. For the time being, the only user performing these tasks is the software architect. The detailed tasks are, respectively: List services; Associate use case(s); Relate goals & rules; Delineate Quality Characteristics; and Define CISQ statement from UC&GR&Srv.

Due to this specification, the activity can be later tailored in a SPEM process, for operationalizing it according to the users' intentions. Each of the first three tasks in the activity can be organized and run in a cascading cycle, handling the elements of the corresponding perspective, preparing the necessary inputs or generating the intended outputs for the final tasks. The organization of the cascading tasks implies a corresponding visualization on the PGR-SOA Cube, as in Fig. 2, with the possibility to rotate each perspective accordingly.

That is, this type of cube-structure and associated tailorable SPEM process adapt to one another. When the cube switches in any of its three axis, the cascading order of the three first tasks reciprocally switches too, in order to conform to the desired processing sequence or to the specific visualization perspective. The two final tasks are the only ones that should not switch, as they are to be processed at the end for each cubie, detailing its CISQ based tuples.

All-in-all there are six possibilities for cube rotations, by performing different rearrangements of the three perspectives (Fig. 5). This cube-structure and its associated method allow handling three one-dimensional perspectives in a three-dimensional reality. Conversely, the opposite is also possible, as for example in the case of generating CISQ measures system documentation specifically by service or use case (a one-dimensional reality), from the complete cube information on the three perspectives.

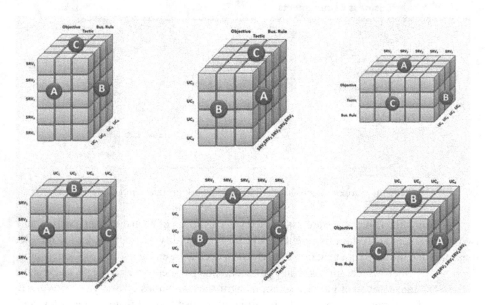

Fig. 5. Cube perspectives (C-CISQ, B-Use Cases, A-Services)

4 Demonstration

Having specified all the elements to be used in the method, the associated process can then be assembled and tailored to the preferences of the team that will be implementing it.

The complete tailored activity 'Generating Services' QC from Business Requirements', as depicted in Fig. 6, receives as input the existing participants' services in the derived logical architecture, is executed by a team of system architects and delivers a set of services' quality characteristics. While the three cycles inside the activity plus the relation of the SQC measures are merely automatic, being suitable for machine processing, the specific task of defining a system/software quality characteristic statement involves all the complexity, being crucial for the successful execution of the process.

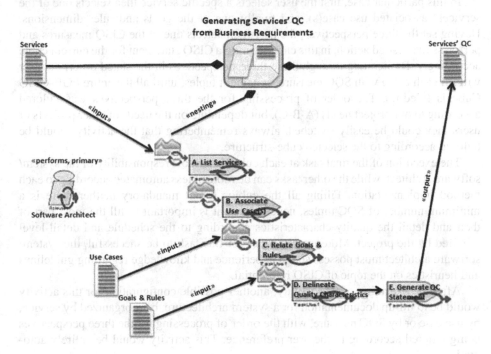

Fig. 6. Example tailored activity for 'Generating Services' QC from business requirements'

Our approach focus is on the initial aggregation and relation of the use cases (plus the goals and rules) information to each service, assured by the three cycles, going through each of the four (or more) quality characteristics, to search and analyze the information in order to generate the intended characteristic issues for the system to-be. This interpretation and adaptation of the business-side goals and rules information directly to the logical architecture quality characteristics is, for now, the sole responsibility of the system/software architects, counting on their own heuristics and specific domain knowledge.

At the end of this process, each service counts with diverse quality characteristic's issues, which later can be transformed in rules for specific system or software solutions, derived from the goals and rules associated to its originating use cases, and so, in a totally traceable and aligned solution. This demonstration allows exploring the possibilities of our three-dimensional, quality-based approach, the PGR-SOA Cube. By using its structures and the associated tailorable method one can obtain the same or even better results than with the previous approach, in a more user friendly way, through an improved, conceptualized, visualization of the entire method.

This activity can be performed by our method through the use of one of the six available cube-structures (Fig. 5) and the corresponding tailored activity (Fig. 6). The chosen activity guides the user through a cascading cycle in the following way: Select a Service; Select an associated Use Case; Select a Goals & Rules dimension; Select a CISQ measure; and Define a CISQ statement.

In this particular case, first the user selects a specific service then selects one of the services' associated use case(s), and finally one of the goals and rules dimensions. Having set the three perspectives, the user then selects one of the CISQ measures and performs the desired action, in this case defining a CISQ statement for the current cubie accordingly. By iterating through these three perspectives in the stated order, the user will fill each cubie with SQC measure, statement tuples, until all the entire PGR-CISQ Cube is filled-up. The order of processing for the three perspectives was tailored according to our project needs (A-B-C), but depending on the needs of other projects or users they could be easily switched, always remembering that the activity should be tailored according to the selected cube-structure.

The execution of the final task at each cubie is the sole responsibility of the system/ software architect, while the other tasks can be more or less automated according to each method implementation. Filling all the cubies is not mandatory neither there is a minimum number of SQC tuples, nevertheless, it is important to fill the most part of then and detail the quality characteristics according to the schedule and detail-level required by the project. Moreover, in order for this task to be successful, the system/ software architect must possess sound experience and knowledge regarding guidelines and heuristics on the topic of CISQ referential.

After the execution of this activity, another possible configuration for this activity would be to fill-up documentation for a system architecture, be it organized by service, by use case or by SQC measure, with the order of processing for the three perspectives being tailored according to the user preference. This activity would be entirely automatic.

5   Discussion

Cube structures are interesting in the way they allow for better perceptions from the users and added flexibility in the techniques to work with them. This is important to aid in the work towards reducing the gap between experts and novices, by supporting practical roadmaps, frameworks, and guidelines that can be more linear and easily taught to students, novices or analysts outside a specific domain. These are key issues, as most approaches are hard to tackle at first and require a significant level of skill and expertise from the analysts to be used effectively.

5.1 Related Research

An example of using three-dimensional perspectives is a generic model termed the "Sustainability Innovation Cube", which consolidated research on sustainability and innovations into a coherent framework clarifying existing relations in the field [8]. Its generic conception facilitates its application to a wide field of businesses and products while at the same time enabling decision-makers to tailor the model by applying existing assessment methods. Another example is our proposal for the specification of a three-dimensional business model, covering the elicitation of business goals and rules from process-level use cases, and their connection to balanced scorecard [15]. It was later explored in a practical application scenario, revisiting a project for elicitation and generation of a business model canvas, where it allowed for the use of different viewpoints to perform diverse business model transformations [9].

Research in quality requirements and architecture is still scarce, with much room for evolution in the coming years. However, there are already sound bases for the early selection of a candidate logical architecture [16], considering known standards as the Unified Process (UP) and the now deprecated ISO 9126-1 quality model framework. By prioritizing use cases, associating quality requirements directly to them, they provide a better justification for the selection of the key use cases relevant to the baseline architecture, where, more recently, a Unified Process for Domain Analysis (UPDA) was proposed [16], based on Aspect and Goal orientations to deal with NFR, already using the latest ISO/IEC 25010 quality standard. Regarding the elicitation and treatment of NFR in architecture design, this is still a very fuzzy topic, as there are many transversal issues involved. Trying to integrate existing research has proven to be difficult [17].

5.2 Contributions and Future Work

As to contributions of this work, the added value of the additional CISQ measures in an existing functional and nonfunctional requirements metamodel specification, previously aligned to a service logical architecture, alongside its cube axis rotations and visualizations, and also the SPEM activity tailoring, count as an innovative step forward regarding existing solutions in this topic. This contributes in advancing the research knowledge, and supplies practitioners with a set of options for processing and visualizing the alignment of services' quality characteristics in more linear ways.

The focus on the alignment between CISQ and the nonfunctional part of a system requirements elicitation allows for a stronger and clearer architecture quality management, enhancing the interconnection between the business and the IS/IT realities. Likewise, existing interconnection of CISQ with both the problem-side elicited functional and nonfunctional requirements, and the technical-side architecture model elements, permits widespread traceability throughout the entire solution and flexibility in applying any of the available transformation perspectives.

Regarding future work, we plan to further detail the proposed tasks, developing guiding heuristics and strategies to guide their operationalization, while exploring other scenarios and comparisons between the user's performance and its adaptability regarding the use of different service model views. Also, an empirical evaluation of this approach in academic/industrial projects, where the plan is to test and evaluate the application of the presented activities in a real setting, is also in our plans. The development of an aiding support tool to explore and process the different perspectives, by taking advantage of the metamodel and SPEM foundations of this work is also essential at this point of this research.

In another direction, the interrelation between business models and enterprise architectures is not so far off as it was in the past. As research from both sides matures, connecting the two worlds becomes a reality, so, a future step will be to relate the PGR-CISQ Cube with our business model elicitation method, the PGR-BSC Cube. This would enable to fully align and trace all elements in the V-Model structure, so they could be stored and used during design, allowing modifying the architecture at run time in configurable systems, according to any specific quality requirements.

The development of early prototypes and execution of architectural evaluations are needed to demonstrate that the delivered system is able to meet its quality goals [3], being part of the ongoing challenges that should be addressed to bridge the gap between requirements and architecture. It also contributes to confirm the iterative nature in which quality requirements are elicited and in making new observations related to current practices in the validation and measurability of quality requirements.

6   Conclusion

Architectures are at the heart of an organizations information system, being closely related to its enterprise. Its interrelation with functional and nonfunctional perspectives, as business processes, and business goals and rules, allows for an expanded three-dimensional view and control over the entire strategy and vision of an organization. With the use of modeling features as well as popular reference models inside the area for this proposal, it allows for further development of the present solution and leaves an open door to future connections to other points of interest.

The alignment between the business requirements and the quality characteristics of logical architectures is present in a wide range of active topics of research, traversing the requirements engineers and software architects competencies. The combination of the different but connected techniques for elicitation of business requirements, derivation of a logical architecture and generation of quality characteristics, seem to be particularly fit to the business and IS challenges posed by modern society.

Our work integrates all of these topics, detailing and proposing a SPEM-tailored quality-based method aligning between requirements and architecture, two different but complementary realities, with the support of a PGR metamodel extension for its representation. The ongoing and planned work with the PGR, 4SRS-SoaML and CISQ referentials, further detailed and analyzed by the PGR-CISQ Cube solution, as well as the development of a support tool prototype, present a promising standpoint from where to further develop, test, evaluate and evolve this research work.

Acknowledgements. This work has been supported by FCT– *Fundação para a Ciência e Tecnologia* in the scope of the project: FCT/MITP-TB/CS/0026/2013.

References

1. Galster, M., Eberlein, A., Moussavi, M.: Comparing methodologies for the transition between software requirements and architectures. In: Conference Proceedings - IEEE ICSMC, pp. 2380–2385 (2009)
2. Yue, T., Briand, L.C., Labiche, Y.: A systematic review of transformation approaches between user requirements and analysis models. Requir. Eng. **16**, 75–99 (2011)
3. Cleland-Huang, J., Hanmer, R.S., Supakkul, S., Mirakhorli, M.: The twin peaks of requirements and architecture. IEEE Softw. **30**, 24–29 (2013)
4. Loniewski, G., Insfran, E., Abrahao, S.: A systematic review of the use of requirements engineering techniques in model-driven development. In: Petriu, D.C., Rouquette, N., Haugen, Ø. (eds.) MODELS 2010, Part II. LNCS, vol. 6395, pp. 213–227. Springer, Heidelberg (2010)
5. Breivold, H.P., Crnkovic, I., Larsson, M.: A systematic review of software architecture evolution research. Inf. Softw. Technol. **54**, 16–40 (2012)
6. Salgado, C.E., Teixeira, J., Santos, N., Machado, R.J., Maciel, R.S.: A SoaML approach for derivation of a process-oriented logical architecture from use cases. In: Nóvoa, H., Drăgoicea, M. (eds.) IESS 2015. LNBIP, vol. 201, pp. 80–94. Springer, Heidelberg (2015)
7. Buglione, L., Abran, A.: QEST nD: n-dimensional extension and generalisation of a software performance measurement model. Adv. Eng. Softw. **33**, 1–7 (2002)
8. Hansen, E.G., Grosse-Dunker, F., Reichwald, R.: Sustainability innovation cube — a framework to evaluate sustainability-oriented innovations. Int. J. Innov. Manag. **13**, 683–713 (2009)
9. Salgado, C.E., Machado, R.J., Maciel, R.S.P.: Exploring a three-dimensional, requirements-based, balanced scorecard business model: on the elicitation and generation of a business model canvas. In: IEEE 17th Conference on Business Informatics, pp. 88–95 (2015)
10. CISQ: Specifications for Automated Quality Characteristic Measures (2012)
11. Salgado, C.E., Machado, R.J., Maciel, R.S.P.: Using process-level use case diagrams to infer the business motivation model with a RUP-based approach. In: Escalona, M.J., Aragón, G., Linger, H., Lang, M., Barry, C., Schneider, C. (eds.) Information System Development, pp. 123–134. Springer, Heidelberg (2014)
12. OMG: Software & Systems Process Engineering Meta-Model Specification (SPEM) (2008). http://www.omg.org/spec/SPEM/2.0/
13. Werneck, V.M.B., Oliveira, A. de P.A., do Prado Leite, J.C.S.: Comparing GORE Frameworks: i-star and KAOS. WER, pp. 1–12 (2009)
14. Salgado, C.E., Machado, R.J., Maciel, R.S.: Aligning Business Requirements with Services Quality Characteristics by Using Logical Architectures. In: Rocha, A., Correia, A.M., Costanzo, S., Reis, L.P. (eds.) New Contributions in Information Systems and Technologies. AISC, vol. 353, pp. 593–602. Springer, Heidelberg (2015)
15. Salgado, C.E., Machado, R.J., Maciel, R.S.P.: A Three-dimensional, Requirements-based, Balanced Scorecard Business Model. In: Proceedings of the 6th International Conference on Information and Communication Systems, pp. 1–6 (2015)
16. Losavio, F., Matteo, A., Camejo, I.P.: Unified process for domain analysis integrating quality, aspects and goals. CLEI Electron. J. **17**, 1–21 (2014)
17. Ameller, D., Ayala, C., Cabot, J., Franch, X.: Non-functional requirements in architectural decision making. IEEE Softw. **30**, 61–67 (2013)

Value Co-creation Through Knowledge Management and User-Centric Services

Framing Meaningful Experiences Toward a Service Science-Based Tourism Experience Design

Jesús Alcoba[1(✉)], Susan Mostajo[2], Rowell Paras[2],
Grace Cella Mejia[2], and Romano Angelico Ebron[2]

[1] Centro Superior de Estudios Universitarios La Salle, Madrid, Spain
jesus@lasallecampus.es
[2] De La Salle University-Dasmariñas, Dasmariñas, Philippines
{stmostajo,rrparas,grmejia,rtebron}@dlsud.edu.ph

Abstract. From a service science approach, this paper describes the use of sentiment analysis technology to analyze visitor's reviews in order to design experiences in the tourism business sector. Despite what the mere accidental observation could show, tourism is one of the significant experiences for human beings and that makes it optimal to test new concepts in service science, such as experience design and sentiment analysis. This is the first time in the literature that both concepts are used in the analysis of a large number of tourist reviews across a whole country. The value of this work lies in providing experience design recommendations on the basis of a systematic study. Thus, the potential of analyzing services through a scientific focus is shown .

Keywords: Tourism · Experience · Design · Service science · Meaning · Narrative · Sentiment analysis

1 Introduction

Pine and Gilmore's groundbreaking work discloses a new stage in the progress of the economic value that customers give to the products and services they acquire. From commodities, there is a move to the consumption of goods and from there to the use of services, and eventually to the search of experiences [1]. In the same way that that service design is central to the services sector, the design of experiences is fundamental to the management of customer experience. Understanding the phenomenological implications of human experiences, as well as the bases for experience design, is vital to work properly in this field. Due to its clearly experiential components, the services sector is a particularly useful field to carry out a research on this area, as this paper proposes.

1.1 Phenomenology of Experiences

A general definition of experience is that provided by Diller, Shedroff, and Rhea [2], for whom this concept represents the conscious feeling that something is changing in

© Springer International Publishing Switzerland 2016
T. Borangiu et al. (Eds.): IESS 2016, LNBIP 247, pp. 129–140, 2016.
DOI: 10.1007/978-3-319-32689-4_10

the interior of the human being; it could be his context, his body, his mind or his spirit. Therefore, an experience is something that happens daily although some experiences can be superficial while others can be more profound. As Coxon details [3], the term can have three different meanings, clarifying that degree of superficiality or profundity: a personal experience (reading a book), an unnoticed everyday experience (catching the bus), or the cumulative sum of the experiences that a human being has and which contributes to his life experience. In general terms, experience design is oriented toward the first group of experiences and, in particular, toward those the customers have with brands. In this way, customer experience can be defined as the sum of the experiences the customer has with a brand through his/her different points of contact, that is, the experiences produced by the customer journey.

The point is that human beings describe their experiences with words and, therefore, after living an experience, it is natural for us to construct a narrative, a means of explaining what has happened. This narrative might or might not match the customer's narrative conceptual framework and, therefore, will or will not generate a meaning. Generally speaking, a customer tends to use products or services that relate with his/her own conception of the world and to reject those that are unrelated or opposed to such conception [4]. If the experience, through its narrative, generates a meaning for the customer, it will then become part of his/her biography. S/he will talk about it to him/herself and to others as something that is part of him/herself. Finally, depending on the extent to which this biographical element becomes emotionally charged, it will end up occupying a significant place in the customer's identity. In sum, the key elements are: experience, narrative, meaning, biography, and identity.

1.2 Experience Design

Experience design is one of the central elements in customer experience management. The key difference between both concepts is that the former refers solely and exclusively to the design of experiences, while the latter is wider and implies the global organizational competence which makes an adequate customer experience possible. Therefore, while customer experience management considers that strategy and implication of the organization, the knowledge of the customer, the metrics, and of course, the creation of experiences, design refers exclusively to this latest competence.

Experience design is based on the concept of customer journey, which is the sum of the points of contact that a customer has, along with his relationship with a brand. In the different stages (initial contact, later interest, discovery and information, acquisition, use and maintenance, and drop out or recycling), the customer enters in contact with different people and systems through which the surface of the brand enters in contact with the ecosystem that constitutes the market.

In each of these points of contact, the aim is to create an unforgettable and positive experience that will become part of the customer's identity, consequently increasing his loyalty. The result of this positive memorability for the company is that the customer has a longer relationship with the brand. It increases its share of wallet with respect to its products and also to the customer's recommendations, which, in turn, decrease the cost of the acquisition of new customers.

Experience design is still an emerging concept; thus, it is important to make clear from the beginning its differences and similitude with other approaches already extant in the business field. One of the most evident is the clear orientation of this discipline toward customer journey in general and toward the points of contact in particular. Experience design is a methodology pertaining to customer experience management, and its essential differential feature is the creation of points of contact that truly shape and give value to the experience that the customer lives with the brand.

Therefore, the most remarkable difference between experience design and other value creation disciplines is that its main aim is the creation of experiences that the customer lives at the different points of contact and which together form the customer's experience. The main concern of experience design is not the elaboration of products, services, processes or systems; and it does not pertain to operations, marketing or information technologies departments, but rather involves all these, aiming to generate an unforgettable experience for the customer. In other words, there can and should be an experience design with relative independence from the fact that products, services, processes, and systems are also usually designed, managed, and assessed.

Within the creation of the sum of experiences that shape the customer journey, one of the important key aspects, which imply a differential aspect deriving from experience design, is the importance given to the emotional aspect. Albeit traditional product design has focused more on sensorial and cognitive aspects, experience design adds up the emotional level to these two dimensions [6].

Nevertheless, the most relevant question is how to carry out the active design of this kind of experiences that become part of the customer's imaginary and are introduced into his biography and identity. Experience design is still a growing area; therefore, any approach made to its structure is necessarily a tentative attempt. In this case, building on Newbery and Farnham's work [5], we propose the simplified outline that is summarized in Fig. 1, which introduces the idea that the distinctive core of experience design is the design of each one of the touch points.

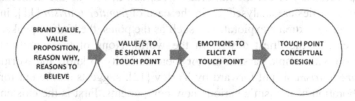

Fig. 1. Experience design.

1. The creation of an experience at a point of contact draws from the mission the company has in the market, and should respond to a reason why. Thus, the first step is the elaboration of a series of conceptual elements that provide the company with an identity. These elements usually have the name of the brand value, the value proposal, the reasons why or reasons to believe, what the company wants to offer to the market, the reason why its products or services exist, and ultimately, the trace they want to leave in its customers.

2. The next step is to determine, for each point of contact, which is/are the value/s the brand wants to transmit to its customers. It is evident that a company envisions several values, but not all of them need to be present at each point of contact with the customer although this could also be the case.

3. Next, the process consists of determining which is/are the emotion/s that the brand wants to evoke in the customers at each point of contact. It should be taken into account that customers are not linked to products or services because of their economic or functional value, but because of what these products and services make them feel [7]; thus, a key value in memorability is emotions. It should also be taken into account that these emotions do not have to be the same at all points of contact. The appropriate emotion for each point of contact does not depend on the values of the company, but also on the specific site of the point of contact within the customer journey, and also on the channel being used.

4. Then comes the design stage itself, in which the goal is to define the series of elements that define each specific point of contact (such as symbols, sounds, typography, photography, graphic forms, color, materials, language, and movement). The aim should be that the point of contact designed from these specific features elicits the intended emotions which, in turn, will transmit the values of the brand. The cumulative sum of all the emotions and value along the touch points will eventually generate the customer experience the brand looks for.

1.3 Tourism as an Experience

As argued in a previous work [8], tourism is an experience that is clearly experiential. Indeed, tourism is one of the most relevant experiences in human life. For decades, it has been noted that tourism means more than just the joy of leisure or the mere curiosity to know other realities, as seen in the works of Allcock [9] or Willson, Mcintosh, and Zahra [10].

It is relatively easy to see the importance tourism has in the life of human beings when certain varieties are analysed, as in the case of *frontier tourism* [11], in which a person embarks on extreme explorations, such as the poles, the highest peaks, the most dangerous seas, or the driest deserts in the world. None of these motivations has anything to do with simple passive rest or mere curiosity to know the world.

Adventure tourism, as put forward by Varley [12], suggests a different form where there is elaboration of tourism's various new components. First is the existence of the responsibility of tourists to assume the consequences of one's own decisions. Second is the confrontation with risks and uncertainty, which implies the confrontation between one's own abilities and the environment. And third is the experience of "transcendence" by crossing the frontier of the everyday life.

Another valuable example that illustrates the connection between tourism and central aspects of human life is *film tourism*, in which the main goal is to visit a site related to the film world. According to Buchmann, Moore, and Fisher [13], these travels are interpreted as expressions of the need to have a meaningful experience and they are connected with religious pilgrimages.

Perhaps, the most evident example of how tourism can constitute essential experience in human life is found in those people who consider travelling as way of life. In his research on this phenomenon, Cohen [14] shows that this way of understanding life is an extension of backpacking tourism, in which tourists eventually turn geographic mobility into their life's axis, whether as backpackers, crossing the ocean on a ship, or travelling in their caravan.

The above considerations lead us to attempt a first approach at the design of tourism experiences from research.

1.4   Experience Design Applied to Tourism

Experience can be attributed as the product of interaction between the individual and the environment. As an interactive process, experience may entail direct observation, participation, and involvement to the event or environment. The quality of experience maybe deep or superficial depending on how the individual takes in and interprets sensory information and the value s/he creates from it to form meaning. Thus, the creation of meaning of an experience is dependent on individual perception relative to his/her needs, interests, values, and culture. When the experience responds to the person's needs and expectations, favorable meaning is elicited. Similarly, when his/her culture and values are congruent to the place visited or with the people s/he interacts with, positive reactions and emotions maybe expected. Thus, the concept of perception in tourism experience design for the creation of a meaningful touristic experience is valuable.

According to Pine and Gilmore [1], customers crave experiences; hence, an escalating number of businesses respond by unequivocally designing and promoting it. Experience is perceived as both process and outcome. It involves a mental journey that leaves the customer with positive memories, leading to a reaction that results in recognition of value that creates a lasting effect in one's memory.

Mansfeldt, Vestager, and Iversen recognize the concept of experience design as a new, not well-explored concept, within tourism as well as in other fields [15]. Thus, the study aimed to examine and incorporate the concept of experience design in tourism industry by mapping and arranging the interaction between the service providers and tourists with innovative processes and methods based on the tourists' experience themselves. Each of these processes has elements that are considered worthy for the experience design.

As shown in Fig. 2, the initial process to consider in tourism experience design is the exposure and actual engagement of the tourist to tourism elements like services, physical and social environments, and attractions of the tourism destination termed as "Tourism Facility Engagement". This stage is crucial because it is here where the tourist personally experiences the tourism elements, thus creating initial impressions of the tourism destination. The "services" are amenities and others of value to the tourist that satisfy his/her expectations and needs while in the venue. The "physical and social environments" refer to the total physical set-up, appearance, facilities, attractions, equipment, and the people whom the tourist interacts with such as staff and other tourists. The physical facilities should be satisfactorily functional, sufficient, safe,

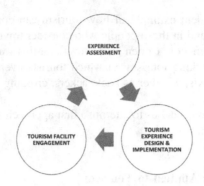

Fig. 2. Tourism experience design framework.

clean, and in order. The social environments, particularly the staff, should have the competencies, attitude, and ability to deliver the services. The "attractions" are the types of tourism facilities visited and which can be natural or built attractions, cultural and religious events, buildings, and places. It is necessary that the tourism facility is desirable, stimulating, and satisfying to the senses of the tourist. Tourists' active participation may lead to a more emotionally meaningful experience.

The next process is "Experience Assessment". In any service, feedback of customers is valuable. This covers the process of measuring the tourist's quality of experience by means of feedback generation. The feedback is analyzed and served as basis in improving the experience design. It undergoes analyses of the cognitive and affective perception of the individual to the touristic experience – how the tourist thinks and interprets the experience, the memories, and learning it creates; and how the tourist feels and reacts to the experience as manifested by his/her behavior toward the tourism destination. In this study, "Experience Assessment" is done by analyzing the tourists' sentiments. This ensures a customer-centered tourism experience design that meets the needs and expectations of the tourist to eventually create a meaningful, worthy experience.

Lastly is the "Design Review and Implementation", which involves identifying the gaps of the experience and addressing them to come up with a tourism experience design that creates a valuable and more psycho-emotionally meaningful one. It is in this process that exploration of potential solutions based on tourists' feedback, design of new solutions, and implementation of the recognized solutions is done. Moreover, the cycle of experience design should not stop in this process but moves continuously for constant and endless improvement of the tourism experience design.

2   Methodology

This research sought to capture the disclosed meaningful experiences of foreign tourists with the end goal of conceptualizing a service science-based tourism experience design. Secondary data from TripAdvisor.com, world's largest travel site, were used. Specifically, reviews of the top eight frequently visited provinces where the tourism destinations

(TD) in the Philippines are located, based on Department of Tourism (DOT) website 2015, namely: Aklan, Bohol, Cebu, Davao, Ilocos, Ifugao, Manila, and Palawan, were considered. Only foreign tourists' online reviews were gathered from 2012 to 2015, with a total of 6371 reviews. The analysis strategy had three steps. Firstly, we identified the most frequent nouns throughout all the opinions. Then, we calculated descriptive statistics of each one of them on the basis of the sentiment analysis created by Bitext, a proprietary deep linguistic analysis platform powered by grammars, dictionaries, and also business rules specific for each case. The sentiment analysis produced 44123 coded lines in total. Finally, we analyzed the most frequent adjectives related to each noun that describe how the tourists perceive the TD and feel about their experience. Data were further analyzed and used as bases in cropping up a specific tourism experience design with the final goal of delivering the optimal customer experience.

3 Results and Discussion

As observed in Tables 1, 2, and 3, the results of the analysis of feelings show that the most commonly used terms in the tourists' assessments for each of the three analyzed categories (hotels, restaurants, and attractions) receive a moderately positive evaluation. Although standard deviations are also moderately high and, thus, the differences between averages may not be significant, the term which receives the highest average across categories is "staff" under the hotel category. Furthermore, the highest combination of mean and mode is found in the terms "hotel", "service", and "breakfast" for the hotel category; "food", "place", and "staff" for the restaurant category; and "view" and "hills" for the attractions category. In a global interpretation, the most commonly used terms relate to service ("staff" and "service") and the most frequent adjectives are "great" and "good". These results reveal that the element in the TD which is remarkably noticeable to foreign tourists is the good or great service of staff.

Table 1 shows the results for the hotel category, which contains 3072 opinions and 30958 sentiment analysis coded lines. The terms tourists use most frequently to express their hotel experience are "room", "hotel", "staff", and "breakfast". It is interesting to remark that, besides finding a positive feeling in all cases, all the adjectives which are most commonly used to describe these nouns are also positive. It is significant that breakfast is so relevant for tourists that it appears among the five most used terms. Moreover, adjectives which can be associated to a person such as friendly, helpful, great, and good are also found in "service" to describe the tourists' experience under hotel category. Data validate that tourists value the staff's traits in delivering remarkable experience. Generally, these positive adjectives used to describe all the frequently identified nouns affirm that the tourists have a pleasing emotional experience in the accommodation facilities of the TDs where they stay.

Table 2 shows the results for the restaurant category, which includes 668 opinions and 3526 sentiment analysis coded lines. In this case, the most commonly used terms are "food", "service", "staff", and "buffet". Interestingly, the term "restaurant" cannot be found among these. It does not appear in the table although it would be next term, right below "buffet". It is presumed, however, that restaurant is associated with food and buffet.

Table 1. Hotels. Sentiment analysis statistics. Most frequent nouns and adjectives.

Most frequent nouns	Frequency	Most frequent adjectives	Frequency
Room	**6569**	Clean	636
Average	2,3	Spacious	374
Standard deviation	2,1	Comfortable	353
Median	2,0/2	Nice	283
Min/max value	−6,00/20,00	Good	246
Hotel	**6369**	Great	225
Average	2,6	Nice	207
Standard deviation	2,3	Good	197
Median/mode	3,0/4	Clean	157
Min/max value	−8,00/15,00	Best	122
Staff	**4097**	Friendly	632
Average	**3,5**	Helpful	417
Standard Deviation	2,0	Great	200
Median/mode	2,0/2	Nice	156
Min/max value	−6,00/20,00	Good	132
Service	**2575**	Good	161
Average	3,0	Excellent	160
Standard deviation	2,3	Great	158
Median/mode	3,0/4	Friendly	96
Min/max value	−7,50/12,00	Helpful	40
Breakfast	**2106**	Good	187
Average	2,3	Great	102
Standard deviation	2,2	Excellent	68
Median/mode	3,0/4	Nice	58
Min/max value	−7,20/15,00	Delicious	41

The evaluations of the analysis of feelings are once again positive and so are the adjectives. Again, it is highly noticeable that traits associated to a person such as good, great, and friendly are used by the tourists to express their experience in non-human tourism elements such as food, service, and place. They additionally use "attentive" to describe service.

Finally, Table 3 shows the evaluations obtained for the attractions category, which contains 2631 opinions and 9639 sentiment analysis coded lines. In this case, meeting also a globally positive feeling and adjectives equally positive to describe the tourists' experience, visitors choose most frequently the terms "place", "view", "hills", and "time".

This reveals that natural attractions and places such as views and hills, which are described as beautiful, amazing, and great, are appreciated by foreign tourists. Furthermore, it can be observed from the adjectives like nice, good, great, and beautiful that the tourists' experience with attractions is meaningful and worthwhile.

Table 2. Restaurants. Sentiment analysis statistics. Most frequent nouns and adjectives.

Most frequent nouns	Frequency	Most frequent adjectives	Frequency
Food	**705**	Good	67
Average	2,6	Great	42
Standard deviation	2,3	Excellent	25
Median/mode	3,0/4	Delicious	18
Min/max value	−5,80/9,00	Friendly	16
Service	**377**	Good	49
Average	2,8	Great	28
Standard deviation	2,4	Excellent	24
Median/mode	3,0/4	Friendly	24
Min/max value	−6,00/11,00	Attentive	11
Place	**271**	Great	26
Average	2,5	Good	18
Standard deviation	2,4	Nice	16
Median/mode	3,0/4	Best	12
Min/max value	−8,00/8,00	friendly	8
Staff	**270**	Friendly	41
Average	**3,0**	Attentive	21
Standard deviation	2,5	Good	20
Median/mode	3,0/4	Great	11
Min/max value	−7,50/12,10	Helpful	11
Buffet	**232**	Best	19
Average	2,4	Expensive	10
Standard deviation	2,4	Good	9
Median/mode	3,0/4	Better	5
Min/max value	−6,00/7,50	Awesome	4

Table 3. Attractions. Sentiment analysis statistics. Most frequent nouns and adjectives.

Most frequent nouns	Frequency	Most frequent adjectives	Frequency
Place	**772**	Nice	51
Average	2,6	Great	40
Standard deviation	2,5	Good	33
Median/mode	3,0/2	Beautiful	26
Min/max value	−6,00/18,00	Amazing	14
View	**553**	Great	51
Average	**3,0**	Amazing	44
Standard deviation	2,4	Beautiful	39
Median/mode	3,0/4	Good	38
Min/max value	−8,00/20,00	Nice	34

(Continued)

Table 3. (*Continued*)

Most frequent nouns	Frequency	Most frequent adjectives	Frequency
Visit	**475**	Worth	23
Average	2,6	Beautiful	7
Standard deviation	2,1	Great	3
Median/mode	3,0/2	Nice	3
Min/max value	−4,00/7,50	Best	2
Hills	**457**	Green	12
Average	2,1	Beautiful	9
Standard deviation	3,4	Brown	9
Median/mode	3,0/4	Great	9
Min/max value	−10,00/14,00	Worth	9
Time	**423**	Great	16
Average	2,1	Best	11
Standard deviation	2,5	Good	9
Median/mode	2,0/2	Long	9
Min/max value	−4,00/11,25	Nice	8

4 Conclusions

Building on the obtained results and taking into account that the terms related to service associated with people traits are most frequently used, and that the adjectives "good" and "great" are the most commonly repeated ones, it could be considered that the tourists' experience in the Philippines could be summarized in a slogan "the country of great service". This motto is undoubtedly different from the one currently used by the DOT of the country ("It's more fun in the Philippines"), but the truth is it is in line with tourists' real perception in the Philippines. Although there are attempts to promote the country as an enjoyable place, the perception that the Philippines is a place which offers great service to visitors weighs heavily on the tourists' experience. It may indeed more appropriate to have a promotional tagline to capture the Filipino nature of service and traits like *"Experience Philippines: Places. Service. People"* The elements of tourism; the Filipino nature of service to visitors as extension of the self [8]; and other Filipino traits like being friendly, helpful, and hospitable are felt and appreciated by foreign tourists. More than the attractions, restaurants, and hotels, it is the people's encounter that seems to create remarkable experience for tourists. In the Philippines, service has the human (Filipino) element of interpersonal connectedness to please and satisfy the visitor, and to make the experience worthy and meaningful to those who engage with it. For example, Filipinos prepare, cook, and serve food to satisfy the visitor; clean and prepare the room to make the visitor feel comfortable; and provide friendly service to show willingness to extend assistance. Thus, service for Filipinos is a "customer-valued service" because they value customers as extension of the self.

The design of narrative elements with which to communicate the touristic value proposition, based on the present analysis, can be expanded to each of the value proposition which conforms to the customer experience of those who visit the Philippines. It has been introduced the concept of *semantic mean* [16], which would be the way in which tourists would explain their experience with a specific service. In the case of hotels, the following statement could be generated: "In the Philippines you will stay in great hotels where the members of staff are nice, helpful, and friendly; the rooms are comfortable, spacious, and clean; the service is excellent and breakfast is delicious". This sentence may sound like any other marketing slogan, but there is an important difference because this motto has been created using the same terms that tourists use most frequently and, even more importantly, it has been created using the terms for which tourists show positive feelings. The theoretical framework that supports this study argues that this kind of sentence is better synchronized with the tourists' interior narrative. Therefore, they can help to construct meaning, making the experience unforgettable and making it likely to be part of the visitor's biographical imaginary. If lived experiences are provided with sufficient intensity, the tourist's experience is likely to become part of the tourist's identity.

One of the great advantages of the analysis of feelings as regards experiences design is that it focuses on the touch points within the customer's journey. For instance, in the case of hotels, it is evident that the contact with staff, rooms, and breakfast are focal points of high interest for the tourists since they are the most commonly used terms. Other touch points can also be interesting, such as the web site or the reception desk, where more design efforts are concentrated on. Because the tourists' feeling as regards these places is positive, it can be relatively easy to increase the quality of their experiences. Each hotel establishment should link its mission statement with the values it wants to highlight for each touch point, and the emotions it wants to foster in the client to create an experience design. Once this task is completed, a second advantage that this approach provides is to map the direction and intensity of the feeling that evolves once the design has been implemented.

Experience design is an emerging research field and a development factor in the business arena. The creation of value from a customer-centered culture is to find out the customer's experience in relation to his interaction with a product or service which eventually would develop an experience that transmits a company's proposal and its brand values. Tourism, due to its experiential essence, is one of the services which can benefit most from this avant-garde approach as the present article has argued.

Acknowledgement. The authors of this paper would like to express their gratitude to Bitext for providing the sentiment analysis technology that made possible the data exploration.

References

1. Pine, J., Gilmore, J.H.: Welcome to the experience economy. Harv. Bus. Rev. **76**(4), 97–105 (1998)
2. Diller, S., Shedroff, N., Rhea, D.: Making Meaning: How Successful Businesses Deliver Meaningful Customer Experiences. New Riders, Berkeley (2008)

3. Coxon, I.: Fundamental aspects of human experience: a phenomenological explanation. In: Benz, P. (ed.) Experience Design: Concepts and Case Studies. Bloomsbury Academic, New York (2015)
4. Alcoba, J.: Beyond the paradox of service industrialization: approaches to design meaningful services. In: Wang, J. (ed.) Management Science, Logistics and Operations Research. IGI Global, Hershey (2014)
5. Newbery, P., Farnham, K.: Experience Design: A Framework for Integrating Brand, Experience, and Value. Wiley, Hoboken (2013)
6. Svabo, C., Shanks, M.: Experience as excursion: a note towards a metaphysics of design thinking. In: Benz, P. (ed.) Experience Design: Concepts and Case Studies. Bloomsbury Academic, New York (2015)
7. Jiwa, B.: The Fortune Cookie Principle: The 20 Keys to a Great Brand Story and Why Your Business Needs One. CreateSpace, North Charleston (2013)
8. Alcoba, J., Mostajo, S., Clores, R., Paras, R., Mejia, G.C., Ebron, R.A.: Tourism as a life experience: a service science approach. In: Nóvoa, H., Drăgoicea, M. (eds.) IESS 2015. LNBIP, vol. 201, pp. 190–203. Springer, Heidelberg (2015)
9. Allcock, J.B.: Tourism as a sacred journey. Loisir et Societé/Society and Leisure 11(1), 33–48 (1988)
10. Willson, G.B., McIntosh, A.J., Zahra, A.L.: Tourism and spirituality: a phenomenological analysis. Ann. Tour. Res. 42, 150–168 (2013)
11. Laing, J.H., Crouch, G.I.: Frontier tourism: retracing mythic journeys. Ann. Tour. Res. 38(4), 1516–1534 (2011)
12. Varley, P.: Confecting adventure and playing with meaning: the adventure commodification continuum. J. Sport Tour. 11(2), 173–194 (2008)
13. Buchmann, A., Moore, K., Fisher, D.: Experiencing film tourism: authenticity and fellowship. Ann. Tour. Res. 37(1), 229–248 (2010)
14. Cohen, S.A.: Lifestyle travellers: backpacking as a way of life. Ann. Tour. Res. 38(4), 1535–1555 (2011)
15. Mansfeldt, O.K., Vestager, E.M., Iversen, M.B.: Experience design in city tourism. Nordic Innovation Centre and Wonderful Copenhagen (2008). http://www.visithelsinki.fi/.../experience_design_in_city_tourism_20080704.pdf. Accessed 24 November 2015
16. Alcoba, J.: The paradox of service industrialization and the creation of meaning. Int. J. Serv. Sci. Manage. Eng. Technol. 3(2), 50–62 (2012)

Personal Service Eco-Environment (PSE²): A User-Centric Services Computing Paradigm

Zhongjie Wang[✉], Dianhui Chu, and Xiaofei Xu

Harbin Institute of Technology, Harbin 150001, Heilongjiang, China
rainy@hit.edu.cn

Abstract. Compared with manufacturing industries, service industries have a distinct characteristic called "heterogeneity", i.e., there is a wide variation in service offerings to different customers due to their individualized demands. Traditional resource-centric services computing paradigm tries to make use of mass customization approaches to fulfill customer demands in a cost-effective way, but sacrifices the personalization degree and decreases customer satisfaction. We propose a user-centric paradigm called "Personal Service Eco-Environment (PSE²)" which plays as a "personal assistant" of each user. PSE² is composed of personal data, services, and social relations around a user, and fully-personalized service/social collaboration solutions are to be planned on the basis of the individualized characteristics extracted from his personal data and the dynamic multi-end context. This paper introduces the high-level architecture and design philosophy of PSE².

Keywords: Services computing · Personal data · Service eco-system · Full personalization · Multi-end context · User-as-a-hub

1 Introduction

With the flourish of cloud computing, mobile computing, social networking and Internet of Things (IoT), massive and diversified real-world things around people have been virtualized as "services" which are deployed on and accessed by Internet and IoT. Life of people depends on these services more and more. Here the *"services"* is a general term, i.e., besides traditional web-based software services (usually called *Web Services*), there are many embedded services in the smart phones, watches, glasses, sports bracelets, wearable healthcare equipments, and so on, that facilitate the anytime-and-anywhere sensing and controlling of the real world around a user, and many online Social Network Services (SNS) that facilitate easy social networking among people. These services mostly follow the "cloud-terminal convergence" architecture style [1], in which users utilize the services in the smart/mobile terminals (e.g., Apps) to access the services and data in the remote clouds, to fulfill their daily personal demands.

It is necessary to organize multiple fine-grained services together and make them collaborate with each other to fulfill the large-grained demand of a user. In

© Springer International Publishing Switzerland 2016
T. Borangiu et al. (Eds.): IESS 2016, LNBIP 247, pp. 141–154, 2016.
DOI: 10.1007/978-3-319-32689-4_11

both research and practices, collaborative service solutions have been promoted as "*first-order entities*" in service systems [2]; in other words, they exist permanently and are managed and provisioned independent of those fine-grained services. Here the "*collaboration*" includes both the collaboration among multiple services and the social collaborations among multiple users (under the support of SNS). Here are two examples:

Example 1 (Healthcare Service Collaboration). There appear some abnormal signals in the physical condition of a person. A set of healthcare services are required to closely collaborate for diagnosis and treatment to make him be recovered from the abnormal situation. Healthcare service providers dynamically organize a collaborative service network in terms of the individualized physical condition, so that a highly personalized composite healthcare service solution is offered to the person [3].

Example 2 (Social Collaboration for Software Development). Open Source Software (OSS) development is a typical social collaborative process [4], e.g., a mass of developers discuss software requirements by mail list and forums, commit their source code via Github, report bugs and submit repairs via Bugzilla, make technical Q&A via StackOverflow, and write documentation by Google Docs. Under the support of these SNS, developers make social collaboration for agile and iterative OSS development of a specific OSS project [5].

Today an important trend of Information Technology is that the *resource-centric* computing paradigm is gradually replaced by the *user-centric* computing paradigm [6,7], and the dominant power in a service relation is transferred from the resource owners to the demand owners, i.e., from service provider side to the customer side. In terms of a customer, various services that he uses, the hardware, mobile terminals and the cloud where these services are deployed, the personal data that these services generate, and other users who have social relations with him, together constituent his Personal Service Eco-Environment (PSE^2). PSE^2 of a specific user can be considered as a convergence of three networks including Personal Service Network (PSvN), Personal Social Network (PScN), and Personal Data Network (PDN). Elements in PSvN and PScN facilitates the fulfillment of personal functional and social demands by close and adaptive collaborations among external services/users, respectively; during the collaboration, a lot of personal data that contains rich personal characteristics and real-time personal states is generated and impacts the emergence of successive demands, and further, the successive decision making on his future's service selection and usage (i.e., his behaviors that he would exhibit in PSvN and PScN).

This paper is a high-level introduction to the idea of PSE^2. In the past year we are working on the architecture of PSE^2, and the objective of this paper is to give an overview on why PSE^2 does really exist around each user, and on the fundamental mechanism of how PSE^2 fulfills the daily demands of a user by dynamically planning the service/social collaboration.

2   Personal Service Eco-Environment (PSE²)

2.1   Architecture of PSE²

Figure 1 shows the high-level architecture of PSE². The human icon on the top is a user u, and the rounded rectangle underneath represents u's PSE². There are three networks in PSE², i.e., PScN, PSvN and PDN. PSvN connects external services from diversified service domains into PSE²; these services are either frequently or occasionally used by u, and there are loose or tight, and, direct or underlying collaboration among them. PScN connects other users from different social network (SN) platforms into PSE². u has a social circle in each SN, and PScN integrates all the users who have social relations with u in each SN into a virtualized social network. There is a Personal Data Cloud (PDC) [8] that stores the personal data generated by external services or external social relations during the service/social collaboration, in the form of PDN that connects potentially semantics-related personal data entities into linked data.

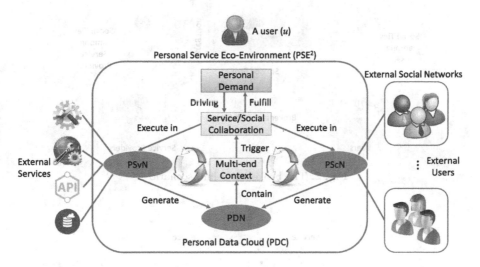

Fig. 1. Personal service eco-environment (PSE²): a user-centric paradigm

Personal data represents the *history* of the user, including his behavior records and behavior results in both real world and online world. Rich context information can be extracted from the personal data and will trigger the collaboration among external services or social collaboration among the user and other external users. If the user explicitly raises his demand, service/social collaboration will also be planned and executed to fulfill the demand. Such process iterates, so that the explicit or implicit demands of the user are fulfilled one by one along with the time.

To note that, in today's dominating third-party-broker based services computing paradigm, there is a broker who is responsible for aggregating external services and composing them into coarse-grained composite services which are then offered to users (see Fig. 2). In our PSE^2 paradigm, it is the user himself that plays the role of broker (see Fig. 3). The philosophy of the broker-as-a-hub scenario is "mass customization oriented services offering", i.e., to use a small number of service solutions to fulfill the demands of massive customers by customization techniques; on the contrary, the one of the user-as-a-hub scenario is "complete personalization", i.e., each customer has his own broker (i.e., his PSE^2) who serves only for himself by exploring the personal data for constructing the personalized service network and social network. This conforms to today's trend in service industries — the deeper personalization the offered service solutions have, the higher satisfaction the customer would have, and the more profit service providers would earn from him.

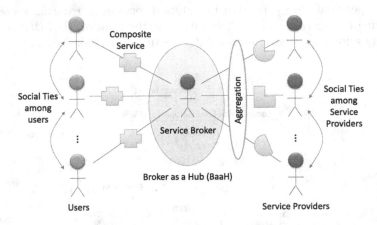

Fig. 2. The broker-as-a-hub scenario

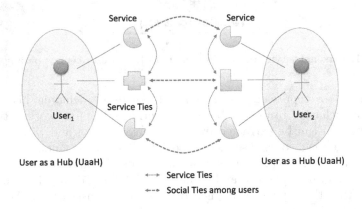

Fig. 3. The user-as-a-hub scenario

2.2   Personal Data

The cornerstone of PSE^2 idea is "personal data". Personal data has another name "small data" and is a hot research issue relative to today's "big data" wave. There are three typical approaches how personal data is collected/generated, i.e., (1) they are generated by the business systems of various service providers; (2) they are created by the user himself; and (3) they are collected by pervasive sensors around the user. Personal data has been the principal part of big data and has been considered as important "assets" of people. Users are the "data subject, data controller, data processor" of personal data [9]. There are four types of personal data, i.e., attribute/profile data, volunteered data, observed data, and inferred data [10], which together delineate the multi-dimensional state of the user, such as location, social, environment, sentiment, financial situation, interests and preferences, and so on [11].

The followings are some examples of personal data:

- The orders and payment data that a user owns in various e-Business services represent his buying habits and consumption preferences;
- The content fragments that a user generates in various SNS represent his social interests and social behavior habits;
- The amount of exercises (walking, running, sleeping, etc.) and the physical states of a user are collected by the sports bracelet and they represent the health condition of the user;
- The location information collected by the GPS sensors in the smartphone of a user represents his physical context, and further, his preferred trace and touring habits.

Estrin [12] thinks that personal data, especially the data change trace along with the time (She called it "personal digital trace"), is a fairly important supplement for the traditional massive data. However, most of personal data is now controlled by service providers and there lacks enough integration due to the barriers such as storage location isolation, technique/format incompatibility, semantics inconsistency, and privacy control. Nevertheless, with a comprehensive personal data view, many valuable predictive and personal analytics applications have been developed [13], and the ultimate goal is to realize "Quantified-Self" [14]. A lot of novel personal data management approaches have been put forward, such as Personal Information Management Systems (PIMS) [15], Personal Data Store (PDS), Personal Data Vault, and Personal Data Inventory [16,17], to help users collect, integrate and control their own data effectively and with rigorous privacy protection.

A key reason why personal data is so important is that personal knowledge, interests, goals, and preferences can all be extracted from the personal data. With rich personal data, service providers could offer to the user more personalized and more accurate service solutions which are much closer to his implicit preferences and value expectations [18].

For example, in healthcare services, the personal data that a user published on social medias, the personal data collected from his wearable equipments, and the personal Electronic Medica Records (EMR) have been combined to analyze personal health situation, and an empirical study has shown that these personal data stemming from different sources are highly correlated and can improve the healthcare service quality [19]. Another example is Netflix – when Netflix recommends movies to its users, various forms of personal data are utilized such as the scoring data (delineating the user's perceptions on movies), behavioral data (delineating the user's actions when he accesses the Netflix movie pages), social data (from user-generated contents from various social media), and personal profiles, and the recommendation accuracy has been greatly improved [20].

Even in government level a lot of actions have been taken, such as the Blue-Button[1] and Smart Disclosure[2] that are both conducted by US government and allow users to export personal data from service systems of various service providers in standardized and machine-readable format. Similar acts includes the MiData[3] conducted by UK government and the Mes Infos[4] by France government. More and more personal data oriented novel Internet services or mobile Apps appear, such as Personal.com, My Eyes Only[5], mHealth[6], etc.

2.3   Multi-end Context

In PSE^2, the context that a user reside in is a mixed "multi-end context". Here the "multi-end" includes four "ends": (1) mobile context, indicating the real-world physical environment information around the user (such as the location and places, speed and acceleration, temperature, etc.); (2) cloud service context, indicating the dynamic situation that an external service exhibits (such as the fluctuant QoS and dynamically updated SLA of the service); (3) personal data context, indicating the past, present and future states and state transitions of the user (such as the orders he placed on e-Business sites, the revenue and payment records of his bank account, the movies he has watched and is going to watch); (4) social context, referring to the shared information that he and other users co-produce and dynamically update during their social collaboration. These types of contexts are not independent with each other but there are underlying correlations. The user, each external service provider, and each socially-connected user make their own decisions in terms of their own context and other types of context, and then the service/social collaborations gradually come into being to fulfill personal demands.

Figure 4 gives an overview of the multi-end context around PSE^2 of a specific user.

---

[1] http://www.healthit.gov/patients-families/your-health-data.

[2] https://www.data.gov/consumer/smart-disclosure-policy.

[3] https://www.gov.uk/government/news/the-midata-vision-of-consumer-empowerment.

[4] http://mesinfos.fing.org/english.

[5] http://myeyesonlyapp.com.

[6] http://openmhealth.org.

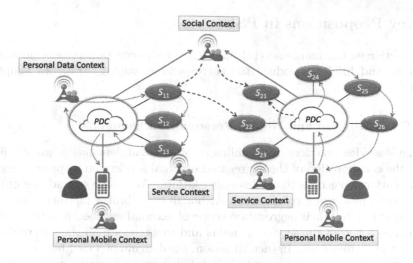

Fig. 4. Multi-end context in PSE²

2.4 Personal Entropy in PSE²

There are "stable" and "unstable" states in PSE². A stable state implies that the personal demands (both explicit and implicit) can be fully satisfied by the services and social relations included in the PSvN and PScN, and an unstable state implies that there are some demands that cannot be satisfied by current configuration of PSE². We prefer to use the "entropy" to measure the stability of PSE² in specific time and call it "personal entropy". Along with the continuously emerging personal demands and the on-going dynamically changed multi-end contexts, personal entropy usually increases along with time. The user-centric service/social collaboration can be considered as the process of "to proactively plan and execute the collaboration relations among a set of selected services, or to plan and execute the social collaborations among the user and a set of other users, with the objective of recovering a user's PSE² from an unstable state (high entropy, in chaos) to a stable state (low entropy, highly ordered)".

A user's PSE² is not static but keeps evolution along with time. For example, a user has different levels of perception on different external services, and over time he might have much deeper awareness on some services and this would update his preferences on these services (e.g., he dislikes some services or is more inclined to use some services); on this occasion, the service collaboration that best fulfills his demands would be changed, too. In this sense, PSE² is very similar as the natural eco-system in which the amount and importance of various species keeps evolution over time, too.

3   Key Propositions in PSE^2

In this section we summarize several challenges of user-centric services computing paradigm, and briefly introduce the corresponding coping strategies adopted in PSE^2.

3.1   Cross-Domain and Highly Personalized Demands

In today's service practices, the fulfillment of personal demands is usually limited in the collaboration of the aggregated external services on a specific service broker platform (such as the e-Business platform Amazon.com and the online travel service platform Expedia.com). Although these broker platforms are continuously extending their aggregation scope of external services, it is impossible for them to cover all the service domains and to aggregate all the external services that users might use. In such situation, the demand of a user has to be split into multiple segments each of which is fulfilled by one specific service broker platform or one specific service provider, and it is the user himself's responsibility to deal with the coordination among these platforms, which is time-consuming and error-prone.

Similarly, in personal social collaborations, the "friends" of a person are distributed in different social network platforms (e.g., some of my friends are using Facebook but they are the users of Twitter, and vice versa). At the same time, each available SNS is tightly bound with a specific SN (e.g., the SNS *Friend Circle* is offered by WeChat, thus it cannot cover the users who have no WeChat account). Thus, a personal social demand have to be cut into multiple segments each of which is conducted in a specific SNS that covers only a part of the user's social relations.

In PSE^2, aforementioned issues are overcome by the approach that both service and social collaboration would break the boundaries among service domains and the ones among social network platforms; in other words, personal demands are fulfilled by the *"cross-domain"* approach. Specifically, the PSvN of a person is regarded as the direct or potential collaborations among the external services around him (i.e., all the services that he knows and uses), no matter which domains they belong to; the PScN of a person is regarded as a virtualized social network among the external users around him (i.e., the users with whom he has social relation in at least one social network platform). The reason why we called PSvN and PScN "personal" is that these service/social collaboration relations are to fulfill the user's OWN functional/social demands, rather than a generalized one that is suitable for all the users.

Figure 5 shows a conceptual example of PSvN/PScN. There are four domain-specific service broker platforms in which each node represents a service. Services belonging to the same domain have more close relations with each other. The central oval represents the cross-domain PSvN of the user and it is composed of a subset of services of the four domains, and they collaborate to fulfill the

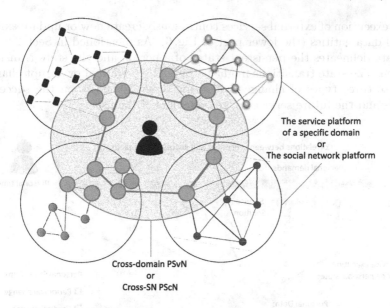

The service platform
of a specific domain
or
The social network platform

Cross-domain PSvN
or
Cross-SN PScN

Fig. 5. Cross-domain PSvN and PScN

personalized demand. This figure can be also used to describe the cross-SN PScN, and the four circles are four SN platforms in which each node represents a user, thus the central oval is regarded as the PScN of the user.

3.2 A User is "Stateful": Service Patternalization and Anchoring

A fundamental assumption of web user behavioral modeling is that the user's behavior is consistent with the Markov process and the user's next behavior only depends on his current behavior regardless of the historical behaviors of the past. However, the latest research has shown that a user's behavior sequence is not a Markov process, but an aperiodic infinitary long-range memory power-law process [21]. Personal demands emerge continuously along with the time, they depends on the subjective willingness, the present and past states, the real-time personal context, and the personalized preferences/interests, of a specific user. Because of the "statefulness" of a user, his demands appearing at different time are not completely independent but are with obvious correlations: during the iterative process of using services to fulfill his personal demands, the content and degree that the personal state is locally or global changed has more or less influence on his successive demands in the future. Considering such underlying correlation between precedent and successive demands, when a service solution for one demand is planned, it should not be considered independently without considering his previous demands and his historical state transitions. For example, in terms of a patient, the treatment plan largely depends on the medical treatments he received before. This idea is described in the upper part of Fig. 6.

The execution of external services continuously create new or update existing personal data entities (the lower part of Fig. 6). As mentioned in Sect. 2.2, personal data delineates the persistent states of a person and the state transitions over time. The state transitions might be periodical, gradual or abrupt changes, and these three types of changes will bring different effects on the successive demands and the future service usage behaviors of the user.

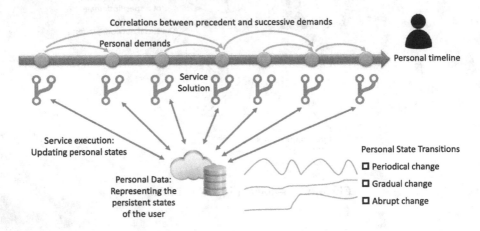

Fig. 6. Persistent states of a person and the potential influence on his demands and service usage

From the perspective of external services, the style that a service participates into the fulfillment of a person's demand might be short-term/one-time temporary (e.g., to randomly select a specific flight of a specific airline for a temporary business trip), or be long-term/multi-time (e.g., if a person has the membership of an airline, he would like to take flights of this airline more frequently than the ones of other airlines). The former is usually under the situation when the user has no enough perception on services, and along with the deeper acknowledgment he has on the services, some satisfying services would be transformed into the latter. Here the "*patternlization effect*" refers that a user prefers to use the services that he previously used so as to avoid the cost of learning about new services, therefore his behaviors shows some specific patterns. The "*anchoring effect*" refers that the contract between the user and the external service provider usually drives the user continuously and chronically use these services to fulfill his similar demands, because the longer a service is used by him, the more rewards he would usually get from the service provider (e.g., the mileage accumulation offered by the airline).

3.3   Information Asymmetry

The information asymmetry [22] between customers and service providers is bi-directional. Firstly, in terms of a user, it is difficult for him to get the dynamic context information of the external services (e.g., the fluctuation of service price and QoS) accurately and timely; thus when the user selects services from candidates, he has a certain limitation to find the most appropriate ones whose current context is in full accordance with his own preferences. Secondly, in terms of an external service provider, it owns only some personal data that is generated and maintained by the service itself, but the amount and diversity of these personal data is insufficient and thus it is difficult to make accurate service recommendation and offering to the user.

In terms of the former, with the flourish of services on the Internet, users play the dominant role in service relations in a highly competitive buyer's market, therefore, if external service providers passively wait for users to come to request their services, it is difficult for them to win the competitive advantages. On the contrary, service providers should proactively approach to look for potential users and offer the services being in accordance with their personal demands and preferences.

In terms of the latter, the possible solution is to extend the scope of personal data that these external service providers can access. Under the strict protection of personal privacy, if a user would like to open some of his personal data to external services, these services could utilize these cross-domain personal data to offer more accurate services. A similar approach can be found in Vescovi et al. [23]: the personal data store is integrated into a framework which enables the development of trusted and transparent (in terms of access and use of personal data) services and Apps, thus an eco-system of personal data based trusted Apps/services is created and potentially allows users to gain direct economic benefit from the disclosure/exchange of their data.

In summary, information asymmetry puts obstacles to the personalized service offering. Our solution in PSE^2 paradigm is two-fold: (1) external services proactively make collaborations and offer services in terms of the personal demands; and (2) users open part of their personal data to external services to improve the accuracy of service offering.

The two perspectives are jointly shown in Fig. 7. The oval is a user's PSE^2, and he publishes his personal demands in the PSE^2. Then, if an external service would like to participate into the fulfillment of the user's demands, it will dispatch an autonomic agent to the PSE^2; the service agent has the responsibilities of (1) to get the real-time service context information from the corresponding external service providers; (2) to collaborate or compete with the agents of other external services and plan a service collaboration solution for the corresponding demand. We will not discuss the details of how to make collaborative decision-making by agents. The right side of the PSE^2 describes the openness of personal data to external services under the privacy control.

4   A Short Summary

The PSE^2 research is to help establish personal computing environment as a "personal assistant" by proactively planning the collaborations around a person,

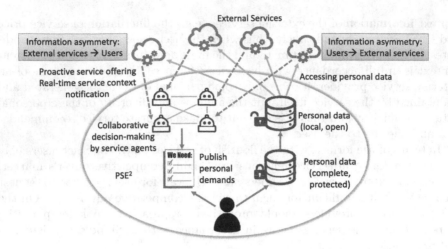

Fig. 7. Two approaches dealing with two types of information asymmetry

with the help of the aggregated personal data delineating the personal life log, trace, and knowledge of the person. The PSE^2 paradigm deals with the continuously emerging personal demands in the personal timeline of a user, and PSE^2 is considered as a virtualized place where the demands are published and fulfilled, with the objective of realizing the extremely personalized service offering for the fulfillment of personal demands.

Specifically speaking, the key techniques of PSE^2 include: (1) to collect and aggregate multi-source heterogeneous personal data; (2) in terms of the semantics correlation, to connect related personal data entities as personal data cloud (in the form of Linked Data); (3) to identify the individualized characteristics, preferences, and patterns of the user based on the historical changes of his personal data; (4) to plan the service/social collaboration under the support of multi-end context information and the distributed decision-making among multi-parties.

To note again, this paper is just a high-level introduction to the PSE^2 idea. More introduction to the detailed techniques will appear in other papers.

Acknowledgment. Work in this paper is funded by the Natural Science Foundation of China (No. 61272187, 61472106) and the Key Project of Science and Technology Development of Shandong Province, China (No. 2015ZDXX0201B02).

References

1. Huang, G., Liu, X.Z., Zhang, Y.: A mobile web application platform with synergy of cloud and client. Scientia Sinica Informationis **43**(1), 24–44 (2013)
2. Murray-Rust, D., Robertson, D.: LSCitter: Building social machines by augmenting existing social networks with interaction models. In: 23rd International World Wide Web Conference, pp. 875–880(2014)

3. Andriopoulou, F., Birkos, K., Lymberopoulos, D.: P2Care: a dynamic peer-to-peer network for collaboration in personalized healthcare service delivery. Comput. Ind. **69**, 45–60 (2015)
4. Crowston, K., Wei, K., Howison, J., Wiggins, A.: Free/Libre open-source software development: what we know and what we do not know. ACM Comput. Surv. **44**(2), 7 (2008)
5. Liptchinsky, V., Khazankin, R., Truong, H.-L., Dustdar, S.: Statelets: coordination of social collaboration processes. In: Sirjani, M. (ed.) COORDINATION 2012. LNCS, vol. 7274, pp. 1–16. Springer, Heidelberg (2012)
6. Xu, Z., Xie, Y., Hai, M., Li, X., Yuan, Z.: Universal compute account and personal information asset algebra in human-cyber-physical ternary computing. J. Comput. Res. Dev. **50**(6), 1135–1146 (2013)
7. Gnesi, S., Matteucci, I., Moiso, C., Mori, P., Petrocchi, M., Vescovi, M.: My data, your data, our data: managing privacy preferences in multiple subjects personal data. In: Preneel, B., Ikonomou, D. (eds.) APF 2014. LNCS, vol. 8450, pp. 154–171. Springer, Heidelberg (2014)
8. Wang, J., Wang, Z.: A Survey on Personal Data Cloud. The Scientific World Journal, Article ID 969150 (2014)
9. Kalapesi, C.: Unlocking the value of personal data: from collection to usage. World Economic Forum Technical Report (2013)
10. Schwab, K., Marcus, A., Oyola, J., et al.: Personal data: The emergence of a new asset class. An Initiative of the World Economic Forum (2011)
11. Vescovi, M., Perentis, C., Leonardi, C., Lepri, B., Moiso, C.: My data store: toward user awareness and control on personal data. In: The 2014 ACM International Joint Conference on Pervasive and Ubiquitous Computing, pp. 179–182 (2014)
12. Estrin, D.: Small data, where n=me. Commun. ACM **57**(4), 32–34 (2014)
13. Regalado, A., Tucker, P., Simonite, T., et al.: Big data gets personal, pp. 1–29. MIT, Technology Review (2013)
14. Rehman, M., Liew, C.S., Wah, T.Y., Shuja, J., Daghighi, B.: Mining personal data using smartphones and wearable devices: a survey. Sensors **15**(2), 4430–4469 (2015)
15. Abiteboul, S.: Andr B., Kaplan, D.: Managing your digital life. Commun. ACM. **58**(5), 32–35 (2015)
16. de Montjoye, Y.-A., Shmueli, E., Wang, S., Pentland, A.: openPDS: Protecting the privacy of metadata through SafeAnswers. PLoS ONE, 9, 7, e98790 (2014)
17. Mun, M.Y., Kim, D.H., Shilton, K., Estrin, D., Hansen, M., Govindan, R.: PDVLoc: a personal data vault for controlled location data sharing. ACM Trans. Sens. Netw. **10**(4), 58 (2014)
18. Kay, J., Kummerfeld, B.: Creating personalized systems that people can scrutinize and control: drivers, principles and experience. ACM Trans. Interact. Intell. Syst. **2**(4), 24 (2012)
19. Haddadi, H., Ofli, F., Mejova, Y., Weber, I., Srivastava, J.: 360 Quantified Self (2015). arXiv:1508.00375
20. Amatriain, X.: Big and personal data: and models behind netflix recommendations. In: The 2nd International Workshop on Big Data, Streams and Heterogeneous Source Mining, pp. 1–6 (2013)
21. Li, Y., Meng, X., Liu, J., Wang, C.: Study of the long-range evolution of online human-interest based on small data. J. Comput. Res. Dev. **52**(4), 779–788 (2015)

22. Aarikka-Stenroos, L., Jaakkola, E.: Value co-creation in knowledge intensive business services: a dyadic perspective on the joint problem solving process. Ind. Mark. Manage. **41**(1), 15–26 (2012)
23. Vescovi, M., Moiso, C., Pasolli, M., Cordin, L., Antonelli, F.: Building an ecosystem of trusted services via user control and transparency on personal data. In: Jensen, C.D., Marsh, S., Dimitrakos, T., Murayama, Y. (eds.) Trust Management IX. IFIP AICT, vol. 454, pp. 240–250. Springer, Heidelberg (2015)

Using User-Generated Content to Explore Hotel Service Quality Dimensions

Vera L. Miguéis[✉] and Henriqueta Nóvoa

Faculdade de Engenharia da Universidade do Porto, Porto, Portugal
{vera.migueis,hnovoa}@fe.up.pt

Abstract. A better evaluation and understanding of the client's perception of the service provided by hotels is critical for hotel managers, especially in the "Travel 2.0" era, where tourists not only access but also actively review the service provided. This paper analyses data automatically collected from TripAdvisor reviews regarding 2 star and 5 star hotels in Porto. TripAdvisor user generated content is explored through text mining techniques with the purpose of creating word clouds, synthesizing and prioritizing the aspects of the service raised by customers. Furthermore, this content is analyzed using the SERVQUAL model to identify the service quality dimensions most valued by guests of the two types of hotels. The results of the preliminary study demonstrate that the methodology proposed allows us to identify service perceptions with reasonable effectiveness, highlighting the potential of the procedure to become a complementary tool for hotel management.

Keywords: Hotel service quality · User-generated content · SERVQUAL · Text mining

1 Introduction

In most industrialised countries we have witnessed an ample shift from the primary and secondary sectors to the tertiary sector in the last decades, with the service sector gaining prominence and becoming a key pillar of these economies. In these highly competitive markets, service industries need to maintain and nurture ongoing relationships with their customers, if they want to keep being competitive and foster growth. Thus, it is mandatory that companies design innovative differentiation strategies and deliver high quality services [1], as it has been proved over and over again that providing an excellent service quality leads to increased customer satisfaction [2–4].

Hospitality industry is one of the service industries that has promoted the development of the economy at a global scale in recent decades [5], and several governments have concentrated their efforts in developing this fast growing industry and, consequently, tourism. This growth has been faster than that observed in other notable industries, such as, for example, manufacturing, financial services or retail [6]. In fact, and according to the World Travel and Tourism

© Springer International Publishing Switzerland 2016
T. Borangiu et al. (Eds.): IESS 2016, LNBIP 247, pp. 155–169, 2016.
DOI: 10.1007/978-3-319-32689-4_12

Council [6], the hospitality industry will triple in size by the year 2020, becoming one of the largest industries in the world.

Similarly to other services settings, in the tourism and hospitality industry, service quality is considered to be a strategic tool for companies to keep their competitive edge, as good quality affects customer satisfaction, motivating customers to return and influencing their behavior regarding future recommendations of the service provider. In this context, it is of utmost importance for companies to clarify what customers perceive as a good service, as different customers have different perceptions of this concept. When asking customers to define a good service, many of them say something like: "get what I want, when I want it" or "being greeted with ..., smile" [2]. It is obvious from these examples the importance of both tangible and intangible aspects in guaranteeing customer's satisfaction. Consequently, service companies' managers and marketers must explore customers' expectations and perceptions concerning the quality of the services provided, as these quality dimensions are crucial to guarantee the company's success. Service quality is conceptualized and measured by several models, the most popular being the SERVQUAL model in almost all of the services industries [7].

In parallel with the development of the tourism and hospitality industry, web 2.0 applications in the tourism sector are growing at an incredible pace, creating a cultural change in the tourism world [8]. By sharing opinions and experiences through text, photos, videos, music, insights and perceptions, social media plays an active role for choosing and preparing a trip, highly influencing the idea or image created about a destination, a hotel or a museum.

The objective of this study is to analyze the User-Generated Content (UGC) available in TripAdvisor concerning 2 and 5 star hotels in Porto during the month of September 2015, as Porto is one of the European capitals where tourism is growing more rapidly. This analysis will be supported by text mining techniques, focusing firstly on the issues highlighted by users when spontaneously describing the quality of the service provided. The SERVQUAL model will be used to classify the dimensions mentioned by guests in their reviews, enabling a better comparison of their perceptions of the two types of hotels.

2   Service Quality in Hospitality

Customer satisfaction is clearly imperative for the success of any type of hotel in the long run. Consequently, customer satisfaction has been adopted frequently as a key performance indicator by those that aim to achieve and maintain competitive advantages over their competitors. In the hotel industry we have witnessed a constant change in customer's demands and expectations, both growing at a fast rhythm. Therefore, hotels need to keep pace in order to measure and establish concrete measures to increase customer satisfaction. Measurement of customer satisfaction has been a note-worthy addition to the ISO 9000:2000 standard, and still is a major requirement of the new ISO 9000:2015. Organizations certified according to this standard are now required to identify what are the parameters subjacent to customer satisfaction and to consciously measure them [9].

Related to customer satisfaction, service quality is crucial to measure the performance in hospitality [10,11]. However, due to the proper nature of this broad concept, there is a lack of a general agreement about what constitutes service quality. Knowing what guests consider important when evaluating the quality of the hotel offerings will help hotel managers know what to improve and whether service quality has been met or not [12]. This knowledge most certainly is a precious help in reducing the gap between guest's expectations and the actual service provided.

In the hospitality industry, several studies have explored hotel attributes that guests find important when evaluating the performed service quality. These studies are mainly based on surveys administered to hotel guests. Literature review suggests that security and safety [13,14], cleanliness [13,15], employees' empathy and competence [16,17], convenient location [18,19], value for money [13,20] and physical facilities [17,20] are attributes that hotel guests perceive as being important.

Several methods have been proposed in the literature to measure service quality. Seth et al. [21] examine the service quality models introduced in the period between 1984-2003. This critical review of the different service quality models did not conclude about one universally accepted model, however emphasizes the positive characteristics of the GAP model of quality and dimensions of quality presented in SERVQUAL model, introduced by Parasuraman et al. [22]. Since its development, SERVQUAL has been extensively applied in a variety of contexts in the service industries, such as retailing [23], banks [24], hospitals [25] and higher education [26]. For this reason, SERVQUAL model remains the best measure for cross-sectional research and industry benchmarking [27]. Despite this, it is important to note that due to both conceptual and methodological concerns, SERVQUAL is also target of some criticism [28,29].

SERVQUAL model measures the difference between customers' expectations about the general quality of a service and the actual performance of a service. The original SERVQUAL model defined service quality using 10 determinants of quality: reliability, responsiveness, competence, credibility, access, courtesy, communication, assurance, empathy and tangibles. Some years later, [30] reduced these dimensions to five dimensions, i.e. tangibles, reliability, responsiveness, assurance and empathy. Tangibles dimension refers to the appearance of physical facilities, equipment, personnel, and communication materials. Reliability concerns the ability to perform the promised service carefully and accurately. Responsiveness is linked with the willingness to help customers by providing a prompt service, and the assurance dimension is concerned with the knowledge, courtesy and trustworthiness of the personnel. Finally, empathy relates to the effort to really know and understand customers and their needs.

SERVQUAL model has been and still is a very popular model in measuring hotels service quality. For example, recently Blei et al. [31] used a questionnaire research aimed at measuring the service quality in spa hotels in Serbia and Sharma [32] has also used the SERVQUAL model through a questionnaire to measure customer satisfaction in an Indian hotel. A similar approach was followed by

Karunaratne and Jayawardena [33] and Mola [34]. Most of the studies available in the literature use questionnaires to support SERVQUAL findings. Therefore, this paper uses a different approach, contributing to the literature by processing natural language in which customers' reviews have been expressed in order to classify hotels according to SERVQUAL.

3   Travel 2.0

The technological advances observed in the last decades enabled the propagation of consumer reviews on social media platforms, where consumers shop for goods and services. Consumer reviews address a wide range of products or services and are becoming a key component of the decision-making process for many consumers [35]. Due to the specific nature of experience goods such as hotel rooms, the potential impact of consumer reviews can be significant. Experience goods are, by definition, intangible products, difficult to evaluate before acquisition, characterized as high involvement and risk considering the personal importance usually involved [36].

Online reviews, that constitute the denominated User-Generated Content (UGC), is notoriously affecting travel consumer decisions. [37] refers that online reviews offer quality information to reduce risk in experience goods. Most consumers perceive UGC as being likely to provide up-to-date and reliable information, in comparison to the more static nature of the information provided by service providers [37]. In fact, online reviews enable consumers to learn about the perception of service quality from previous consumers without experiencing the service themselves. UGC demonstrates also the evaluation level and feedback of experience goods, thus providing an important reference for new buyers to help them make decisions and choose the service that best match their requirements or preferences.

Currently, about 92 % of consumers consider UGC when purchasing travel services [38]. In fact, online consumer reviews have become an important source of information for consumers, replacing the offline word-of-mouth (WOM) communication about the quality of service providers [39]. According to [38], 80 % of consumers trust reviews as much as personal recommendations.

Several studies have explored UGC, namely from TripAdvisor content, as a source of valuable information in the analysis of tourism and hospitality industry. For example, [40] estimates the effect of factors of online consumer review, including quantity, quality and consistency, on the offline hotel occupancy. Similarly, [41] analyzes the impact of online user-generated reviews on business performance. [42] examines online travelers' perceptions of the credibility of UGC sources and how these perceptions influence attitudes and intentions toward UGC utilization in the travel planning process. Finally, [43] explores the motivation of users from different countries to share information regarding their recent trips.

4 Methodology

The objective of this preliminary study is to use an automated procedure to extract knowledge from hotel's reviews available in TripAdvisor. This was the platform chosen due to the fact that currently this platform is the largest travel site in the world [44]. Text mining techniques are used to create an image resulting from the aggregation of opinions expressed online by tourists after experiencing 2 star or 5 star hotels, the extremes of the hotels rating. Furthermore, the SERVQUAL model will be used to stratify the service quality dimensions mostly mentioned and, consequently, mostly valued by hosts of the two types of hotels.

After reviewing about one hundred papers about destination image analysis, Pike [45] concludes that less than half of them used any type of qualitative information. However, with travel 2.0, the amount of textual data increased exponentially [46] and has promoted the use of quantitative methods, such as, for example, text mining techniques. In tune with this idea, this study is based on a random sample of textual reviews automatically extracted from TripAdvisor concerning 2 star hotels and 5 star hotels. Only reviews in English were selected in order to further apply text mining techniques.

Text mining refers to the process of parsing unstructured text in order to derive high quality information. In this study, text mining tools are used to compute word's frequency used by consumers in their reviews. For a more complete analysis, the most frequent bigrams are identified. A bigram is a pair of consecutive words that allows to find more complete ideas included in the reviews. Furthermore, sometimes some of the interpretations are based on the context involving the words directly in the reviews text.

The pipeline for the information extraction tool is depicted in Fig. 1.

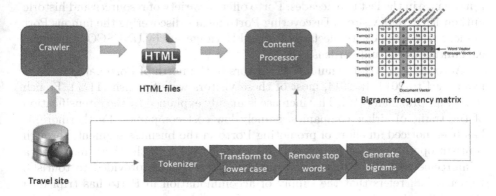

Fig. 1. Pipeline for the information extraction.

The first component of the pipeline is a crawler that retrieves the web pages we want to collect data from. In this particular case we were interested in crawling the pages referring to the hotel reviews. The html pages collected are initially stored and, afterwards, each of them is sent to a natural language processor. This processor first breaks the review into pieces, called tokens. This process usually involves removing certain characters, such as punctuation characters, resulting in sets of individual words. The next step involves converting all words to lower case, which is followed by the removal of stopwords of the English dictionary, i.e. ordinary words such as "the" and "a" that are not significant. Having excluded the stopwords, this process implies the identification of bigrams. This is the basis for the construction of a document-term matrix that describes the frequency of bigrams that occur in each review. In this particular case, the columns of the document-term matrix correspond to the reviews in the collection and the rows correspond to the bigrams identified in the complete set of reviews.

In this paper we construct a document-term matrix for 2 star hotels and another one for 5 star hotels. These matrices enable to compute the bigrams frequency observed in the reviews of the two categories of hotels. Based on this information we construct two words clouds that are a powerful visual representation of the words frequency. Furthermore, we analyze SERVQUAL dimensions more frequently addressed in the UGC, in order to identify the hospitality characteristics more frequently quoted.

5 Case Study

5.1 Setting

The Portuguese northern city of Porto, the second largest city in the country, has become one of the most attractive tourism destinations in Europe. In 2012 and 2014, Porto was elected the "Best European Destination", winning the title over 19 major European cities. Porto, located at the mouth of the Douro river and with a population of about 300,000 inhabitants, has undergone a remarkable renaissance in the last two decades. Porto offers a variety of resources and historic authenticity to its visitors. Discovering Porto means discovering the famous Port Wine, a Historical Center declared a World Heritage site by UNESCO, museums, enchanting parks and gardens.

According to [47], the number of visitors in the north of Portugal grew 66 % from 2004 to 2014. In 2014, most of these visitors were Spanish (11 %), French (6 %) and Brazilian (4 %). This increase is mainly explained by the intensification of the traffic of airline companies, namely low cost companies. Furthermore, it has been noticed an effort of promoting Porto in the business segment, through tourism operators. Resulting from this tendency of growth, there has been a reinforcement of the diversity and quality of the services provided to tourists. Pimenta [48] refers that the supply of accommodation in Porto has tripled in the last decade.

Porto offers very distinct accommodation solutions. Guests can choose among hotels, hostels, guest houses, and apartments. The exact number of tourist accommodations is not known precisely. However, according to the director of the Tourism of Porto and North of Portugal, from the 570 tourist accommodations, only 80 are hotels [49].

5.2 Synthesis of Hotel Reviews

This study is based on reviews generated by guests' reviews available on TripAdvisor in September 2015. This website included 22 hotels classified as 2 star and 7 hotels classified as 5 star. We collected 938 TripAdvisor reviews referring to the 2 star hotels and 350 reviews referring to the 5 star hotels.

Following the methodology introduced in Sect. 4, we constructed two word clouds, illustrated in Figs. 2 and 3. The size of the words is closely related to the frequency of the bigrams used by TripAdvisor users. In dark grey, it is represented the most used set of two words. The subsequent levels of importance are represented in different shade. Table 1 shows the relative frequency of the bigrams referring to 2 star hotels and 5 star hotels.

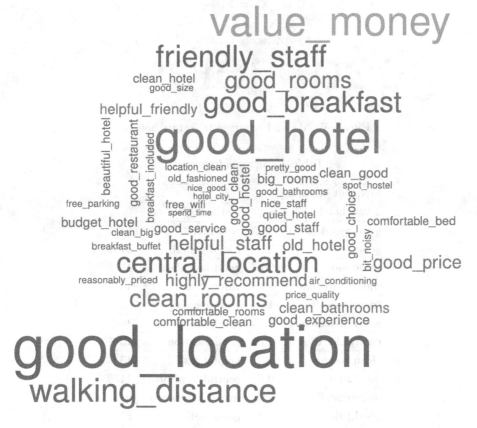

Fig. 2. Word cloud referring to 2 star hotels.

By analyzing the word clouds, it is possible to verify that the overwhelming majority of bigrams represent positive feelings about the service provided by both classes of hotels. The negative aspects mentioned for both 2 star and 5 star

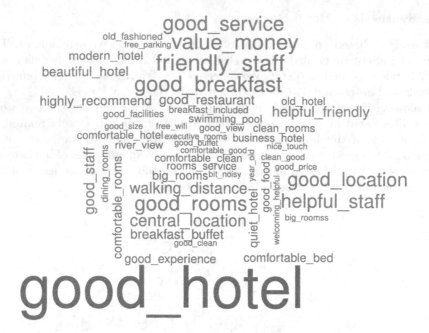

Fig. 3. Word cloud referring to 5 stars hotels.

Table 1. Bigrams frequency.

Frequent bigrams			
2 star hotels		5 star hotels	
good_location	30 %	good_hotel	54 %
good_hotel	23 %	friendly_staff	17 %
value_money	20 %	good_breakfast	15 %
walking_distance	15 %	value_money	15 %
friendly_staff	14 %	good_rooms	15 %
good_breakfast	13 %	good_service	14 %
central_location	13 %	good_location	13 %
clean_rooms	10 %	helpful_staff	13 %
good_rooms	9 %	central_location	11 %
helpful_staff	7 %	walking_distance	9 %
good_price	7 %	good_staff	8 %
highly_recommend	5 %	helpful_friendly	7 %
old_hotel	5 %	breakfast_buffet	7 %
helpful_friendly	4 %	highly_recommend	7 %
clean_bathrooms	4 %	beautiful_hotel	6 %

(*continued*)

Table 1. (*continued*)

Frequent bigrams			
2 star hotels		5 star hotels	
big_rooms	4 %	good_restaurant	6 %
budget_hotel	4 %	comfortable_bed	6 %
good_experience	4 %	comfortable_rooms	6 %
good_staff	4 %	modern_hotel	6 %
clean_good	3 %	quiet_hotel	5 %
good_hostel	3 %	big_rooms	5 %
clean_hotel	3 %	good_experience	5 %
comfortable_bed	3 %	business_hotel	4 %
good_restaurant	3 %	clean_rooms	4 %
beautiful_hotel	3 %	comfortable_clean	4 %
comfortable_clean	3 %	old_hotel	4 %
good_service	3 %	good_food	4 %
good_choice	3 %	river_view	4 %
good_clean	3 %	swimming_pool	4 %
bit_noisy	2 %	comfortable_hotel	3 %
breakfast_included	2 %	rooms_service	3 %
comfortable_rooms	2 %	good_facilities	3 %
nice_staff	2 %	breakfast_included	3 %
quiet_hotel	2 %	dining_rooms	3 %
free_wifi	2 %	good_view	3 %
free_parking	2 %	old_fashioned	2 %
air_conditioning	1 %	big_rooms	2 %
old_fashioned	1 %	clean_good	2 %
pretty_good	1 %	executive_rooms	2 %
clean_big	1 %	nice_touch	2 %
reasonably_priced	1 %	bit_noisy	1 %
breakfast_buffet	1 %	comfortable_good	1 %
good_bathrooms	1 %	free_parking	1 %
good_size	1 %	free_wifi	1 %
spot_hostel	1 %	good_buffet	1 %
location_clean	1 %	good_price	1 %
price_quality	1 %	good_size	1 %
basic_clean	1 %	welcoming_helpful	1 %
clean_spacious	1 %	air_conditioning	1 %
good_bed	1 %	buffet_style	1 %

hotels are related to noise issues and the antiquity of the hotels. The positive aspects cover a considerable diversity of issues. However, it is interesting to verify that most of these aspects are highlighted for both classes of hotels, which might mean that, in general, the service dimensions valued by guests are independent of the category of the hotel.

Regarding 2 star hotels, the good location of the hotels is the issue more frequently mentioned by TripAdvisor's users (30 % of the reviews). Furthermore, other expressions related to the location, such as central location and walking distance are fairly common. Concerning 5 stars hotels, a generic characterization of the hotels as good is the most frequent idea conveyed (54 % of the reviews). It is interesting to note that this is the second idea most frequently mentioned when reviewing 2 star hotels (23 % of the reviews). This difference between the perceptions of the two types of hotels is in line with their category level. Location is also mentioned by guests of 5 stars hotels, but with less representativeness (13 %).

Both 2 star and 5 star hotels are considered to have friendly staff, offer good breakfast and are considered to be value for money hotels. These bigrams are referred with a similar frequency when reviewing the two classes of hotels. A distinctive point between the reviews is the repetitiveness of expressions concerning the cleanliness of the rooms. In fact, concerning 2 star hotels, about 10 % of the reviews mention this issue, while only 4 % of the reviews of 5 stars hotels mention this issue. This fact suggests that cleanliness is a concern mainly in lower class hotels, an aspect that is taken for granted in higher class hotels. The price is considered to be good by 7 % of the guests of 2 star hotels, while this is also mentioned by 1 % of 5 stars hotel's guests. This may reveal either that the price of 5 stars hotels is not reasonable or that most of its guests are not price sensitive, which is not the case for 2 star hotel's guests. Other aspects that distinguish this type of hotels from 2 star hotels, often referred by guests, include the quality of the breakfast buffet offered by the 5 stars hotels, the modernity of the hotels, the fact of being business oriented, the river view and the existence of a swimming pool.

5.3   Analysis of Service Quality

Aiming at understanding the perceptions of hotel guests based on the UGC in TripAdvisor, it was conducted an analysis of the five dimensions of the SERVQUAL model for the two classes of hotels, i.e. 2 star and 5 star hotels. Tables 2 and 3 summarize the categorization of the aspects mentioned by TripAdvisor users about hotels' service.

The dimension empathy encompasses all service characteristics that complement the core service. When comparing 2 star hotels and 5 star hotels, both are considered to have friendly staff, who provide an attentive and personalized service. Furthermore, both offer complementary services, such as car parking and wi-fi. Regarding 5 stars hotels, guests highlight the view of the hotels and the existence of swimming pools, giving a particular emphasis to the quality of the breakfast buffet.

Regarding reliability, this dimension refers to the ability to perform the promised service. Analyzing guests' reviews, the reliability of both 2 star and 5 star hotels is addressed mainly through a general characterization of the facilities and location as "good". Moreover, UGC includes a general description of the staff as being "good". Within the reliability dimension, the cleanliness of the hotel is another aspect that is frequently stressed out. Although the aspects highlighted about 2 star hotels' guests and 5 stars hotels' guests are about the same, if we consider the frequency of reviews mentioning each aspect as a proxy for their weight in the assessment of the reliability of the service, we obtain two distinct pictures. For example, expressions related to the cleanliness of the hotel are more frequent when reviewing 2 star hotels which, as mentioned before, seems to suggest that in the case of the top level hotels, cleanliness is not an issue, as it is taken for granted.

Assurance is one of the dimensions less frequently addressed by TripAdvisor users. We consider that the knowledge and education of the staff is assessed when there is a general characterization of the staff. The staff of the two types of hotels is generally characterized as good. We consider that assurance also includes the price fairness and both types of hotels are considered to be good value money, and 2 star hotels are even considered to have good, low or reasonable prices by a considerable number of guests.

Responsiveness evaluates the willingness to help customers and this is the SERVQUAL dimension less frequently addressed by TripAdvisor users. According to TripAdvisor reviews, both categories of hotels are considered to have helpful staff and, more generally, are considered to have good staff. However, the frequency of reviews in which these responsiveness aspects are included is higher for 5 stars hotels.

Tangibles dimension is the most frequently dimension addressed in guests' reviews. Generally, guests refer the good quality of beds, rooms and bathrooms. Furthermore, reviews of both types of hotels include aspects related to the location, parking facilities and wi-fi. The reviews of 2 star hotels also stress the relevance of cleanliness issue in this type of hotel. The reviews of 5 stars hotels highlight the view of the hotels and the existence of swimming pool. These aspects are common to the empathy dimension.

Summing up, the characteristics of the service provided by hotels mostly mentioned for 2 star hotels are also mentioned for 5 stars hotels. However, in most cases, the weight of each service characteristic in the total set of reviews is different. This means that some aspects are more relevant for the assessment of 2 star hotels service than for the 5 star hotel service and the other way around. It is important to note that particularly in the case of 5 stars hotels, some important characteristics of the service, e.g. cleanliness, are not mentioned that frequently, as in this category of hotels these characteristics are taken for granted.

6   Conclusions and Future Research

In the past, hotel quality models were mainly supported by the information collected through surveys that had the primary aim of estimating the gap between

Table 2. SERVQUAL - 2 star hotels

Empathy
Friendly staff, Breakfast included, Free wi-fi, Free parking, Breakfast buffet

Reliability
Good location, Good hotel, Good breakfast, Clean rooms, Good rooms, Clean bathrooms, Good staff, Good hostel, Clean hotel, Comfortable bed, Good restaurant, Good service, Bit noisy, Comfortable rooms, Air-conditioning available, Good bathrooms, Good size, Spacious rooms

Assurance
Value money, Good price, Budget hotel, Good staff, Reasonably priced

Responsiveness
Helpful staff, Good staff

Tangibles
Good location, Walking distance, Central location, Clean rooms, Good rooms, Old hotel, Clean bathroom, Big rooms, Clean hotel, Comfortable bed, Beautiful hotel, Good restaurant, Comfortable rooms, Quiet hotel, Free wi-fi, Free parking, Air-conditioning available, Old fashioned, Big hotel, Good bathrooms, Spacious rooms, Good bed

Table 3. SERVQUAL - 5 stars hotels

Empathy
Friendly staff, Breakfast buffet, River view, Swimming pool, Breakfast included, Good view, Free parking, Free wi-fi, Good buffet, Buffet style

Reliability
Good hotel, Good breakfast, Good rooms, Good service, Good location, Good staff, Good restaurant, Comfortable bed, Comfortable rooms, Quiet hotel, Clean rooms, Comfortable hotel, Clean hotel, Old hotel, Good food, Good facilities, Bit noisy, Good buffet, Good size, Air-conditioning available

Assurance
Good staff, Value money, Good price

Responsiveness
Helpful staff, Good staff

Tangibles
Good rooms, Good location, Central location, Walking distance, Beautiful hotel, Good restaurant, Comfortable bed, Comfortable rooms, Modern hotel, Quiet hotel, Clean rooms, Clean hotel, Old hotel, Good food, Swimming pool, River view, Comfortable hotel, Good facilities, Old fashioned, Big rooms, Free parking, Free wi-fi, Good size, Air-conditioning available

customer's perceptions and expectations. Right now, with the widespread use of internet technologies in multiple platforms, hotels service quality might be assessed using more efficient approaches. Guests' reviews are at the leading edge of e-business in the hospitality industry, being a primary source of valuable information to evaluate hotels service quality.

In this paper we develop a preliminary analysis of online consumer reviews based in TripAdvisor, referring to 2 star hotels and 5 star hotels in Porto. For this purpose we use an automatic process to collect these reviews using text mining to extract the ideas most frequently mentioned by guests. Furthermore, we use the SERVQUAL model to explore the service quality dimensions addressed more frequently by guests' reviews. The knowledge acquired through this process may provide useful and timely information for management of the two types of hotels, constituting an inexpensive mechanism for hotel managers to get feedback of the service provided from UGC.

From this initial study it is evident that, in general, Porto visitors have a very positive feeling about the hotels where they stayed. The negative aspects mentioned for both 2 and 5 stars hotels are the existence of noise and the age of the hotels. The positive aspects encompass a considerable diversity of points and most of them are common to both hotels' categories. However, it is interesting to observe that some service aspects are more frequently mentioned in the case of 2 star hotels and others in the case of 5 stars hotels. Moreover, we believe that, in the particular case of 5 stars hotels, some important aspects of the service are taken for granted as these are not mentioned that frequently when comparing with 2 star hotels.

SERVQUAL model constructed from TripAdvisor reviews reveals that assurance and responsiveness are the dimensions less frequently addressed by users. On the other hand, tangibles and reliability dimensions are those more frequently addressed. These dimensions are clearly linked, demonstrating that the physical features are still critical when measuring the quality of the service provided.

In the future, it would be relevant to extend the sample of the reviews analyzed and to use additional sources of information, such as hotel ratings. Furthermore, since the techniques used account only for one part of the potential emotion-expressing kinds of sentences, future work should consider more advanced techniques to account diverse types of expressions. Furthermore, in the future it would be interesting to use natural language processing for extracting knowledge regarding the quality of the experience instead of quality of service.

References

1. Combe, I.A., Rudd, J.M., Leeflang, P.S., Greenley, G.E.: Antecedents to strategic flexibility: management cognition, firm resources and strategic options. Eur. J. Mark. **46**(10), 1320–1339 (2012)
2. Martin, W.B.: Quality Service: What Every Hospitality Manager Needs to Know. Prentice Hall, Upper Saddle River (2002)
3. Kumar, M., Kee, F.T., Manshor, A.T.: Determining the relative importance of critical factors in delivering service quality of banks: an application of dominance analysis in SERVQUAL model. Manag. Serv. Qual. Int. J. **19**(2), 211–228 (2009)
4. Lewis, B., Varey, R.: Internal Marketing: Directions for Management. Routledge, London (2012)

5. Kuo, C.M.M.: Service attitude is crucial element to the successful tourism and hospitality industries. J. Tour. Hosp. **2**(2), e127 (2013)
6. World Travel & Tourism Council: Travel & tourism: Economic impac. Tech. rep. Romania (2013)
7. Amin, M., Yahya, Z.: Service quality dimension and customer satisfaction: an empirical study in the malaysian hotel industry. Serv. Mark. Q. **34**(2), 115–125 (2013)
8. Miguens, J., Baggio, R., Costa, C.: Social media and tourism destinations: TripAdvisor case study. In: Advances in Tourism Research, vol. 26, no. 28 (2008)
9. Rai, A.K.: Customer Relationship Management: Concepts and Cases. PHI, New Delhi (2013)
10. Bowen, J.T., Chen, S.L.: The relationship between customer loyalty and customer satisfaction. Int. J. Contemp. Hosp. Manage. **13**(5), 213–217 (2001)
11. Pizam, A., Ellis, T.: Customer satisfaction and its measurement in hospitality enterprises null. Int. J. Contemp. Hosp. Manage. **11**(7), 326–339 (1999)
12. Blešić, I., Ivkov-Džigurski, A., Dragin, A., Ivanović, L., Pantelić, M.: Application of gap model in the researches of hotel services quality. Turizam **15**(1), 40–52 (2011)
13. Gundersen, M.G., Heide, M., Olsson, U.H.: Hotel guest satisfaction among business travelers: what are the important factors? Cornell Hotel Restaur. Adm. Q. **37**(2), 72–81 (1996)
14. Lockyer, T.: Business guests accommodation selection: the view from both sides null. Int. J. Contemp. Hosp. Manage. **14**(6), 294–300 (2002)
15. Teare, R., Olsen, M.D. (eds.): International Hospitality Management: Corporate Strategy in Practice. Financial Times Prentice Hall, London (1992)
16. Enz, C.A.: Hospitality Strategic Management: Concepts and Cases, 2nd edn. Wiley, Hoboken (2009)
17. Marković, S.: Measuring service quality in the croatian hotel industry: a multivariate statistical analysis. Our Economy (Nase Gospodarstvo) **50**(1/2), 27–35 (2004)
18. Callan, R.J., Kyndt, G.: Business travellers' perception of service quality: a prefatory study of two european city centre hotels. Int. J. Tour. Res. **3**(4), 313–323 (2001)
19. LeBlanc, G., Nguyen, N.: An examination of the factors that signal hotel image to travellers. J. Vacat. Mark. **3**(1), 32–42 (1996)
20. Choi, T.Y., Chu, R.: Determinants of hotel guests satisfaction and repeat patronage in the Hong Kong hotel industry. Int. J. Hosp. Manage. **20**(3), 277–297 (2001)
21. Seth, N., Deshmukh, S.G., Vrat, P.: Service quality models: a review. Int. J. Qual. Reliab. Manage. **22**(9), 913–949 (2005)
22. Parasuraman, A., Zeithaml, V.A., Berry, L.L.: A conceptual model of service quality and its implications for future research. J. Mark. **49**(4), 41–50 (1985)
23. Naik, C.N.K., Gantasala, S.B., Prabhakar, G.V.: Service quality (servqual) and its effect on customer satisfaction in retailing: introduction measures of service quality. Eur. J. Soc. Sci. **16**(2), 231–243 (2010)
24. Ilyas, A., Nasir, H., Malik, M.R., Mirza, U.E., Munir, S., Sajid, A.: Assessing the service quality of Bank using SERVQUAL model. Interdisc. J. Contemp. Res. Bus. **4**(11), 390–400 (2013)
25. Al-Borie, H.M., Damanhouri, A.M.: Patients' satisfaction of service quality in Saudi hospitals: a SERVQUAL analysis. Int. J. Health Care Qual. Assur. **26**(1), 20–30 (2013)

26. Yousapronpaiboon, K.: SERVQUAL: measuring higher education service quality in Thailand. Procedia Soc. Behav. Sci. **116**, 1088–1095 (2014)
27. Grönroos, C.: Service Management and Marketing: A Customer Relationship Management Approach. Wiley, Chichester (2000)
28. Carman, J.M.: Consumer perceptions of service quality: an assessment of the SERVQUAL dimensions. J. Retail. **66**, 33–55 (1990)
29. Buttle, F.: SERVQUAL: review, critique, research agenda. Eur. J. Mark. **30**(1), 8–32 (1996)
30. Parasuraman, A., Zeithaml, V., Berry, L.: SERVQUAL: a multiple-item scale for measuring consumer perceptions of quality. J. Retail. **64**(1), 12–40 (1988)
31. Blešić, I., Ivkov-Džigurski, A., Stankov, U., Stamenkoviæ, I., Bradiæ, M.: Research of expected and perceived service quality in hotel management. Revista de turism - studii si cercetari in turism/J. Tour. Stud. Res. Tour. **11**(11), 6–14 (2011)
32. Sharma, H.: A service quality model applied on indian hotel industry to measure the level of customer satisfaction. Int. J. Sci. Res. **3**(3), 2319–7069 (2014)
33. Karunaratne, W.M.K.K., Jayawardena, L.N.a.C.: Assessment of customer satisfaction in a five star hotel - a case study (2010)
34. Mola, F., Jusoh, J.: Service quality in penang hotels: a gap score analysis. World Appl. Sci. J. **12**, 19–24 (2011)
35. Mauro, P.: The Effects of Corruption on Growth, Investment, and Government Expenditure. Tech. Repp. 96/98, International Monetary Fund (1996)
36. Papathanassis, A., Knolle, F.: Exploring the adoption and processing of online holiday reviews: a grounded theory approach. Tour. Manage. **32**(2), 215–224 (2011)
37. Gretzel, U., Yoo, K.H.: Use and impact of online travel reviews. In: OConnor, D.P., Hpken, D.W., Gretzel, D.U. (eds.) Information and Communication Technologies in Tourism 2008. Springer, Vienna (2008)
38. BrightLocal: Local Consumer Review Survey. BrightLocal (2015)
39. Lewis, D., Bridger, D.: The Soul of the New Consumer: Authenticity - What We Buy and Why in the New Economy. Nicholas Brealey Publishing, London/Boston (2001). rev upd edition
40. Xie, K.L., Chen, C., Wu, S.: Online consumer review factors affecting offline hotel popularity: evidence from tripadvisor. J. Travel Tour. Mark. **33**(2), 211–223 (2016)
41. Ye, Q., Law, R., Gu, B., Chen, W.: The influence of user-generated content on traveler behavior: an empirical investigation on the effects of e-word-of-mouth to hotel online bookings. Comput. Hum. Behav. **27**(2), 634–639 (2011)
42. Ayeh, J.K., Au, N., Law, R.: Do we believe in tripadvisor? examining credibility perceptions and online travelers attitude toward using user-generated content. J. Travel Res. **52**(4), 437–452 (2013)
43. Wilson, A., Murphy, H., Fierro, J.C.: Hospitality and travel the nature and implications of user-generated content. Cornell Hosp. Q. **53**(3), 220–228 (2012)
44. comScore: Media Metrix for TripAdvisor Sites Report. Tech. rep. (2015)
45. Pike, S.: Destination image analysisa review of 142 papers from 1973 to 2000. Tour. Manage. **23**(5), 541–549 (2002)
46. Luca, M.: User-Generated Content and Social Media. SSRN Scholarly Paper ID 2549198, Social Science Research Network, Rochester, NY (2015)
47. INE: ProTurismo. Tech. rep. (2014)
48. Pimenta, P.: Há um buzzá volta do Porto. PúBLICO (2014)
49. Pires, S.: Porto: o destino da moda faz multiplicar hotéis. OJE Digital (2015)

How Service Innovation Contributes to Co-Create Value in Service Networks

Maria Vincenza Ciasullo[✉], Francesco Polese, Orlando Troisi, and Luca Carrubbo

Department of Business Science - Management and Information System, University of Salerno,
Via Giovanni Paolo II, 132, 84084 Fisciano, SA, Italy
{mciasullo,fpolese,otroisi,lcarrubbo}@unisa.it

Abstract. The purpose of this paper is to investigate how service innovations (in a living lab context) contribute to co-create value in a service network. Exploratory research is developed using a qualitative approach and case study on mobility services in Bologna. Our findings reveal that the involved entities are able to recombine their existing resources and design a new value proposition based on the ICT solution. Theoretical and empirical research suggests that collaboration and participation in decision making are critical to service system reconfiguration. The study shows the importance of including insights from Service Science Management and Engineering and Design (SSMED) in the management of network theory. Moreover, the research paves the way for new perspectives on analysis of local governance issues based on value co-creation processes in the ICT service solution context. Using this perspective, service innovations in the overall management of public services view a city as a Smart Local Service System (SLSS), whose competitiveness depends on its ability to access and share common resources to create mutual value.

Keywords: Service Science Management and Engineering (SSME) · Living lab · Value co-creation · Service innovation

1 Introduction

Currently, cities are viewed as complex service systems. Urbanization is emblematic of Twenty-first century economic and social progress, which evidences that cities are engines of economic growth, as well as the *milieux* of research, innovation, participation, coexistence, culture and education. At the same time, cities create new problems, such as air pollution and traffic congestion. When considered as complex systems, cities are based on the involvement of multiple stakeholders and characterized by intense interdependence, competitiveness, shared and non-shared objectives and values and social and political complexity. In this sense, city-related problems are becoming intertwined. The complexity involved in such systems imposes the need to constantly interpret the emerging socio-economic dynamics (e.g., safety issues, traffic and immigration) on institutional governing bodies. At the same time, further research is needed to identify adequate governance mechanisms that are able to add value and create system viability to these key factors. Based on consensus and public and private actors' participation in

© Springer International Publishing Switzerland 2016
T. Borangiu et al. (Eds.): IESS 2016, LNBIP 247, pp. 170–183, 2016.
DOI: 10.1007/978-3-319-32689-4_13

decisions regarding issues of common interest, the transition from a transactional to a relational vision is characterized by a strategic importance. Agranoff and McGuire [1] state that the use of networks in public management is increasing; moreover, the value for the individual customer and network as a whole is created in co-operation with different network actors. Currently, most cities are involved in multiple networks with different purposes: strategy creation, resource exchange and promotion of specific projects based on ICTs innovation. Cities are also encouraged to relinquish old hierarchical service systems and configure new service systems characterized by innovative approaches; accordingly, new technologies offer interesting insights into a service oriented economy [2]. From the service science perspective, in this paper, we present a new service innovation mechanism in the context of a value network in which all involved entities are able to recombine existing resources to design a new value proposition based on ICTs solution. In the next section, we explore some important contributions on service science and service innovation. Then, we develop a case study in which we describe how the service innovation has been designed. Finally, we discuss the main findings and theoretical and managerial implications from this perspective.

2 Literature review

2.1 Service Systems

The attention given to the complexity of modern economies emerges from service management studies, which are centered on closely linked concepts, such as service, service systems and, more recently, complex service systems. The current literature has provided different and wide interpretations of service, underlining its multidimensional and more systemic nature. The literature on service systems has emphasized a systemic vision of service, aiming to develop a wider multidisciplinary knowledge of service management, engineering and design [3, 4]. According to Maglio and Spohrer [4], a service system is defined as "a configuration of people, technologies, organizations and shared information, able to create and deliver value to providers, users and other interested entities through service". This integration of needs, resources, informations and objectives among providers and users stimulates co-creation processes that dominate the developed economies of the world [5]. At the same time, every service system represents a service supplier and user, which is structured, according to its necessity, as a value chain, a value network, or a value system [6]. If the smallest service system centers on an individual as he or she interacts with others, then, the largest one comprises the entire global economy. The history of a service system can be defined as a sequence of interactions with other service systems in which service systems, through their decision makers, act as integrators of operant and operand resources [7], provided either from within an organization or through networks [8]. In service systems, interaction becomes the driver of value or the mean through which service systems develop a joint process of value creation [9]; hence, service systems can create competitive advantages and improve reticular relationships. Recently, researchers have highlighted the complexity surrounding service systems [10, 11]. As socio-technical systems, people are at the core of the organizational structure, which emphasizes the importance of the human aspect and uncertainty associated with service exchanges [5]. In this perspective, service systems are generally characterized by open and emergent interactions that may result in complex conditions [12]. Literature focuses on the modern, intelligent and smart-type service systems, with particular regard to those ones that are encouraged by the international progress of ICTs. In today's highly dynamic innovation landscape, literature calls for investigating and understanding the intersection of ICTs and service innovation [13, 14].

2.2 Service Innovation Through Networks

In corporate activities, the paradigm which considers the customer as an active part of the process, along with the development of ICTs, has promoted the democratization of value creation process and is considered the main enabler of innovation in a service context [15]. Moreover, the concept of "prosumer" highlights how the participation of consumers in operations, as well as in the development of innovative products and services, is becoming essential for the viability of any social and business organization. Recent paradigms, such as open innovation and open business models [16], Web 2.0 [17] and the Living Labs, currently viewed as user-driven open innovation ecosystems, are driving consumers toward more proactive and co-creative roles of users in the research and innovation processes. Referring to the digitization of progressive services, public service systems have begun to implement user-led innovation processes, particularly user-driven innovation in a value co-creation context. The focus is gradually shifting toward the search for service innovations with high technological content able to adapt supply to growing demand from citizens and businesses and to ensure productivity and social cohesion at the same high employment levels.

A living lab is a social environment in which consciously built indeterminate and uncontrollable dynamics of everyday life are accepted as part of an innovation allowing designers and users to co-produce new products and services. In this sense, a living lab is a platform that aggregates and involves all stakeholders (such as end-users, researchers, industrialists and policy makers) at the earliest stage of the innovation process, to test breakthrough concepts and their potential value for both society (citizens) and individual users that will lead to innovative developments. According to the living lab concept, the lab environment is introduced to the users and experiments are validated in the context of real life. Schaffers et al. [18] stress that networking is an integral part of the living lab model, which allows a focus on value generation and distribution in a network of cooperating partners, including customers and users. In the same way, Ramaswamy and Gouillart [19] state that network relationships are one of the main components of the co-creation principle. Network configurations are dynamic; therefore, potential changes over time that reflect the requirements of both the involved actors and the (social) context [20] are normal. Vargo and Lusch [21] agree that networks are complex and dynamic systems of actors. They also note that not only companies learn in dynamic and changing environments but that value co-creation takes place in what they call "service ecosystems" too. These systems are defined as "spontaneously sensing and responding spatial and temporal structure of largely loosely coupled, value-proposing social and economic actors interacting through institutions, technology and language to (1) co-produce service offerings, (2) engage in mutual service provision and (3) co-create value". Therefore, these ecosystems require adaptability and agility. Ecosystems are comparable to a living lab because they are continuously learning, evolving and adapting; in other words, they are able to reconfigure themselves to generate better innovative outcomes.

3 Research Methodology

In the City of Bologna study, we focus our attention on mobility services. Key questions are "how do complex service systems contribute to value co-creation?" and "how do ecosystems support service innovation?"

The exploratory research is developed by using a qualitative approach and a case study methodology [22].

The qualitative research methodology involves the following activities:

- The content analysis of documents produced during the focus groups and design/ planning tables;
- The data collection from interviews with project managers and mobility managers of Bologna City and Emilia Romagna Region;
- The secondary data collection from the Metropolitan Strategic Plan of Bologna (PSM) and reports completed by project managers during the SmartIP project implementation.

The primary sources of qualitative data comes from documents and design tables produced during the focus groups. Overall, these documents are analyzed to reflect the attitude of participants in value co-creation and how project managers have integrated the mobility service information and suggestions that emerge during meetings. Interviews help to acquire detailed knowledge of the involved processes and interactions. The interviews range from 1 to 3 h in length. All interviews are audio-recorded and transcribed. A semi-structured guide supports the interviewing process. Empirical data were collected at regular intervals over a ten-month period to capture the elements of change and development according to a longitudinal perspective. Data analysis provides a better understanding of the following elements:

- the nature of value co-creation process between Bologna City and its citizens;
- service innovation mechanisms of value co-creation;
- IT solutions generated to achieve innovative outcomes.

4 Case study

4.1 Background to the Case Study

Bologna represents a highly attractive area in terms of structural endowment for industrial, commercial and, above all, cultural (university) components, as well as national and international transport infrastructures. Changes induced by socio-economic transformations have complicated the issue of mobility. However, Bologna has not reacted or adjusted to the value of infrastructure and related mobility services in a timely manner. Thus, the outcome has been the difficulty in satisfying relevant needs through traditional public transport.

A survey (source: Metropolitan Strategic Plan) issued by the city of Bologna has measured the citizens' sentiments regarding their perceptions of the daily strengths and weaknesses of urban life. The most relevant issues relate to mobility services and the perceived quality of life. The results have highlighted the annoyance of citizens in terms of the effectiveness of the railway station; access to the historical center; parking difficulties; delays in public transport timetables; poor connections; a lack of bicycle lanes and shared means of travel; and safety and reliability conditions for pedestrians. These issues have resulted in a state of anxiety and discontent among the community, which is confirmed by the reported low level of satisfaction with living conditions; consequently, only 4.2 % of the respondents have indicated improvement in their quality of life over the last three years. Changes in behavioral dynamics by collective entities (e.g., citizens, individual, tourists and students), induced by emerging economic, social and cultural factors, have imposed a need to re-contextualize, through which conditions of harmony, empathy and dialogue within the reference context can be preserved, on government. In terms of mobility services, the local authority has initiated a cooperation process with citizens, as well as public and private partners, to find common solutions for redesigning services and making them coherent with the context. This cooperation aims to improve the mobility system of management and monitoring and encourage alternative transport solutions that have a reduced environmental impact. Co-designing methods have been put in place for this purpose.

4.2 The Project SmartIP: Actors and Resources

The redesign of mobility services is placed in the context of the European project SmartIP - Smart Metropolitan Areas Realized Through Innovation and People. The five pilot cities are Manchester, Ghent, Cologne, Oulu and Bologna.

The project has been implemented in an interactive manner through dynamic interactions and cooperation among the following actors: mobility managers of Bologna and the Emilia Romagna Region, two companies specializing in the application of information technology in the field of mobility, police officers/traffic wardens, transport companies, individuals, citizens, local communities and research centers (e.g., Politecnico di Milano). A networked ecosystem has enabled the actors to share valuable resources in terms of knowledge and expertise to improve mobility in Bologna in terms of value co-creation [23]. In this context, it is important to highlight that the role of the actors is determined by their actions and based on openness and the common goals of the network. The network is coordinated by two project managers (employees working in Bologna and the Emilia Romagna Region) in their roles of enabler and orchestrator in terms of accomplishing new ways of dealing with the challenges from a mobility service innovation perspective; the role of providers is assumed by the research center that brings knowledge of user-centric methods for design; by the information technology companies, which are involved as providing service management; and by police officers/ traffic wardens, transport companies that bring their knowledge in terms of security, control and management mobility. Finally, individuals, citizens and local communities play a role as users. In particular, users are viewed as informants when they produce in-depth knowledge of most everyday life problems and needs in terms of opinions, experience and perceptions about the mobility services as a whole; they are co-creators and testers in the overall co-design process. Therefore, the reorganization of service mobility is influenced by the degree of intensity with which each actor participates in transforming and updating services based on their shared experiences. Living labs and social networks have enabled the network to co-design smart mobility solutions, while innovation has been achieved from a citizen/user driven approach.

4.3   The Process Involving Citizens

The citizens/individuals in their roles of users are directly involved in co-creating, exploring, experimenting and evaluating new ideas. In particular, these fundamental operant resources have contributed to the value co-creation process of the network as described in the following sections.

Identification of Needs. In this phase, information needs, relative to mobility service, are identified through a questionnaire and a CATI survey (computer-assisted telephone interviewing). The citizens of Bologna indicate their routine activities in terms of mobility - moving within the city, using technology, information services and public transport, accessing information channels and expressing their personal ideas for mobility services improvement. The CATI survey comprises interviews of 1,400 citizens, while the questionnaire is submitted to 10 online communities, two of a general nature that operate in the city (Tagbolab and Hyperbole) and eight that are related to mobility themes (Free to move, Along The Way, Bike Pride Bologna, Bologna pedestrian, bike in Bologna, La Consulta of the Bicycle, Gomypass, Open Bike). The analysis results highlight several gaps in terms of information related to existing mobility services.

In particular, citizens complain about the lack of detailed information (see Fig. 1) for their journeys on public transport (50 %), cycling themes (50 %), inter-modality (41 %) and shared transport (40 %). In terms of channels to access information on mobility (see Fig. 2), 85 % of the sample identifies the Internet as their preferred tool, followed by e-mail (47 %), information points (44 %) and mobile applications (42 %). Finally, the information tools that are considered most effective (see Fig. 3) in terms of timely information on mobility include: websites (64 %), geo-located maps (58 %), social networks (43 %) and e-mail (43 %). The information that is acquired focuses on citizen needs and highlights the malfunctioning scenarios affecting their daily lives.

Co-Design Applications. The co-design application phase is developed in living labs. The workshops are conducted during the months of March and September 2012 at the Bologna municipal seat. The workshops are used to encourage people to speak about a topic of personal interest. The main advantage is that the process of reflection by a group of people on a particular problem takes place in a synergistic environment, which enables project managers to collect opinions and ideas about innovative mobility services.

During the participants' interactions, ideas are exchanged, which have the potential to create an effect that enables them to develop new thoughts that cannot occur independent of the process.

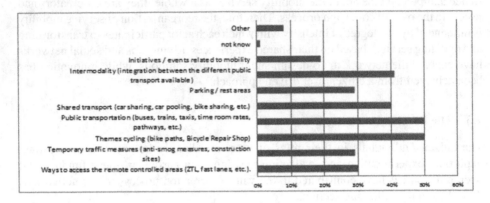

Fig. 1. Information requirements on mobility services (Source: Adapted by the authors from empirical data)

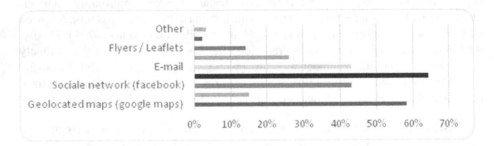

Fig. 2. Preferred information channels (Source: Adapted by the authors from empirical data)

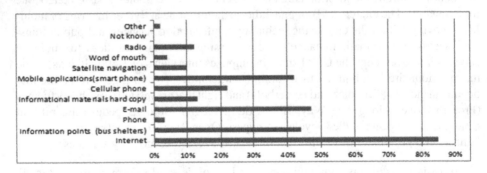

Fig. 3. Main tools for information on mobility choices (Source: Adapted by the authors from empirical data)

54 citizens and all of the actors that are involved in the network have participated in this phase. The phase envisions:

- an initial session in which project managers describe the state of the art of mobility in Bologna, paying particular attention to public transport: bus services, routes, etc.;
- a focus group during which participants take part in hour-long discussions about city's daily transport problems. The problems relating to public transportation (buses) comprise most of the meetings. At the end of each meeting, project managers invite participants to summarize three or four problems of greatest importance on an index card. The resulting information is crucial to understanding how new technologies can be incorporated into citizens'/individuals' daily routines:
- co-designing workshops, during which citizens are given the tools to make sense of their experiences and transform them into concrete issues. In particular, four discussion tables, each one with its own subject of debate: biking trails, shared media (e.g., car / bike sharing and carpooling), car parks, public transport (e.g., train and bus) are utilized. On each topic, participants are asked to provide 10 ideas for service reorganization. At the end of each meeting, a spokesman communicates the conclusions from each table to the project managers. The quality of information obtained during the meetings largely depends on the coordination and management of the project managers. Exalting the sense of belonging to a group, the informal meetings help to foster a climate of empathy and trust among people who share a common problem. The inclusive nature of the meetings stimulates citizens to become active participants, which results in the generation of new ideas in developing new mobility services. Co-creative efforts have produced 40 ideas around reorganizing service mobility, which have been subsequently transformed into several applications by IT service providers and presented in a public meeting. The IT service provider and mobility managers have collaborated to design a prototype and integrate many of the elements suggested by citizens.

Testing the Identified Solution. The experimental phase is conducted on two prototypes during the months of November and December 2012, involving:

- 54 beta-testers (individuals who are experts in the use of information technology) and 8 citizen testers and
- 79 employees of the Region of Emilia Romagna.
- The beta testers (users of smart phones and mobility services) commute daily for a week to use the prototype and provide feedback on
- general service design;
- effectiveness of prototype for everyday mobility using media (mobile, desktop, SMS);
- effectiveness of each service (SMS service, map, widget) in everyday routines; and
- -usability (icons, smooth navigation) in daily routines.

The services with the ability to satisfy the beta testers' need for mobile information (see Fig. 4) are bike paths (58 %) and information on traffic, parking and routes (33 %).

The 8 citizens who have tested the prototype using computer equipment (PC, Mobile, Tablet) report:

- use of service methods;
- differences in prototype usability, based on functional devices;
- improvements for existing services; and
- new service ideas.

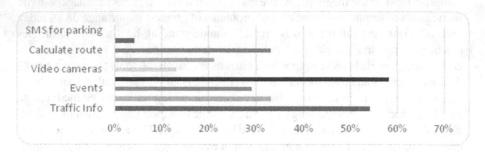

Fig. 4. Ratings that are provided by the beta testers on the utility of each service which is activated within the prototype (Source: Adapted by the authors from empirical data)

The overall feedback of 8 citizens regarding the prototype (see Fig. 5) is positive. They consider parking as the most efficient and complete service (42 %), followed by driving (29 %) and traffic (23 %).

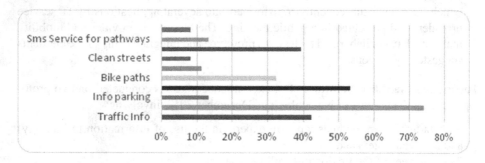

Fig. 5. Services that have the highest satisfaction among the eight citizens (Source: Adapted by the authors from empirical data)

The second test involves the employees of the Emilia Romagna Region, who are frequent users of public transport. Regarding the considered sample (see Fig. 6), the service info on buses is the most effective (74 %), followed by info on events (53 %) and traffic (42 %). The employees also provide information on margins for improvement of the prototype (see Fig. 7).

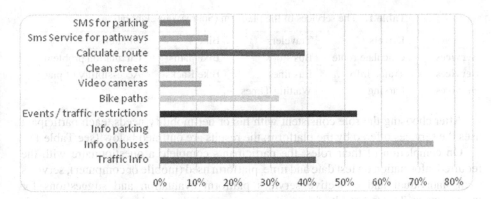

Fig. 6. Rating by Emilia Romagna employees (Source: Adapted by the authors from empirical data)

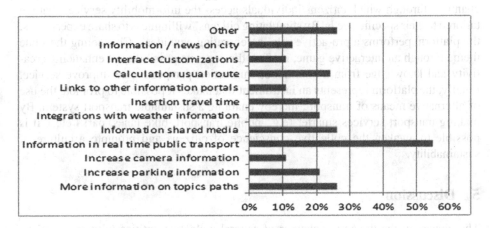

Fig. 7. Margin of Improvement (Source: Adapted by the authors from empirical data)

The testing phase is completed with the creation of a prototype consisting of 10 innovative mobile information services. In this phase, project managers and service providers, supported by several other actors, such as transport companies, policemen and the Politecnico di Milano, assume a central role.

Validation of Results. The result validation includes 250 citizens. Each participant is asked to play a part, which is outlined below and corresponds to a potential user of the platform:

- drivers (whoever drives, cars, motorcycles, vans, any motor);
- travelers (whoever travels on public transport);
- bikers (whoever uses bikes for travelling);
- "umarells" (citizens/individuals observing).

Table 1. The services of the platform (Source: our elaboration)

	Drivers	Travelers	Bikers	Umarells
Services	Calculate route	Bus stops	Bike paths	Circulation problems
Services	Traffic Info	Bus lines	Bike Racks	Accessibility of places
Services	Parking	Waiting Times		

After choosing the role consistent with his or her mobility needs, each participant uses the services offered by the platform; the results are outlined below (see Table 1):

On completion of their roles, the participants complete a questionnaire with the required information on test date and time, platform used (mobile or computer), services used, individual and collective services platform evaluation and suggestions for improvement. The end result of the entire process has led to the development and installation of "I move Smart", a highly innovative platform that is customized to the need of the citizens. The platform is configured as an aggregator of services and integrated channels, through which citizens/individuals access the info-mobility services that are tailored to their specific needs. By stimulating citizens' willingness to share experiences, the platform performs a pro-active role in generating new ideas. Channeling the same theme through an interactive game, it offers the concrete possibility of enhancing creativity and knowledge from a continuous innovation perspective to improve service. Finally, the platform represents an instrument that makes it possible to promote the use of alternative means of transport, thereby enabling a sustainable transport system. By making transport services smarter (e.g., public transport, bike lanes, parks etc.), it is possible to awaken the collective conscience of citizens and promote a culture of sustainability.

5   Discussion

The change in the dynamic behavior of several collective entities (citizens, tourists, students, etc.) of the city of Bologna have led to an emergence of new needs related to mobility service by requiring decision-makers to re-contextualize their decision making processes. From this perspective, using a win-win logic, the government has initiated cooperation with citizens, as well as public and private partners, to co-create solutions to redesign the services with the aim of improving the management and monitoring of the mobility system, as well as encouraging alternative transport solutions. Through living labs and social networks, it has been possible to design and implement customized service innovations that meet the needs of the citizens. All of the actors have been involved in a service experience capable of satisfying both their subjective and specific needs. The citizens, or customer systems, are involved in both the co-production of value (in terms of value proposition) and the co-creation of value (in terms of value in use). In this context, the role of information technology in service innovation is of particular interest because the intensity of the growing information services is transformed into value for users. Service providers can also benefit from the growing volume and speed of information while improving their own operations through the effective management of service related information. The efficiency of the internal structure has been pursued through the implementation of flexible service platform, which has led to a recovery of the effectiveness of a dynamic external environment in the municipality of Bologna. Flexibility in the technological and organizational environment has enhanced human creativity toward finding better solutions, which has stimulated ongoing interaction between technology design choices and organizational practices.

Our study yields highly detailed qualitative data, which are appropriate for exploration and theory building but which may limit the generalizability of our conclusions. In this respect, it is necessary to extend the study to other contexts.

6 Theoretical and Managerial Implications

From a theoretical perspective, our paper contributes to highlight the importance of the service science perspective. In fact, taking a service system view has enabled us to understand how service innovations are able to co-create value in a service network [24]. In particular, service innovation requires a service system reconfiguration in terms of the living lab, in which all of the actors involved create a new value proposition by accessing resources to the mutual benefit of all entities. From this perspective, rules are not formalized, rather, social interactions arise from networks, which are based on the operant and operand processes of ongoing access and sharing. The IT platform is based on a combination of multiple resources; in other words, it can be considered a collaborative technology that allows individuals to easily share their information and experiences. The platform offers new opportunities for the exchange of expertise between providers and users and between users and other members, which facilitates connections between people and the recombination of intra and inter organizational value propositions [6].

The service network proactively aims to uncover, understand and satisfy latent needs rather than to simply react to existing or currently expressed needs. In other words, the focus of a service system is not only on its entities but also on the interactions between these entities that use all of the available resources. The service science perspective may support the development of industrial research projects by enabling the access and the dynamic reconfiguration of resources, in particular, by guiding operant resources toward a shared goal.

In terms of managerial implications, the previously described process may support managers in identifying those specific actions and tools which are aimed at encouraging real and particular users' involvement in each phase of the process. Particularly in co-design, specific actions that facilitate the emergence of innovation from the traditional focus groups and workshops that have the latest storyboard can be used. For the city of Bologna, these instruments represent the winning cards to achieving citizens' involvement in co-design process. In co-delivery, the creation of intelligent platforms aims to promote citizens' inclusion in providing services to create a real information network among the various stakeholders (e.g., customers, providers and institutions), which accelerates the value of the processes used. Another managerial implication pertains not only to citizen relations management but also to the definition of differing degrees of involvement, which are possible thanks to the segmentation of preferences. In fact, public services managers should aim to enhance the delivery of emotional aspects, as well as work to offer vital core functional attributes, in line with the needs of today's consumer and the concept of experiential service. The involvement of citizens in the value creation process is also revealed in the sphere of political decision-making. In this context, the role that is played by local governance has to involve the establishment of visions and shared paths that are in line with stakeholder expectations. If this is true, the satisfaction of a public need is the result of a joint action by a network of specialized and interdependent actors that individually contribute to satisfying the need; it is also true that government action is expressed in the governance of complex system networks. Using such a logic, the government has to create and foster the development of conditions needed to enrich the culture of the territory as a whole in harmony with the socio-economic dynamics of the local community in which it is placed. In essence, the governance model has to encourage profitable interaction among the actors in the field while circulating ideas, initiatives and knowledge. Through ongoing involvement, the government cannot simply provide services; in terms of shared values, it has to respond, guide and stimulate society. In this context, service innovations for the overall management of public service systems (i.e., mobility; water; health; education; lighting; etc.) can conceptualize a city as a Smart Local Service System (SLSS), whose competitiveness depends on the ability to create mutual value by accessing and sharing common resources and in which partners' resources are orchestrated into a new value proposition, through a dynamic relationship, that incorporates the needs and expectations of users and is increasingly based on IT solutions.

References

1. Agranoff, R., McGuire, M.: Big questions in public network management research. J. Public Adm. Res. Theory 11(3), 295–32 (2001)
2. Maglio, P.P., Breidbach, C. F.: Service science: toward systematic service system innovation. In: Newman, A., Leung J., Smith, J.C., Catonsville, M.D.: INFORMS Tutorials Series, Bridging Data and Decisions, pp. 161-170 (2014)
3. Maglio, P.P., Srinivasan, S., Kreulen, J.T., Spohrer, J.: Service systems, service scientists, SSME and innovation. Commun. ACM 49(7), 81–85 (2006)
4. Maglio, P.P., Spohrer, J.: Fundamentals of service science. J. Acad. Mark Sci. 36(1), 18–20 (2008)
5. Qiu, R.G.: Computational thinking of service systems: dynamics and adaptiveness modeling. Service Science 1(1), 42–55 (2009)
6. Vargo, S., Maglio, P.P., Akaka, M.A.: On value and value co-creation: a service systems and service logic perspective. Eur. Manag. J. 26(3), 145–152 (2008)
7. Lusch, R.F., Vargo, S.L.: The Service-Dominant Logic of Marketing: Dialog, Debate, and Directions. Routledge, London (2014)
8. Spohrer, J., Anderson, L., Pass, N., Ager, T.: Service science and service dominant logic. Proc. Otago Forum 2, 4–18 (2008)
9. Polese, F.: The influence of networking culture and social relationships on value creation. Sinergie 16, 193–215 (2009)
10. Barile, S.: Towards qualification of the concept of systemic complexity. Sinergie rivista di studi e ricerche 79 (2011)

11. Miller, J.H., Page, S.E.: Complex Adaptive Systems: an Introduction to Computational Models of Social Life: an Introduction to Computational Models of Social Life. Princeton University Press, Princeton (2009)
12. Sawyer, R.K.: Social Emergence: Societies as Complex Systems. Cambridge University Press, Cambridge (2005)
13. Maglio, P.P., Breidbach, C.F.: Service Science: Toward Systematic Service System Innovation, Tutorials in Operations Research, pp. 161–170 (2014). http://pubsonline. informs.org/doi/book/10.1287/educ
14. Breidbach, C.F., Maglio, P.P.: A Service Science Perspective on the Role of ICT in Service Innovation. ECIS 2015 Research-in-Progress Papers. Paper 33 (2015)
15. Bitner, M.J., Zeithaml, V.A., Gremler, D.D.: Technology's impact on the gaps model of service quality. In: Maglio, P.P., Spohrer, J., Kieliszewski, C.A. (eds.) Handbook of Service Science, pp. 197–218. Springer, Berlin (2010)
16. Chesbrough, H.: Open Innovation. Harvard Business School Press, Boston (2003)
17. O'Reilly, T., Battelle, J.: Web squared Web 2.0 five years on. O'Reilly Media Inc, Newton (2009)
18. Schaffers, H., Cordoba, M. C., Hongisto, P., Kallai, T., Merz C., Van Rensburg, J.: Exploring Business Models for Open Innovation in Rural Living Labs. In: Proceedings of the 13th International Conference on Concurrent Enterprising (ICE). Sophia-Antipolis (2007)
19. Ramaswamy, V., Gouillart, F.: The Power of Co-Creation. Free Press, New York (2010)
20. Koch, C.: Innovation networking between stability and political dynamics. Technovation **24**(9), 729–739 (2003)
21. Vargo, S.F., Lusch, R.F.: It's all B2B…and beyond: toward a systems perspective of the market. Industrial Marketing Management **40**(2), 181–187 (2011)
22. Yin, R.K.: Case Study Research: Design and Methods. Sage Publications, Thousand Oaks (2003)
23. Tommasetti, A., Vesci, M., Troisi, O.: The internet of things and value co-creation in a service-dominant logic perspective. In: Colace, F., De Santo, M., Moscato, V., Picariello, A., Schreiber, F.A., Tanca, L. (eds.) Data Management in Pervasive Systems, pp. 3–18. Springer, Switzerland (2015)
24. Barile, S., Polese, F.: Linking the viable system and many-to-many network approaches to service-dominant logic and service science. Int. J. Qual. Serv. Sci. **2**(1), 23–42 (2010)

Service Design Methodologies
and Patterns

Needmining: Towards Analytical Support for Service Design

Niklas Kuehl[(✉)]

Karlsruhe Service Research Institute (KSRI),
Karlsruhe Institute of Technology (KIT), Englerstr. 11, 76131 Karlsruhe, Germany
kuehl@kit.edu

Abstract. The identification of customer needs is an important task for Service Design. The paper proposes an approach for automatically detecting customer needs from micro blog data (e.g. Twitter). It shows first results on identification models and lays the foundation for future research in this field.

Keywords: Service design · Need elicitation · Customer requirement analysis · Machine learning · Method evaluation

1 Introduction

Identifying the needs and demands of (potential) customers is an important task in order to design new market-driven services [1–3]. In the field of *Service Design* there are different methods on how to identify those needs. Typically used methods can be generally grouped into observations [4], surveys [5] or interviews [6], whether it is in the area of research [7] or in the industry [8]. Those methods are either time-consuming (if done by the researcher/ or employee) or cost-intensive (if outsourced). The proposed approach of this paper evaluates the alternative to use popular and available micro blog data (e.g. Twitter) as a source for identifying customer needs. This approach is called "Needmining". One of its advantages is the automatic aggregation of needs. These needs are expressed autonomously by the customer, for example in a moment of dissatisfaction or inconvenience with the underlying demand for a certain (service) solution. The goal is to generate a list of the most frequently expressed and most important needs posted by (potential) customers out of huge data sets (e.g. > 5 million tweets) for a certain topic. With this information white spots can be identified and service innovations can be developed. To achieve this goal the following research questions have to be answered:

1. **Identification of Micro Blog Instances containing Needs:** Is it possible to train a machine learning model to identify micro blog instances containing customer needs on an unseen test set with superior statistical performance?
2. **Identification and Quantification of Needs:** With those instances at hand—Is is possible to identify and/or quantify the needs themselves?

© Springer International Publishing Switzerland 2016
T. Borangiu et al. (Eds.): IESS 2016, LNBIP 247, pp. 187–200, 2016.
DOI: 10.1007/978-3-319-32689-4_14

3. **Approach Evaluation:** What are currently used methods in *Service Design* and related fields to identify and quantify customer needs and how well does the proposed approach of Needmining perform against them? In which case would which approach be preferable?

The central contribution of this research-in-progress paper is twofold: First, it proposes an approach to automatically identify customer needs with the advantages of being easily scalable and applicable to all domains with available micro blog data. Secondly, it delivers first results by showing how micro blog data instances containing needs can be identified and how a possible clustering could be conducted.

2   Related Work

Concerning the definition of *customer needs*, the state of the art definitions use the differentiation into *needs*, *wants* and *demands* [9–11]. Since there is little benefit in distinguishing between those terms for a first proof of concept study, for the sake of this paper the term need contains all three aspects (needs, wants and demands).

In general, the work is multidisciplinary, touching the disciplines of Service Science, Marketing, Statistical and Machine Learning. In terms of an overall research discipline it is highly related to Service Engineering [12], Service Design [4] and the development of new services and products (NSD/NSP, [13]). There are different approaches and pieces of literature on the topic of need identification in Service Design. Need elicitation and a good understanding of the customer in general are of high importance to companies [14]. First insights about measuring external customer needs and integrating them into the company's internal (quality) improvement was shown by Hermann et al. (2000) [2]. On the matter of analytical support for this process, Big Data is helpful with capturing customer needs [15]. Text Analysis is an important method in achieving this, often realized by analyzing customer reviews [16]. For those reviews, a Sentiment Analysis (also called Opinion Mining) allows to identify subjective opinions and aggregate them [17]. Needmining has similarities to such customer review analyses, the most relevant being Zhuo et al. (2015), who propose a new paradigm of customer needs elicitation based on Sentiment Analysis of online product reviews with a Machine Learning approach [18]. Needmining differs in some aspects, most notably by not regarding product review forums, but a large, not product specific micro blogging platform, which is important to cover a domain holistically.

In some cases, the process of need elicitation is very similar to the so-called *customer requirement elicitation*. Summarizing customer requirement management in general and focusing on requirement elicitation and analysis was shown in Jiao (2006) [19].

To the knowledge of the author, there is no publication on the topic of how to identify customer needs in micro blog data as a method of need elicitation in order to design new services. The most comparable approach would be the work of Misopoulus et al. (2014), who conducted a sentiment analysis with Twitter data in order to aggregate customer needs for the airline industry [20]. While this work also analyzes Twitter data, it uses sentiment analysis methods, whereas Needmining first uses Machine Learning models to identify if a tweet contains a need or not and then applies different approaches for clustering.

3   Research Design and Methodology

The following section explains the general methodology of this approach. As shown in Fig. 1, the first step is to retrieve relevant micro blog data and store it. To enhance the data, existing enrichment algorithms allow to predict personal data (like age or gender). In order to focus on relevant customer needs out of the micro blog data, data has to be pre-processed and then classified on whether or not it contains customer needs, elaborated in Sect. 3.1. With only data containing customer needs at hand, different approaches on how need identification and quantification can be realized is shown in Sect. 3.2. Apart from the process of the Needmining approach itself, it is important to evaluate it against existing methods of need elicitation, illustrated in Sect. 3.3.

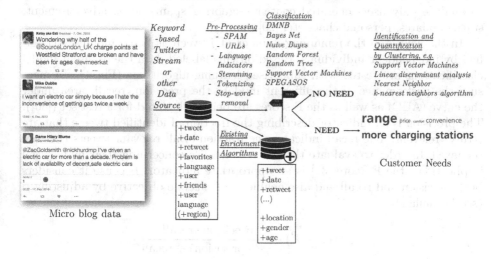

Fig. 1. General approach of Needmining for the exemplary domain of eMobility

3.1   Identification of Micro Blog Instances Containing Needs

Possible sources for user content on social media in general are the two major and mainly text-based social media networks Facebook and Twitter [21]. Only a minority of Facebook posts is publically available and most interactions occur in seperated communites and circles of friends [22]. Twitter is selected as a source of publicly available micro blog data since it is the largest and most popular micro blog service with over 500 million user messages per day [23]. To harvest Twitter for relevant micro blog instances (tweets), an appropriate ontology for the domain of interest has to be created or identified. This ontology will result in a list of suitable keywords and hashtags, which will be placed on a white list. It is important to note that some of the identified keywords might resemble features of already existing products—which might be desired, but has to be accounted for when interpreting the results at a later point in time. By using the Twitter Streaming API [24], the tool will record all available tweets which contain the keywords on the white list over a certain period of time (t). Other Twitter data sources can also be used. The tool will use existing enrichment algorithms to identify gender [25], age [26], location [27] and more in order to get approximations of the personalities who authored the tweets. This information will later be needed for drawing conclusions and rating their significance (e.g. regarding age, gender, income etc.).

After retrieving a total amount of n tweets, a random pick of k tweets is being analyzed by using a Descriptive Coding approach [28]. Each of the k tweets is manually coded by a team of researchers. Afterwards low correlations between all identified codes and the *need*-code are excluded in order to only consider relevant tweets in the following steps. By applying this identified rule set to the total number of n tweets, a data set of j tweets remains. This is necessary in order to analyze only user-generated content—ignoring spam, news, advertisement, status updates, personal chats etc. [29].

In the next step the remaining number of j tweets is being manually classified by independent individuals. Based on this labeled data the different model classifications are tested with supervised learning algorithms (Fig. 1). To measure the performance of the different models, the precision, recall, area under the curve (AUC) as well as the F-scores are being calculated for a test set ([30]). The precision is an indicator describing the fraction of identified tweets that are (truly) relevant. The recall indicates the fraction of all relevant tweets that are retrieved. In order to evaluate the different models concerning their managerial implications, the F-Score [31] is an appropriate indicator, because it considers both precision and recall and also enables to focus one objective by adjusting β (see Formula 1).

$$F_\beta = (1 + \beta^2) \cdot \frac{\text{precision} \cdot \text{recall}}{(\beta^2 \cdot \text{precision}) + \text{recall}} \tag{1}$$

As a result, tweets containing customer needs are being identified.

3.2   Identification and Quantification of Needs

By choosing an adequately trained model (even out of unseen data sets) only those tweets are regarded that contain customer needs. In this case it is made possible by choosing a model with a high precision and $F_{0.5}$-score—and therefore a high probability for a tweet containing a need. The next step is to identify and/or quantify the needs themselves. Table 1 shows a comparison of the different

Table 1. Comparison of different application possibilities once only tweets containing needs are aquired.

	Needs known	Needs unknown
Qualitative	Not applicable	*Detect unknown customer needs:* For example, a strategic manager can find out what needs are expressed in general in an unknown domain
Quantitative	*Quantify already known needs:* For example, an innovation manager can find out how many customers express which need in order to prioritize upcoming services or service improvements	*Detect and quantify (previously) unknown customer needs:* For example, the company can find out what needs are expressed by how many (potential) customers in order to prioritize new business areas

approaches and applications for the next steps by contrasting the knowledge of needs (known/unknown) with the expected result (qualitative/quantitative).

The first approach is to *quantify already known needs*. These needs might be either familiar because of the experience of a person (e.g. an innovation manager), by conducting a literature research or by applying other means of needs identification (see Sect. 3.3). With these needs at hand, there are two suggestions on how to quantify them by using the available data set:

- Out of the known needs, keyword-based white lists representing categories can be created and then occurrences of relevant keywords can be identified within the single tweets. In an aggregated list the occurrences can be presented to illustrate the quantity of each need. The performance of this method can be evaluated by manually assigning tweets to the identified categories and measuring the performance of the automated assignments with precision and recall. An advantage of this possibility is that it can easily be implemented. A disadvantage is that it depends heavily on the quality of the selection of the underlying keywords or ontology.
- The data set or a subset can be labeled by researchers to determine which tweets contain which specific needs. With the addition of these features (responses), supervised machine learning algorithms can be trained to identify the specifically addressed need. The advantage of this possibility is a higher reliability of the results since the model was evaluated (e.g. in terms of accuracy, precision and recall). A disadvantage is that the model is not flexible for additional needs at a later point in time as well as the necessity to label data beforehand.

A more complex and more contributing application is to *detect unknown customer needs*. There are two different suggestions on how to approach this challenge:

– First, the tweets containing needs are coded manually in a descriptive way to build semantically-meaningful clusters. Then unsupervised machine learning algorithms are applied to the data to cluster the tweets and compare the results of the different models with the human-based clustering. One challenge of this approach are missing performance indicators on how good a clustering is in terms of meaningfulness and content. Literature suggests evaluation criteria, which have to be checked for their suitability [32].
– Apply unsupervised learning algorithms to the tweets containing needs and evaluate the results in terms of semantic meaningfulness by experts in a workshop.

The most sophisticated application would be the combination of *detecting and quantifying (previously) unknown needs*. In order to achieve this, a combination of the previously proposed suggestions will be applied.

Depending on the chosen approach and its results, the customer needs are either identified and/or quantified, which is the final step of the proposed approach.

3.3   Approach Evaluation

To evaluate Needmining against existing methods, at first a systematic literature review based on Brocke et al. (2009) [33] is conducted in order to gain knowledge of a state of the art, interdisciplinary understanding of needs identification and quantification methods as well as possible comparison criteria. On the basis of these criteria the methods are compared and evaluated in the future. The goal is to gain an overview of the advantages and disadvantages of the individual methods as a baseline for Needmining to determine which approach is preferable depending on the conditions. A throughout literature review revealed ten different methods to identify and/or quantify customer needs from the fields of Product Design, Service Design and Marketing. Figure 2 shows those methods based on their usage in the design process. For the (mostly) qualitative identification of needs—needs elicitation—there are different methods available: *1-to-1 Interviews* are individual interviews with usually 10 to 30, in exceptional cases also a few hundred, (potential) customers [34]. In the *Lead User* method specific customers/users are selected, to whom a certain need is very important, which is usually not satisfied. Those users are then interviewed. In some cases those customers already started developing their own solutions, which might be of help [35]. A different approach are so-called *Focus Groups*, where up to twelve selected (potential or representative) customers discuss certain needs with a moderator [36]. While the first three mentioned approaches mostly aim at identifying needs known to the customer, *Empathic Design* is a set of techniques aiming at identifying needs either unknown to the customer or thought to be unsatisfiable [37].

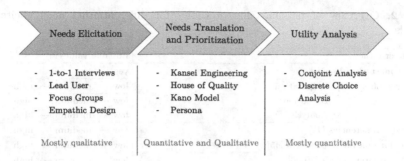

Fig. 2. Overview of existing methods for need identification and quantification

Concerning the translation and prioritization of needs, four different methods can be identified. *Kansei Engineering* deals with the translation of feelings and/or images of a product into the design process to directly address (emotional) needs of a customer. It offers a complete tool set to implement this approach for a specific problem [38]. The *House of Quality* is part of the Quality Function Deployment (QFD) and confronts the customer needs with the company's capabilities to account for the "Voice of the Customer" [39]. The *Kano Model* differentiates customer needs into three fundamental categories (exciters, satisfiers, dissatisfiers) and aims at helping companies to prioritize those aspects that are noticed by the customer [40]. The *Persona* method suggests creating a fictional "persona" to represent a typical customer segment with typical customer needs to simulate possible solutions for this persona [41].

Regarding the—mostly quantitative—utility analysis the two methods of *Conjoint Analysis* and *Discrete Choice Analysis* can be identified. The central question of the Conjoint Analysis is why a customer chooses one product or brand over another product or brand [42]. While the Conjoint Analysis focuses on comparable attributes of an offering, Discrete Choice also considers offerings that are not simply comparable by specific attributes [43]. Concerning the comparison and evaluation of the different mentioned methods and the Needmining approach, possible criteria are shown in Table 2. These criteria reflect the current status of the literature review and may be refined in the future. The combination of the different methods with the criteria results in an evaluation framework. To perform the evaluation and comparison, experts will be invited to discuss the values for each method as part of future research.

4   First Results

By applying the methodology in a first proof of concept study, the following results are achieved and described as part of ongoing research. While the classification of tweets containing needs is already completed (see Kuehl et al. (2016) [48,49]) and is briefly summarized, the identification and quantification of needs themselves are still research in progress and show preliminary findings. As a

Table 2. Overview of possible characteristics for differentiating need elicitation methods

Possible criteria		Possible values
Product must already exist		yes — no
Expense / Effort [34]	Preparation	low — medium — high
	Execution	low — medium — high
	Analysis	low — medium — high
Required competencies [44]		low — medium — high
Suitable for innovative products [45]		low — medium — high
Suitable for latent needs [39,46]		low — medium — high
Findings transferable to target group [47]		low — medium — high
Activity of participant [44]		active — passive
Increase of expenses with increasing number of participants [34]		below proportional — proportional — disproportional

domain of application for the study, the field of electric mobility (e-mobility) is selected. E-mobility is defined as "*a highly connective industry which focuses on serving mobility needs under the aspect of sustainability with a vehicle using a portable energy source and an electric drive that can vary in the degree of electrification.*" ([50, p. 25]) As one outcome of recent studies on the acceptance of e-mobility [51,52] the relevancy of innovative e-mobility services as means to further foster the acceptance of e-mobility in society is getting more and more obvious among industry and science. The necessity of offering complementary mobility services (as proposed in [53,54]) however, is a relatively new branch of research. In order to create new innovative services for e-mobility it is therefore important to gain knowledge about the customers needs first. To narrow down the geographic area, only the German market will be regarded in the first study.

Identification of Micro Blog Instances Containing Needs. At first, a workshop with e-mobility experts is conducted to generate a keyword list of 23 terms for the tweet streaming. A tool for saving all relevant tweets based on the Twitter Streaming API, which allows to capture all relevant tweets for a set of keywords—as long as there are less than 400 keywords and the fetched data does not exceed more that 1 % of all tweets [55])—is implemented and runs for six months in 2015. With the addition of more tweets from before 2015 by using IBM Insights for Twitter, a data set of $n = 645,226$ tweets is acquired. Out of a random pick of this data ($k = 200$), two independent researchers apply descriptive codes. Code-correlations are analyzed and as a result tweets containing a URL are excluded for future processing because of the low correlation of "URL" with "need" (3.64 %). After excluding duplicates, non-German tweets and tweets containing URLs, $j = 2,396$ relevant tweets are left for the machine learning model training. The remaining tweets are labeled for their feature of containing a need or not by 35 (paid) individuals. Each tweet is being labeled three times independently to minimize errors and subjectiveness. As a basis for the classification algorithms, only tweets with consensus are regarded

(1928, excluding 468). The tweets are stemmed, tokenized and stop-words are removed. Since the data set is imbalanced and only 17.21 % of the tweets contain customer needs, different sampling techniques (Undersampling, Oversampling, SMOTE [56]) may be applied for the training set. These are then combined with the following classification algorithms: Discriminative Multinomial Naive Bayes (DMNB) [57], Bayes Net [58], Naive Bayes [59], Random Forests [60], Random Trees [60], Support Vector Machines [61] and SPEGASOS: Stochastic variant of Pegasos (Primal Estimated sub- GrAdient SOlver for SVM) [62]. More details on the classification are elaborated in Kuehl et al. (2016) [49].

The best overall performance in detecting tweets containing needs as a compromise between precision and recall (F_β-score with $\beta = 1$) is achieved by a model combining undersampling and SPEGASOS with $F_1 = 0.466$. The precision of identifying a need is 42 %, the recall (over all tweets containing needs) is 52.4 % with an AUC of 0.687. If the emphasis is on a higher precision—meaning that the probability of identifying a tweet as containing need, although it does not (false positives) decreases ($\beta = 0.5$)—the combination of no sampling with SVM delivers the best result with $F_{0.5} = 0.522$, a precision of 68.5 %, a recall of 26.8 % and an AUC of 0.621. If the aim is to achieve the highest precision possible with disregarding the recall, the best performing model is a combination of no sampling and Random Forests, achieving a remarkable precision of 93.3 % with a poor recall of 4.2 % and an AUC of 0.739. Depending on the intention of the person applying these models, one can be selected. While these results show that an identification of needs within tweets is possible in general, the models still lack either precision or recall [49]. Future research will focus on improving those models, for example by using different pre-processing techniques (eg. n-grams) or different algorithms (eg. neural networks). The implementation and evaluation of enrichment algorithms as mentioned in Sect. 3.1 is part of future research.

Identification and Quantification of Needs. Going forward, it is required to select a model with highest possible precision. The following sections assume that such a model could be trained and applied to large, unseen data sets to identify tweets containing needs in order to then detect and quantify the needs themselves.

As a first proof of concept, major needs in the field of e-mobility are identified from recent literature to approach the first quadrant of Table 1 (needs known/quantitative). Four major categories of needs could be identified: *Cost-related, car-related, charging-related* and *social-related* needs. By generating four disjunctive white lists containing stemmed key words with terms from the previous literature review, a foundation for the need quantification in the data is laid. From the previous data set (2,396 relevant tweets) only those tweets are selected which were labeled as expressing a need (332 relevant tweets). The need-containing tweets are then labeled again to be assigned to one of the four major categories or "other" as a test set for the white list-based classification. A first calculation shows that based on the (rather simple) white lists, a high precision in the categories cost (82.8 %) and charging (95 %) can be achieved

Table 3. Precision, Recall and Accuracy of first classification attempt based on need white lists

	Cost	Car	Charging	Social	Other
Recall	0.483	0.131	0.705	0.448	0.891
Precision	0.828	0.5	0.95	0.722	0.256
Accuracy	0.888	0.816	0.837	0.936	0.626

(Table 3). The recall is unsteady between poor 13.1 % (car-related needs) and solid 70.5 % (charging-related needs). As of now, these are only first prototypical attempts of identifying and/or quantifying needs themselves in the data. Nonetheless, the results show that cost-related and charging-related needs can already be identified precisely out of the tweets—and therefore, even this simple model can be used to quantify needs for the two mentioned categories. Future research will apply more elaborate ways of quantifying known needs in the data. To achieve this, more sophisticated white lists can be created automatically by harvesting synonym/similarity APIs and compare the results for improvements. Additionally, other clustering approaches will be tested on their performance as mentioned in Sect. 3.2.

5 Conclusion and Outlook

In conclusion, the described approach called Needmining could be a valuable alternative to established need identification methods. It allows the identification of customer needs for a topic of interest, represented (preferably) by an ontology or a list of keywords to start with. It considers already available (micro blog) data and classifies this data with the application of supervised learning algorithms. The relevant data sets are then used to either quantify already known needs or identify new ones as well as the combination of both. Needmining has the advantage of looking at data that customers willingly expressed and therefore having a high value to innovation managers and potential businesses. After the successful analysis of customer needs in the field of e-mobility, identified customer needs can be satisfied by creating according business models and the acceptance of electric vehicles can be increased.

It was shown that it is possible to identify tweets containing needs with different models—the choice of the model however depends on the scope: If the focus is to only regard tweets with a very high probability of being a need, a model with high precision can be selected. This results in a lower recall, meaning only a fraction of the tweets containing a need is shown. Concerning the identification and quantification of needs as well as the evaluation, first elaborations are shown, but are mostly subject to future work.

The approach has limitations since it only regards customer needs expressed by Twitter users. Nonetheless, by applying enrichment algorithms to determine personalities, gender, age etc. conclusions concerning the representativeness can be drawn. Another limitation is that the approach is tested for a specific domain (e-mobility) and it has to be checked which of the mentioned steps can be directly applied to a different domain (e.g. health care).

The managerial implications are, however, already remarkable. The approach is at this stage able to detect tweets containing needs (in e-mobility) and can help to gain a better understanding of (potential) customers. The next steps are to do further work on tuning the need-tweet-detection models for delivering better performances as well as evaluating different approaches for identifying and quantifying the needs themselves—without having to look at the tweets. Additionally, it would be of interest to collect data of the same domain with different keywords and compare the results. Other areas of work are the application to a different domain of interest as well as the evaluation of this method compared to already established methods of need identification and quantification. A promising field of research lies ahead.

Acknowledgments. The author would like to thank Lisa Schmittecker for her support in the field of need elicitation, Jan Scheurenbrand for his support in implementing the Needmining tool, Marc Goutier for his support with first clustering attempts as well as Gerhard Satzger for his general support.

References

1. Goldstein, S.M., Johnston, R., Duffy, J., Rao, J.: The service concept: the missing link in service design research? J. Oper. Manage. **20**(2), 121–134 (2002)
2. Herrmann, A., Huber, F., Braunstein, C.: Market-driven product and service design: bridging the gap between customer needs, quality management, and customer satisfaction. Int. J. Prod. Econ. **66**(1), 77–96 (2000)
3. Teare, R.E.: Interpreting and responding to customer needs. J. Workplace Learn. **10**(2), 76–94 (1998)
4. Brown, T., et al.: Design thinking. Harvard Bus. Rev. **86**(6), 84 (2008)
5. Victorino, L., Verma, R., Plaschka, G., Dev, C.: Service innovation and customer choices in the hospitality industry. Managing Serv. Qual.: Int. J. **15**(6), 555–576 (2005)
6. Reynolds, T.J., Gutman, J.: Laddering theory, method, analysis, and interpretation. J. Advertising Res. **28**(1), 11–31 (1988)
7. Driscoll, D.L.: Introduction to primary research: observations, surveys, and interviews. Writ. Spaces: Read. Writ. **2**, 153–174 (2011)
8. Kärkkäinen, H., Elfvengren, K.: Role of careful customer need assessment in product innovation management? empirical analysis. Int. J. Prod. Econ. **80**(1), 85–103 (2002)
9. Line, M.B.: Draft definitions: information and library needs, wants, demands and uses. In: Aslib Proceedings, vol. 26, p. 87. MCB UP Ltd (1974)
10. Arndt, J.: How broad should the marketing concept be? J. Mark. **42**(1), 101–103 (1978)
11. Armstrong, G., Adam, S., Denize, S., Kotler, P.: Principles of Marketing. Pearson Australia, Sydney (2014)
12. Bullinger, H.J., Scheer, A.W.: Service engineering - Entwicklung und Gestaltung innovativer Dienstleistungen. Springer, Heidelberg (2006)

13. Cowell, D.W.: New service development. J. Mark. Manage. **3**(3), 296–312 (1988)
14. Dieste, O., Juristo, N., Shull, F.: Understanding the customer: what do we know about requirements elicitation? IEEE Softw. **25**(2), 11–13 (2008)
15. van Horn, D., Olewnik, A., Lewis, K.: Design analytics: capturing, understanding, and meeting customer needs using big data. In: Proceedings of the ASME 2012 International Design Engineering Technical Conferences and Computers and Information in Engineering Conference, pp. 1–13 (2012)
16. Hu, M., Liu, B.: Mining and summarizing customer reviews. In: Proceedings of the Tenth ACM SIGKDD International Conference on Knowledge Discovery and Data Mining, pp. 168–177. ACM (2004)
17. Pang, B., Lee, L.: Opinion mining and sentiment analysis. Found. Trends Inf. Retrieval **2**(1–2), 1–135 (2008)
18. Zhou, F., Jiao, R.: Latent customer needs elicitation for big-data analysis of online product reviews. In: 2015 IEEE International Conference on Industrial Engineering and Engineering Management (IEEM), pp. 1850–1854. IEEE (2015)
19. Jiao, J.R., Chen, C.H.: Customer requirement management in product development: a review of research issues. Concurrent Eng. **14**(3), 173–185 (2006)
20. Misopoulos, F., Mitic, M., Kapoulas, A., Karapiperis, C.: Uncovering customer service experiences with twitter: the case of airline industry. Manage. Decis. **52**(4), 705–723 (2014)
21. Statista.com: Leading social networks worldwide as of January 2016, ranked by number of active users (in millions). www.statista.com/statistics/272014/global-social-networks-ranked-by-number-of-users/. Last Accessed on 16 February 2016
22. Wilson, R.E., Gosling, S.D., Graham, L.T.: A review of facebook research in the social sciences. Perspect. Psychol. Sci. **7**(3), 203–220 (2012)
23. Twitter: About the company. https://about.twitter.com/company. Last Accessed on 15 December 2015
24. Bifet, A., Frank, E.: Sentiment knowledge discovery in twitter streaming data. In: Pfahringer, B., Holmes, G., Hoffmann, A. (eds.) DS 2010. LNCS, vol. 6332, pp. 1–15. Springer, Heidelberg (2010)
25. Miller, Z., Dickinson, B., Hu, W.: Gender prediction on twitter using stream algorithms with n-gram character features. Int. J. Intell. Sci. **2**(4A), 143–148 (2012)
26. Nguyen, D., Smith, N.A., Rosé, C.P.: Author age prediction from text using linear regression. In: Proceedings of the 5th ACL-HLT Workshop on Language Technology for Cultural Heritage, Social Sciences, and Humanities, pp. 115–123. LaTeCH 2011, Association for Computational Linguistics, Stroudsburg (2011)
27. Compton, R., Jurgens, D., Allen, D.: Geotagging one hundred million twitter accounts with total variation minimization. In: 2014 IEEE International Conference on Big Data (Big Data), pp. 393–401. IEEE (2014)
28. Saldaña, J.: The Coding Manual for Qualitative Researchers. Sage, London (2012)
29. Egger, M., Lang, A., Schoder, D.: Who are we listening to? detecting user-generated content (ugc) on the web. In: ECIS 2015 Proceedings (2015)
30. Hastie, T., Tibshirani, R., Friedman, J., Franklin, J.: The elements of statistical learning: data mining, inference and prediction. Math. Intelligencer **27**(2), 83–85 (2005)
31. van Rijsbergen, C.J.: Information Retrieval, 2nd edn. Butterworths, London (1979)
32. Halkidi, M., Batistakis, Y., Vazirgiannis, M.: Clustering algorithms and validity measures. In: Thirteenth International Conference on Scientific and Statistical Database Management, SSDBM 2001. Proceedings, pp. 3–22. IEEE (2001)

33. Brocke, V., Simons, A., Niehaves, B., Riemer, K., Plattfaut, R., Cleven, A.: Reconstructing the giant: on the importance of rigour in documenting the literature search process. In: Proceedings of the 17th European Conference On Information Systems, Verona, pp. 2206–2217 (2009)
34. Griffin, A., Hauser, J.R.: The voice of the customer. Mark. Sci. **12**(1), 1–27 (1993)
35. Von Hippel, E.: Lead users: a source of novel product concepts. Manage. Sci. **32**(7), 791–805 (1986)
36. Töpfer, A., Silbermann, S.: Einsatz von kunden-fokusgruppen. In: Handbuch Kundenmanagement, pp. 267–279. Springer (2008)
37. Leonard, D., Rayport, J.F.: Spark innovation through empathic design. Harvard Bus. Rev. **75**, 102–115 (1997)
38. Nagamachi, M.: Kansei engineering: a new ergonomic consumer-oriented technology for product development. Int. J. Ind. Ergonomics **15**(1), 3–11 (1995)
39. Herstatt, C., Verworn, B.: Management der frühen Innovationsphasen. Springer (2007)
40. Sauerwein, E., Bailom, F., Matzler, K., Hinterhuber, H.H.: The kano model: how to delight your customers. In: International Working Seminar on Production Economics, vol. 1, pp. 313–327. Innsbruck (1996)
41. Pirola, F., Pezzotta, G., Andreini, D., Galmozzi, C., Savoia, A., Pinto, R.: Understanding customer needs to engineer product-service systems. Advances in Production Management Systems. Innovative and Knowledge-Based Production Management in a Global-Local World. IFIP Advances in Information and Communication Technology, vol. 439, pp. 683–690. Springer, Heidelberg (2014)
42. Green, P.E., Krieger, A.M., Wind, Y.: Thirty years of conjoint analysis: reflections and prospects. Interfaces **31**(3-supplement), S56–S73 (2001)
43. Polaine, A., Løvlie, L., Reason, B.: Service Design. From Implementation to Practice. Reosenfeld Media, New York (2013)
44. Edvardsson, B., Kristensson, P., Magnusson, P., Sundström, E.: Customer integration within service development a review of methods and an analysis of insitu and exsitu contributions. Technovation **32**(7), 419–429 (2012)
45. Cooper, R.G., Kleinschmidt, E.J.: Success factors in product innovation. Ind. Mark. Manage. **16**(3), 215–223 (1987)
46. Hanski, J., Reunanen, M., Kunttu, S., Karppi, E., Lintala, M., Nieminen, H.: Customer observation as a source of latent customer needs and radical new ideas for product-service systems. In: Engineering Asset Management 2011, pp. 395–407. Springer (2014)
47. Bryman, A., Bell, E.: Business Research Methods. Oxford University Press, USA (2015)
48. Kuehl, N., Scheurenbrand, J., Satzger, G.: "needs from tweets": towards deriving customer needs from micro blog data. Multikonferenz Wirtschaftsinformatik (MKWI) 2016 (2016)
49. Kuehl, N., Scheurenbrand, J., Satzger, G.: Needmining: identifying customer needs in micro blog data: karlsruhe Institute of Technology. Karlsruhe Service Research Institute, Discussion Paper (2015)
50. Scheurenbrand, J., Engel, C., Peters, F., Kuehl, N.: Holistically defining e-Mobility: a modern approach to systematic literature reviews. In: 5th Karlsruhe Service Summit, Karlsruhe, Germany, pp. 17–27 (2015)
51. Pfahl, S., Jochem, P., Fichtner, W.: When will electric vehicles capture the german market? and why?. In: Electric Vehicle Symposium and Exhibition (EVS27), 2013 World, pp. 1–12. IEEE (2013)

52. Sierzchula, W., Bakker, S., Maat, K., Van Wee, B.: The influence of financial incentives and other socio-economic factors on electric vehicle adoption. Energy Policy **68**, 183–194 (2014)

53. Stryja, C., Fromm, H., Ried, S., Jochem, P., Fichtner, W.: On the necessity and nature of e-mobility services? towards a service description framework. Exploring Services Science. Lecture Notes in Business Information Processing, vol. 201, pp. 109–122. Springer International Publishing, Switzerland (2015)

54. Hinz, O., Schlereth, C., Zhou, W.: Fostering the adoption of electric vehicles by providing complementary mobility services: a two-step approach using best-worst scaling and dual response. J. Bus. Econ. **85**(8), 921–951 (2015)

55. Twitter: Twitter   streaming   api.   https://twittercommunity.com/t/best-solution-for-fetching-tweets-mentioning-hundreds-of-terms/28294.   Accessed on 18 December 2015

56. Chawla, N.V., Bowyer, K.W., Hall, L.O., Kegelmeyer, W.P.: SMOTE: synthetic minority over-sampling technique. J. Artif. Intell. Res. **16**, 321–357 (2002)

57. Su, J., Zhang, H., Ling, C.X., Matwin, S.: Discriminative parameter learning for bayesian networks. In: Proceedings of the 25th International Conference on Machine Learning, ICML 2008, NY, USA, pp. 1016–1023. ACM, New York (2008)

58. Cooper, G., Herskovits, E.: A Bayesian method for constructing Bayesian belief networks from databases. In: Proceedings of the Conference on Uncertainty in AI, pp. 86–94 (1990)

59. John, G.H., Langley, P.: Estimating continuous distributions in bayesian classifiers. In: Proceedings of the Eleventh Conference on Uncertainty in Artificial Intelligence, pp. 338–345 (1995)

60. Breiman, L.: Random Forrest. Mach. Learn. **45**(1), 5–32 (2001)

61. Platt, J.C.: Fast Training of Support Vector Machines Using Sequential Minimal Optimization. Advances in kernel methods, pp. 185–208. MIT Press, Cambridge (1998)

62. Shalev-Shwartz, S., Srebro, Y.S., N.: Pegasos: primal estimated sub-grAdient sOlver for SVM. In: 24th International Conference on Machine Learning, pp. 807–814 (2007)

An Efficient Procedure to Determine the Initial Basic Feasible Solution of Time Minimization Transportation Problem

Aminur Rahman Khan[1,2(✉)], Adrian Vilcu[2], Md. Sharif Uddin[1], and Cristiana Istrate[2]

[1] Department of Mathematics, Jahangirnagar University, Dhaka, Bangladesh
aminurju@yahoo.com, msharifju@yahoo.com
[2] Department of Management Engineering, "Gheorghe Asachi" Technical Universsity of Iasi, Iasi, Romania
adrian_vilcu@yahoo.com, cristianagr@yahoo.com

Abstract. To meet the challenge of delivering products to the customers in a minimum time, Time Minimization Transportation Problem (TMTP) provides a powerful framework to determine the better ways to deliver products to the customer. In this paper, we present a new procedure for determining an initial basic feasible solution of TMTP. Comparative study is accomplished between the presented procedure and the other existing procedures in virtue of sample examples which demonstrate that the presented procedure requires less number of iterations to reach the optimal transportation time.

Keywords: Time minimization transportation problem · Feasible solution · Pointer cost · Optimum solution

1 Introduction

Transportation problem (TP), one of the simplest combinatorial problems in Operations Research, deals with the circumstance in which a single identical vendible is transported from a number of sources to a number of destinations in such a way so that the total transportation cost is minimized while fulfilling all supply and demand limitations. The basic TP was originally developed by Hitchcock [1]. Efficient methods of solution derived from the simplex algorithm were flourished, primarily by Dantzig [2] and then by Charnes *et al.* [3]. This type of problem is known as cost minimizing TP, which has been deliberated since long and is famous by many researchers [4–26].

Again, the process of transporting exigent material, such as weapons used in military operations, salvage equipments, equipments used for dealing with emergency, people or medical treatment things and the fresh food with short storage period, where the speed of delivery is more important than the transportation cost, is known as TMTP. This problem was first addressed by Hammer [27]. An initial basic feasible solution for minimizing the time of transportation can be obtained by using any existing methods such as, North West Corner Method (NWCM) [11], Least Cost Method (LCM) [11], Vogel's Approximation Method (VAM) [11], Extremum

© Springer International Publishing Switzerland 2016
T. Borangiu et al. (Eds.): IESS 2016, LNBIP 247, pp. 201–212, 2016.
DOI: 10.1007/978-3-319-32689-4_15

Difference Method (EDM) [12], Highest Cost Difference Method (HCDM) [5, 6] and Average Cost Method (ACM) [4]. Extensive work has also been done on TMTPs by several researchers [17, 28–34]. They introduced various algorithms for solving TMTPs. Garfinkel and Rao [29] solved time minimization transportation problems. Hammer [27] and Szwarc [34] used labeling techniques to solve such kind of problems respectively. Ilijia Nikolic [30] presented an algorithm to minimize the total transportation time to TMTPs. Md. Main Uddin *et al.* [32] reduced the total transportation cost on the basis of time using VAM, M Sharif Uddin [31] used the HCDM whereas Mollah Mesbahuddin Ahmed used HCDM [17, 33] on Modified Transportation Cost Matrix (MTCM) to minimize the transportation time. Very recently Mollah Mesbahuddin Ahmed also introduced Allocation Table Method (ATM) [19] to do the same.

In this paper, we define and calculate the pointer cost by subtracting the time units of every cell of total opportunity time matrix from the sum of respective row and column highest and allocate to the cell corresponding to the maximum pointer cost. Finally we use the optimality test of time minimizing transportation problem.

2 Formulation of Time Minimization Transportation Problem

A general time minimization transportation problem is represented by the network in the following Fig. 1.

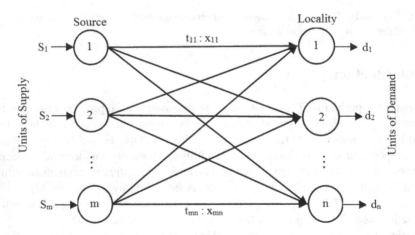

Fig. 1. Network representation of time minimization transportation problem

There are m sources and n destinations, each represented by a node. The arrows joining the sources and the localities represent the route through which the single identical vendible is transported. Suppose S_i is the availability of the same at ith ($i = 1$, $2, \ldots \ldots, m$) source, d_j is the availability of the same at jth ($j = 1, 2, \ldots \ldots, n$) destination, t_{ij} denotes the unit transportation time from ith source to jth destination, x_{ij}

represents the amount is transported from ith source to jth destination. Then the LPP model of the balanced time minimization transportation problem is:

Minimize: Max $t_{ij} \mid x_{ij} > 0$

$$\text{s/t,} \sum_{j=1}^{n} x_{ij} = s_i \quad i = 1, 2, \ldots\ldots, m$$

$$\sum_{i=1}^{m} x_{ij} = d_j \quad j = 1, 2, \ldots\ldots, n \tag{1}$$

$$x_{ij} \geq 0 \text{ for all } i, j.$$

3 Algorithm of Presented Method

The proposed algorithm for determining initial basic feasible solution consists of the following steps:

Step 1: Choose the smallest entry of every row and subtract it from each elements of the corresponding row of the TMTP and put them on the right-top of the corresponding elements.

$$t_{ij}^{t_{ij} - t_{ik}}, \text{ where } t_{ik} = \min(t_{i1}, t_{i2}, \ldots\ldots, t_{in})$$

$$i = 1, 2, \ldots\ldots, m$$

Step 2: Apply the same process on each of the columns and put them on the left-bottom of the corresponding elements.

$$t_{ij - t_{kj}} t_{ij}, \text{ where } t_{kj} = \min(t_{1j}, t_{2j}, \ldots\ldots, t_{mj})$$

$$j = 1, 2, \ldots\ldots, n$$

Step 3: Form the TOTM whose entries are the summation of right-top and left-bottom elements of Steps 1 and 2.

$$t_{ij} = (t_{ij} - t_{ik}) + (t_{ij} - t_{kj})$$

Step 4: Select the largest time element of every row, $\bar{u}_i$ and place them on the right besides corresponding row.

Step 5: Select the largest time element of every column, $\bar{e}_j$ and place them below the corresponding column.

Step 6: Determine the pointer cost, Δ_{ij} for each cell by subtracting the unit time of each cell from the sum of corresponding row and column highest time.

Step 7:   Allocate maximum possible amount to the cell having largest value of the pointer cost, Δ_{ij}. If tie occurs, select the cell where the allocation is maximum.

Step 8:   No further consideration is required for the row or column which is fulfilled. If both the row and column are fulfilled at a time, delete a row or a column randomly.

Step 9:   Continue Step 4 to Step 8 for the remaining sub-matrix until all rows and columns are satisfied.

Step 10:   Shift all the allocations to the original transportation matrix.

Step 11:   Determine the largest time T_k corresponding to basic cells.

Step 12:   Cross off all the non-allocated cells for which $t_{ij} \geq T_k$.

Step 13:   Construct a loop associate with largest time T_k including a non-allocated cell in such a way that the allotment in the cell with T_k is shifted to the non-allocated cell in the loop. If no such loop can be formed, the solution under test is optimum. Otherwise move to the next step.

Step 14:   Repeat Step 12 and 13 until an optimum basic feasible solution is obtained.

4   The Novelty of Our Algorithm

Here we have used TOTM proposed by Kirca and Satir in our presented algorithm, and we define and calculate the pointer cost (in step 6) by subtracting the time units of every cell of TOTM from the sum of respective row and column highest. We allocate maximum possible amount to the cell corresponding to the highest pointer cost.

5   Numerical Illustration

The proposed algorithm for finding an initial basic feasible solution of time minimizing transportation problem is illustrated by the following two randomly selected examples.

5.1   Example 1 (Table 1)

Iteration 1: 3 is the minimum element of the first row, so we subtract 3 from each elements of the first row. In a similar fashion, we subtract 6 and 5 from each elements of the 2nd and 3rd row respectively and place all the differences on the right-top of the corresponding elements in Table 2.

Iteration 2: In the same way, we subtract 4, 15 and 3 from each elements of the 1st, 2nd and 3rd column respectively and place the result on the left-bottom of the corresponding elements in Table 2.

Iteration 3: We add the right-top and left-bottom entry of each element of the transportation table obtained in Iteration 1 and Iteration 2 and formed the TOTM as following (Table 3)

Table 1. Time minimizing transportation problem for the numerical example

		Destination			
		1	2	3	Supply
Factory	1	4	15	3	80
	2	27	23	6	120
	3	7	26	5	300
Demand		140	90	270	

Table 2. Formation of total opportunity time matrix

		Destination				
		1	2	3	t_{ik}	Supply
Factory	1	$_0 4^1$	$_0 15^{12}$	$_0 3^0$	3	80
	2	$_{23} 27^{21}$	$_8 23^{17}$	$_3 6^0$	6	120
	3	$_3 7^2$	$_{11} 26^{21}$	$_2 5^0$	5	300
t_{kj}		4	15	3		
Demand		140	90	270		

Table 3. Total opportunity time matrix

		Destination			
		1	2	3	Supply
Factory	1	1	12	0	80
	2	44	25	3	120
	3	5	32	2	300
Demand		140	90	270	

Iteration 4: Select the largest time element of every row, $\bar{u}_i$ and place them on the right besides corresponding row. Also select the largest time element of every column, $\bar{e}_j$ and place them below the respective column (Table 4).

Iteration 5: Here, c_{11} is 1, largest unit time in the first row, $\bar{u}_i$ is 12 and in the first column, $\bar{e}_1$ is 44, so $\Delta_{11} = \bar{u}_1 + \bar{e}_1 - c_{11} = 12 + 44 - 1 = 55$. In a Similar fashion, we

Table 4. Largest time unit of every row and column

		Destination			$\bar{u}_i$	Supply
		1	2	3		
Factory	1	1	12	0	12	80
	2	44	25	3	44	120
	3	5	32	2	32	300
$\bar{e}_j$		44	32	3		
Demand		140	90	270		

calculate all the values of Δ_{ij}. Since the cell (3, 1) contains the largest value of Δ_{ij}, we allocate 140 units (minimum of 300 and 140) to this cell (Table 5).

Table 5. Initial basic feasible solution after Iteration 5

		Destination			$\bar{u}_i$	Supply
		1	2	3		
Factory	1	55 / 1	32 / 12	15 / 0	12	80
	2	44 / 44	51 / 25	44 / 3	44	120
	3	140 / 71 / 5	32 / 32	33 / 2	32	300
$\bar{e}_j$		44	32	3		
Demand		140	90	270		

Iteration 6: We adjust the supply and demand requirements corresponding to the cell (3, 1). Since the demand for this cell is satisfied, we delete the first column and calculate all the values of Δ_{ij} again for the resulting reduced transportation table. Since the cell (3, 3) contains the largest value of Δ_{ij}, we allocate 160 units (minimum of 160 and 270) to this cell (Table 6).

Iteration 7: We adjust the supply and demand requirements again corresponding to the cell (3, 3). Since the supply for this cell is satisfied, we delete the third row and

Table 6. Initial basic feasible solution after Iteration 6

Factory		Destination			$\bar{u}_i$	Supply
		1	2	3		
	1		32 / 12	15 / 0	12	80
	2		32 / 25	25 / 3	25	120
	3	140	32 / 32	160 · 33 / 2	32	160
$\bar{e}_j$			32	3		
Demand			90	270		

calculate all the values of Δ_{ij} again for the resulting reduced transportation table. Since the cell (1, 2), (2, 2) and (2, 3) contains largest value of Δ_{ij}, we allocate 110 units (minimum of 120 and 110) to the cell (2, 3) because the allocation in this cell is maximum corresponding to other cell (Table 7).

Table 7. Initial basic feasible solution after Iteration 7

Factory		Destination			$\bar{u}_i$	Supply
		1	2	3		
	1		25 / 12	15 / 0	12	80
	2		25 / 25	110 · 25 / 3	25	120
	3	140		160		
$\bar{e}_j$			25	3		
Demand			90	110		

Iteration 8: We adjust the supply and demand requirements again corresponding to the cell (2, 3). Since the demand for this cell is satisfied, we delete the third column and calculate all the values of Δ_{ij} again for the resulting reduced transportation table. Since

Table 8. Initial basic feasible solution after Iteration 8

		Destination				
		1	2	3	$\bar{u}_i$	Supply
Factory	1		80 | 25 12		12	80
	2		10 | 25 | 110 25		25	10
	3	140		160		
$\bar{e}_j$			25			
Demand			90			

only the second column is remaining with two unallocated cell in this case, we allocate 80 units (minimum of 80 and 90) to the cell (1, 2) and 10 units (minimum of 10 and 10) to the cell (2, 2) (Table 8).

Iteration 9: We adjust the supply and demand requirements again and we see that all supply and demand values are exhausted. Since all the rim conditions are satisfied and total number of allocation is 5.

Therefore, the initial basic feasible solution for the given problem is

$$x_{12} = 80, \ x_{22} = 10, \ x_{23} = 110, \ x_{31} = 140 \text{ and } x_{33} = 160.$$

Iteration 10: We shift all the allocations to the original matrix and see the time of basic cells is

$$t_{12} = 15, \ t_{22} = 23, \ t_{23} = 6, \ t_{31} = 7, \text{ and } t_{33} = 5.$$

Therefore, the total transportation time required

$$
\begin{aligned}
T_0 &= \max\{t_{12}, t_{22}, t_{23}, t_{31}, t_{33}\} \\
&= \max\{15, 23, 6, 7, 5\} \\
&= 23
\end{aligned}
$$

Optimality Test: Now largest time is $T_0 = 23$ in the cell (2, 2), therefore we cross off the non-basic cells (2, 1) and (3, 2) which contain larger time units than T_0 (Table 9).

Table 9. Optimality test

		Destination			
		1	2	3	Supply
Factory	1	4	80 5	3	80
	2	27	10 23	110 6	120
	3	140 7	26	160 5	300
Demand		140	90	270	

Now we cannot form any loop originating from the cell (2, 2). Thus the obtained solution $x_{12} = 80$, $x_{22} = 10$, $x_{23} = 110$, $x_{31} = 140$ and $x_{33} = 160$ is optimum and the optimum time of shipment is max $\{15, 23, 6, 7, 5\} = 23$ time units and iteration no. is 0.

5.2 Example 2

Table 10. Time minimizing transportation problem for the numerical example

		Destination				
		1	2	3	4	Supply
Factory	1	3	6	8	4	20
	2	6	1	2	5	28
	3	7	8	3	9	17
Demand		15	19	13	18	

6 Result

Table 11 shows a comparison for minimum time and no. of iteration required among the solutions obtained by our proposed method and the other existing methods and also with the optimum solution by means of the above sample examples and it is seen that our proposed procedure requires less number of iterations to reach the optimal transportation time.

Table 11. A comparative study of different solutions

No.	Methods Name	Time		No. of iteration	
		Ex. 1	Ex. 2	Ex. 1	Ex. 2
1	Proposed Method	23	7	0	0
2	North West Corner Method	27	9	2	3
3	Row Minimum Method	26	9	2	2
4	Column Minimum Method	23	9	0	2
5	Least Cost Method	27	9	2	2
6	Vogel's Approximation Method	26	9	1	1
7	Extremum Difference Method	26	7	1	0
8	Highest Cost Difference Method	27	9	2	2
9	Average Cost Method	26	8	1	1
10	TOTM-MMM	27	9	2	1
11	TOTM-VAM	26	9	1	1
12	TOTM-EDM	26	9	1	1
13	TOTM-HCDM	27	9	1	1
14	TOTM-SUM	26	7	1	0
15	MTCM-HCDM	27	9	3	3
16	Allocation Table Method	27	9	1	1
	Optimum Solution	23	7	0	0

7   Conclusion

A new procedure for finding an initial basic feasible solution of time minimization transportation problem is presented and also illustrated numerically to test the efficiency of the method. Comparative study among the solution obtained by presented method and the other existing methods is also carried out by means of sample examples and it is seen that our proposed procedure requires less number of iterations to reach the optimal transportation time. Therefore, the algorithm claims its wide application in the field of optimization in solving the time minimization transportation problem.

Acknowledgement. The first author acknowledges the financial support provided by the EU Erasmus Mundus Project-cLINK, Grant Agreement No: 212-2645/001-001-EM, Action 2.

References

1. Hitchcock, F.L.: The distribution of a product from several sources to numerous localities. J. Math. Phy. **20**, 224–230 (1941)
2. Dantzig, G.B.: Application of the simplex method to a transportation problem. In: Koopmans, T.C. (ed.) Activity Analysis of Production and Allocation, pp. 359–373. Wiley, New York (1951)
3. Charnes, A., Cooper, W.W., Henderson, A.: An Introduction to Linear Programming. Wiley, New York (1953)
4. Rashid, A., Ahmed, S.S., Uddin, Md.S.: Development of a new heuristic for improvement of initial basic feasible solution of a balanced transportation problem. Jahangirnagar Univ. J. Math. Math. Sci. **28**, 105–112 (2013)
5. Khan, A.R.: A re-solution of the transportation problem: an algorithmic approach. Jahangirnagar Univ. J. Sci. **34**(2), 49–62 (2011)
6. Khan, A.R.: Analysis and re-solution of the transportation problem: a linear programming approach. M. Phil. thesis, Department of Mathematics, Jahangirnagar University (2012)
7. Khan, A.R., Vilcu, A., Sultana, N., Ahmed, S.S.: Determination of initial basic feasible solution of a transportation problem: a TOCM-SUM approach. Bul. Ins. Pol. Din Iasi, Romania, Secția Automatica si Calculatoare **LXI**(LXV), 1, 39–49 (2015)
8. Khan, A.R., Banerjee, A., Sultana, N., Islam, M.N.: Solution analysis of a transportation problem: a comparative study of different algorithms. Accepted for publication in the Bul. Ins. Pol. Din Iasi, Romania, Section Textile. Leathership (2015)
9. Khan, A.R., Vilcu, A., Uddin, Md.S., Ungureanu, F.: A competent algorithm to find the initial basic feasible solution of cost minimization transportation problem. Bul. Ins. Pol. Din Iasi, Romania, Secția Automatica si Calculatoare **LXI**(LXV), 2, 71–83 (2015)
10. Russell, E.J.: Extension of Dantzig's algorithm to finding an initial near-optimal basis for the transportation problem. Ope. Res. **17**(1), 187–191 (1969)
11. Hamdy, A.T.: Operations Research: An Introduction, 8th edn, pp. 193–220. Prentice Hall, Upper Saddle River (2007)
12. Kasana, H.S., Kumar, K.D.: Introductory Operations Research: Theory and Applications, pp. 221–243. Springer, Heidelberg (2004)
13. Uddin, Md.S., Anam, S., Rashid, A., Khan, A.R.: Minimization of transportation cost by developing an efficient network model. Jahangirnagar J. Math. Math. Sci. **26**, 123–130 (2011)
14. Islam, Md.A., Khan, A.R., Uddin, Md.S., Malek, M.A.: Determination of basic feasible solution of transportation problem: a new approach. Jahangirnagar Univ. J. Sci. **35**(1), 101–108 (2012)
15. Babu, Md.A, Das, U.K., Khan, A.R., Uddin, Md.S.: A simple experimental analysis on transportation problem: a new approach to allocate zero supply or demand for all transportation algorithm. Int. J. Eng. Res. App. (IJERA) **4**(1), 418–422 (2014)
16. Uddin, Md.M., Khan, A.R., Roy, S.K., Uddin, Md.S.: A new approach for solving unbalanced transportation problem due to additional supply. Accepted for publication in the Bul. Ins. Pol. Din Iasi, Romania, Section Textile. Leathership (2015)
17. Ahmed, M.M.: Algorithmic approach to solve transportation problems: minimization of cost and time. M. Phil. thesis, Department of Mathematics, Jahangirnagar University (2014)
18. Ahmed, M.M., Tanvir, A.S.M., Sultana, S., Mahmud, S., Uddin, Md.S.: An effective modification to solve transportation problems: a cost minimization approach. Ann. Pure Appl. Math. **6**(2), 199–206 (2014)

19. Ahmed, M.M., Khan, A.R., Uddin, Md.S., Ahmed, F.: A new approach to solve transportation problems. Open J. Opt. **5**(1), 22–30 (2016)
20. Ahmed, N.U., Khan, A.R., Uddin, Md.S.: Solution of mixed type transportation problem: a fuzzy approach. Bul. Ins. Pol. Din Iasi, Romania, Secţia Automatica si Calculatoare, **LXI**(LXV), 2, 19–31 (2015)
21. Kirca, O., Satir, A.: A heuristic for obtaining an initial solution for the transportation problem. J. Oper. Res. Soc. **41**, 865–871 (1990)
22. Reinfeld, N.V., Vogel, W.R.: Mathematical Programming. Prentice-Hall, Englewood Cliffs (1958)
23. Anam, S., Khan, A.R., Haque, Md.M, Hadi, R.S.: The impact of transportation cost on potato price: a case study of potato distribution in Bangladesh. Int. J. Manag. **1**(3), 1–12 (2012)
24. Shenoy, G.V., Srivastava, U.K., Sharma, S.C.: Operations Research for Management, 2nd edn. New Age International (P) Limited Publishers, New Delhi (1991)
25. Das, U.K., Babu, Md.A., Khan, A.R., Helal, Md.A, Uddin, Md.S.: Logical Development of Vogel's Approximation Method (LD-VAM): an approach to find basic feasible solution of transportation problem. Int. J. Sci. Tech. Res. (IJSTR) **3**(2), 42–48 (2014)
26. Das, U.K., Babu, Md.A., Khan, A.R., Uddin, Md.S.: Advanced Vogel's Approximation Method (AVAM): a new approach to determine penalty cost for better feasible solution of transportation problem. Int. J. Eng. Res. Tech. (IJERT) **3**(1), 182–187 (2014)
27. Hammer, P.L.: Time minimizing transportation problems. N. Res. Log. Q. **16**(3), 345–357 (1969)
28. Sharma, A., Verma, V., Kaur, P., Dahiya, K.: An iterative algorithm for two level hierarchical time minimization transportation problem. Eur. J. Oper. Res. **246**, 700–707 (2015)
29. Garfinkel, R.S., Rao, M.R.: The bottleneck transportation problem. N. Res. Log. Q. **18**, 465–472 (1971)
30. Nikolic, I.: Total time minimizing transportation problem. Yugosl. J. Oper. Res. **17**, 125–133 (2007)
31. Uddin, Md.S.: Transportation time minimization: an algorithmic approach. J. Phys. Sci. **16**, 59–64 (2012)
32. Uddin, Md.M., Rahaman, Md.A., Ahmed, F., Uddin, Md.S., Kabir, Md.R.: Minimization of transportation cost on the basis of time allocation: an algorithmic approach. Jahangirnagar J. Math Math. Sci. **28**, 47–53 (2013)
33. Ahmed, M.M., Islam, Md.A., Katun, M., Yesmin, S., Uddin, Md.S.: New procedure of finding an initial basic feasible solution of the time minimizing transportation problems. Open J. Appl. Sci. **5**, 634–640 (2015)
34. Szwarc, W.: Some remarks on the transportation problem. N. Res. Log. Q. **18**, 473–485 (1971)

The Possible Evolution of the Co-operative Form in a Digitized World: An Effective Contribution to the Shared Governance of Digitization?

Paolo Depaoli[1(✉)] and Stefano Za[1,2]

[1] CeRSI – LUISS Guido Carli University, Rome, Italy
{pdepaoli,sza}@luiss.it
[2] eCampus University, Novedrate, CO, Italy
stefano.za@uniecampus.it

Abstract. This conceptual paper considers the cooperative enterprise model in the light of how it can be affected by the digital world and - at the same time - of how it can positively affect both the Internet and its users. The aim of the paper is therefore twofold: (i) to consider the extent and the way in which cooperative principles are going to be affected by the transition of these firms towards 'digital materiality' [1]; (ii) to outline the potential implications of a diffusion of cooperative forms to Internet organizations and users. Based on the traits of this enterprise model, an emerging perspective is described whereby the 'cooperative' (especially if considered as a 'service system') has an interesting potential both as a competent actor in the domain of virtual enterprises and as a possible driver for safeguarding Internet users.

Keywords: Cooperative enterprise · Digital world · Federated system · Virtual enterprise · Service system · Shared governance

1 Introduction

According to the United Nations Committee for the Promotion and Advancement of Cooperatives [2] the cooperative sector worldwide has about 800 million members in over 100 countries. Cooperatives contribute to GDP from 45 % in Kenya to 25 % in New Zealand. They are present in all industries and in some of them their weight is overwhelming: e.g. 80 to 99 % of milk production in Norway, New Zealand and the USA. Consumer cooperatives are market leaders in Italy, Switzerland, Singapore, and Japan. The European bank cooperatives have shown better performance than other types of financial institutions in the present unstable financial systems [3]. In general, cooperatives have shown resilience to the world economic crisis [4].

The evolution of cooperative enterprises has been regarded with fluctuating interest (and favour) by famous economists [5] from Adam Smith (who thought that this form was bound to decline) and Karl Marx (who sympathized with producers cooperatives) to Alfred Marshall (who considered cooperation a "difficult thing but worth doing") and to John Maynard Keynes who showed broad sympathy for co-ops and mutuals.

© Springer International Publishing Switzerland 2016
T. Borangiu et al. (Eds.): IESS 2016, LNBIP 247, pp. 213–220, 2016.
DOI: 10.1007/978-3-319-32689-4_16

They certainly pointed out the potential weaknesses of this model but also its positive effects due to its basic traits. To-day they are summarized in the definition of a cooperative which can be found on the site of the International Cooperative Alliance [6]:

"An autonomous association of persons united voluntarily to meet their common economic, social and cultural needs and aspirations, through a jointly owned and democratically controlled enterprise."

In fact, differently from profit seeking companies where shareholders mainly pursue a pecuniary gain from the employment of capital, cooperatives basically aim at satisfying the common socio-economic needs of their members [7]. Furthermore, in the cooperative organization members can play multiple roles, for example acting both as suppliers and clients. By combining the internal and external networks, this characteristic emphasizes the potential for an active and effective participation in the production and commercialization processes. In other words, since members can be both buyers and sellers of their products and services, the decision making process concerning the cooperative goals is better suited than in other types of firms to be democratically oriented, i.e. to take into account different needs thus achieving its social objectives [7]. These distinctive traits identify the cooperative as a different organizational form compared to the 'company', the 'civil organization', and the 'public organization'. They converge to build the three pillars upon which the performance of a cooperative can be based: its economic capacity, its organizing capacity, and its capacity for change [8]. For example, recent research has shown that cooperatives have a driving role not only in the traditional industries mentioned above but also in emerging areas such as the diffusion of renewable energy technologies in highly developed countries such as Canada, the US, UK, Denmark, and Germany. They successfully overcome barriers to adoption by means of community-based social marketing initiatives [9, 10].

Given the spreading of digitization, the research question addressed in this conceptual paper is therefore: what are the implications of digitization for cooperatives?

The aim of the paper is twofold: (i) to consider the extent and the way in which cooperative principles are going to be affected by the transition of these firms towards 'digital materiality' [1]; (ii) to outline the potential implications of a diffusion of cooperative "modes of production" to Internet organizations and users.

2   The Research Strategy Adopted

At the 'macro' level one of the consequences of the information revolution is the 're-ontologization' of the world, a neologism introduced by Luciano Floridi [11] "to refer to a very radical form of re-engineering that not only designs, constructs or structures a system (e.g. a company, a machine or some artefact) anew, but one that also fundamentally transforms its intrinsic nature, that is, its ontology or essence". At both macro and micro level the work by Wanda Orlikowski is relevant because her research has convincingly shown the entanglement of technology (including information technology) and organization: "Materiality is not an incidental or intermittent aspect of organizational life; it is integral to it" [12]. Furthermore, building on the concept of generativity put forth by Jonathan Zittrain, which "denotes a technology's overall capacity to produce unprompted change driven by large, varied, and uncoordinated audiences" [13], Hanseth and Nielsen [14] show that platforms can both limit and spur innovation according to the aims and strategies of their promoters and, of course, on the programmability of terminals (to harness the so called end-to-end principle). Here we refer to their work to show that if the promoter of a platform is a cooperative, then (because of its characteristics) it is more likely (in comparison with other organizational forms) that it is designed both to promote and protect the interests of its members in an "open" way. Thus, exactly because Lawrence Lessig [15] envisages the hampering of innovation and creativity through a de facto regulation of the Internet by governments and by large, powerful commercial enterprises, Yochai Benkler [16] supports the idea that an effective alternative to strict cyberspace regulation can come from solutions "commons based". Indeed, protection of rights (e.g. personal data and intellectual property) and security can come from participating to a commons where relevant tools and information are managed collectively by members who have free access to what has been generated individually.

This short paper is divided into two main parts. In the first, building on the preceding research of one of the two co-authors of this work [17], we examine the literature on virtual enterprises (VEs) so that both the consequences of the 'entanglement' of technology and organization and the traits of cooperative firms are considered with respect to the challenges raised by virtualization ('digital materiality'). In the second part, we explore and outline the potential implications of a diffusion of cooperative "modes of organizing" to Internet organizations and users.

3   First Results and Implications

3.1   The Cooperative Form and the Challenges Posed to Virtual Enterprises

A virtual enterprise (VE) can be defined as "a temporary alliance of enterprises that come together to share skills, core competencies and resources in order to better respond to business opportunities, and whose co-operation is supported by computer networks" [18]. Basically, the strengths of a VE are related to the complementary expertise of the firms involved. Such capabilities can be organized to exploit an emerging temporary opportunity in a given market without the constraints of geographical proximity and by leveraging appropriate communication technologies and techniques. VEs potential weaknesses (risks) are the reverse of the coin. They have to do, mainly, with: (i) the organization and integration of different competences, resources and management styles from creation to decommission (relying fundamentally on 'diffused leadership' rather than authority); (ii) the probably different familiarity of members with a set of production and communication technologies to be shared.

Given the decisive character of coordination and integration of resources, to avoid the risks of excessive centralization (one partner that becomes indispensable), of inefficiencies in the exploitation of the market (only one associate searches the market looking for new opportunities), and of heterogeneous activities conducted by one actor (marketing and production management), further research [19] has proposed a 'multi-role architecture'. Besides a 'broker' (which still controls and manages the virtual process enactment and coordinates tasks and applications) the new venture should be based on a 'catalyst' (in charge of new business scouting and relations with customers) and on an 'enabler' (responsible of supporting workflow schema design, of building inter-organizational trust and negotiation, and of VE reconfiguration for new businesses). The challenges faced by VEs can be facilitated if the VE partners are cooperatives because of the principles inspiring these firms: voluntary and open membership, democratic member control, member economic participation, autonomy and independence, education, training and information, co-operation among cooperatives, concern for the community (as stated by ICA). Yet, some specific difficulties come from how digital technology is conceived and developed by the parties involved. This brings our discourse to the second part of the issue addressed in this paper.

3.2   The Cooperative Form: A Possible Driver for Safeguarding Internet Users

Besides the inefficiency of their organizational configurations, one obstacle to the development of VEs has been identified in the limits of their supporting cooperation platforms [20]. Indeed mechanisms aimed at increasing trust and security in these online communities are not sufficient [21]. In general, trust has to do with the identification of the information to be shared, a critical element in the implementation process of inter-organizational systems. Further, since the Internet is considered to be an insecure environment [22, 23], information security plays a crucial role as an enabler of trust [24]. This issue is particularly relevant when there are no ownership relations among the partners, and a strong integration is required [25–29]. Here, the concept of trust is multidimensional: a combination of social, institutional, and technological trust [23]. In such cases the use of 'federated systems' (for providing federated authentication and authorization) is considered to be an appropriate solution to support digital transactions among the actors involved. In these systems each partnering enterprise has the control of what kind of information is to be shared by the other partners. This solution allows a shared view only of certain "data" concerning relevant sources such as, for example, customers and employees. [20]. It is thus apparent that the handling of (and the access to) information is one of the main assignments of information security. This concerns also what users do in a digital environment: an emerging problem is in fact related to 'profiling'. Some research has highlighted that "potential consumers are increasingly profiled to detect their habits and preferences in order to provide for targeted services" [30]. It is becoming common for governments, service providers, and specialized data aggregators to systematically collect this kind of information without the user's knowledge or approval [31]. Therefore, because of the discourse developed above, cooperative contexts seem to be effective also in protecting these crucial data (real assets, actually). Of course, this happens only if: (i) data collection and use are governed by means of pertinent agreements among all the actors involved and (ii) a 'federated system' is adopted throughout the partnering organizations (Fig. 1). Hence, within a cooperative system decisions concerning how and for what purposes the information generated can be used, can be discussed and supported in an organized way. For example, should a commercial exploitation be envisaged, the members of a digital environment cooperative are able to define what relationships should be established with their service providers (SP), thus regulating the quality and the costs of the services on the basis of the amount and of the kind of personal information shared with them.

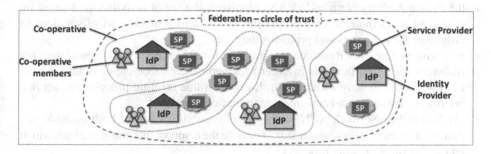

Fig. 1. Federated system - circle of trust

In sum, when considering an active participation in the digital world, the characteristics of the cooperative form seem to contribute to further develop digital networks by exploring and exploiting the opportunities that have been highlighted by Benkler's The wealth of Networks [16] and which can be grouped in 'information sharing', 'collective action', and 'collaboration' [32].

4 Implications and Conclusions

Bringing together digitization and the cooperative form of organizing, this paper marks a first step in showing that, because of their specific traits, cooperatives are appropriate ways to explore both the opportunities offered (and the drawbacks entailed) by the 're-ontologization' of the world that digital technologies are bringing about. Cooperatives are well suited to face the challenges concerning VEs and they can also be drivers for enhancing the security and protection of personal data. While there is an extensive literature concerning the cooperatives present in traditional industries such as banking, agriculture, or retail, new fields and sub-fields where they are emerging (e.g. microfinance, fair trade, renewable energy) need to be given appropriate attention [33]. The digitized world affects both old and new areas of interest for cooperatives because its artifacts cut across sectors and change the environment where these organizations operate, cooperate, and compete by innovating processes, products and services [34]. A further interesting implication emerges here: cooperative organizations in a digitalized world can be understood also as 'service systems'.

4.1 The Cooperative Form as a 'Service System'

Service systems are defined as dynamic, value co-creation configurations of resources (people, technology, organizations, and shared information) [35]. Among the different definitions present in the literature, here the one proposed by Kim and Nam [36] is adopted because it appropriately supports our discourse. They define a service system as the ensemble of three components, i.e. a 'value activity network', a 'resource integrator network', and a 'capability network':

- the 'Value Activity Network' (VAN) represents the set of activities performed by customers and suppliers; their purposeful interactions provide a set of solutions to customers for the issues and problems they face;
- as a primary role, the 'Resource Integrator Network' (RIN) provides and organizes resources for all participants in order to support their value creation activities; it represents several actors with their roles in the value creating process: e.g. service providers, customers and customer communities, suppliers;
- the 'Capability Network' (CN) is the set of capabilities and of both tangible and nontangible resources present inside or outside the resource integrator network which enable the value creating process.

Cooperative organizations can be seen as service systems, where: (i) the VAN is formed by all the actors' interactions taking place within the cooperative system; (ii) the RIN is represented by all the members involved in the service provision, and (iii) the CN consists of a variety of resources such as tools (operand resources) and skills and knowledge (operant resources) which are owned by external service providers and/or by members of the cooperative. Since the main objective of service systems is to provide high quality and innovative services in an interactive and productive way [37], they contribute to the growth of organizations [38]. When growth has a socio-economic nature, the service system can serve as an effective model for the evolution of a cooperative organization within a digitized world.

4.2   Emerging Areas of Interest

The development of new breeding grounds for cooperatives was mentioned in the introduction to this paper (e.g. the field of renewable energy). Awareness is being built within the cooperative practice, community, and movement concerning the challenges posed by digitization. For example, recent research has shown the relevance and vitality of the Italian cooperative sector [39]. Within this lively context, the institution that represents at the national level the cooperative movement (Legacoop) has started to evaluate the opportunities linked to the 're-ontologization' of cooperatives entailed by digitization processes [40]. This example shows the relevance of further investigations in this research area to gain a specific understanding of cooperators when they deal with designing and redesigning cooperatives within a digital materiality perspective.

References

1. Leonardi, P.M.: Digital materiality? How artifacts without matter, matter. First Monday **15**, 1–15 (2010)
2. COPAC: Background paper on cooperatives (2008)
3. Ayadi, R., Llewellyn, D.T., Schmidt, R.H., Arbak, E., De Groen, W.P.: Investigating Diversity in the Banking Sector in Europe - Key Developments. Performance and Role of Cooperative Banks, Brussels (2010)

4. Birchall, J., Ketilson, L.H.: Resilience of the Cooperative Business Model in Times of Crisis. International Labour Organization, Geneva (2009)
5. Whyman, P.B.: Co-operative principles and the evolution of the "dismal science": the historical interaction between co-operative and mainstream economics. Bus. Hist. **54**, 833–854 (2012)
6. International Co-operative Alliance. http://www.ica.coop
7. Bruque, S., Moyano, J., Vargas, A., Hernandez, M.J.: Ownership structure, technological endowment and competitive advantage: do democracy and business fit? Technol. Anal. Strateg. Manag. **15**, 65–79 (2003)
8. van Oorschot, K., de Hoog, J., van der Steen, M., van Twist, M.: The three pillars of the co-operative. J. Co-op. Organ. Manag. **1**, 64–69 (2013)
9. Viardot, E., Wierenga, T., Friedrich, B.: The role of cooperatives in overcoming the barriers to adoption of renewable energy. Energy Policy **63**, 756–764 (2013)
10. Nolden, C.: Governing community energy—feed-in tariffs and the development of community wind energy schemes in the United Kingdom and Germany. Energy Policy **63**, 543–552 (2013)
11. Floridi, L.: Ethics after the information revolution. In: Floridi, L. (ed.) The Cambridge Handbook of Information and Computer Ethics, pp. 3–19. Cambridge University Press, New York (2010)
12. Orlikowski, W.J.: Sociomaterial practices: exploring technology at work. Organ. Stud. **28**, 1435–1448 (2007)
13. Zittrain, J.: The generative internet. Harward Law Rev. **119**, 1974–2040 (2006)
14. Hanseth, O., Nielsen, P.: Infrastructural innovation: flexibility, generativity and the mobile internet. Int. J. IT Stand. Stand. Res. **11**, 27–45 (2013)
15. Lessig, L.: Code, version 2.0. Basic Books, New York (2006)
16. Benkler, Y.: The Wealth of Networks: How Social Production Transforms Markets and Freedom. Yale University Press, New Haven (2006)
17. Depaoli, P., D'Atri, A., De Marco, M.: "Industrial districts enterprises" and "virtual enterprises": proximity and distance, ICT-IS, and organizational learning. In: Proceedings of the Ninth Wuhan International Conference on E-Business, pp. 1323–1333. China University of Geosciences, Wuhan (2010)
18. Camarinha-Matos, L.M., Afsarmanesh, H.: The virtual enterprise concept. In: Camarinha-Matos, L.M., Afsarmanesh, H. (eds.) Infrastructures for Virtual Enterprises: Networking Industrial Enterprises, vol. 25, pp. 3–14. Springer, New York (1999)
19. D'Atri, A., Motro, A.: VirtuE: a formal model of virtual enterprises for information markets. J. Intell. Inf. Syst. **30**, 33–53 (1999)
20. Spagnoletti, P., Za, S.: Securing virtual enterprises: requirements and architectural choices. Int. J. Electron. Commer. Stud. **4**, 327–336 (2013)
21. Spagnoletti, P., Resca, A.: A design theory for IT supporting online communities. In: Sprague, R.H. (ed.) Proceedings of the 45th Hawaii International Conference on System Sciences, pp. 4082–4091. IEEE Computer Society Press, Los Alamitos (2012)
22. Ratnasingam, P.: The importance of technology trust in web services security. Inf. Manag. Comput. Secur. **10**, 255–260 (2002)
23. Olden, M., Za, S.: Biometric authentication and authorization infrastructures in trusted intra-organizational relationships. In: D'Atri, A., De Marco, M., Braccini, A.M., Cabiddu, F. (eds.) Management of the Interconnected World, pp. 53–60. Physica-Verlag HD, Heidelberg (2010)

24. Za, S., D'Atri, E., Resca, A.: Single sign-on in cloud computing scenarios: a research proposal. In: D'Atri, A., Ferrara, M., George, J.F., Spagnoletti, P. (eds.) Information Technology and Innovation Trends in Organizations, pp. 45–52. Physica-Verlag HD, Heidelberg (2011)

25. Bachmann, R., Inkpen, A.C.: Understanding institutional-based trust building processes in inter-organizational relationships. Organ. Stud. **32**, 281–301 (2011)

26. Ford, W., Baum, M.: Secure Electronic Commerce: Building the Infrastructure for Digital Signatures and Encryption. Prentice Hall, Upper Saddle River (1997)

27. McKnight, D., Cummings, L., Chervany, N.: Initial trust formation in new organizational relationships. Acad. Manag. Rev. **23**, 473–490 (1998)

28. Pavlou, P., Liang, H., Xue, Y.: Understanding and mitigating uncertainty in online exchange relationships: a principal-agent perspective. MIS Q. **31**, 105–136 (2007)

29. Ray, S., Ow, T., Kim, S.S.: Security assurance: how online service providers can influence security control perceptions and gain trust. Decis. Sci. **42**, 391–412 (2011)

30. Hildebrandt, M.: The dawn of a critical transparency right for the profiling era. Digit. Enlight. Yearb. **2012**, 41–56 (2012)

31. Brecht, F., Fabian, B., Kunz, S., Mueller, S.: Are you willing to wait longer for internet privacy? In: ECIS 2011 Proceedings, pp. 1–12, Paper 36 (2011)

32. Shirky, C.: Here Come Everybody: the Power of Organizing without Organizations. Penguin Press, New York (2008)

33. Huybrechts, B., Mertens, S.: The relevance of the cooperative model in the field of renewable energy. Ann. Public Coop. Econ. **85**, 193–212 (2014)

34. Yoo, Y., Boland, R.J., Lyytinen, K., Majchrzak, A.: Organizing for innovation in the digitized world. Organ. Sci. **23**(5), 1398–1408 (2012)

35. Maglio, P.P., Spohrer, J.: Fundamentals of service science. J. Acad. Mark. Sci. **36**, 18–20 (2007)

36. Kim, Y.J., Nam, K.: Service systems and service innovation: toward the theory of service systems. In: AMCIS 2009 Proceedings, pp. 1–6, Paper 1 (2009)

37. Prahalad, C.K., Ramaswamy, V., Innovation, E.: The new frontier of experience innovation. MIT Sloan Manag. Rev. **44**, 12–18 (2003)

38. Sawhney, M., Balasubramanian, S., Krishnan, V.V.: Creating growth with services. MIT Sloan Manag. Rev. **45**, 34–43 (2004)

39. Battilani, P., Zamagni, V.: The managerial transformation of Italian co-operative enterprises 1946–2010. Bus. Hist. **54**, 964–985 (2012)

40. Cooperative Commons. http://www.cooperativecommons.coop

A Service-Value Approach to Mobile Application Valuation

Maurizio Cavallari[✉] and Roberto Moro Visconti

Department of Business Administration, Università Cattolica del Sacro Cuore,
Largo Gemelli 1, 20123 Milano, Italy
maurizio.cavallari@unicatt.it,
roberto.morovisconti@morovisconti.it

Abstract. Mobile Application Software (M-Apps) is increasingly popular and by now represents the interactive trendiest software. Investigations about their valuation paradigms are so increasingly common. Even if M-Apps belong to the broad category of Intellectual Property assets, underlying business model is so innovative and different from traditional intangibles that they require new valuation paradigms. The main research question of this paper is to investigate about Service as a primary value driver of M-Apps. A Service-Value-Approach is proposed as a new appraisal method, which embodies customers' perception of M-Apps service value. The empirical evidence fully confirms the hypothesis of the mediating role of Service Quality on application value. This study has practical implications for both scholars and professionals as it provides significant empirical evidence of the role of Service Quality into M-Apps valuation, and value co-creation between providers and users.

Keywords: M-Apps · Valuation · Technology value · Service quality · Application value

1 Introduction

M-Apps, (a shortening of the term "Mobile Application Software") represent a computer program (software) designed to run on mobile devices such as smart-phones, tablet computers, phablets, smart watches or other mobiles, such as notebooks (with specific extensions).

M-Apps are increasingly popular and by now represent the trendiest software device. Investigations about their valuation paradigms are so increasingly common. Even if M-Apps belong to the broad category of Intellectual Property (IP) assets, their underlying business model is so innovative and different from traditional intangibles (such as patents, brands, etc.) that standard appraisal patterns, normally used for IP, may only be used as a starting point for valuation.

The research question of this paper is to investigate about Service Quality as the main value driver propositions in banking/payment M-Apps valuation, to introduce an innovative valuation approach. The paper is organized as follows: after an introduction about the different M-Apps typologies, traditional IP valuation methods are proposed and challenged. A Service Value Approach (SVA) is then theoretically presented as an

© Springer International Publishing Switzerland 2016
T. Borangiu et al. (Eds.): IESS 2016, LNBIP 247, pp. 221–234, 2016.
DOI: 10.1007/978-3-319-32689-4_17

innovative valuation method. An empirical investigation is then conducted considering key parameters such as technological value and service quality. The proposed valuation model embeds literature gaps and trendy scenarios, even considering Internet of Things. Network theory, linking developers with users, is also briefly considered, leaving room for further research avenues. Hypotheses about Service value significance into banking/payment M-Apps are developed and tested. An empirical investigation is then pursued to verify the SVA model and determinants.

2 Definition and Typologies

From a legal point of view, a M-Apps is a piece of software. Computer software is any set of instructions that directs a computer to perform specific operations. Computer software consists of computer programs, libraries and related non -executable data (such as online documentation or digital media). M-Apps are to be included within the software system, since they are embedded in hardware devices (albeit different from PCs), to perform some defined tasks, linked to the Web.

Some companies offer M-Apps as an alternative method to deliver content (media) with certain advantages over an official website. Platforms (stores) represent a key value driver in the industry, becoming central nodes (hubs) within the networks that link different stakeholders, such as users and developers. Sale of M-Apps through stores represents a typical e-commerce transaction. When platforms become dominant, they represent industry standards (as it happened with MS Windows) and generate scalable returns, since their fixed costs can easily reach a break even point, being complemented by negligible variable costs, associated with additional users. M-Apps can be sold for free (freemium = free + premium) or paid. Some 90 % of the M-Apps downloaded tend to be freemium. Revenue streams for freemium app providers follow different patterns and are mainly represented by following premium services (e.g., a free app that introduces to paying services). Even paid M-Apps earn much or their revenues from accessories (on-line advertising; B2B or B2C e-commerce; web customer profile to be sold, etc.). Paid M-Apps are normally cheap (from 0.99 $ up to few $) and their revenue model also relies on high volumes of customers and users. Since the M-Apps market is becoming increasingly crowded, with million M-Apps competing, their added value is growing as the industry is becoming saturated and mature. For instance, popular weather M-Apps find it increasingly difficult to differentiate from others, and they tend to be all freemium. M-Apps are increasingly connected with the Internet of Things (IoT). IoT is a novel paradigm that is rapidly gaining ground in the scenario of modern wireless telecommunications [1].

3 From Standard Intellectual Property Appraisal to Customized M-Apps Valuation

The economic valuation of M-Apps has to follow methodological criteria that are partially different from those traditionally used by established firms or classic intangible assets such as trademarks or patents.

3.1 Traditional Valuation Approaches

Being intangible resources, M-Apps may be valued with the same complementary methods (cost-based; income-based or market-based), whose practical implications go well beyond traditional appraisals, also concerning proper accounting or ability to serve promptly debt.

Issues relating to the valuation of intangibles are surfacing with unprecedented regularity and posit an intriguing challenge for the accounting fraternity that is entrenched in the traditional ascendancy of "reliability" over "relevance". Intangible assets, such as patents or trademarks, are particularly difficult to evaluate [2], due to their intrinsic "immaterial" nature and many different - complementary - quantitative and qualitative valuation methods [3, 4] are traditionally used within the business community. Valuation issues are even more complicated for non-tradable or not deposited non-routine intangibles [5], characterized by limited if any marketability, higher and pervasive information asymmetries and less defined legal boundaries, especially within increasingly specific businesses. The main financial/market methods used for intangibles' fair pricing, with an appropriate rating and ranking, selectively applicable to intangible assets, are the following:

1. **cost-based methods**, with an estimate of the "what-if" costs to reproduce or replace intangibles from scratch.
2. **income methods**, based on the estimate of past and future economic benefits, assessing the ability of the intangible to produce licensing income (royalties, which etymologically derive from "sovereign rents") or sale of the intangible.
3. **market-based methods**, evaluating an intangible asset by comparing it with sales of comparable/similar assets (considering their nature; using functional analysis...).

3.2 Beyond Standard Intellectual Property: The Need of a Service-Value Approach

All the standard Intellectual Property (IP) valuation methods have shown limited validity while dealing with emerging technologies such as M-Apps [6, 7]. Even if they provide some interesting appraisal clues, these approaches are hardly applicable to App valuation services [8, 9].

One of the main differentiating characteristics of M-Apps is based on the interaction between developers and users. Users are not to be considered as typical customers who are provided with IP products and services (buying branded goods; using patented technological devices, etc.), with little if any interaction with the provider. On the contrary, end users are now fully involved in the game, continuously interacting with suppliers and contributing, with their feedbacks, to reshape products and services. ICT scalability is also embedded in these services, allowing for economies of scale that create shareable added value, to the benefit of the whole value chain and its stakeholders. Those are the main reasons why traditional IP appraisal methods, while being of some use, are not fit for M-Apps valuation. Cost-based valuation provides useful information about incurring expenses to develop similar M-Apps, with break-even scenarios for incumbents and new competitors.

However, costs may not represent M-Apps service value [10], which depends on other parameters. Competition-based valuation (included in market-based paradigms) employs competitors' prices as a benchmark for fixing prices. It is used mainly in oligopolistic companies, or for valuation of commodities and standardized M-Apps services. However, if M-Apps service companies have lower non-monetary costs than competitors (e.g. lower waiting times, drawbacks or times for M-Apps service selection) a competition-based approach is unsuitable to price such difference of non-monetary costs [10]. The M-Apps market is far from being oligopolistic, especially from the side of developers. The only oligopolistic component of the value and supply chain is nowadays represented by platforms, which are however in constant evolution. Service-based valuation complements traditional IP valuation paradigms since it takes into account customers' perceptions of M-Apps service value and their willingness to pay; it fixes price according to M-Apps service value provided and communicated to clients. Service-based valuation allows earning higher margins than other valuation methods. It is positively related to the profitability of new M-Apps services, while such relation is neither proved for cost-based nor for competition-based valuation.

Besides, Service-based valuation is suitable for value-added M-Apps services and for communicating M-Apps service quality to customers. Whenever customers perceive a higher Value for Money, if compared to traditional services, they are more willing to pay a premium, which increases economic and financial margins of the App provider. To the extent that these extra margins are duly captured by innovative valuation paradigms, traditional IP valuation models, such as those synthetically illustrated in Sect. 3.1., may be adapted to App valuation paradigms.

To apply Service-based valuation effectively a company has: to be aware of its M-Apps services' value; to employ an effective communication of such a value to customers; to know customers' expectations and perceptions about its M-Apps services [10]. Once a M-Apps service has been designed and its value for customers has been determined, marketing techniques can improve communication of such a value; accordingly, a M-Apps service price can be determined. Despite benefits awarded to Service-based valuation, it is not widely adopted by companies yet [11, 12]: in a summary about valuation models, over the period 1983–2006, only 17 % of M-Apps service companies employ Service-based valuation, as reported by Hinterhuber [8]. Such limited use is surprising given the benefits ascribed to it [10, 13, 14]. The authors of the present paper had reviewed current scientific research to verify if a new approach and model might support overcoming of such implementations difficulties and, accordingly, enhancing Service-based valuation.

4   Service-Value Approach

The Service Value Approach (SVA) is an approach elaborated by authors within this paper, for representing consequential activities of a M-Apps service process. SVA summarizes M-Apps service operations from a customer's perspective; it allows understanding the whole M-Apps service process and its support systems, and improving M-Apps service quality provided to clients.

The main factors to detect in a SVA are the combinations of customers' actions (or employees), onstage and backstage activities supporting M-Apps service provisioning. Customers' and employees' ongoing activities have to be separated from backstage customers' activities; finally, backstage activities and support activities have to be highlighted [7, 10].

4.1 The Theoretical Background

SVA provides a common ground for identifying and managing contact points between a company and its customers. Using this it allows to improve customers' perceived quality, on the one hand, and the company's awareness of the service perceived value by customers. Besides, SVA supports M-Apps service innovation [7] or detection of organizational problems. SVA allows building a shared M-Apps service vision [10, 15].

To the authors' knowledge, in the extant literature no research explores approaches like SVA and service-based valuation jointly. Nevertheless, according to the reviewed literature, it is possible to state that SVA is a technique capable of providing parameters on which fixing service-based valuation. Actually, SVA by mapping a M-Apps service process allows identifying its main value-added activities and its shortages. SVA provides companies with information for valorising its strengths and for managing its inadequacies. Customers base their value assessment and their willingness to pay mostly on these strengths and pitfalls. The conjecture that SVA can be an enabling factor of service-based valuation, is then worthy to be investigated.

4.2 Empirical Evidence

Since significant differences exist between various categories of M-Apps services, traditional demand-based valuation is not suitable to all of them.

Several classification matrixes have been developed for categorizing M-Apps services. The most widely used is the Schmenner's [16] framework: it is a matrix for classifying M-Apps services according to their production attributes [17]. Particularly, M-Apps services can be categorized in four typologies, according to intensity degree (low-high) of both human labour and customization/interaction: mass M-Apps services (e.g. retailing, wholesaling), M-Apps service factories (e.g. airlines, hotels), M-Apps service shops (e.g. hospitals, banking) and professional M-Apps services (e.g. doctors, lawyers). Professional M-Apps services are the most suitable M-Apps service typologies for employing service-based valuation. These two types of M-Apps services provide value-added and highly customized M-Apps services. Therefore, the cost-based valuation does not allow a fair appraisal of added value [10, 18].

Service-based valuation, i.e. customers' perceptions of M-Apps service value, is suitable for M-Apps services characterized by: high customization; significant interaction; great value-added attributes; high operating margins. In the light of the above, the present research focuses on payment and on-line banking applications, as they represent a significant example of service-based applications, i.e. dealing with customers' money, in fact, banks rely heavily on service levels when it comes to process payments and customers' resources [6].

4.3 The Model

The transition from goods-based to the service-oriented economy and the corresponding opportunities for service enhancement, driven by technology innovation, has been much debated in the literature, as in Faria and Nóvoa [19], in Borangiu et al. [20] and in Militaru et al. [21].

This research calls for a service-oriented logic to reflect the multifaceted value service related to technology. M-Apps are no exception from this value service approach for designing and delivering services. Service Value Approach logic sees services as an exchange process in which one party may also benefit itself by applying specialized competencies for the sake of another party. That is, the service value logic shifts the focus from value distribution to value co-creation, a collaborative process in which customers play the role of collaborative partners in producing and sustaining value as in Vargo and Lusch [22–24].

Prior research on mobile service adoption and continuance mainly focuses on Technology value factors, including perceived usefulness, perceived ease of use, system quality, and service usefulness [25]. These determinants reflect the goods-dominant logic view and suggest that if technology developers and service providers can design these qualities into the "products" they offer high adoption or continuance intentions can be expected. The notion of value-in-use requires the integration of the service-dominant logic view into mobile service research to identify the role of service value [22]. Therefore, whereas the technology factors provide high explanatory power in prior research models, considering the role of service value in the context of SVA would further our understanding of factors leading to Service Value [26]. Drawing on the service-dominant logic perspective, the present research thus aims to bridge the gap between the growth potential of M-Apps and the limited understanding of what service experience is and how it affects the overall Service Value.

4.4 Technology Value

Technology can be defined in a broad variety of ways, though we focused on M-Apps technologies. The goods-dominant logic considers technology as a tangible product. Users continue using a technology if the technology is perceived to be superior in user friendliness, performance enhancement, reliability, and responsiveness [6, 12]. Given that perceived ease of use, perceived usefulness, system quality, and reliability reflect these important user perceptions regarding service value of M-Apps technology, the current study conceives technology as a multidimensional construct consisting of the following four sub-constructs that represent users experience and cognitive beliefs.

Perceived ease of use and perceived usefulness are two basilar user experience factors that lead to technology value, as in Borgianu et al. [27]. As the original definition of Davis [28], this study defines perceived ease of use as the degree to which a user believes that using a M-Apps would be of little effort. Besides, perceived ease of use is defined as the extent of one's perception that using a M-Apps would enhance the performance of his/her task. Usually discrepancies exist between people's judgments and actual performance. This entails a possible bias because users do not know the significance of this discrepancy. If a technology fails to deliver its expected outcome, it will result in a loss to the user (e.g. payment M-Apps).

System Quality has to do with interface design, functionality, and response time, reflecting the technical level of success of a system concerning information production [29]. The definition of Reliability, derived from Varian [30] is how well the delivered service level of M-Apps matches expectations, and M-Apps' error rate. This study conceptualizes Technology Value (i.e. TV) as a multidimensional construct that has a formative relationship with the four sub-constructs is the first Latent Variable taken into account for the SVA model [31].

4.5 Service Quality

Vargo and Lusch [24] consider service quality to be highly dependent on experience. Although there are many definitions and conceptualizations of service experience, it is considered the result of the interaction and the important process of co-creation among the service provider, the customer, and other value-creation partners that can occur at any conscious moment. Service quality has received researchers' attention in areas such as marketing, information systems, service design and management. In Drăgoicea et al. [32], researchers have proposed and discussed some feelings and sensation elements that reflect the essence of service quality; other studies include functions, interaction [33] and system security [34, 35]. The current study conceptualizes service quality as a superordinate second-order construct reflected by the following three first-order determinants.

Functions factor is related to peak performance, meaning full use of one's potential to behave efficiently and achieve optimal functioning. Excellent functions have two distinguishing characteristics, namely, a sense of self in clear process and full focus; they are used for investigating a range of research issues about human performance. Examples of research issues include productivity, excellence, and creativity [36].

Interaction is one of the important elements of experience. Earlier research has indicated that positive interaction captures one's emotional response to a place [35]. Stimulation of interest or of positive feelings is an essential aspect of the experience to encourage continuing motivation and following involvement. Prior research has argued that interest sets the foundation to be engaged in a topic or event [37].

Perceived security (as the complement of perceived risk) affects people's confidence in their decisions [35]. Risky situations can be those where the probabilities of outcomes are not known and the outcome is known or unknown, and users want to feel security (risks are taken into account and mitigated by M-Apps developers/bank/systems). In previous studies on consumer research, Perceived Security was defined as the perceived certainty in a purchase situation [38]. Service Quality (SQ) is the second Latent Variable taken into account for the SVA model.

4.6 Hypothesis Development

Gefen and Straub theorized that the effect of technology excellence determinants on Value would be affected by the nature of the service [39]. A recent study demonstrated that Technology value had greater effects on Value for a service technology [25]. At this point we can consider a third Latent Variable as the Application Value (AV), dependent from the above mentioned, first (TV) and second (SQ), latent variables that serve as antecedents of 3rd Latent Variable: Application Value (AV).

So we can expose the following Hypothesis 1: **H1**. Technology value is positively associated with the Application Value. One difference between the service-dominant logic and the goods-dominant logic is that the former values the interaction between the service provider and the customer and places high priority on the importance of understanding and delivering customer experience because it affects users' experience, whereas the latter focuses on the transfer of ownership of output [23, 24].

A favourable experience not only creates positive outcomes but also opens up further opportunities because customers want to continue the service experience unavailable from other companies/banks. Prior research has illustrated the influence of service quality on value. For example, cognitive and emotional responses associated with a positive experience increase consumers' intentions to return to a service or to repurchase [26]. Confirmation of service quality with user expectations positively contributes to service continuance because users are satisfied with the service [18]. Moreover, a positive service quality contributes to customer loyalty and further leads to customers' willingness to develop a continuing relationship with the service provider [10, 12]. Service quality is crucial in the service provision process because the phenomenological nature of service value indicates that it is often uniquely and subjectively interpreted. Service providers build relational ties with customers by offering unique and quality service experiences so that M-Apps users are willing to become continual "beneficiaries" of the service [14]. We can draw then the following Hypothesis 2: **H2**. Service Quality is positively associated with the Application Value. The key is whether user perceptions can be used to foster the creation of positive experiences leading to M-Apps value. The significance of such good creation lies in servicing the needs of the users in their unique contexts [26].

The above discussion suggests the critical role of service quality in which M-Apps serve as a vehicle to convey value. Based on the debate above, Hypothesis 3 is proposed as follows: **H3**. Service Quality mediates the relationship between Technology Value and Application Value.

5 Research Methodology

This paper presents a new method for Service Value Appraisal, in the field of M-Apps for e-banking. The particular domain is addressed by questionnaires belonging to Quality of Experience. Likert scale is going to be used for opinion scores.

The research methodology is going to be adapted to statistic structural modelling, performing validity analysis. The research constructs in this study were measured using validated items from prior studies. Technology value is formed by four first-order indicators: Perceived Ease of Use (PEoU), Perceived Usefulness (PU), System Quality (SQ), and Reliability (REL). Service Quality is defined by three first-order indicators: Functions (FUN), Interaction (INT) and Perceived Security (PS). The second order variable Application Value is defined by App Need (AN), Availability to Pay (AtP) and App Fidelity (AF).

5.1   Construct Operationalization

Perceived ease of use was adapted from Davis [28] and the scale of perceived usefulness was derived from Vargo and Lusch [24]. System quality and reliability were measured using items adapted from Zhou et al. [26] and Ahn et al. [29]. The measurement items for functions were adapted from Petter et al. [31] and Shin [33].

The items for Interaction and Perceived security were measured using items adapted from Varian [30] and from Cavallari [34, 36]. All items were measured using seven-anchor Likert scales, ranging from strongly disagree (1) to strongly agree (7). Control variables in the research model were: respondents' age and gender.

5.2   Data Gathering and Method

This study conducted an online survey for the data collection to reach a wide group of banking/payment M-Apps users. The population was all Italian although the questionnaire was provided in English. Italy has proven to be an excellent environment for banking/payment M-Apps, as the are about 4 million users registered. The survey was posted on a dedicated portal in Italy to a banking/payment M-Apps users community in Italy (http://www.quantitative-research.org/limesurvey/index.php), between 21/09/2015 and 25/10/2015. For privacy reasons no identification was required to complete the questionnaire and the IP address of each respondent was not recorded for any filtering purpose. A total of 179 valid responses were collected. Among the valid respondents, 71 were female (39.67 %), and 108 were male users (60.33 %). Most of the respondents were in their 30's, with ages 31–45 accounting for 59.25 %, and ages 46–over for 27.41 %; the minor part were younger than 31 (13.34 %). Partial Least Squares (PLS) method was chosen for the data analysis because it is prediction-oriented and thus recommended for early stages of theory development [38, 39]. SmartPLSv. software vers. 3.2.3, was a valuable instrument for our research model, Ringle et al. [40]. The possibility to have formative, as well as reflective constructs made PLS suitable for our research [39, 41].

Remark 1. Column (1) represents path coefficients that are estimated for patterns A., B. and C. independently for the given independent variable (iv); column (2) represents

Table 1. Measurement Items (Variables) and Loadings (not including control variables)

Variable	Mean	STD	Loadings
Technology Value	6.374	1.345	0.962
Service Quality	6.701	1.882	0.970
Application Value	6.812	1.572	0.941

Table 2. Mediation Analysis

Pattern	Service Quality	
	column (1)	column (2)
A. Technology Value $\rightarrow$ Service Quality	.467*	.455*
B. Service Quality $\rightarrow$ Application Value	.297*	.340*
C. Technology Value $\rightarrow$ Application Value	.223*	.211*
*p < 0.01	(partial) mediation confirmed!	

path coefficients that are estimated simultaneously for all of the patterns (i.e., A., B. and C.) for the given (iv). If pattern C. is significant (i.e. p < 0.01) both in column (1) and (2), with column (1) greater than column (2), then Service Quality partially mediates the impact of the corresponding (iv), on Application Value (dv), as stated in Baron and Kenny [42] (Table 2).

5.3   Construct Validity

To assess the measurement properties of the SVA model and the instruments proposed, a thorough construct validity analysis was conducted.

Confirmatory Factor Analysis. A confirmatory factor analysis (CFA) was carried out by utilizing individual level data to test the construct distinctiveness of the two predictors variables of Technology Value and Service Value. The hypothesis of two factors model provided good fit indexes, all within acceptable levels: $\chi^2 = 2.54$, df = 39, p < .001; RMSEA = .069; GFI = .95; CFI = .91 [41]. To validate the hypothesis of the proposed model (Fig. 1), we tested two alternative two-factor models utilizing different aggregations of the predictors. Validation-varied-model 1 utilized the factors: Perceived Ease of Use and Perceived Usefulness, as one single factor; it showed $\Delta\chi^2 = 1.63$. Validation-varied-model 2 was a two-factor model with Functions and Interactions grouped as one factor ($\Delta\chi^2 = 1.19$). This test confirmed that the two-factor predictors model had a consistently better fit than the alternative models, based on χ^2 difference test. Acceptable ranges, in adherence with Straub et al. [41], are considered: GFI $\geq$ .90, CFI $\geq$ .90, Adjusted Chi-square $\leq$ 3.0, RMSEA $\leq$ .08.

Common method. As all variables considered are coming from the same sources and because they are not evaluated in different contexts, common method bias can occur. Following the approach suggested by Podsakoff et al. [43] we included a common method factor into the model, which linked to all of the single-indicator constructs converted from observed indicators. Because the factor loadings were insignificant and the indicators' substantive variances were substantially greater than their method variances, common method bias is not likely to represent a problem.

Convergent validity and Discriminant validity. To ensure the individual item reliability and convergent validity of constructs, we examined the average variance extracted (AVE) and the factor loadings of individual measures on their corresponding constructs. All loadings on relative constructs were above the recommended minimum value of 0.707, indicating that at least 50 % of the variance was captured by the construct, as Chin [44]. Square root of the average variance extracted (AVE) for each construct was compared with the other correlation scores. The square root of the AVE was higher than the corresponding off-diagonal correlations of the constructs to their latent variables. Cross-loadings of the items on other constructs show that all of the measurement item loadings were above 0.82 and were at least 0.1 less on their load-ings, as recommended by Gefen and Straub [39].

5.4 Analysis

We used a latent variables model to verify the hypotheses and to check the mediating effect of one the independent variable (Service Quality), on dependent variable (Application Value). Table 1 shows the measurement items scores (we averaged all constructs' items to facilitate the readability and because of constraints on paper length). The results of the model estimation (including standardized path coefficients, the significance of the paths based on a two-tailed t-test, and the variances explained (R^2), are presented in Fig. 1. The significant path coefficients of all hypotheses were supported (i.e. $p < 0.01$ or $p < 0.001$, see Fig. 1). Control variables had no role, as they don't explain additional correlation (i.e. 0.2 %).

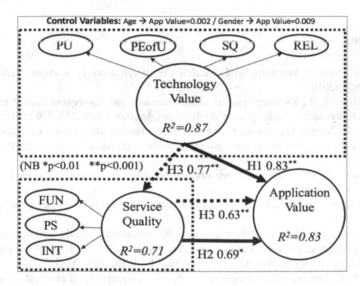

Fig. 1. The SVA: Model, Relationships, Path Coefficients, Variance Explained (R^2).

6   Conclusion and Research Recommendations

This paper has shown that Service-Value M-Apps represent a peculiar intangible asset. M-Apps are so different from traditional Intellectual Property products and services, that standard IP valuation approaches can be used only to provide some auxiliary information (e.g. about break-even costs or market comparables). New business models, based on innovative value chains, require unprecedented appraisal paradigms and approaches, such as the one tentatively presented in this paper.

Hypotheses **H1**, **H2** were fully confirmed, and partially confirmed was **H3**, the (partially) mediating role of Service Quality on Application Value. It emerged that coefficients in column (1) for the independent variable (iv) were significant, satisfying initial conditions to test mediation role of Service Quality. Mediation analysis confirmed that Service Quality partially mediates effect on Application Value. The results of our study offer important practical implications for both scholars and professionals/ banks/mobile payment institutions as it provides significant empirical evidence of the role of Service into App Valuation. This gives scholars in Service Science a significant contribution regarding research scope and significance of Service appraisal in Application Valuation. New research avenues, which go far beyond the targets of this paper, may, for instance concern the interaction of M-Apps business paradigms with the new interactions among the stakeholders that rotate around these innovative supply and value chains. These continuous feedbacks may be conveniently examined and eventually analysed within a sharing economy framework, where stakeholders continuously collaborate. Interaction among stakeholders may be modelled with Service Theory paradigms, considering relationships among different nodes (represented by App developers, intermediating platforms and interactive end users), through their linking edges.

References

1. Atzori, L., Iera, A., Morabito, G.: The internet of things: a survey. Comput. Netw. **54**(15), 2787–2805 (2010)
2. Moro Visconti, R.: Exclusive patents and trademarks and subsequent uneasy transaction comparability: some transfer pricing implications. Intertax **40**(3), 212–219 (2012)
3. Lagrost, C., Martin, D., Dubois, C., Quazzotti, S.: Intellectual property valuation: how to approach the selection of an appropriate valuation method. J. Int. Cap. **11**(4), 481–503 (2010)
4. Andriessen, D.: IC valuation and measurement: classifying the state of the art. J. Int. Cap. **5**(2), 230–242 (2004)
5. Moro Visconti, R.: Evaluating know-how for transfer price benchmarking. J. Fin. Acc **1**(1), 27–38 (2013)
6. Hussain, A., Abubakar, H.I., Binti Hashim, N.: Evaluating mobile banking application: Usability dimensions and measurements. In: International Conference on Information Technology and Multimedia (ICIMU), pp. 136–140. IEEE, New York (2014)
7. Bitner, M.J., Ostrom, A.L., Morgan, F.N.: Service blueprinting: a practical technique for service innovation. Calif. Manage. Rev. **50**(3), 66–94 (2008)
8. Hinterhuber, A.: Customer value-based pricing strategies: why companies resist. J. Bus. Strat. **29**(4), 41–50 (2008)
9. Anderson, C.K., Xie, X.: Improving hospitality industry sales twenty-five years of revenue management. Cornell Hosp. Q. **51**(1), 53–67 (2010)
10. Zeithaml, V.A., Bitner, M.J., Gremier, D.D.: Service Marketing: Integrating Customer Focus across the Firm. Irwin McGraw-Hill, New York (2006)

11. Kimes, S.E., Wirtz, J.: Has revenue management become acceptable? findings from an international study on the perceived fairness of rate fences. J. Serv. Res. **6**(2), 125–135 (2003)
12. Avlonitis, G.J., Indounas, K.A.: Pricing objectives and pricing methods in the services sector. J. Serv. Mark. **19**(1), 47–57 (2005)
13. Beldona, S., Kwansa, F.: The impact of cultural orientation on perceived fairness over demand-based pricing. Int. J. Hosp. Manage. **27**(4), 594–603 (2008)
14. Chiang, W.C., Chen, J.C., Xu, X.: An overview of research on revenue management: current issues and future research. Int. J. Rev. Manage. **1**(1), 97–128 (2007)
15. Coenen, C., von Felten, D., Schmid, M.: Managing effectiveness and efficiency through FM blueprinting. Facilities **29**(9/10), 422–436 (2011)
16. Schmenner, R.W.: How can service business survive and prosper? Sloan Manage. Rev. **27**(3), 21–32 (1986)
17. Tinnilä, M.: Efficient service production: service factories in banking. Bus. Proc. Manage. J. **19**(4), 648–661 (2013)
18. Docters, R., Reopel, M., Sun, J.M., Tanny, S.: Capturing the unique value of services: why pricing of services is different. J. Bus. Strat. **25**(2), 23–28 (2004)
19. Faria, J.A., Nóvoa, H.: An agile BPM system for knowledge-based service organizations. In: Nóvoa, H., Drăgoicea, M. (eds.) Exploring Services Science. IESS 1.5. LNBIP, vol. 201, pp. 65–79. Springer, Heidelberg (2015)
20. Borangiu, T., et al.: Service Oriented Architecture for Total Manufacturing Enterprise Integration. In: Nóvoa, H., Drăgoicea, M. (eds.) Exploring Services Science. IESS 1.5. LNBIP, vol. 201, pp. 95–108. Springer, Heidelberg (2015)
21. Militaru, G., Purcărea, A.-A., Borangiu, T., Drăgoicea, M., Negoita, O.D.: How social responsibility influences innovation of service firms: an investigation of mediating factors. In: Nóvoa, H., Drăgoicea, M. (eds.) Exploring Services Science. IESS 1.5. LNBIP, vol. 201, pp. 135–151. Springer, Heidelberg (2015)
22. Vargo, S.L., Lusch, R.F.: Evolving to a new dominant logic for marketing. J. Mark. **68**(1), 1–17 (2004)
23. Vargo, S.L., Lusch, R.F.: From goods to service(s): divergences and convergences of logics. Ind. Mark. Manage. **37**(3), 254–259 (2008)
24. Vargo, S.L., Lusch, R.F.: Service dominant logic: continuing the evolution. J. Acad. Mark. Sci. **36**(1), 1–10 (2008)
25. Hong, S.-J., Thong, J.Y.L., Tam, K.Y.: Understanding continued information technology usage behavior: a comparison of three models in the context of mobile Internet. Decis. Supp. Syst. **42**(3), 1819–1834 (2006)
26. Zhou, T., Lu, Y.: Examining mobile instant messaging user loyalty from the perspectives of network externalities and flow experience. Comput. Hum. Behav. **27**(2), 883–889 (2011)
27. Borangiu, T., Oltean, V.E., Drăgoicea, M., Cunha, J., Jacob, I.: Some aspects concerning a generic service process model building. In: Snene, M., Leonard, M. (eds.) Exploring Services Science. IESS 1.5. LNBIP, vol. 169, pp. 1–16. Springer, Heidelberg (2014)
28. Davis, F.D.: Perceived usefulness, perceived ease of use, and user acceptance of information technology. MIS Q. **13**(3), 319–339 (1989)
29. Ahn, T., Ryu, S., Han, I.: The impact of web quality and playfulness on user acceptance of online retailing. Inf. Manage. **44**(3), 263–275 (2007)
30. Varian, H.: System reliability and free riding. Adv. Inf. Sec. **12**, 1–15 (2003)
31. Petter, S., Straub, D., Rai, A.: Specifying formative constructs in information systems research. MIS Q. **31**(4), 623–656 (2007)

32. Drăgoicea, M., Borangiu, T., Falcão e Cunha, J., Oltean, V.E., Faria, J., Radulescu, S.: Building an extended ontological perspective on service science. In: Snene, M., Leonard, M. (eds.) Exploring Services Science. IESS 1.4. 169, pp. 17–30. Springer, Heidelberg (2014)

33. Shin, N.: Online learner's 'flow' experience: an empirical study. Br. J. Educ. Technol. **37**(5), 705–720 (2006)

34. Cavallari, M., Adami, L., Tornieri, F.: Organisational aspects and anatomy of an attack on NFC/HCE mobile payment systems. In: ICEIS 2015 − 17th International Conference on Enterprise Information Systems, Proceedings, vol. 2, pp. 685–700 (2015)

35. Cavallari, M.: A conceptual analysis about the organizational impact of compliance on information security policy. In: Snene, M. (ed.) Exploring Services Science. IESS 1.2. LNBIP, vol. 103, pp. 101–114. Springer, Heidelberg (2012)

36. Cavallari, M.: The role of extraordinary creativity in organizational response to digital security threats. In: D'Atri, A., Ferrara, M., George, J.F., Spagnoletti, P. (eds.) Technology and Innovation Trends in Organizations, pp. 479–486. Springer, Heidelberg (2011)

37. Carver, C.S., Scheier, M.F.: Attention and Self-Regulation: A Control-Theory Approach to Human Behavior. Springer, Heidelberg (2012)

38. Gefen, D., Straub, D.W.: The relative importance of perceived ease-of-use in IS adoption: a study of e-commerce adoption. JAIS **1**(8), 1–28 (2000)

39. Gefen, D., Straub, D.W.: Structural equation modeling and regression: guidelines for research practice. CAIS **4**(7), 1–77 (2000)

40. Ringle, C.M., Wende, S., Becker, J.M.: SmartPLS 3. SmartPLS GmbH, Boenningstedt (2015). http://www.smartpls.com

41. Straub, D.W., Bourdeau, M.C., Gefen, D.: Validating guidelines for IS positivist research. CAIS **13**(24), 380–427 (2004)

42. Baron, R.M., Kenny, D.A.: The moderator-mediator variable distinction in social psychological research: conceptual, strategic and statistical considerations. J. Person. Soc. Psychol. **51**(6), 1173–1182 (1986)

43. Podaskoff, P., Mackenzie, S., Lee, J., Podaskoff, N.: Common Method Biases in Behavioral Research: A Critical Review of the Literature and Recommended Remedies. J. App. Psychol. **88**(5), 879–903 (2003)

44. Chin, W.W.: Issues and opinion on structural equation modeling. MIS Q. **22**(1), 7–16 (1998)

Service Innovation and Strategy

The Assessment of Municipal Services: Environmental Efficiency of Buildings Construction

Isabel M. Horta[1(✉)], Ana S. Camanho[1], Teresa G. Dias[1], and Samuel Niza[2]

[1] Faculdade de Engenharia, Universidade do Porto, Porto, Portugal
{imhorta, acamanho, tgalvao}@fe.up.pt
[2] Instituto Superior Técnico - Universidade de Lisboa,
Campus Taguspark, Lisboa, Portugal
samuel.niza@dem.ist.utl.pt

Abstract. This paper develops an innovative methodology to assess municipal performance concerning the environmental efficiency of new buildings construction, focusing on the consumption of different types of materials. This study aims to support local governments in the definition of policies for improvements in service provision based on the results of a benchmarking study. The methodology developed includes two stages. The first step concerns the evaluation of municipal environmental efficiency using Data Envelopment Analysis and the identification of factors that may explain different levels of performance. The second step enables the classification of municipalities in terms of the efforts required to achieve environmental efficiency. For this purpose, we used clustering analysis, namely the k-means algorithm. To illustrate the methodology developed, we analyzed the data of the major materials used in the construction of new buildings (metals, non-metallic minerals, fossil fuels, and biomass) in the municipalities of Lisbon metropolitan area between 2003 and 2009. The study revealed that the environmental efficiency of new buildings construction varies considerably among municipalities, suggesting a high potential for performance improvement.

Keywords: Municipal services · Public sector · Buildings · Data envelopment analysis · Clustering

1 Introduction

The efficient provision of public services has gained increased attention in recent years. This is mainly motivated by citizens' demand for high quality and cost effective public services, and also by municipal scarce resources and budget constraints. This opened a research agenda focused on the assessment of municipal performance. The literature on municipal performance includes studies that evaluate the performance of local governments in the provision of several services under their responsibility (see [1] for more details), or studies that assess the performance of specific services (e.g., waste management, transportation, water services). The literature has only recently started to

© Springer International Publishing Switzerland 2016
T. Borangiu et al. (Eds.): IESS 2016, LNBIP 247, pp. 237–250, 2016.
DOI: 10.1007/978-3-319-32689-4_18

study municipal services related to the construction industry (CI). The topic of CI performance at municipal level was first considered by [2], focusing on the consumption of resources in residential buildings.

CI is the major consumer of natural resources of all industries worldwide. It accounts for almost half of the total resources used and approximately 40 % of the total energy consumed. It is also responsible for generating a considerable amount of waste streams and gas emissions [3]. In particular, CI is estimated to generate around 30 % of CO_2 emissions, and 40 % of human-produced waste. As a large share of CI activities are under the responsibility of local governments, it is crucial to develop models for the assessment of municipal performance concerning building construction, adopting an environmental perspective.

The concept of sustainable construction was first introduced by [4] that defined it as "the creation and responsible management of a healthy built environment based on resource efficient and ecological principles". Nowadays, sustainable construction relies on four main pillars: environmental, social, economic, and technical [5]. The assessment of construction sustainability with an environmental focus has been subject to a considerable amount of research in recent years. The studies conducted mostly focus on the evaluation of buildings (see [6] for a literature review).

Traditionally, the evaluation of buildings from an environmental perspective was based on a single criterion, such as water, energy, or materials usage. [7] reviews the main issues in terms of water conservation to be considered in buildings' environmental evaluations. [8] performs a critical review of the life cycle energy analyses (embodied and operation energy) of buildings resulting from 73 cases across 13 countries. [9] reviews the life cycle assessment of 13 buildings in different countries identifying which phase of the life cycle and which type of building consumes more energy and has more greenhouse gas (GHG) emissions. [10] assesses the most appropriate energy performance indicators to model the performance of the residential building envelope. [11] presents the results of a life cycle assessment by comparing the most commonly used building materials and some eco-materials using three different impact categories. Other studies focused on the environmental impact of specific building materials, such as concrete [12], clay bricks [13], marble [14], facade materials [15], and insulating stone wool [16].

However, sustainability issues are multidimensional and monitoring housing performance merely based on a single criterion may limit the evaluation. Following this concern, comprehensive assessment systems were developed in the last few decades to certify the environmental/sustainability performance of buildings. These systems typically comprise a set of environmental criteria assessed by performance indicators. The scope of the analysis frequently covers different types of buildings (e.g. residential or industrial), and various phases of the buildings life cycle (e.g. design, construction or operation). The first building assessment method was launched in 1990, in the United Kingdom, and is called the BRE Environmental Assessment Method (BREEAM). It includes the assessment of new and existing buildings of any type (e.g. supermarkets, offices, light or heavy industrial buildings). Currently, the BREEAM serves as a support to the development of various building assessment systems in different countries, such as in Australia, Canada, and Hong Kong. A few other tools to assess building projects appeared later. For instance, the Leadership in Energy and Environmental Design Green

Building Rating System (LEED) was developed in 2002 in the United States, the Comprehensive Assessment System for Building Environmental Efficiency (CASBEE) was developed in 2004 in Japan, and the Sustainable Building Tool (SBTool) was developed in 1995 to provide an international tool for building assessment.

In the last decade, these systems broadened the scope and developed evaluations at the neighborhood or block scale as a way to contribute to sustainable urbanization which requires adequate facilities, buildings and utilities leading to improvements in environmental quality, quality of life, and urban governance. The best known tools are typically extensions of the building assessment tools (BREEAM Communities, SBTool Generic, LEED for Neighborhood Development, and CASBEE for Urban Development). As the development of these tools is recent, the number of scientific publications related to this topic is still very scarce [17].

The purpose of this paper is to assess municipal performance concerning the environmental efficiency of new buildings construction, which is a critical issue worldwide. Note that the entire life cycle of buildings includes an initial phase of materials production or extraction, followed by the design, construction, operation and maintenance, and demolition or rehabilitation phases. Herein, we focus on the quantities of materials used in the construction of new buildings.

The methodology developed involves two main steps. The first stage evaluates municipal performance, using the Data Envelopment Analysis (DEA) technique, and explores factors that may explain the spread in efficiency levels. DEA has the ability to derive a single summary measure of efficiency for each municipality in a given year, based on the comparison with the other municipalities in the sample. In this context, a high efficiency score for a particular municipality indicates that the municipality is able to use fewer materials per square meter built than its peers.

The second stage classifies the municipalities into groups according to the efforts required to achieve an efficient level of materials usage. The k-means clustering algorithm was used to identify groups of similar municipalities in terms of resource consumption for new buildings construction. With this approach, municipalities in the same cluster can collaborate in the design of policies to address the common inefficiency features detected in their group by learning from practices adopted in other groups.

The methodology proposed was applied to the municipalities of Lisbon metropolitan area between 2003 and 2009. The input variables included in the DEA model relate to the major materials used in the construction of new residential buildings (fossil fuels, metallic materials, non-metallic materials, and biomass), and the output is the floor area built of new residential buildings in a municipality in a given year.

The remainder of this paper is organized as follows. Section 2 describes the methodology proposed in the paper. Section 3 presents the data used in the empirical analysis and describes the sample analyzed. Section 4 discusses the results obtained for the case study of Lisbon municipalities. The last section concludes and provides recommendations for future research.

2 Methodology

2.1 Data Envelopment Analysis

DEA, first introduced by [18], is a linear programming model that can be used to assess relative efficiency. Typically, the construction of buildings involves the use of multiple resources/inputs (e.g. tonnes of wood or concrete) to produce the output (i.e., square meters of floor area built). DEA enables the estimation of an efficiency measure for each municipality in a given year based on a comparison with the other municipalities in the sample, which are examples of best practices. These best practice municipalities are located on the frontier of the production possibility set and are assigned an efficiency score equal to one. For the municipalities deemed inefficient, their efficiency score is lower than one and is an estimate of the distance to the best practice frontier.

One of the main advantages of DEA is that it is based on an optimization procedure that allows each municipality to be shown in the best possible light. This means that the set of weights to aggregate the multiple input and output dimensions is calculated in order to give higher importance to the areas where the municipality performed better. This flexibility in the choice of weights makes the assessments less prone to controversy, as it does not require the use of a unique set of weights that could put some municipalities in disadvantage.

Consider a set of n municipalities ($j = 1,\ldots,n$), each consuming m resources x_{ij} ($i = 1,\ldots,m$) to produce s outputs y_{rj} ($r = 1,\ldots,s$). Herein, the resources correspond to four categories of construction materials (fossil fuels, metallic materials, non-metallic materials, and biomass) and the output is the floor area built of new residential buildings in each municipality and year. The DEA model used to calculate the relative efficiency of a municipality j_0 is presented in (1). It corresponds to a standard formulation with an input minimizing perspective and constant returns to scale (CRS).

The variables of model (1) are u_r and v_i, which correspond to the weights attached to the outputs and inputs, respectively. The optimal solution of model (1), $e_{j0}{}^*$, is the efficiency score of the municipality j_0 under evaluation, which reflects the proportion by which all materials can be proportionally reduced without decreasing the floor area built.

$$e_{jo} = \max \sum_{r=1}^{s} u_r y_{rjo}$$

$$\sum_{i=1}^{m} v_i x_{ijo} = 1$$

$$\sum_{r=1}^{s} u_r y_{rj} - \sum_{i=1}^{m} v_i x_{ij} \leq 0, \quad j = 1,\ldots,n \tag{1}$$

$$v_i \geq 0, \quad i = 1,\ldots,m$$

$$u_r \geq 0, \quad r = 1,\ldots,s$$

Note that prior to the estimation of municipal performance, we explored whether they were operating under constant or variable returns to scale. The issue of returns to scale is a crucial question in any efficiency study. The returns to scale measures the response of output to equal proportional changes in all inputs. The bootstrapping procedure proposed by [19] was used to test the hypothesis regarding returns to scale. Bootstrapping was first introduced by [20] and it is a resampling method, with replacement, for statistical inference. For a sample with n observations, bootstrap involves to generate a large number of samples, each with n observations randomly drawn from the original data. In particular, we tested for evidence against the null hypothesis that the consumption of construction materials in the municipalities occurs under CRS. The p-value obtained for the entire period was 0.610 indicating that the best practice frontier globally exhibits CRS for the period analyzed. In the context of this study, this could be expected as it is likely that the floor area built (the output variable of DEA model) increases proportionally to the increase in the materials used (the inputs) in buildings construction.

2.2 Clustering Analysis

Clustering is a data mining technique that was used to group municipalities with similar resource consumption features in new buildings construction. [21, 22] provide an overview on several clustering algorithms. In this study, we applied the k-means algorithm, introduced by [23], which is a widely used partitional clustering algorithm. Partitional clustering techniques enable the division of the municipalities into non-overlapping groups (i.e., clusters) such that each municipality belongs to exactly one cluster. The k-means algorithm, suitable for continuous variables, partitions a set of n municipalities into k clusters in order to achieve high intra-cluster similarity and low inter-cluster similarity. First, it randomly selects k of the municipalities, each of which initially represents a cluster mean. Each of the remaining municipalities is then assigned to the most similar cluster, based on the distance (e.g. Euclidean distance) between the municipality and the cluster mean. Then, it determines the new mean for each cluster. The process iterates until the criterion function (e.g. square error) converges to a value close to the minimum.

The k-means algorithm has two primary advantages. It is easy to implement and is not computationally demanding. One of the major limitations of the algorithm relates the prior specification of the number of clusters. As it is not possible to theoretically determine the optimal number of clusters, several methods were proposed (see [24] for a review). In this paper, we used the well-known Bayesian Information Criterion (BIC) developed by [25] to find the number of clusters to retain. BIC identifies a model that optimally balances model fit and complexity. The appropriate number of clusters corresponds to the clustering model with the smallest BIC value.

3 Data and Sample

The sample analyzed in this paper included 17 municipalities from the metropolitan area of Lisbon (the Portuguese capital). The longitudinal assessment covered the period between 2003 and 2009. The Lisbon region can be considered a medium-sized

European metropolitan area, with more than 2.8 million residents according to the 2011 census. At a national level, about 26 % of Portugal habitants are in the Lisbon region, and it assumes a central role in the economic activity of the country. The data used in this paper came from the study carried out by [26] that analyzed the urban metabolism of Lisbon. The data used by [26] was collected from two distinct databases: the National Statistics Institute (INE) and the Studies, Statistics and Planning General Directorate from the Ministry of Labor and Social Security.

Table 1 presents descriptive statistics for each municipality during the period analyzed, namely the population, the municipality area, the ratio between the number of new apartment buildings, the total number of new residential buildings, including new apartment buildings and detached houses (named apartment buildings hereafter), the ratio between the number of new dwellings owned by private entities and the total number of new dwellings owned by public and private entities (named private ownership hereafter), the average value of bank evaluation (measured in euros per square meter) to proxy building quality, the ratio between the number of rehabilitated buildings and the total number of new and rehabilitated buildings (named rehabilitation level hereafter), and the floor area built of new residential buildings (measured in square meters). This information was collected from the INE.

As we can observe in Table 1, Lisbon municipalities are quite diverse in terms of population and geographic area. In particular, there are municipalities, such as Montijo, Alcochete and Palmela with low population density, whereas municipalities such as Odivelas and Amadora are highly populated. It is interesting to observe that in most municipalities the majority of new residential buildings are detached houses, owned by private entities. In addition, the average value of bank evaluation is around 1400 €/m^2 in the Lisbon region, with the highest average values observed in Loures and Palmela and the lowest value observed in Montijo.

Rehabilitation projects have a relatively small expression in Lisbon municipalities (average proportion of rehabilitation is around 7.5 %), although a few municipalities exhibit higher levels of rehabilitation activity such as Cascais. The municipalities with high floor area built of new residential buildings correspond to Cascais and Loures, and the municipalities of Alcochete and Moita exhibited low new construction activity. According to INE database, the data available concerning the floor area built of new residential buildings for the Lisbon city is underestimated, so this municipality was not included in this study.

Table 1. Municipalities descriptive indicators, mean 2003–2009.

Municipality	Population (hab)	Municipality area (sq.km)	Apartment buildings (%)	Private ownership (%)	Building quality (€/m^2)	Rehabilitation level (%)	Floor area (sq.m)
Alcochete	18113	100.3	23.7	98.8	1423.5	2.0	23886
Almada	165991	69.7	16.3	99.6	1402.7	0.0	63728
Amadora	170828	23.8	82.4	99.4	1503.7	0.0	62923
Barreiro	77529	32.1	40.9	100.0	1238.2	10.4	39593
Cascais	189606	96.9	24.7	99.9	1225.2	48.6	128935
Loures	193630	167.6	27.2	99.6	1833.1	0.8	127885

(Continued)

Table 1. (*Continued*)

Municipality	Population (hab)	Municipality area (sq.km)	Apartment buildings (%)	Private ownership (%)	Building quality ($€/m^2$)	Rehabilitation level (%)	Floor area (sq.m)
Mafra	73061	290.9	16.9	99.7	1469.0	17.6	107959
Moita	71844	44.1	27.1	98.3	1331.5	3.7	27173
Montijo	41623	343.3	44.6	89.6	1127.0	4.1	65585
Odivelas	155827	26.5	19.5	100.0	1282.1	5.8	99447
Oeiras	172609	45.7	35.3	100.0	1456.2	0.3	78723
Palmela	63861	458.3	14.0	95.4	1641.1	8.7	60011
Seixal	178332	88.8	18.9	99.9	1228.0	2.0	79182
Sesimbra	54525	193.3	12.6	98.7	1355.6	0.6	40602
Setúbal	125293	175.1	11.8	99.0	1422.6	9.1	65542
Sintra	454188	318.3	17.8	99.0	1242.3	10.8	119010
V. F. Xira	144123	267.9	39.0	100.0	1279.8	3.1	95117

Based on the review of literature [27–29], it can be concluded that the materials most used in the construction of residential buildings include: concrete, steel, wood, glass, tiles, plaster and aluminum. Thus, the performance assessment model was specified including variables representing the major construction materials identified. The categories considered are those proposed by [30] for a Material Flow Analysis: metals, non-metallic minerals, fossil fuels and biomass.

In terms of variables definition, metals include steel, light metals, other ferrous and non-ferrous metals. Non-metallic minerals include sand, cement, clay, stone, and other non-metallic minerals. Fossil fuels include fossil fuels, lubricants, oils, solvents, plastic and rubbers. Biomass includes wood, fuels, paper, board, and textile biomass. All these variables are measured in tonnes. Table 2 reports the mean values of the inputs used in the DEA assessment for each municipality over the period analyzed.

From Table 2, it is possible to observe that non-metallic minerals are the materials most used in buildings construction in all municipalities, followed by metals and fossil fuels.

Table 2. Material flows descriptive statistics, mean 2003–2009.

Municipality	Fossil fuels (t)	Metals (t)	Non-metallic (t)	Biomass (t)
Alcochete	903	952	15652	138
Almada	5994	6279	103996	911
Amadora	8300	8703	144054	1262
Barreiro	1302	1382	22663	200
Cascais	3844	3908	65939	574
Loures	8265	8685	143563	1257
Mafra	1932	2018	33481	293
Moita	1904	1993	33030	289

(*Continued*)

Table 2. (*Continued*)

Municipality	Fossil fuels (t)	Metals (t)	Non-metallic (t)	Biomass (t)
Montijo	1646	1725	28534	250
Odivelas	5168	5448	89803	787
Oeiras	9068	9517	157416	1378
Palmela	2831	2941	49119	428
Seixal	6471	6806	112466	985
Sesimbra	3517	3689	61054	535
Setbal	3257	3394	56308	494
Sintra	12562	13162	218341	1906
V. F. Xira	4660	4861	80694	707

To verify the adequacy of using the set of input and output variables in the DEA model, an isotonicity test was conducted [31]. This involved the determination of correlation coefficients between the inputs and the output to identify whether increasing amounts of inputs lead to greater output. The Pearson correlation coefficients estimated are positive (ranging between 0.43 and 0.45) and significant at a 1 % level for all relationships between each input and the output variable, so the principle of isotonicity is satisfied. This shows that the inclusion of all variables in the DEA model is a consistent option.

4 Empirical Results

In this section, we first present the municipal performance in terms of the environmental efficiency estimates of new residential buildings construction. The efficiency scores for each municipality were estimated based on a comparison with a pooled frontier representing the best practices observed in the 7 years analyzed. Table 3 reports the efficiency scores obtained using model (1), as well as the grand mean for each year and municipality. Table 3 also specifies the cluster attributed to each municipality in a given year inside the square brackets.

To test the robustness of the DEA efficiency estimates in relation to outliers, we applied the jackknifing procedure. Jackknifing was first introduced by [32] and it is a resampling method. For a sample with n observations, jackknife involves the construction of n samples each with n-1 observations, omitting a different observation in each sample. As proposed by [33, 34], DEA models were run dropping one efficient municipality each time. As we only have one efficient observation in the sample, the jackknife procedure involved running an additional DEA model that excludes Mafra in 2003 from the assessment. Following the procedure adopted by [33, 34], we conducted the Spearman rank correlation test to evaluate the similarity of performance rankings between the DEA model with all municipalities and with the removal of the efficient municipality. The correlation coefficient is equal to 0.97 and is significant at a 1 %

level, which indicates that the ranking is not affected by the removal of the efficient municipality. This indicates that Mafra in 2003 should not be considered an outlier.

Looking at the results reported in Table 3, we can observe considerable variability in performance trends over the years. Some municipalities show an improvement trend (e.g. Odivelas), others a declining trend (e.g. Almada), but most municipalities appear to have an irregular pattern. This suggests that keeping consistently high environmental efficiency levels for long periods is arduous. Based on these results, we recommend the promotion of self-diagnosis in each municipality. This would enable the identification of the best practices implemented over the years in order to improve performance in the future.

Analyzing the efficiency estimates in more detail, it is possible to verify that some municipalities, such as Mafra and Montijo, achieved significantly higher environmental efficiency scores than others, such as Amadora and Oeiras. This means that there is a large gap in municipal performance levels, suggesting a high potential for improvement in most municipalities.

A few factors could potentially explain the spread in the performance levels observed in Lisbon municipalities. First, the municipalities that construct more apartment buildings than detached houses may be able to be more efficient in terms of materials usage. Apartments within a building are constructed using a repeated process that tends to be less demanding in terms of resource consumption than detached houses. Second, the average quality levels of buildings in different municipalities may be different. The building quality is typically associated with the exterior and interior finishing materials, as they enable to enhance the usability and aesthetic features of the building. Third, the proportion of private vs public ownership buildings constructed in each municipality may also explain the spread in environmental efficiency. For instance, [35]

Table 3. Environmental efficiency results.

Munici-pality	2003		2004		2005		2006		2007		2008		2009		Mean
Alcochete	0.43	[C1]	0.29	[C1]	0.21	[C1]	0.36	[C1]	0.27	[C1]	0.31	[C1]	0.33	[C1]	0.31
Almada	0.17	[C1]	0.12	[C2]	0.14	[C2]	0.10	[C2]	0.11	[C2]	0.14	[C2]	0.08	[C3]	0.12
Amadora	0.06	[C3]	0.06	[C3]	0.08	[C3]	0.10	[C2]	0.13	[C2]	0.13	[C2]	0.09	[C3]	0.09
Barreiro	0.44	[C1]	0.31	[C1]	0.26	[C1]	0.31	[C1]	0.50	[C1]	0.36	[C1]	0.26	[C1]	0.35
Cascais	0.13	[C2]	0.38	[C1]	0.48	[C1]	0.56	[C1]	0.38	[C1]	0.61	[C1]	0.56	[C1]	0.44
Loures	0.19	[C1]	0.17	[C1]	0.10	[C2]	0.15	[C2]	0.22	[C1]	0.24	[C1]	0.24	[C1]	0.19
Mafra	1.00	[C1]	0.60	[C1]	0.60	[C1]	0.60	[C1]	0.53	[C1]	0.60	[C1]	0.70	[C1]	0.66
Moita	0.35	[C1]	0.10	[C2]	0.13	[C2]	0.13	[C2]	0.11	[C2]	0.19	[C1]	0.21	[C1]	0.17
Montijo	0.34	[C1]	0.37	[C1]	0.30	[C1]	0.48	[C1]	0.52	[C1]	0.88	[C1]	0.55	[C1]	0.49
Odivelas	0.05	[C3]	0.14	[C2]	0.19	[C1]	0.30	[C1]	0.25	[C1]	0.31	[C1]	0.40	[C1]	0.23
Oeiras	0.12	[C2]	0.10	[C2]	0.05	[C3]	0.08	[C3]	0.12	[C2]	0.15	[C2]	0.11	[C2]	0.10
Palmela	0.32	[C1]	0.20	[C1]	0.27	[C1]	0.27	[C1]	0.12	[C2]	0.31	[C1]	0.25	[C1]	0.25
Seixal	0.13	[C2]	0.09	[C2]	0.11	[C2]	0.16	[C1]	0.15	[C2]	0.22	[C1]	0.20	[C1]	0.15
Sesimbra	0.28	[C1]	0.11	[C2]	0.10	[C2]	0.13	[C2]	0.10	[C2]	0.10	[C2]	0.14	[C2]	0.14
Setúbal	0.32	[C1]	0.18	[C1]	0.14	[C2]	0.23	[C1]	0.22	[C1]	0.28	[C1]	0.39	[C1]	0.25
Sintra	0.19	[C1]	0.08	[C3]	0.09	[C2]	0.12	[C2]	0.09	[C2]	0.10	[C2]	0.11	[C2]	0.11
V.F. Xira	0.28	[C1]	0.27	[C1]	0.16	[C2]	0.22	[C1]	0.29	[C1]	0.22	[C1]	0.24	[C1]	0.24
Mean	0.28		0.21		0.20		0.25		0.24		0.30		0.29		

concluded that private projects outperformed public projects in terms of cost and schedule deviations, and also implemented a higher number of best practices.

In order to guide environmental efficiency improvements, it is important to quantify the impact of these factors on environmental efficiency. For this purpose, we conducted a truncated regression as proposed by [36]. The model specified for the analysis was formulated using the environmental efficiency score as the dependent variable, and the apartment buildings, private ownership, and building quality as regressors (see the descriptive statistics of regressors in Table 1). We also included time and municipality dummies in the model to control for year and municipality effects.

Table 4 reports the estimates from the panel data truncated model, the coefficients, standard errors and p-values. The total number of observations included in the model was 119, corresponding to the 17 municipalities analyzed in the 7 years. The overall regression model was found to be statistically significant (χ_2 test with p-value < 0.0001, with a pseudo R^2 equal to 0.80).

From the analysis of the results reported on Table 4, we can conclude that building type is an important factor to explain municipal performance. The positive coefficient indicates that apartment buildings have higher environmental efficiency, meaning that fewer materials are consumed per square meter built. Although the literature suggests that private projects outperform public projects in terms of cost and schedule deviations, we have found no significant relationship between environmental efficiency levels of new buildings construction and ownership type. Similarly, we found no evidence that building quality has a significant impact on environmental efficiency levels. Note that this result should be interpreted with caution due to the limitation associated to the measurement of the building quality variable. This variable was measured by a proxy, corresponding to the average value of bank evaluation, which depends not only on the quality of the construction and materials used but also on the location of the buildings.

Based on these results, benchmarking efforts to improve environmental efficiency should take into account the profile of the municipality in terms of the type of buildings constructed (apartments vs. detached houses).

Table 4. Truncated regression results.

Variable	Coefficient	Standard error	p-value
Apartment buildings	0.004	0.001	0.000
Private ownership	−0.002	0.003	0.520
Building quality	−0.027	0.109	0.805
Constant	0.421	0.293	0.151

Next, the k-mean algorithm was used to identify groups of municipalities with similar levels of environmental efficiency and comparable profiles in terms of materials' consumption per square meter built. Therefore, the segmentation of municipalities was based on five variables: environmental efficiency score, fossil fuels per square meter, metals per square meter, non-metallic minerals per square meter, and biomass per square meter.

Using the Bayesian Information criterion (BIC), the most appropriate number of clusters was found to be three. Tables 3 and 5 provide a comprehensive characterization of the clusters identified. Table 5 presents the distribution of the 119 observations analyzed, the mean efficiency score and the mean consumption of each type of construction material for the three clusters.

Table 5. Clusters' description.

Cluster	No. obs.	Mean efficiency	Mean fossil fuels per m^2	Mean metals per m^2	Mean non-metals per m^2	Mean biomass per m^2
C1	71	0.35	0.04	0.04	0.69	0.01
C2	39	0.12	0.10	0.11	1.76	0.02
C3	9	0.07	0.18	0.17	3.07	0.03

From Table 5, we can observe that cluster C1, with 71 observations, is constituted by the best municipalities (mean efficiency equals 0.35) with low materials' consumption per square meter. Cluster C2, with 39 observations, includes the municipalities with intermediate consumption levels for all materials (mean efficiency equals 0.12). Cluster C3, with 9 observations, is composed by the municipalities with the worst performance levels (mean efficiency equals 0.07), where the highest levels of materials consumption per square meter were observed.

Municipalities belonging to cluster C3 should be given priority in the implementation of performance improvement practices. In turn, it is important to highlight that four municipalities (Alcochete, Barreiro, Mafra, Montijo) managed to belong to cluster C1 in all years analyzed (see clusters in Table 3). Therefore, municipalities from cluster C3 could learn with the best practices adopted by this subset of four municipalities in order to improve environmental efficiency. For instance, in year 2009, Almada and Amadora could focus their attention in municipalities such as Montijo or Mafra.

5 Conclusions

This paper develops an innovative methodology to evaluate municipal performance concerning the environmental efficiency of new buildings construction focusing on the usage of construction materials. The methodology proposed identifies the municipalities that urge environmental efficient improvements. The methodology developed combines the use of DEA with clustering analysis. It provides new insights for the definition of strategies leading to efficient materials' use. This objective is aligned with the provision of efficient services.

The empirical study revealed that the environmental efficiency in the construction of new buildings varies considerably among Lisbon municipalities, suggesting a wide potential for performance improvement. The exploratory study of the factors that can explain the differences in environmental efficiency levels revealed that building type can affect significantly the level of materials' usage. In particular, it was observed that improvements in the use of materials in detached houses can lead to considerable environmental efficiency enhancements.

In addition, it was found that the municipalities can be classified into three groups according to the efforts required to achieve environmental efficiency: some can be regarded as examples of best practices, others exhibit intermediate levels of environmental efficiency, and others need considerable improvements. This subset of municipalities should join synergies in the definition of policies towards the reduction of materials' use in new buildings construction. This can be supported by learning from the best performing municipalities.

Finally, other interesting avenues for future research could include the application of this methodology to evaluate municipal performance in terms of the efficiency of materials' consumption in industrial sectors (e.g. manufacturing), as well as in different metropolitan areas in order to disseminate best practices. The environmental efficiency evaluation could also be extended to other aspects of buildings life cycle, such as energy used in construction and operation phases. Furthermore, the study of other factors affecting environmental efficiency levels can be useful for the design of improvement policies promoted by regional authorities.

Acknowledgments. The authors are grateful to Leonardo Rosado from Chalmers University, Gothenburg, for compiling some of the data used in this study. The authors also acknowledge the financial support of the Portuguese Foundation for Science and Technology (FCT) through iTEAM project (MIT-Pt/SES-SUES/0041/2008) and MeSUr project (PTDC/SEN- ENR/111710/2009).

References

1. Cruz, N.F., Marques, R.C.: Revisiting the determinants of local government performance. Omega **44**, 91–103 (2014)
2. Horta, I.M., Camanho, A.S., Dias, T.G.: Residential building resource consumption: a comparison of Portuguese municipalities' performance. Cities **50**, 54–61 (2016)
3. CIB and UNEP-IETC: Agenda 21 for sustainable construction in developing countries. Technical report Bou/E0204 (2002)
4. Kibert, C.: Principles of sustainable construction. In: Proceedings of the First International Conference on Sustainable Construction, Tampa (1994)
5. Vatalis, K.I., Manoliadis, O.G., Charalampides, G.: Assessment of the economic benefits from sustainable construction in Greece. Int. J. Sustain. Dev. World **15**(5), 377–383 (2011)
6. Ding, G.K.: Sustainable construction: the role of environmental assessment tools. J. Environ. Manage. **86**(3), 451–464 (2008)
7. Ilha, M.S.O., Oliveira, L.H., Goncalves, O.M.: Environmental assessment of residential buildings with an emphasis on water conservation. Build. Serv. Eng. Res. Technol. **30**(1), 15–26 (2009)
8. Ramesh, T., Prakash, R., Shukla, K.K.: Life cycle energy analysis of buildings: an overview. Energy Build. **42**, 1592–1600 (2010)
9. Sharma, A., Saxena, A., Sethi, M., Shree, V.: Life cycle assessment of buildings: a review. Renew. Sustain. Energy Rev. **15**, 871–875 (2011)

10. Mwasha, A., Williams, R.G., Iwaro, J.: Modeling the performance of residential building envelope: the role of sustainable energy performance indicators. Energy Buildings **43**(9), 2108–2117 (2011)
11. Bribián, I., Capilla, A., Alfonso, U.: Life cycle assessment of building materials: comparative analysis of energy and environmental impacts and evaluation of the eco-efficiency improvement potential. Build. Environ. **46**, 1133–1140 (2011)
12. Bjorklund, T., Tillman, A. M.: LCA of building frame structures environmental impact over the life cycle of wooden and concrete frames. Technical Environmental Planning Report. Chalmers University of Technology, Uppsala, (1997)
13. Koroneos, C., Dompros, A.: Environmental assessment of brick production in Greece. Build. Environ. **42**(5), 2114–2123 (2007)
14. Traverso, M., Rizzo, G., Finkbeiner, M.: Environmental performance of building materials: life cycle assessment of a typical Sicilian marble. Int. J. Life Cycle Assess. **15**(1), 104–114 (2010)
15. Kim, K.H.: A comparative life cycle assessment of a transparent composite facade system and a glass curtain wall system. Energy Build. **43**(12), 3436–3445 (2011)
16. Schmidt, A.C., Jensen, A.A., Clausen, A.U., Kamstrup, O., Postlethwaite, D.: A comparative life cycle assessment of building insulation products made of stones wool, paper wool and flax. Int. J. Life Cycle Assess. **9**, 122–129 (2004)
17. Haapio, A.: Towards sustainable urban communities. Environ. Impact Assess. Rev. **32**(1), 165–169 (2012)
18. Charnes, A., Cooper, W.W., Rhodes, E.: Measuring efficiency of decision making units. Eur. J. Oper. Res. **2**(6), 429–444 (1978)
19. Simar, L., Wilson, P.: Non-parametric tests of returns to scale. Eur. J. Oper. Res. **139**(1), 115–132 (2002)
20. Efron, B.: Bootstrap methods: Another look at the jackknife. Ann. Stat. **7**(1), 1–26 (1979)
21. Cheng, Y.-M., Leu, S.S.: Constraint-based clustering and its applications in construction management. Expert Syst. Appl. **36**(3), 5761–5767 (2009)
22. David, G., Averbuch, A.: SpectralCAT: categorical spectral clustering of numerical and nominal data. Pattern Recognit. **45**(1), 416–433 (2012)
23. MacQueen, J. B.: Some methods for classification and analysis of multivariate observations. In: Proceeding of the fifth Berkeley Symposium on Mathematical Statistics and Probability. University of California Press, vol. 1, pp. 281–297 (1967)
24. Tibshirani, R., Walther, G., Hastie, T.: Estimating the number of clusters in a data set via the gap statistic. J. Roy. Stat. Soc.: Ser. B (Stat. Methodol.) **63**(2), 411–423 (2001)
25. Schwarz, G.: Estimating dimension of a model. Ann. Stat. **6**(2), 461–464 (1978)
26. Rosado, L., Niza, S., Ferrão, P.: A new method for urban material flow accounting: UMAn - a case study of the lisbon metropolitan area. J. Ind. Ecol. **18**(1), 84–101 (2014)
27. Asif, M., Muneer, T., Kelley, R.: Life cycle assessment: A case study of a dwelling home in Scotland. Build. Environ. **42**(3), 1391–1394 (2007)
28. Bastianoni, S., Galli, A., Pulselli, R.M., Niccolucci, V.: Environmental and economic evaluation of natural capital appropriation through building construction: practical case study in the Italian context. Ambio **36**(7), 559–565 (2007)
29. Shin, S., Tae, S., Woo, J., Roh, S.: The development of environmental load evaluation system of a standard Korean apartment house. Renew. Sustain. Energy Rev. **15**(2), 1239–1249 (2011)
30. EUROSTAT: Economy-wide material flow accounts and derived indicators: a methodological guide. Technical report, Statistical Office of the European Union, Luxembourg (2001)
31. Avkiran, N.: Productivity Analysis in the Service Sector with Data Envelopment Analysis. Camira, Queensland (1999)

32. Quenouille, M.: Approximate tests of correlation in time series. J. Roy. Stat. Soc. **11**(Series B), 68–84 (1949)
33. Charles, V., Kumar, M., Kavitha, S.I.: Measuring the efficiency of assembled printed circuit boards with undesirable outputs using data envelopment analysis. Int. J. Production Economics **136**(1), 194–206 (2012)
34. Mostafa, M.M.: Does efficiency matter?: examining the efficiency-profitability link in the US specialty retailers and food consumer stores. Int. J. Prod. Performance Manage. **59**(3), 255–273 (2010)
35. Hwang, B.G., Liao, P.C., Leonard, M.P.: Performance and practice use comparisons: public vs. private owner projects. KSCE J. Civil Eng. **15**(6), 957–963 (2011)
36. Simar, L., Wilson, P.: Estimation and inference in two-stage, semi-parametric models of production processes. J. Econometrics **136**(1), 31–64 (2007)

"Agile Adoption" in IT Companies - Building a Change Capability by Qualitative Description of Agile Implementation in Different Companies

Barbora Moravcová and Filip Legény[✉]

Department of Information Systems, Faculty of Management,
Comenius University in Bratislava,
Odbojárov 10, 820 05 Bratislava 25, Slovakia
barbora.moravcova@fm.uniba.sk, filip@legeny.sk

Abstract. As the interest in "Agile" Adoption continues to grow, there is an increasing need for organizations to understand how to adopt it successfully. This study has as objective to identify the concerns of deployment of agile practices and provide insight into existing challenges of adopting "Agile". First, the existing literature and case studies are reviewed. A definition of "Agile" Adoption is then formed based on the literature by breaking down the concept. The work deepens the understanding of the complex issue associated with "Agile" Adoption, contributes to the knowledge of "Agile" Adoption and improvement of the software development processes. We surveyed 5 companies, in total 200 employees. Finally, we present 25 impediments for the company's "Agile" Adoption that were identified based on the interviews. Software companies, who plan their current strategy for "Agile" Adoption, might use the processed output.

Keywords: Agile · Change · Challenges · Impediments · Change capability

1 Introduction

Organizations use various approaches to project management and to the models of conducting the development activities. Throughout history, these models of management have had various forms. The best known since the second part of 20th century up to now is the advance planning and strict adherence with the plan. This model is suitable for developing products in a stable and predictable environment, which however, is not typical for many companies [1]. As the interest in market continues to grow, companies are confronted with three fundamental problems of the product development as (1) continuous acceleration of market evolvement, (2) ability to change, and (3) the increasing complexity of the product [2]. The Fig. 1 below depicts the conditions [3, 4] for the development of products and services in the current unstable environment.

The speed of development activities is a major challenge for the development teams. The urgency to accelerate the development activities is advocated as well by

© Springer International Publishing Switzerland 2016
T. Borangiu et al. (Eds.): IESS 2016, LNBIP 247, pp. 251–262, 2016.
DOI: 10.1007/978-3-319-32689-4_19

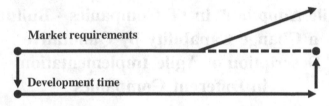

Fig. 1. Current state of the conditions for the development of products and services (own creation according to [3, 4])

Menon from a perspective of competitive economy. Menon argues [5] that a shortened product development cycle of a product will result in a competitive advantage. This argument corresponds with a contribution of J.T.Vesey's, an author of the idea [6] that traditional management practices were based on an idea of "comfortable time constraints". Experts in such practices were able to consider options and operate on the projects within a budget with low risk. With regards to the global competitive tender, a pressure is being put on managers to shorten the time for introduction of the products to the market.

A change creates new opportunities and it is often a cause for the development of new products. The market during the development of a new product may change. As a consequence of changes, the original specifics of the new product may become obsolete. After launching of a new product on market the other competing companies are forced to revise their plans. In the relation to the product development Stacey proposed a definition of complexity [7]. He claims, "(...) the nature and the number of sub-tasks, their organization and interrelationships, determine the complexity of the project". He is assessing a certainty of the predictability of the activities needed to carry out the work. The Fig. 2 indicates the three dimensions of the product development:

- Requirements scale from the very exact, with low risk of changes to vague requirements, followed by expected changes.
- Technology; very well known and understood and unknown, involving use of multiple technologies and products.
- People: verified and regular, including a small number of people in the team and the projects with more than five people, sometimes hundreds, that constantly changing [7].

While advance planning and strict adherence to the plan is suitable for projects from the simple quadrant from Stacey's graph as their exact requirements are known, "Agile" Approach is suitable for solving complicated projects. Agile manifesto [11] presents 12 principles, which should be respected by any agile framework, and considers (1) satisfaction of any customer with the early and continuous delivery of valuable software and (2) responding to change over following a plan. Continuous delivery and response to change is assured by iterative and incremental planning, with product cycles (3) from a couple of weeks to a couple of months, with a preference to

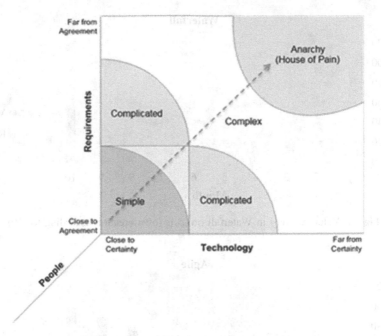

Fig. 2. Stacey's Graph (own creation regarding to [7])

the shorter timescale. Agile approach can be mapped to Menon's [5] argument for shorter product cycles and therefore, its application on value delivery should result in a competitive advantage.

One of the main drivers of "Agile" Adoption Approach is the need to accelerate time to reach the market. Traditional projects struggle to reach the market fast due to their waterfall approach; the funding is ongoing, but the value, in the form of actual product, is delivered only at the end of the project (Figs. 3, 4). The risk of project failure is accumulating and reaching the highest point at the time of the delivery, when the customer gets to review the finished product. Waterfall approach fixes the project scope in the beginning phases of development, which leads to a higher chance of discrepancy between customer expectations and the actual product. In contrary to the waterfall model, agile projects deliver value in iterations and increments and open up the possibility of scope adoption between each increment. Ongoing feedback loop prevents deviations between customer's expectations and the actual product and thus, the risk of project with each iteration failure is decreasing [8].

Accordingly, software applications development supported through the agile process have three times the success rate of the traditional waterfall approach, and a much lower percentage of time and cost overruns. The adaptive nature of agile development and openness to changes of the original scope is one of the factors why finished agile projects may rest classified as "challenged" and not be considered "successful" following the methodology used by Standish Group [8–10].

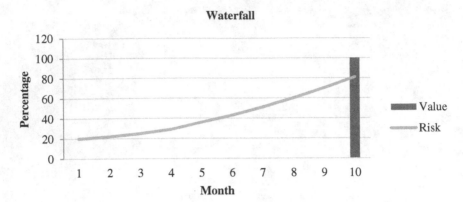

Fig. 3. Value delivery in Waterfall projects (own creation according to [10])

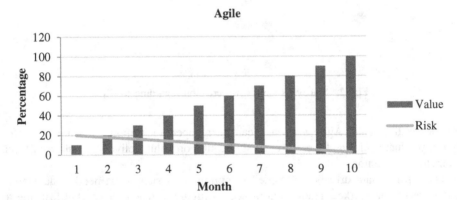

Fig. 4. Value delivery in agile projects (own creation according to [10])

2 The Concerns of Agile Practices Deployment

Change Management methods and tools during an Agile Adoption can play an important role to facilitate changes, in processes as well as in the corporate culture. According to the Lean Change Management [12, 13] the early involvement of people affected by the changes and the barriers between departments and companies have to be addressed by Organizational Change Management. However, the most important factor for success can be found in the role of senior management.

2.1 The Agile Adoption Reasons

The Agile Adoption might address the three challenges mentioned in introductory section [14]. Following statistics are based on the data in the "State of Agile 2015" annual report. The majority of respondents aim to focus on customer and to increase the predictability by the Agile Adoption. The results indicate [15] that after the transition to Agile up to 70 % of the projects got delivered to the customer and reached the market. Earlier than planned by adopting the Agile Adoption a 5 % of the projects reached the market later than by adopting the traditional approach. The Fig. 5 indicates three of the most frequently mentioned benefits of the Agile Adoption, which are (1) accelerate time to reach the market, (2) simplify a management of the changes prioritization, (3) align the IT with the business goals.

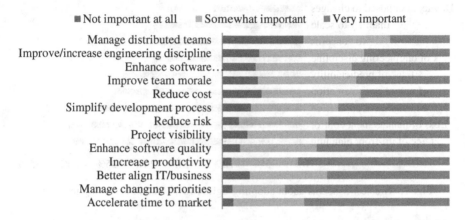

Fig. 5. Reason cited for Agile Adoption (own creation according to [15])

2.2 The Agile Adoption Failures

A traditionalist mindset [15] was indicated as the greatest barrier in the adoption process, followed by a resistance to change and the implementation of Agile practices in a traditional environment (Fig. 6). A time required to transition to Agile and the budgetary constraints have the negligible impact on the Agile Adoption.

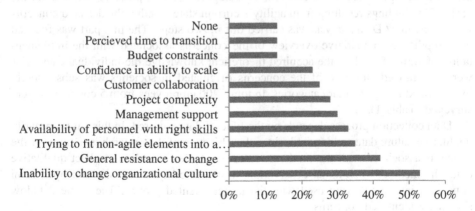

Fig. 6. Barriers to further Agile Adoption (own creation according to [15])

The most frequently recorded concern associated with the Agile Adoption, represented by 34 % was the absence of the one-off planning at the beginning of the project. Of losing their position feared 31 % of respondents (Fig. 7).

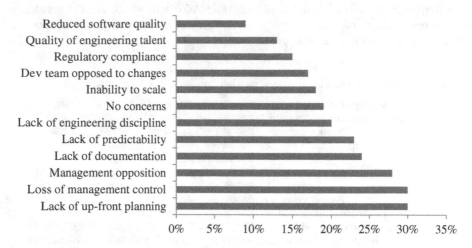

Fig. 7. Greatest concerns about adopting agile (own creation according to [15])

3   Empirical Data Gathering

The initial phase of the research was based on generalizations of the observed reality for the purpose of gaining a deeper insight of the essence of issues. As an outcome of the initial phase an early draft of research questions was created about Agile Adoption and the Agile practices in the software companies. Later on, by logical deductions based on the interviews conducted with the experts in Agile a formation of research questions was instanced as follows; what kind of concerns have you came across when transiting to Agile? Can these concerns be categorized? Is it possible to assess on the basis of the findings resulting from agility's current state whether the detected concerns were overcame? Data analysis was carried out in two steps. The first part was focused on compiling a comparative overview of the concerns associated with the implementation of Agile. Based on the acquired theoretical knowledge the individual categories were generalized and each of the concerns originated in societies was subsequently incorporated into particular categories. In total, 200 employees from 5 companies were surveyed (Table 1).

Data collection process depends on the type of data required. In this case, primarily qualitative nature data are required, since the objective of the research is to uncover the concerns associated with the implementation of Agile. In order to collect qualitative data, the methods such as an observation, a structured questionnaire and open semi structured interviews were used with the target-oriented groups. The Table 2 below shows the identified concerns.

Table 1. Overview of 5 surveyed companies (own creation)

	Company				
	A	B	C	D	E
Number of employees	500	More than 1000	50	500	100
Product and market	Offshore model – company provides human resources that are allocated into team based on customer requirements. A company is product-oriented.	Production system, tailored application development product service	Tailored Software development	ERP systems, cloud solutions, economic software	Navigation system
Location	A team distributed across 5 locations	Teams distributed across more than 5 locations in Slovakia	Teams are distributed within 1 location in Slovakia	Teams are distributed across 4 locations in Slovakia	1 Location
Target group	B2B, B2C	B2B, B2C, state listed companies	B2B	B2B, B2C, B2G	B2B, B2C, B2G, distributor, integrators
Adoption Duration	1 year	11 months	8 months	9 months	1 year
Agile practices	Scrum, Kanban	Scrum, Kanban	Scrum, Kanban	Scrum	Scrum

4 Post-analysis of Detected Concerns

The cases below represent the challenges identified in Chapter 3. The challenges from each case are listed in the Table 2. All challenges are analyzed according to the (1) organizational perspective and (2) viable solutions.

4.1 Case Company A

While the Agile Adoption in company A was the longest from the group, it was still very brief considering the number of employees impacted by the transition. The fear of changing tasks on the fly was based on the lack of understanding of Agile method-ologies and self-organizing teams. At the end of adoption, continuous change of tasks was adopted with positive feedback by the team and leaders. Embracement of self-organizing practices leads to a lower workload on managers outside the team and did not lead to a complete loss of control. In the opinion of management and subse-quent confirmation of the team members, successful change of the traditionalist

Table 2. The identified concerns categorized and mapped into dimensions (own creation)

Concerns...	Company				
	A	B	C	D	E
Existence of both traditional and Agile roles in company			X	X	
Creating of new roles can produce a fear of loss of the status within the company					X
By implementing of Agile the existing company rule swill be broken			X		
Time spent to familiarize with Agile and a training	X				X
Development teams haven't got sufficient knowledge of the business			X		
Loss of relaxed work atmosphere					
An organizational units allocation will not be based on the roles					
A changes of tasks on the fly	X		X		
Adjustment of the processes	X	X	X	X	
Decreased number of projects per one employee	X				
Results will not be achieved through selected method (Scrum, XP, Kanban)			X		
Incapability to implement the transparency into processes					
Agile practices adversaries	X		X	X	
Team stabilization without a change during the project					X
Inability to maintain motivation in the large multi-functional teams	X		X	X	
Management of the team will be outside of the team	X		X		
Increase in demand for social skills of developers			X	X	
Increase in demand for analytical skills of developers			X		
Change of mind set of the work force	X		X		
Increase in demand for presentation skills of developers			X		
A need to estimate the resources needed for development activities in the beginning of the process	X			X	
Prioritization of the tasks			X		
Management of the offshore teams					
The requirements will not be split into smaller parts prior the implementation (beginning of the project)		X			

thinking of people was achieved thanks to an extensive mentoring program executed by an external coach. External partner was able to dismantle most of the prejudices, and also provide enough clout to navigate around Agile practice adversaries. Since team members were able to see positive results of the change, their motivation was kept high.

Number of projects per employee was decreased as the company feared, but it did not resulted in decreased productivity. Survey showed that self-organized teams were able to focus more on tasks on hand, and were able to work more effectively with less context switching. At the end of the adoption, the company is able to deliver more projects in a year than it was able to deliver in previous period of the same length. Resource management was adjusted according to agile practices, and the company moved from fixed scope to fixed resources budgeting. Contracting practices were also transferred from fixed price contracts to time and means or fixed units where applicable.

4.2   Case Company B

Similar to the case of Company A, presence of a coach on board ensured a smooth transition to Agile and was cited as one of the key factors of success by the management of Company B. Concerns about errors resulting from not splitting requirements into smaller parts prior to the implementation was also based on previous development methodologies, and was proven as unjustified after the transition was complete. Management adapted multi-level planning process, where high-level planning happens on a change advisory board level. Weekly and daily planning activities fall into the competence of assigned product owner, who is also reporting to the CAB if necessary.

Currently the company is going through a phase where if the upper management helps the teams below to adapt mentally to the open culture and survive, and the company slowly begins to move towards enterprise agility.

4.3   Case Company C

Despite its smaller size, Company C was one of the most conservatives in the sample and presented most fears of them all. The young team enthusiastically supported Agile Adoption, but due to continuous malfunction of performed processes, this motivation started to decline. They are currently at the stage where the motivation is being re-gained by the help of an external coach who helps eliminate any discovered issues of concern, which have been confirmed. Initial concerns the management of the freedom of the teams were overcome, and teams are able to organize their work independently without the intervention of higher hierarchy levels. Team leader confirmed that young age of employees is seen as a benefit as it is relatively easy to steer in the right direction as far as for example presentation and social skills are concerned.

Company C was unique where fear of development teams' insufficient knowledge of the business was presented, but post-implementation survey showed that this fear was not justified. The company was small enough for information to propagate via osmotic methods of communication, and all teams and their leaders confirmed that understanding of the business in not a problem during planning of sprints or during execution of any related planning tasks.

4.4   Case Company D

An initial fear of coexistence of both traditional and agile roles in the company was confirmed. Company D is still dominated by a traditionalist and conservative thinking attitude of individuals, which complicates the deployment of agile frameworks. Strong support of the management board, however, may gradually steer the teams in accordance with agile values and transform the company as a whole. Head of development thinks that promoting positive attitude towards learning on mistakes can motivate all teams to embrace change and reduce the number of opponents to the idea of Agile Adoption on enterprise scale. Teams that started transitioning have mixed feelings, and lack of cooperation and ability to keep the pace up from non-Agile teams is cited as a dominant factor contributing to the decrease of motivation. Actions are to be taken by the head of the development in order to address the issue. Some team leaders are also considering calling on an external partner to help team better organize and reduce the impact of external environment on their work.

Help of external partner is also considered due to increased exposure of team members to external environment. Many team members feel that they are not well prepared to actively participate and give demonstrations during Review ceremonies. The fear of increase in demand for social skills was indeed confirmed in these cases, but new head of development is willing to invest in the employees once the environment is prepared to absorb these changes. Estimation and planning process underwent only minor changes at the moment, as majority of the organization is still running with fixed scope projects in mind. Agile teams see this as a roadblock, as their projects can't be considered Agile when parts of the scope are fixed beforehand.

4.5   Case Company E

Company E was a very strong organization with a clear direction and very clear vision of enterprise agility and along with Company B lowest number of fears of the implementation. Transition to Agile has lead to the shifting of roles, but did not result in employee dismissals. Leaders became scrum masters, or were assigned different duties in supporting teams. Those who did not possess sufficient knowledge required for the servant-leader role participated in training and coaching programs. As management stated, the overall training time was longer than expected and indeed confirmed their initial fear, but trainings provided by an external partner proved to be very effective and were one of the key factors that helped them achieve positive adoption results.

5   Conclusion

The answers to the research questions are not trivial, because they contain several aspects, which are tied up to each other. Diversity of the detected fear of Agile Adoption carries in itself a meaning in relation to the development teams and the company as a whole. Some sections are explicitly linked to the activities of the development teams and the others are linked to the implementation of Agile into the traditional environment. For the purpose of understanding the complex diversity of the detected concerns, these were categorized into dimensions. After mapping all the concerns there was created a separate category "Agile in the traditional organization", which is not included in and does not explicitly flow from the Agile Manifesto. The existence of the mentioned concerns relevant from the perspective of individual companies have been demonstrated. Although their occurrence in organisation in some cases has slowed or interrupted Agile Adoption, it was not a barrier that would stop this adoption process. A systematic cooperation of a coach and a management teams bridged almost all arising conflicts of the Agile Adoption process.

References

1. Moravcova, B., Gregus, M.: Agile adoption in IT companies. In: Theory and Practice in Management. Slovakia, pp. 113–121 (2013)
2. Cohn, M.: Succeeding with Agile, Software Development Using Scrum. Addison-Wesley Professional, Michigan (2010)
3. Smith, P.G.: Flexible Product Development – Building Agility for Changing Markets. Wiley, California (2007)
4. Kryvinska, N.: Building consistent formal specification for the service enterprise agility foundation - the society of service science. J. Serv. Sci. Res. 4(2), 235–269 (2012)
5. Menon, A., Chowdhury, J., Lukas, B.A.: Antecedents outcomes of new product development speed: an interdisciplinary conceptual framework. Ind. Mark. Manag. 31(4), 317–328 (2002)
6. Vesey, J.T.: The new competitors: they think in terms of 'speed-to-market'. Society for the Advancement of Management, Ocean Drive (1991)
7. Stacey, R.D.: Complexity and Management: Fad or Radical Challenge to Systems Thinking (Complexity and Emergence in Organizations). Routledge (2010)
8. Urikova, O., Ivanochko, I., Kryvinska, N., Strauss, C., Zinterhof, P.: Consideration of aspects affecting the evolvement of collaborative eBusiness in service organizations. Int. J. Serv. Econ. Manag. 5(1/2), 72–92 (2013)
9. Boehm, B.W.: Software Engineering Economics. 767. Prentice Hall, New Jersey (1981)
10. Verheyen, G.: Measuring Success, Measuing Value (2014). https://www.scrum.org/
11. Agile Manifesto (2001). http://agilemanifesto.org/
12. Little, J.: Lean Change Management - Innovative Practices For Managing Organizational Change. Happy Melly Express, Austria (2014)
13. Stoshikj, M., Kryvinska, N., Strauss, C.: Project management as a service. In: The 15th International Conference on Information Integration and Web-based Applications & Service, Austria, pp. 220–228 (2013)
14. Apello, J.: Management 3.0, Leading Agile Developers, And Developing Agile Leaders. Addison-Wesley Professional, Boston (2011)
15. 8th Annual state of Agile Development Survey, Versionone (2015). https://www.versionone.com/
16. Highsmith, J.: Agile Project Management. Addison-Wesley Professional, Boston (2009)
17. Jongbae, K., Wilemon, D.: The learning organization as facilitator of complex NPD projects. Creativity Innov. Manag. 16, 176–191 (2007)

18. McConnell, S.: Code Complete: A Practical Handbook of Software Construction. 960, 2nd edn. Microsoft Press, Southpark Place Grove (2004)
19. Snowden, D.: A Leader's Framework for Decision Making. Harvard Bus. Rev. **85**, 20–30 (2007)
20. Stoshikj, M., Kryvinska, N., Strauss, C.: Efficient managing of complex programs with project management services. Glob. J. Flex. Syst. Manag. **15**(1), 25–38 (2014). Special Issue on Flexible Complexity Management and Engineering by Innovative Services

Technology for Soccer Sport: The Human Side in the Technical Part

Luisa Varriale[✉] and Domenico Tafuri

University of Naples "Parthenope", via Medina, N. 40, 80132 Naples, Italy
{luisa.varriale,domenico.tafuri}@uniparthenope.it

Abstract. This paper aims to analyze how new technologies are applied in the sport field with specific focus on soccer sport and the related training process. Recently, different areas in the sport sector have been deeply changed thanks to technology, mainly information technology (IT) and internet, with relevant social and economic effects. Starting from the different sub-organizational areas identified in the literature (sport management, sport medicine, athletes' performance improvement, disability and social integration, sporting event management process), this paper focuses on the soccer sport, evidencing the main effects derived from the technology in terms of the cohabitation of human side and technical part in this specific team sport. This phenomenon is still under searched, so this theoretical study, conducted through a deep review of the literature, aims to propose a more clear picture of the social, economic and technical implications of technology in the soccer area, also identifying new research perspectives.

Keywords: Technology · Sport · Soccer · Training · Performance improvement

1 Introduction

In the last decades, thanks to the support of technology individuals tend to significantly reduce the physical interactions in many processes which historically required direct and in person collaborations between participants. Consequently people tend to adopt virtual means in their daily life, such as e-commerce, ATMs automatic teller machines, online distance learning systems [1, 2], and so forth [3]. Thus, an increasing use of the Internet and all the other innovative technologies has characterized the world economy, especially the services industry [4], e.g. educational, tourism and sport fields; individuals tend to use more and more on line programs, all e-learning and e-training programs in order to save time and money [5, 6]. Similarly, the world economy, because of high levels of competiveness, innovativeness, and globalization, is deeply changed.

In this scenario briefly described, the adoption of IT is remarkably changing and transform all the main aspects of human life thanks to the contribution of human-computer interaction (HCI) involving specific fields, such as sport setting, which traditionally was not recognized very relevant in terms of economic impact but only recently it plays a crucial role as significant business. The sport field has been also characterized from important changes for the technology arousing the increasing interest by scholars

© Springer International Publishing Switzerland 2016
T. Borangiu et al. (Eds.): IESS 2016, LNBIP 247, pp. 263–276, 2016.
DOI: 10.1007/978-3-319-32689-4_20

and practitioners who are searching for more effective and efficient tools to manage this business.

In this paper, the authors want to investigate the main application areas and challenges of new technologies in the sport field with specific focus on soccer training area. More specifically, drawing from previous studies in the literature on this topic, this paper aims at investigating the specific sub-organizational area of the soccer sport, mainly soccer training. The main IT applications have been identified and investigated in the soccer team sport for the training process outlining the relevant changes with consequent effects in terms of final performance for the athletes. Hence, we analyze the main insights and challenges concerning the application of IT in the area of soccer training. Indeed, we propose to exam in which way IT can affect the soccer training without missing the human side of this process because of the increasing attention paid to the technical part. Lately the introduction of internet or IT has contributed to promote the development of the sport field thanks to the search of strategies to improve athletes' performance or manage a broad range of information and data. Relevant implications of IT and internet applications concern specific sport disciplines areas, such as the soccer team sport, and, specifically, its training process.

Thanks to computer-mediated-communication (CMC) and, in general, HCI, technology can significantly affect sport in its facts. Although numerous technologies have been introduced in sport, in terms of software, technical instruments or digital programs to support the athletes' performance, this phenomenon is still underrepresented in the literature especially with reference to the specific soccer discipline, with focus on the training process.

This is a theoretical study conducted through a deep and systematic review of the literature aimed to identify and analyze the main insights and challenges related the new technologies application, specifically innovative digital programs and technical instruments, in the soccer training and to propose new research perspectives. The structure of paper is as follows: in the Sect. 2 the sport context is briefly described and also the role played by technology has been investigated, observing the interesting increase of HCI in many application areas. In the Sect. 3 the specific application areas of new technologies in the sport field have been described starting from previous studies on the issue evidencing the main related challenges. The Sect. 4 is focused on the specific soccer discipline sport area with concern to the training process of athletes analyzing the main innovative technologies introduced and applied with their implications. Finally, the Sect. 5 shows some final remarks about the phenomenon investigated.

2   Sport and Role of Technology

Different perspectives and various ways of interpreting sport have been adopted in defining sport in the most contributions in the literature. In some definitions physical and competitive elements inside sport issue have been emphasized, while in others the cultural determinants have been considered.

Moreover, other definitions tend to consider the institutionalization of sporting forms and the increasing significance of rewards, largely financial, that overcome the personal satisfaction, in order to identify broader factors which contribute to make a clear definition of the contemporary sporting landscape. In this direction, scholars and practitioners pay their attention to the codification process of sport evidencing the need of an organizational formal structure that governs its development. For instance, sport concept has been closely associated by North-Americans with competitive game applying some main elements, such as time, space, formalized rules [7]. Additional definitions enrich the sport concept incorporating non-competitive elements, such as recreation and health, so it is possible to have a more comprehensive and clear interpretation of the phenomenon [8–11].

The slogan "Sport for All" is very popular in the global world giving a clear message about the chance that individuals have to be engaged in any kind of physical activity, both passive and active forms, that is passive forms concern mobilization or postural passive alignment, while more highly active forms regard walking or playing competitive football [12].

In addition, in the last three decades, numerous contributions in the literature have focused on the sport issue considered as the expression of physical and cultural phenomenon. According to the several studies on sport field which cross traditional disciplinary boundaries, e.g. history, sociology or socio-political science, some authors argue that the sport term can be used "to describe a wide spectrum of culturally defined physical activities with considerable variation in the level and nature of organization and competition" [13: 5].

Furthermore, in the last decades sport phenomenon has deeply enriched its meaning with new elements, keeping the 'fun' element as a central characteristic, more related to the developed societies, with an increasing attention paid to the political and economic changes occurred.

In this direction, technology represents one interesting theme widely discussed and investigated in the academic and practical sport literature, mainly the link between sport and new technologies, that is information technology and all the innovative technological tools.

Loland [14] has argued that the sport technology term can assume different expressions on the basis of the different philosophical perspectives. "Sport technology represents a certain type of means to realize human interests and goals in sport. Such technology ranges from body techniques, via traditional sport equipment used by athletes within competition, to performance-enhancing machines, substances, and methods used outside of the competitive setting" [14: 1]. In competitive sport all the discussions on the theme consider several interpretations in terms of practices, such as athletic performance [14]. Loland [14] identified three ideal-typical theoretical frameworks to evidence the main implications: the non-theory (that is to find the way to achieve the goals through the sport), the thin theory (in this case sport is conceived as an arena for testing out the performance potential of the humans); the thick theory of athletic performance that is based on equality of opportunity and conceives sport as an arena for moral values and for human self-development and enrichment [14].

In addition, several information technologies, such as systems, vision, audition, and proprioception, have been applied to give feedback to the athletes with the aim to improve their performance [15].

Academics and practitioners widely recognize the role of technology in the sport field with its different applications and functions. In this broad range of applications and ways to consider the link between sport and technology we aim to clarify and systematize the existing studies on the phenomenon in the soccer discipline.

3   Application Areas and Challenges of Sport Technology

A recent depth review of the literature focused on the role of technology in the sport setting [16] has identified five different areas of application of IT and all the innovative technologies.

The following five application areas for the new technologies applied in the sport field have been distinguished [16: 209]:

- "Sport Management (that concerns all studies aimed to investigate the following themes in the sport field: ethics, media and communication, infrastructures, gender diversity, sport infrastructures, innovation systems, sport programs and computer processing. All these issues have been analyzed with reference to the technology, hence, its specific impact on them);
- Sport Medicine (that includes studies focused on the link between technology and sport adopting a medical perspective, that is features as the impact of technology on the athletes' health, the innovative discovering of techniques to support individuals, also seniors, and so forth. The presence of the words medicine, medical, health, wellness allow to identify this application area);
- Sport Disability (that is referred to all the applications of new technologies for allowing people with disability to practice sport or in general physical activities, and also innovative instruments to acquire major autonomy);
- Sport Events (which consists of all the studies on sport events only if they represent innovative events thanks to the adoption of new and more interesting technologies to manage data and information or to realize spectacular ceremonies, and also to monitor, control and measure the results related to all the aspects and phases of sport events);
- Athletes' performance (this area regards all the technologies, like prosthesis or specific innovative equipments, that can really produce an high impact on the athletes' performance; in fact, some useful technological instruments find application to improve continuously the athletes' performance, searching for the best result)".

The Social-Cognitive Theory and the Transtheoretical Model represent the most theoretical frameworks applied in the prevalent studies on the topic with reference mainly to the athletes' performance research area, and the broader Social Marketing model that has been linked to physical activity programs and campaigns.

The Sport Management represents the main search area, considering several interesting sub-themes, "such as how the new technologies impact on the definition of the rules of the game (see e.g. the deep changes occurred in the regulatory system of the Football competitions), on the coaching practices for athletes with the adoption of ad hoc sports management softwares (see e.g. the case of the German Football Team at the

2014 World Football Cup), on the leisure and entertainment (see e.g. the development of the innovative channels for the communication, that is electronic mass media able to show the sport competitions in real time), and on the ethical relevance of the issue" [17–22]. "Considering the athletes' performance, diverse information technologies used to provide relevant feedback to the athletes have been investigated" [15: 209–210].

With reference to the sport events application area, IT plays a key role especially in the sport event management process because it can facilitate and control information and data sharing, especially because of the economic, social, environmental and organizational effects difficult to predict. In this case several and readable applications of IT and control tools in many areas can be applied, such as transportation service, security, health care assistance, financial, socio-economic and cultural impact analysis, communication service, tourism, and so forth.

For instance, in the 2002 Winter Olympic Games in Salt Lake City becomes was applied ICT in the health care service for athletes, event participants, organizers, volunteers, and tourists. Indeed, an "information service system" was implemented to assist hospitals in the medical surveillance [23]. Also, another information service system, named COMPASS2008, was used as software for planning the 2008 Olympic Games in Beijing, considering the mobile digital, multilingual and multimodal companion for participants and visitors [24]. Within each OCOG (Organizing Committee for the Olympic Games), the Olympic Knowledge Service (OKS), uses the TOK (Transfer of Olympic Knowledge), a specific software to manage all data and information regarding sport events, which was implemented in the Sydney Olympic Games 2000 [25–27]. Besides, another sophisticated system, PLATO (Process Logistics Advanced Technical Optimization), was developed in the Athens 2004 Olympic Games for using innovative techniques in all the phases and services related to the planning, design and operation of venues [28].

In the Sport Disability area, people with disabilities can perform sport activities without high risks or any difficulties using innovative and advanced technological instruments (high quality standard prosthesis, software to monitor athletes with disabilities) [29–32]. Thus, the new technologies with all its forms in the sport field significantly affects the traditional development of the sport activities, changing deeply the human interactions because of the increasing attention to the "technical part" of the sport.

Moreover, scholars have increasingly investigated the impact of technologies on the athletes' performance to highly improve it [15, 32–35]. Also, the training process for athletes has been analyzed, in fact, Bettoli [36] has outlined the useful support provided by information technology and computers in sport teaching situations, helping to simplify and increase the efficiency of working procedures, enhance professionalism and provide a platform for effective team work; while, Ross [37] investigated computer programs useful to sports and recreation instruments, including important features, such as team capacity, league formation, scheduling conflicts, scheduling formats, master schedule, team schedules, reports, team rosters, standings, and optical scanning.

In this wide range of applications and ways to consider the technology and its implications in the sport field, we consider specific innovative technological tools applied in the soccer sport, paying more attention to training area.

4   Technology for Soccer Sport

In this theoretical study, we conducted a broad review of the literature considering only published studies in the sport field clearly focused on the new technologies in the soccer sport, mainly training for athletes, from a 30-year period (1985 to 2015). In details, we conducted a search on line adopting the key words "soccer", "technology", "athletes", "training", "IT", "soccer performance", "soccer competition" in Google Scholar, one main freely accessible web search engine specialized in academic literature, and in the ISI Web of Knowledge, in the category of management, medicine, educational, and so forth. We briefly read the abstract of each paper resulting in the search on line and went through the complete reading of the paper, after evidencing its relevance in order to evidence the role of IT in managing, monitoring, measuring and controlling the performance and training process of athletes and all the actors involved in the soccer sector.

Soccer is the most popular sport in the world, and almost every nation on the planet has a national team that regularly plays in international competition. Soccer represents one of the most profitable business, recognized as a rich industry which makes substantial profits, consequently it has very significant economic and social effects at local, national and international level given its large economic induction. For this reason scholars and practitioners are paying an increasing attention to this sport, searching for and investigating innovative practices and tools, also thanks to the support of the technology, IT and internet, to facilitate its development achieving important goals in any ways and application areas. Indeed, drawing from the five different application areas already outlined in previous studies (sport management, sport medicine, sport disability, sport events, and athletes' performance), we can observe regarding soccer sport interesting contributions focused on athletes' performance, specifically how to use technology and which new technologies can improve soccer players' performance making the soccer team more competitive, or how innovative tools can improve the rehabilitation of soccer players, and so forth.

Hence, nowadays technology in any forms offers to soccer sport new ways to improve the players' performance obtaining competitive advantage over the opponents.

In particular, in recent years, there is still an opened debate about convergence GDP instrument with mixed findings considering national team soccer results. In fact, some scholars have examined the results of national soccer teams between 1950 and 2010 and found that, whether measured by the percentage of games won or by goal difference (goals scored minus goals conceded), there is a significant evidence of convergence [38].

Besides, scholars have developed and investigated new technologies, such as the e-book, imposing a new reality on the methods of teaching and learning for soccer. In this direction, an electronic booklet was also built and designed to soccer basics for first year students at the faculty of physical education [39]. The positive design for substance basics of football to the first year students at the Faculty of Physical Education, University of Al-Azhar, was developed from the point of view of faculty members and mentors and students [39].

One interesting application of technology in soccer sport concerns the chance to measure and control the locations of players and of the ball. Thus, the locations of the players and ball are measured and monitored and logs of such locations are created thanks to the adoption of specific tactics supported by sophisticated technological advises. Indeed, it is possible to measure and monitor the trajectories the ball takes on the field and the location of players on field. The most relevant challenge faced by soccer players concerns taking the reverse path, that is given the trajectories of the ball the aim is to identify possible ways to infer the underlying strategy/tactic of teams. Most soccer coaches and professional soccer teams tend to adopt match analysis, in which they can exam and make the visualization of the plays. For instance, recently FC Bayern Munich soccer club shared the own view and data analysis.

In the last decade, most soccer team clubs provide quantitative performance analysis making possible the availability of sport related datasets but these systems present several limitations. First, these systems focus still on descriptive statistics without capturing entirely the strategy of the players and teams, e.g. the average number of shots, goals, fouls, passes are derived both for the teams and the players [40], and they are not able to extract the key components of the strategies to achieve the outcomes identified and evaluated [41–43]. Second, they cannot completely address the dynamic aspect of games, so they are not able to fully process temporal patterns, but only they can show results using small databases [44, 45]. These systems are more computation intensive not able to process large trajectory logs. Some scholars have proposed one method based on Dynamic Time Warping to reveal the tactics of a team through the analysis of repeating series of events, i.e., the positions of the ball, comparing 111 match performances of a Spanish "La Liga" team during the 2010–2011 and 2011–2012 per-seasons [46]. Monitoring an entire season of Spanish first division, the authors have evidenced relevant insights such as passing strategies regarding ball possession or counter attacks, and previous styles focusing on skills and abilities of single players or the entire team [46]. This method is very innovative because it allows to find fine-grained, reoccurring patterns across complete seasons. In add, other studies have analyzed, monitored, and tracked the movements of all the soccer players during a match, in order to build databases able to contain relevant physical performance indicators from the players of a squad [47–52]. In this case global positioning system (GPS) technology has been used for examining the physical demands imposed on professional soccer players during training sessions and also friendly matches [47]. GPS technology has been recognized a portable and economic procedure for monitoring workloads [49, 50]. In addition, thanks to GPS it is possible for coaches to obtain almost immediate feedbacks straight after the training session conclusion. Currently, the most relevant and spread procedure adopted by sports scientists and performance analysts in elite soccer consists in "the strategy of evaluating physical performance in competition with semi-automatic video capture systems and physical training workloads with the GPS" [47: 179–180]. In this direction, scholars have investigated and proposed several effective models to automatically detect event in soccer sport; hence, numerous machine learning algorithms were broadly applied, such as Dynamic Bayesian Network (DBN) model, Hidden Markov Model (HMM), Conditional Random Fields model, Support Vector Machine (SVM) model, and Hidden Conditional Random Field (HCRF) [53–55]. Otherwise, although these machine learning algorithm models play a crucial role in the contemporary soccer sport there are still limitations. For instance, it is necessary a complete sample space for applying HMM whose model construction is very complex [56, 57]. Moreover, also due to the broad computational amount of the model, when the model is created, conditional independence assumption, not easily description of events, is required [58, 59]. Other machine learning methods are based on different models, such as SVM in which semantic event detection is directly classified to solve, instead, or Conditional Random Fields (CRF) model, which defines hidden state variables in creating event model [60, 61]. Another innovative machine learning method (HCRF) is based on hidden conditional random fields model and it has been successfully applied in soccer sport for gesture, voice and action recognition [62–64]. In this model, according to video multigranularity, through the overall analysis and description of video semantic events in terms of video images and audios, an innovative and flexible framework has been developed to detect wonderful episodes in football videos [65]. Hence, research on methods for detecting and acknowledgment of events is paying an increasing attention in field of image processing in soccer sport. However, various techniques and methodologies have been proposed for satisfying different needs. For example, one method for event detection in soccer game broadcasted video comprehending aspects [66].

In this scenario briefly described, one very innovative and interesting application area of technology in soccer sport regards the development and implementation of methods, machines and instruments to detect specific events in order to monitor all the games and prevent any specific circumstances. In fact, during the Football World Cup in 2014 there was still a great debate within FIFA, started for over a decade, about the opportunity to implement specific technologies, like goal-line technology (GLT) [67]. These technologies can manage incorrect calls made on goals, fouls, and offside, especially prevent mistakes made by referees. In particular, GLT is a technological system able to monitor the ball's path to automatically detect when the ball passes over the goal line [67]. In this case, the attention is focused on the search of systems and technologies which act in the regulatory, monitoring and evaluation of soccer game. Furthermore, as already outlined, some methods and technologies have been developed and applied in order to design, implement and evaluate the sport tactics, in fact it has been proposed a soccer tactics analysis supporting system in order to deeply display the players' actions in virtual space [68]. The soccer tactics analysis is conducted using data from multiplayer games and this database is managed thanks to new technologies [68]. Thus, in recent years, soccer video processing and analysis to find critical events such as occurrences of goal event have been considered interesting issues and topics of active researches. Bayat and colleagues [69] have developed a new role-based framework for goal event detection in which it is possible to use the semantic structure of soccer game. Also, considering match analysis, different technologies applications have been developed in order to generate a huge amount of data and process that providing important information to the coach and all the soccer professionals, such as the FootData-Social, that is a computer vision based web application for tracking and analyzing soccer players' movements and team tactics [70], or the professional component (FootData-PRO) considered as a Soccer Resource Planning (SRP), that is a software for acquiring and processing information to meet all the soccer management needs. On the other hand, recently we observe that Enterprise Resource Planning (ERP) applications are widely known and spread in soccer industry, e.g. in Football Club Manchester United, Real Madrid, Barcelona, in order to measure performance and provide opportunities in optimization through benchmarking, allowing to develop performance indexes, e.g. OPTA index, to evaluate, measure and monitor the management quality linked to variables like the team success and club success [71]. In the literature on the issue, it is also interesting to mention some studies mostly focused on the search and development of more sophisticated objects for making soccer more spectacular and successful, for instance, numerous studies have paid their attention to the adoption of technology for producing soccer-balls [72–74]. Likewise, thanks to the new technologies significant improvements in elite soccer have been recorded in terms of performance of individual players and teams that can be analyzed in extreme detail.

In recent years, research in sport science has considerably advanced supported by new technologies which develop our knowledge of various training and testing modalities to optimize performance [74]. Among these technologies, one very relevant consists in semi-automated monitoring by means of video, a technique that initially was used for motion analysis of objects and/or animals. Thus, in the last decade, the computerized video tracking system represents one of the most effective technologies used in elite soccer that quantifies and collect technical and physical performance parameters. This technique, known as video tracking, has been significantly changed evolving in depth since the study by Van Gool and colleagues [75], who first used it at the end of the 1980s to analyze a non-competitive soccer match. Because of "the numerous limitations associated with this manual video tracking technique, elite soccer teams now use expensive and sophisticated semi-automated measurement systems, which are able to track all players on a pitch, as well as the ball and the referee, and this enables an almost automatic analysis of match-play [76]. Although this is an 'indirect' means of quantifying physical performance, it still provides some information on the time–motion characteristics of players, but more development is needed so additional measures such as directional changes, jumps, and accelerations can be quantified accurately" [77: 702]. Thanks to the video tracking system "the volume and immediate availability of this information allows coaches and sports scientists to make more informed decisions about current and future needs, thus increasing the teams' potential to perform" [77: 701–702]. Castellano and colleagues [77] conducted a systematic review to evaluate the pertaining research literature that has specifically used the Amisco and Prozone Computerized video tracking systems to analyze the physical performance of elite players. "Current Computerized tracking systems in elite soccer still provide adequate detail on the physical and technical performances of players but must develop further to compete with the array of additional parameters offered by new technologies such as global or local positioning system technology. However, physical parameters are highly dependent on the role played by technical and tactical factors, and thus improved knowledge of these parameters is needed to allow a more complete understanding of their impact on physical demands" [77: 701].

In summary, studies in the literature on the issue, specifically technology applications and their impact on soccer sport, mainly soccer training, can be categorized following the five application areas identified by scholars in previous research [16]. Hence, in soccer sport research we can distinguish specific contributions focused on sport management, mainly research addressed to investigate specific themes like ethics, media and communication, innovation systems and sport infrastructures in soccer sport. Also, other studies concern sport medicine area, that is the main effects of technology on the athletes' health, the development of techniques to support individuals, and so forth. Researchers have paid their attention also to sport disability, and how technology can make able also people with disability to practice soccer sport. Regarding sport events, the last soccer world competitions, such as the Football World Cup 2014, have shown the crucial role played by new and more interesting technologies to manage data and information or to realize spectacular ceremonies, and also to monitor, control and measure the results related to all the aspects and phases of games. In this categorization the most relevant research area for soccer sport concerns the athletes' performance, where scholars and practitioners look for and investigate most innovative technologies and also equipments, that can really impact on the athletes' performance, improving it.

According to this categorization, we can specifically observe, analyzing the link between technology and soccer sport, mainly soccer training, that four further application sub-areas of new technologies can be distinguished, especially in the area concerning athletes' performance and less sport medicine: 1. Individual player and team performance improvement starting from training process; 2. Injuries prevention for improving performance; 3. Regulatory system, that is using technology to control and monitor all the competitions, so, e.g. to reduce mistakes made by referees and support their decision-making process, 4. Soccer players' performance evaluation and measurement, through the development of tracking player system or other techniques able to monitor all the player performance to improve it.

5   Concluding Remarks

The development and adoption of new technologies in any forms and tools have significantly changed relevant aspects of the traditional sport field, especially soccer sport. Technology can provide positive effects, such as to improve soccer players' performance, thanks to the innovative understanding, monitoring and evaluation performance software, or to overcome geographic and cultural barriers thanks to the new mass media. Although all these recognized benefits, the technology impact on soccer sport, especially soccer training, is sometimes alarming, contributing to deeply change the human interactions concerning the traditional soccer sport competition. Technological innovation in soccer sport is still unsearched and underrepresented in the literature, either by scholars on sport or technology. The findings of our theoretical study can confirm that the interest in this topic is still limited, even though it is increasing in the last two decades and there are not specific theoretical frameworks developed to investigate how technology is deeply changing the overall soccer sport, especially soccer training. This theoretical study, providing a review of the contributions on the soccer sport, mainly training related to technology, presents some limitations, of course, for the methodology adopted and the need to deeply investigate the theme. In the future, considering this starting research point, it might be interesting to investigate the implications of new technologies in the traditional soccer sport relationships, such as the coach-soccer player relation or the assessment and measurement of soccer players' performance. In many of these processes, new technologies can deeply change the way of their development with negative or positive effects. Next step of the study might conduct a meta-analysis, to identify in a wide research design the main variables of the impact of technology on the soccer training trying to develop and adopt effective tools based on interesting theoretical frameworks.

References

1. Spagnoletti, P., Za, S., North-Samardzic, A.: Fostering informal learning at the workplace through digital platforms and information infrastructures. In: Proceedings of 24th Australasian Conference on Information Systems, ACIS2013, Melbourne, pp. 1–11 (2013)
2. Za, S., Spagnoletti, P., North-Samardzic, A.: Organisational learning as an emerging process: The generative role of digital tools in informal learning practices. Br. J. Educ. Technol. 45(6), 1023–1035 (2014)
3. Overby, E.: Process virtualization theory and the impact of information technology. Academy of Management Best Conference Paper 2005 OCIS:G1 (2005)
4. Ricciardi, F., De Marco, M.: The challenge of service oriented performances for chief information officers. In: Snene, M. (ed.) IESS 2012. LNBIP, vol. 103, pp. 258–270. Springer, Heidelberg (2012)
5. Imperatori, B., De Marco, M.: E-work and labor processes transformation. In: Bondarouk, T., Ruel, H., Guiderdoni-Jourdain, K., Oiry, E. (eds.) Handbook of Research on E-Transformation and Human Resources Management Technologies: Organizational Outcomes and Challenges, pp. 34–54. Information Science Reference, Hershey (2009)
6. Dobbs, K.: Too much Learning.com. Training 37(2), 10–12 (2000)
7. Mullin, B.J., Hardy, S., Sutton, W.A.: Sport Marketing. Human Kinetics, Champaign (1993)
8. Chu, D.: Dimensions of Sports Studies. Wiley, New York (1982)
9. Zeigler, E.F.: Ethics and Morality in Sports and Physical Education– An Experimental Approach. Stripe, Chicago (1984)
10. Goldstein, J.H.: Sports, Games, and Play: Social and Psychological Viewpoints. Hillsdale Lawrence Erlbaum, NJ (1989)
11. Brooks, C.M.: Sports Marketing: Competitive Business Strategies for Sports. Prentice Hall, Englewood Cliffs (1994)
12. Palm, J.: Sport for all: Approaches from Utopia to Reality. Hofmann, Schorndorf (1991)
13. Read, L., Bingham, J.: Preface UK sport. In: Levermore, R., Beacom, A. (eds.) Sport and International Development London, pp. 26–54. Palgrave Macmillan, London (2009)
14. Loland, S.: Technology in sport: three ideal-typical views and their implications. Eur. J. Sport Sci. 2(1), 1–11 (2002)
15. Liebermann, D.G., Katz, L., Hughes, M.D., Bartlett, R.M., McClements, J., Franks, I.M.: Advances in the application of information technology to sport performance. J. Sports Sci. 20(10), 755–769 (2002)
16. Varriale, L., Tafuri, D.: Technological trends in the sport field: which application areas and challenges? In: Nóvoa, H., Drăgoicea, M. (eds.) IESS 2015. LNBIP, vol. 201, pp. 204–214. Springer, Heidelberg (2015)
17. Rintala, J.: Sport and technology: human questions in a world of machines. J. Sport Soc. Issues 19(1), 62–75 (1995)
18. Gelberg, J.N.: Technology and sport: the case of the ITF, spaghetti strings, and composite rackets. In: Proceedings and Newsletter-North American Society for Sport History, pp. 77-87 (1996)

19. Marcus, B.H., Owen, N., Forsyth, L., Cavill, N.A., Fridinger, F.: Physical activity interventions using mass media, print media, and information technology. Am. J. Prev. Med. **15**, 362–378 (1998)
20. Wilson, B.: Believe the hype? the impact of the internet on sport-related subcultures. Tribal Play Subcultural J. Sport **4**, 135–152 (2008)
21. Gallardo-Guerrero, L., García-Tascón, M., Burillo-Naranjo, P.: New sports management software: a needs analysis by a panel of Spanish experts. Int. J. Inf. Manage. **28**(4), 235–245 (2008)
22. Coutts, A.J., Duffield, R.: Validity and reliability of GPS devices for measuring movement demands of team sports. J. Sci. Med. Sport **13**(1), 133–135 (2010)
23. Gundlapalli, A.V.: Hospital electronic medical record–based public health surveil-lance system deployed during the 2002 Winter Olympic Games. Am. J. Infect. Control **35**(3), 163–171 (2007)
24. Uszkoreit, H., Xu, F., Aslan, I., Steffen, J.: COMPASS 2008: an intelligent multilin-gual and multimodal mobile information service system for beijing olympic games. In: Proceedings of KI2006 Demo Collection, Germany (2006)
25. Toohey, K.: The Sydney olympics: striving for legacies-overcoming short-term disappointments and long-term deficiencies. Int. J. Hist. Sport **25**(14), 1953–1971 (2008)
26. Bovy, P.: Olympic Games Transport Transfer of Knowledge. HITE/Ol.transp/Bovy-version XYZ. 1 22.4.2008, HITE-ATHENS, IOC Transport Advisor (2008)
27. Halbwirth, S., Toohey, K.: The olympic games and knowledge management: a case study of the sydney organising committee of the olympic games. Eur. Sport Manag. Q. **1**(2), 91–111 (2001)
28. Beis, D.A., Loucopoulos, P., Pyrgiotis, Y., Zografos, K.G.: PLATO helps athens win gold olympic games knowledge modeling for organizational change and resource management. Informs **36**(1), 26–42 (2006)
29. Lane, A.: Relationships between perceptions of performance expectations and mood among distance runners: the moderating effect of depressed mood. J. Sci. Med. Sport **4**(1), 116–128 (2001)
30. Burkett, B.: Technology in Paralympic sport: performance enhancement or essential for performance? Br. J. Sports Med. **44**(3), 215–220 (2010)
31. Burkett, B.: Paralympic sports medicine—current evidence in winter sport: considerations in the development of equipment standards for Paralympics athletes. Clin. J. Sport Med. **22**(1), 46–50 (2012)
32. Burkett, B., McNamee, M., Potthast, W.: Shifting boundaries in sports technology and disability: equal rights or unfair advantage in the case of Oscar Pistorius? Disabil. Soc. **26**(5), 643–654 (2011)
33. Cronin, J., Sleivert, G.: Challenges in understanding the influence of maximal power training on improving athletic performance. Sports Med. **35**(3), 213–234 (2004). (Auckland, NZ)
34. Haake, S.J.: The impact of technology on sporting performance in Olympic sports. J. Sports Sci. **27**(13), 1421–1431 (2009)
35. Dwyer, D.B., Gabbett, T.J.: Global positioning system data analysis: velocity ranges and a new definition of sprinting for field sport athletes. J. Strength Conditioning Res. **26**(3), 818–824 (2012)
36. Bettoli, B.: Data processing: working procedures made easier: sport information technology and team work. Magglingen **54**(11), 18–19 (1997)
37. Ross, C.M.: Computer technology and its impact on recreation and sport programs. In: Annual Conference of the Midwest AAHPERD, Fort Wayne (1998)

38. Szymanski, S.: Convergence and soccer: testing for convergence. Harvard Int. Rev. **36**(1), 41–55 (2014)
39. Los Arcos, A., Yanci, J., Mendiguchia, J., Salinero, J.J., Brughelli, M., Castagna, C.: Short-term training effects of vertically and horizontally oriented exercises on neuromuscular performance in professional soccer players. Int. J. Sports Physiol. Perform **9**(3), 480–488 (2014)
40. Duch, J., Waitzman, J.S., Amaral, L.A.N.: Quantifying the performance of individual players in a team activity. PloSone **5**(6), e10937 (2010)
41. Narizuka, T., Yamamoto, K., Yamazaki, Y.: Statistical properties of position-dependent ball-passing networks in football games (2013). arXiv:1311.0641
42. Gyarmati, L., Kwak, H., Rodriguez, P.: Searching for a unique style in soccer. In: Proceedings KDD Workshop on Large-Scale Sports Analytics (2014)
43. Lucey, P., Oliver, D., Carr, P., Roth, J., Matthews, I.: Assessing team strategy using spatiotemporal data. In: Proceedings 19th ACM SIGKDD, pp. 1366–1374. ACM (2013)
44. Gudmundsson, J., Wolle, T.: Football analysis using spatio-temporal tools. In: International Conference on Advances in Geographic Information Systems. ACM (2012)
45. Mutschler, C.: Online data–mining of interactive trajectories in real time location systems. Friedrich-Alexander-University of Erlangen-Nuremberg (2010)
46. Gyarmati, L., Anguera, X.: Automatic Extraction of the Passing Strategies of Soccer Teams. arXiv preprint (2015) arXiv:1508.02171
47. Mallo, J., Mena, E., Nevado, F., Paredes, V.: Physical demands of top-class soccer friendly matches in relation to a playing position using global positioning system technology. J. Hum. Kinet. **47**(1), 179–188 (2015)
48. Carling, C., Bloomfield, J., Nelsen, L., Reilly, T.: The role of motion analysis in elite soccer: contemporary performance measurement techniques and work rate data. Sports Med. **38**, 839–862 (2008)
49. Witte, T.H., Wilson, A.M.: Accuracy of non-differential GPS for the determination of speed over ground. J. Biomech. **37**, 1891–1898 (2004)
50. MacLeod, H., Morris, J., Nevill, A., Sunderland, C.: The validity of a non-differential global positioning system for assessing player movement patterns in field hockey. J. Sports Sci. **27**, 121–128 (2009)
51. Randers, M.B., Rostgaard, T., Krustrup, P.: Physical match performance and yo-yo IR2 test results of successful and unsuccessful football teams in the Danish premier league. J. Sports Sci. Med. 6(10), 16, 345–352 (2007)
52. Harley, J.A., Lovell, R.J., Barnes, C.A., Portus, M.D., Weston, M.: The interchangeability of global positioning system and semiautomated video-based performance data during soccer match play. J. Strength Cond. Res. **25**, 2334–2336 (2011)
53. Quatton, A., Wang, S., Morency, L.P.: Hidden conditional random fields. IEEE Trans. Pattern Anal. Mach. Intell. **29**(10), 1848–1852 (2007)
54. Yedidia, J.S., Freeman, W.T., Weiss, Y.: Generalized belief propagation. In: Advances in Neural Information Processing Systems, pp. 689–695 (2001)
55. Wang, Y., Cao, Y., Wang, M., Liu, G.: Multi-mode semantic cues based on hidden conditional random field in soccer video. Int. J. Multimedia Ubiquitous Eng. **10**(10), 47–56 (2015)
56. Liwei, M.D., Chan, M.J.: Soccer video highlights the fusion of HCRF and AAM detection. J. Comput. Res. Dev. **1**, 225–236 (2014)
57. Xiping, D., Jiafeng, L., Jianhua, W., Dragon, T.: A semantic level collaborative text image recognition method. J. Harbin Inst. Technol. **3**, 49–53 (2014)
58. Minghao, Y., Jianhua, T., Hao, L.: Nest forest at multi-channel man-machine dialogue system for natural interaction. Comput. Sci. **10**, 18–35 (2014)

59. Lian, W.: And realize multimode teaching video semantic analysis. Nanjing University of Science and Technology (2014)

60. Tian, T.: Study on construction of spatial knowledge obviously multi modal based on information fusion. Huazhong Normal University (2014)

61. Yucheng, H., Junqing, Y., Xianqiang, H., Yunfeng, H.: Tao: user preference mining pipe in the engine of the soccer video search. China J. Image Graph. **4**, 622–629 (2014)

62. Junqing, Y., Qiang, Z., Zengkai, W., Yunfeng, H.: Using the playback scene and emotion encouragement detection in soccer video highlights. Chin. J. Comput. **6**, 1268–1280 (2014)

63. Yanjiao, Z.: Regional map of target detection of video abstract Gauss. Hebei Normal University (2014)

64. Yafei, L.: Study on detection of pedestrian tracking and abnormal motion video surveillance. China Jiliang University (2014)

65. Chenhan, S.: Methods and annotation of video structure extraction. Comput. Knowl. Technol. **26**, 6178–6180 (2014)

66. Arbat, S., Sinha, S.K., Shikha, B.K.: Event-detection-in-broadcast-soccer-video-by-detecting-replays. Int. J. Sci. Technol. Res. **3**(5), 282–285 (2014)

67. Bojanova, I.: IT enhances football at world cup 2014. IT Prof. **4**, 12–17 (2014)

68. Gondo, S., Tarukawa, K., Inoue, T., Okada, K.I.: Soccer tactics analysis supporting system displaying the player's actions in virtual space. In: Proceedings of the 18th International Conference on Computer Supported Cooperative Work in Design (CSCWD) pp. 581–586. IEEE (2014)

69. Bayat, F., Moin, M.S., Bayat, F.: Goal detection in soccer video: role-based events detection approach. Int. J. Electr. Comput. Eng. (IJECE) **4**(6), 979–988 (2014)

70. Rodrigues, J., Cardoso, P.J., Vilas, T., Silva, B., Rodrigues, P., Belguinha, A., Gomes, C.: A computer vision based web application for tracking soccer players. In: Stephanidis, C., Antona, M. (eds.) UAHCI 2014, Part I. LNCS, vol. 8513, pp. 450–462. Springer, Heidelberg (2014)

71. Salimi, F.: Conceptualizing ERP application for soccer industry. Asian J. Bus. Manage. **2**(4), 358–366 (2014)

72. Wright, T.: Pakistan Defends Its Soccer Industry, Wall Street Journal, 26 April 2010

73. Atkin, D., Chaudhry, A., Chaudry, S., Khandelwal, A.K., Verhoogen, E.A.: Organizational barriers to technology adoption: evidence from soccer-ball producers in Pakistan. IZA Discussion Papers, No. 9222, pp. 1–87 (2015)

74. Di Salvo, V., Modonutti, M.: Integration of different technology systems for the development of football training. J. Sports Sci. Med. **11**(3), 205–212 (2009)

75. Van Gool, D., Van Gerven, D., Boutmans, J.: The physiological load imposed on soccer players during real match-play. In: Reilly, T., Lees, A., Davis, K., Murphy, W.J. (eds.) Science and football, vol. I, pp. 51–59. E. & F.N. Spon, London (1988)

76. Carling, C., Bloomfield, J., Nelsen, L., et al.: The role of motion analysis in elite soccer: contemporary performance measurement techniques and work rate data. Sports Med. **38**(10), 839–862 (2008)

77. Castellano, J., Alvarez-Pastor, D., Bradley, P.S.: Evaluation of research using computerised tracking systems (Amisco® and Prozone®) to analyse physical performance in Elite soccer: a systematic review. Sports Med. **44**(5), 701–712 (2014)

Service Operations Decisions in Hybrid Organizations: Towards a Research Agenda

Liliana Ávila[✉] and Marlene Amorim

Department of Economics, Management, Industrial Engineering and Tourism
(DEGEIT), University of Aveiro, Campus Universitário de Santiago,
3810-193 Aveiro, Portugal
{liliana.avila,mamorim}@ua.pt

Abstract. In the last years, are emerging new hybrid structures in the organizational landscape that combine characteristics from different sectors. Social enterprises are a particular type of organization whose operations address social and economic concerns. These organizations face many challenges once mission and profit aims are integrated in the same strategy. In this paper are identified the main operations decisions in social enterprises and is drafted a research agenda for service operations decisions in hybrid organizations. Are pointed four main topics that claim more research efforts: (1) Goals of operations strategy; (2) Mix owned versus external resources; (3) Integration of resources for social versus income generating activities; (4) Performance management.

Keywords: Operations strategy · Hybrid organizations · Social enterprises · Social entrepreneurship

1 Introduction

Operations strategy is a well-explored and mature topic in Operations Management literature. In an exhaustive historical analysis of articles, service and management strategy have emerged among the most addressed topics [1], therefore acknowledging the importance of the decision making concerning the allocation of resources for supporting infrastructure and production. The decisions concerning the specification of an operations strategy are typically driven by the business strategy of the organization, and aim at improving the effectiveness of production while minimizing costs.

The prevalent knowledge on operations strategy is facing new challenges due to the proliferation of a particular kind of organization with a hybrid nature, adopted by many social enterprises. This is attracting a growing interest from academics and practitioners [2]. The emergence of this research field is to a great extent arising from contextual circumstances, notably due to the economic crisis once non-profit organizations receive less financial support from State and see their financial sustainability at risk, being pushed to find alternative ways to generate revenues while pursuing their social mission [3, 4].

Social enterprises face many challenges once they try to conciliate social and economic concerns in the same extent. To be successful, they need to do a great job managing limited resources. Commonly, these enterprises provide services, involving

© Springer International Publishing Switzerland 2016
T. Borangiu et al. (Eds.): IESS 2016, LNBIP 247, pp. 277–286, 2016.
DOI: 10.1007/978-3-319-32689-4_21

their beneficiaries as co-creators or co-producers of the solutions they deliver for a social problem or need [5]. In the last years, studies on social enterprises mainly focused on their definition and description. However, it is important to study these enterprises from the point-of-view of their operations management. How do they manage their operations and limited resources in order to maximize the social and economic impact? How do they organize to achieve their goals?

This article aims to contribute to answer these questions, identifying key strategic decisions that concern the management of hybrid organizations for the definition of their service operations strategy. This is done in line with those which have been recognized as the main structural and infrastructural operations decisions in the prevalent literature on operations management in manufacturing and services firms. The present paper also proposes some directions for future research. It is organized as follows: in the first section are briefly described the main insights from the review of some literature on operations strategy in manufacturing and services firms. After that, are explored the social enterprises as hybrid organizations and the main challenges faced by them in terms of the definition of an operations strategy due to their hybrid nature. Finally, is proposed a research agenda composed by four topics that claim future research: (1) Goals of operations strategy; (2) Mix owned versus external resources; (3) Integration of resources for social versus income generating activities; (4) Performance management.

2 Operations Strategy

Operations strategy is an important domain within the operations management literature. Slack et al. [6] argue that an 'operations strategy concerns the pattern of strategic decisions and actions which set the role, objectives and activities of operations'. It can be conceptualized as a set of decisions or practices with regard to structure and infrastructure variables [7]. Several authors emphasize the effects of the operations strategy on firm's performance [7–9].

Operations strategy can be viewed from four different perspectives: (a) Top-down perspective (*What the business wants operations to do?*); (b) Bottom-up perspective (*What day-to-day experience suggests operations should do?*); (c) Market requirements perspective (*What the market position requires operations to do?*); and (d) Operations resources perspective (*What operations resources can do?*) [6]. The operations resources perspective focus on operations resources, capabilities and processes to make strategic decisions [10].

These strategic decisions influence the ability of one company to successfully reach some competitive priorities such as cost, quality or flexibility and to obtain the expected performance [7] (Fig. 1). These decisions can be classified as structural and infrastructural. Structural decisions have strategic implications, require significant investment and have a long-term impact. They include decisions regarding some aspects such as the manufacturing process technology, the vertical integration degree, facilities and plant location. On the other hand, infrastructural decisions have short-term impact because they do not require large investments. They are related to operational practices and decisions, such as the planning and control systems, organizational structure, workforce management and quality management [7, 8].

Strategic decisions in services are very similar to the structural and infrastructural decisions presented in the literature on the manufacturing field [8, 11]. However, when we are talking about services, structural decisions also include those related to the touch points with clients, such as the relative allocation of service tasks to the front- and back-office and number and types of distribution channels [11].

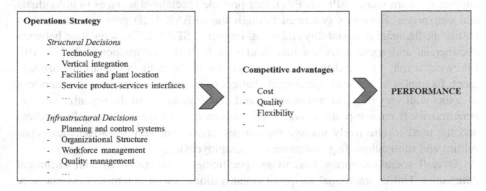

Fig. 1. An overview to operations strategy (Source: elaborated by the authors)

Any organization should define its operations strategy taking into account its competitive priorities. According to a literature review conducted on typologies and taxonomies of operations strategy, three generic operations strategies for industrial companies are commonly accepted in the literature: strategies aiming to minimise costs, strategies focusing on the highest quality products and strategies of organisations that implant new technologies and new operations processes with great flexibility as a way to differentiate [9].

3   Social Enterprises as Hybrid Organizations

Social enterprises are a particular type of organization whose operations address social and economic concerns, i.e. organizations that pursue a social mission while engaging in commercial activities [3, 12]. Social enterprises are labelled as hybrid organizations because they often incorporate characteristics from the private and social sector [4, 12–15]. Some authors also consider that social enterprises incorporate characteristics from the public sector and civil society [2, 5, 16]. In the organizational landscape, they are positioned between traditional non-profit and for-profit organizations [15, 17]. There is a wide range of hybrid business models in this spectrum. Battilana et al. [18] define the hybrid ideal as a fully integrated organization. Everything the enterprise does produces both social value and commercial revenue. Mission and profit aims are integrated in the same strategy. However, a key challenge of hybrid organizations is precisely how to reconcile the management of operations associated to the activities that aim to fulfil its social mission, which often do not generate (enough) revenues, with other commercial activities. An illustrative example is the case of SPEAK.

SPEAK is a linguistic and cultural service offer, created by a Portuguese non-profit, whose objective is to bring people of different origins together, in order to help solving the problem of social exclusion of migrants and contribute to their integration in the cities where they live. Anyone can apply to learn or teach any language or culture including those of the country where migrants are residing. Teachers work in a volunteer basis. At the same time, the same organization also runs other activities, under another program named SPEAK PRO, that provide specialized services to individuals and enterprises. Revenues generated through the SPEAK PRO program are used to ensure the financial sustainability and social impact of SPEAK. The separation between commercial and social activities may lead to a high risk of mission drift [13, 19]. Likewise, it may also lead to some ambidexterity in the domain operations management. Examples of potential operational challenges include the need to deliver services to actors with very different requirements and expectations about the organization (i.e. beneficiaries from non-profit activities vs. customers from the commercial activities) and the need to effectively manage human resources with very heterogeneous capabilities and motivations (e.g. volunteers vs. employees).

Overall, social enterprises have many specificities when compared with traditional companies. Unlike traditional for-profit organizations, social enterprises do not seek valuable, rare, inimitable and non-substitutable resources in order to ensure a competitive advantage and overcome their competitors. According to Glavas and Mish [20], "triple bottom line" firms (those aiming to become more responsive ecologically and socially while prospering economically) strive to have resources that are sustainable and therefore imitable, commonly found and substitutable. This is a necessary condition to assure that the model is scalable and easily replicable in other contexts, perhaps by other individuals or organizations. Rather than focusing on a competitive advantage, they focus on collaborative advantage. Their processes are transparent and they collaborate with others in the value chain, in their sector and also from different sectors.

The following section is therefore devoted to the identification and characterization of key challenges faced by social enterprises in the light of those which have been recognized as the main the structural and infrastructural operations decisions in the literature on Operations Management.

4 Service Operations Decisions in Social Enterprises

The literature on social enterprises to this date has essentially focused on the definition of their boundaries in the organizational landscape, notably by discussing what distinguishes social enterprises from non-profit and for-profit organizations, in order to identify the main challenges arising from their hybrid nature.

However, the existence of a wide variety of social enterprises leads us to think that there are significant differences in the way they organize their operations, once they respond to different social problems and needs and aim to achieve different levels of social impact. According to Smith and Stevens [21] there are three types of social entrepreneurship. In the first one, the focus is on local concerns and the solutions developed are often rather small in scale and scope. The second type of social entrepreneurship identified by these authors focus on issues that are relevant to local concerns but the solution may be applicable to many different contexts. The last one focus on large-scale issues. Social entrepreneurs seek to implement social enterprises to replace the solutions currently provided by the existing institutions. The case of SPEAK, referred in Sect. 3, could be classified in the second category.

Social enterprises, likewise traditional companies, should make some strategic design choices when defining their operations management strategy according to their goals and priorities. This includes long-term decisions, often related to physical aspects of the social enterprise in terms of facilities and the points of contact with stakeholders, such as the beneficiaries. Some social enterprises like SPEAK involve their beneficiaries as co-producers and co-creators of the solution to the social problem. In the same extent, in some cases due to the existence of scarce resources and the impossibility to have their own resources, social enterprises can also opt to incorporate external resources in their delivery system of the solution, for example through the use of facilities owned by other organizations (e.g. public entities) or the involvement of volunteers throughout the process [2, 22]. This can also be a strategy to scale, reach more people and create more impact.

Other decisions have an impact in the short-term. The hybrid nature of social enterprises leads to several internal and external tensions arising from the desire to generate social impact and meet market demands. In the last years, several authors have identified some critical domains for social enterprises to balance social and commercial goals, some of them with implications in terms of operations management. According to Doherty et al. [2] there are two operational mechanisms to manage these tensions which are the use of social mission as a force for strategic direction and find the optimum conditions where the generation of commercial revenue can be linked successfully to the creation of social value. In this article we identify three main critical domains for strategic operations decision in hybrid organizations: governance, human resources management and performance measurement.

Regarding governance, social enterprises may adopt different strategies. When they are acting in different locations, they can decide if they want to involve local actors in the decision making as experts on local issues or to centralize decisions, for example, at the national level, given to experts the legitimacy to address the organizational and strategic challenges of the social enterprise [12]. In the case of SPEAK, as it acts at the community level, probably it involves some local actors, not only in the delivery of the solution, but also in the governance of the social enterprise and decisions at the local level.

The human resources management is another area of tension for social enterprises. According to the level of integration between social and commercial activities, managers may choose by a differentiated workforce to social and commercial activities or a workforce able to perform both. In less integrated social enterprises, it is expected to find a structure composed by people with "social" background to perform social activities and people with commercial expertise allocated to commercial activities [2, 3]. They may also opt by more or less specialized staff, namely through the involvement of volunteers as part of their workforce [2, 3, 12]. For example, teachers in the SPEAK program working directly with the beneficiaries of the social enterprise are volunteers but those integrating the SPEAK PRO program are high qualified professionals. Social enterprises with a more integrated approach should have a workforce that combine skills from the social and private sector. Once this is an emerging field and it is difficult to find human resources with a "hybrid" profile, some authors suggest that social enterprises may choose to hire people with no work experience and train them in order to have a workforce aligned with the dual concerns of the organization [3].

Finally, it is important to define metrics for the performance monitoring and identification of opportunities to the continuous improvement of operations. This could be especially challenging in social enterprises because social indicators have distinct characteristics when compared with financial indicators. Social activities usually have a long-term impact, difficult to measure with quantitative metrics [4, 13].

Table 1 presents an overview of some of the main structural and infrastructural decisions in social enterprises discussed previously, by linking them with those that have been studied in the prevalent literature on operations management in manufacturing and services firms.

5   Research Agenda for the Study of Service Operations Decisions in Social Enterprises

Building on the discussion of key service operations decisions for social enterprises to achieve a successful alignment between their social and commercial activities, a research agenda can be drafted with four topics that claim more research efforts.

5.1   Goals of Operations Strategy

In the context of for-profit organizations, operations decisions are a mean to achieve a competitive advantage that should be aligned with organizational goals. One question that was not answered yet is: what are the competitive advantages that social enterprises pursue? It is clear in the literature that the main focus of these entities is to propose a solution to a social problem that is at least economically sustainable and replicable. They do not intent to have the highest market quote or overcome the competition. Do they work to achieve a collaborative advantage as suggested by Glavas and Mish [20]? Therefore, more research is needed to understand what are the main goals and strategic priorities pursued by social enterprises (e.g. Do social enterprises aim to solve a social problem minimizing costs? Do social enterprises intend to provide products and services adapted to the needs of each beneficiary or client?).

5.2   Mix Owned Versus External Resources

Social enterprises face resources constraints and often spend a big effort on resources mobilization [12], combining their own resources with external resources provided by partners such as public and private entities (e.g. city councils or foundations). Another question that relies without an answer is: what is the ideal mix of owned versus external

Table 1. Structural and infrastuctural operations decisions in for-profit organizations vs. social enterprises.

	For-profit organizations	Social enterprises
Structural decisions	What is the right mix of permanent versus temporary workers?	What is the right mix of employees versus volunteers?
	Does the organization prefer to have a great variety of products for different segments or a great level of homogeneous products?	Does the organization prefer to have an impact at the individual's level or to have an impact in the society as a whole?
	Does the organization prefer to increase their existent plants or to build other new ones in different places?	Does the organization use their own resources or rely on resources of others (e.g. public entities)?
	What are the customer contact touch points and the number and types of distribution channels?	Are the beneficiaries involved in the process as co-producers or co-creators or are they not involved in the delivery of the solution to the social problem?
Infrastructural decisions	What is the preferred decision system: centralization or decentralization to middle managers?	What is the level of involvement of local actors in the governance of the social enterprise?
	What are the recruitment, selection, and formation processes, and how is the person-to-job assignation?	Does the social enterprise prefer to have human resources with a commercial or social background or both?
	How will service/product standards be set?	Will the social enterprise give preference to social or financial indicators?

resources for each social enterprise? Should social enterprises adopting a more integrated approach (i.e. non-profit activities integrated with commercial activities) use more own resources than those that manage their social and commercial activities separately? Shall the mix of resources differ according to the strategic priorities the social enterprise pursues?

5.3 Integration of Resources for Social Versus Income Generating Activities

As mentioned previously, the management of human resources has been identified by several authors as an area of tension for social enterprises, critical to their success. More empirical evidences are needed in order to explain what are the strategies adopted by social enterprises in this matter. Do social enterprises have a workforce with prior work experience in the social sector, the private sector or both? In which extent are the human resources able to perform social, income generating activities or both? Do social enterprises adopting less integrated approaches include more volunteers in their workforce?

5.4 Performance Measurement

Performance measurement is the last topic we identify as an opportunity for conduct future research. Due to their dual and in most of time conflicting objectives, social enterprises need to have metrics for measure their social impact and financial performance. Business metrics tend to be clear, quantitative and short-term, whereas social mission metrics tend to be ambiguous, qualitative, and long-term [4]. Do social enterprises measure their performance differently according to their strategic priorities? Do social enterprises with more integrated approaches have a performance measurement system that balances social and business metrics?

6 Conclusion

Currently, we are assisting to the proliferation of examples of organizations from different sectors adopting hybrid structures, i.e. combining an offer of non-profit activities with commercial operations. Notably, in the last decade, hybrid business models have emerged such as social enterprises, pursuing social objectives while conducting commercial activities. In this paper we provided an exploratory analysis and discussion about key decisions faced by social enterprises regarding the definition of a service operations strategy. When compared with for-profit organizations, social enterprises face many challenges arising from their hybrid nature, due the combination of social and business goals. These challenges have a translation into structural and infrastructural decisions related for example to the involvement of beneficiaries and volunteers in the delivery of services, the management of heterogeneous human resources or the specification of adequate performance measurement indicators.

The wide variety of social enterprises make us believe that they present differences in terms of these operations decisions according to the services they offer and the strategic priorities they choose to pursue. Further research is needed to improve the understanding of how social enterprises organize their operations based on empirical evidence. This will serve both academics and practitioners. For academics, it is important to explore in what extent the literature on operations management fits these new business models and systematize the knowledge about social enterprises. On the other hand, for practitioners is urgent to learn from the best practices in order to make better decisions and ensure the survival and sustainability of their social businesses.

To this end a research agenda was drafted putting forward some topics that may help researchers to identify new opportunities to advance knowledge in this field. First of all, it seems very important gather more information about the goals of social enterprises when they decide to organize their operations in a particular way, once these goals are at the origin of a set of decisions with an impact in the short and long term. Moreover, there are other questions without answer in the literature concerning the way social enterprises are managing their scarce resources in order to deliver their services to customers and/or beneficiaries and the metrics they use to measure performance, analyzing these issues from the point-of-view of operations management.

References

1. Rungtusanatham, M.J., Choi, T.Y., Hollingworth, D.G., Wu, Z., Forza, C.: Survey research in operations management: historical analyses. J. Oper. Manag. **21**, 475–488 (2003)
2. Doherty, B., Haugh, H., Lyon, F.: Social enterprises as hybrid organizations: a review and research agenda. Int. J. Manag. Rev. **16**, 417–436 (2014)
3. Battilana, J., Lee, M.: Advancing research on hybrid organizing – insights from the study of social enterprises. Acad. Manag. Ann. **8**, 397–441 (2014)
4. Smith, W.K., Gonin, M., Besharov, M.L.: Managing social-business tensions. Bus. Ethics Q. **23**, 407–442 (2013)
5. Evers, A., Laville, J.-L.: The Third Sector in Europe. In: Evers, A., Laville, J.-L. (eds.) The Third Sector in Europe, pp. 237–255. Edward Elgar Publishing Ltd., Cheltenham (2004)
6. Slack, N., Chambers, S., Johnston, R.: Operations managment. Financial Times Prentice Hall, Harlow (2001)
7. Díaz-Garrido, E., Martín-Peña, M.L., García-Muiña, F.: Structural and infrastructural practices as elements of content operations strategy. the effect on a firm's competitiveness. Int. J. Prod. Res. **45**, 2119–2140 (2007)
8. Espino-Rodriguez, T.F., Gil-Padilla, A.M.: The structural and infrastructural decisions of operations management in the hotel sector and their impact on organizational performance. Tour. Hosp. Res. **15**, 3–18 (2014)
9. Martín-Peña, M.L., Díaz-Garrido, E.: Typologies and taxonomies of operations strategy: a literature review. Manag. Res. News. **31**, 200–218 (2008)
10. Gagnon, S.: Resource-based competition and the new operations strategy. Int. J. Oper. Prod. Manag. **19**, 125–138 (1999)
11. Roth, A.V., Menor, L.J.: Insights into service operations management: a research agenda. Prod. Oper. Manag. **12**, 145–164 (2003)
12. Pache, A.-C., Santos, F.: Inside the hybrid organization: selective coupling as a response to competing institutional logics. Acad. Manag. J. **56**, 972–1001 (2012)
13. Ebrahim, A., Battilana, J., Mair, J.: The governance of social enterprises: mission drift and accountability challenges in hybrid organizations. Res. Organ. Behav. **34**, 81–100 (2014)
14. Jäger, U.P., Schröer, A.: Integrated organizational identity: a definition of hybrid organizations and a research agenda. Volunt. Int. J. Volunt. Nonprofit Organ. **25**, 1281–1306 (2013)
15. Wilson, F., Post, J.E.: Business models for people, planet (& profits): exploring the phenomena of social business, a market-based approach to social value creation. Small Bus. Econ. **40**, 715–737 (2011)
16. Brandsen, T., Karré, P.M.: Hybrid Organizations: No Cause for Concern? Int. J. Public Adm. **34**, 827–836 (2011)
17. Neck, H., Brush, C., Allen, E.: The landscape of social entrepreneurship. Bus. Horiz. **52**, 13–19 (2009)
18. Battilana, J., Lee, M., Walker, J., Dorsey, C.: In Search of the Hybrid Ideal. Stanford Soc. Innov. Rev. **10**, 51–55 (2012)

19. Santos, F.M., Pache, A.-C., Birkholz, C.: Making hybrids work: aligning business models and organizational design for social enterprises. Calif. Manage. Rev. **57**, 36–58 (2015)
20. Glavas, A., Mish, J.: Resources and capabilities of triple bottom line firms: going over old or breaking new ground? J. Bus. Ethics **127**, 623–642 (2014)
21. Smith, B.R., Stevens, C.E.: Different types of social entrepreneurship: the role of geography and embeddedness on the measurement and scaling of social value. Entrep. Reg. Dev. **22**, 575–598 (2010)
22. Fazzi, L.: Social enterprises, models of governance and the production of welfare services. Public Manag. Rev. **14**, 359–376 (2012)

Automated Business Process Management

Carlos Mendes[1(✉)], Nuno Silva[2], Marcelo Silva[1], and Miguel Mira da Silva[2]

[1] INOV INESC INOVAÇÃO, Rua Alves Redol, Lisbon, Portugal
{carlos.mendes,marcelo.silva}@ist.utl.pt
[2] Instituto Superior Técnico, Rua Alves Redol, Lisbon, Portugal
{nuno.silva,mms}@ist.utl.pt

Abstract. Business process management (BPM) activities can be divided into categories such as design, modelling, execution, monitoring, and optimization. Some of these activities are usually automated, mainly the first ones, where Automated Business Process Discovery (ABPD) solutions, also know as process mining, can automatically find process models (using unstructured, event-level logs). However, BPM usually involves several activities that are executed in different applications, which are not integrated with each other, or are even manually executed. This may involve the waste of resources and time, and eventually not applying BPM with full potential. We propose an integrated solution, that allows to complete the BPM cycle in a single application and with most of the steps automatically. This proposal was applied in practice in the context of a research project and the results are being integrated into a commercial product.

Keywords: Business process management · Process mining · Process execution · Process improvement

1 Introduction

Business Process Management (BPM) is an operations management field focused on improving the performance of organization's business processes by managing and optimising them [1]. BPM enables organizations to be more efficient, more effective and more capable of change than the traditional hierarchical management approach, therefore impacting organization's costs and revenues [2]. This field considers business processes as relevant assets of an organization that must be understood, managed, and developed in order to support the creation of products and services of added value to the organization's clients. The BPM groups its activities into six main categories: *design*, *modelling*, *execution*, *monitoring*, *optimization* and *reengineering* [3].

The first two categories can use Process Mining, a powerful technique for automatically construct a workflow model given a workflow log (provided by workflow management systems) with all the instances (cases), activities, timestamps, resources and other significant data used within a process. This technique is particularly useful for discovering the way people and/or procedures work in reality and for performing Delta analysis, i.e., comparing the actual process model with some predefined, normative process model. Such a model specifies how people and organizations are assumed/expected to work. By comparing the descriptive or prescriptive process model with the discovered model, one can detect discrepancies between both models making it easier for process improvement [4].

However, the activities involved in BPM should maintain a coherent context. For instance, the process instances that are executed should be compliant with the process models achieved in the design and modelling phases, or at least, these incoherencies should be noted in the monitoring phase. This is not always the case and these incoherencies may be caused by the fact that BPM activities are usually executed in different applications that are not integrated with each other, or are even manually executed.

To overcome this problem, we propose to automate the activities involved in BPM in a unique solution. This research was done in the context of the First Sight Model (FSM) project. FSM has the objective to improve GENIO with a new layer of models capable of describing processes and the connection of those with software objects. GENIO is the rapid development solution from Quidgest, the FSM project promoter. In this context, we integrated into GENIO a solution to automate BPM. Therefore, the applications that are developed using GENIO are now able to discover their own processes, to model them graphically, to execute them, and to improve them based on the executions.

This research was conducted by using Design Science Research Methodology (DSRM) that aims at creating a commonly accepted framework for research in Information Systems as well as creating and evaluating artefacts to solve relevant organization problems [5]. In our research, we propose as artefact a method that will give answers and solutions for the encountered problem. The solution is an integrated solution that allows to complete the BPM cycle in a single application and with most of the steps automatically.

The paper is structured as follows. We start by describing the related work of this research (Sect. 2). In Sect. 3, we describe our proposal - Automated Business Process Management - with all phases detailed, including screens of the implementation that was already done. In Sect. 4, we analyse the results of applying our proposal in an incident management application: QUIGENIO. Finally, we present our conclusions and our proposed future work (Sect. 5).

2   Related Work

In this section we describe the related work concerning the context of this research, namely Business Process Improvement, Workflow Mining and Rapid Software Development solutions.

2.1   Business Process Improvement

Processes are in constant change due to new contextual factors and business requirements. By following a reference process model inside a Process-aware information system, when these business changes arise, process workers start to deviate from that reference model. Buijs [6] proposed a Process Mining technique that automatically provides support for updating the reference model to remain aligned with these changes.

This new technique uses traditional process mining discovery approaches to discover a process model, however, it takes into consideration the similarities between the discovered process and the reference process model. Besides the four quality dimensions of the process model (*replay fitness, precision, simplicity* and *generalization*), a new dimension was proposed by the authors: *similarity* to a given process model [6]. This dimension allows for a maximization of the four main quality dimensions and at the same time, alignment with the elements composing the reference model [6].

The *Similarity Boundary* is necessary for restraining the search for a model that balances the four quality dimensions. This makes it possible for discovering a new reference model version that is similar to the initial one and yet, enhanced with respect to the current process behaviour and changes. Depending on the boundary relaxation a more optimal process model can be discovered. However, this may not be a desirable approach since it becomes harder to recognize the original process set-up by analysts and end users.

In order to obtain a good process model quality balance of the four dimensions, a flexible evolutionary algorithm was used [6]. This algorithm focuses on *process trees* structures to represent process models that combined with the *Evolutionary Tree Miner* (ETM) genetic algorithm seamlessly balance the different quality dimensions of the discovered process model [6].

For the ETM algorithm to consider the similarity dimension it had to be extended by adding a metric of similarity. Two types of similarity were considered: *behavioural similarity* [7–12] and *structural similarity* [12]; however only the last one is used by the algorithm since the event log already captures the behaviour of the process model. This type of similarity is then used to quantify the new fifth dimension.

2.2 Workflow Mining

There are some solutions of workflow engines (ex. Bizagi, Oracle BPM, Kissflow, etc.). The main objective of this type of engines is to run processes that were previously defined, with well-defined activities and with tasks related to each activity. These engines can be more or less restricted in allowing non-usual actions.

But we did not find any integration of Process Mining in this type of workflow engines. When some workflow is not working, the workflow has to be reconstructed manually, the engine cannot learn automatically or simply show why the users are not following the defined workflow. Probably Process Mining techniques are being used to define better workflows by analysing data previously, but even for that case, we did not found any evidences.

2.3 Rapid Software Development Solutions

There are solutions on the market that allow to model and execute business processes. These are summarized in the table below using the following criteria:

- **Process definition:** define and model processes;
- **Process integration:** relate processes models with software entities (tables, forms and menus);
- **Process mining:** generate processes using event logs and/or software entities;
- **Process monitoring:** monitor the execution of process instances.

As illustrated by the Table 1, we did not identified in the market a solution that allows to completely automate Business Process Management.

Table 1. Rapid software development solutions

	Process definition	Process integration	Process mining	Process monitoring
Outsystems	Manually	Each activity can be associated with a page	No	Yes
Genexus	Manually	Each activity can be associated with a page	No	Yes
Joget	Manually	Each activity can be associated with a page	No	Yes
Ebase Xi	Manually	Each activity can be associated with a page	No	Yes
Salesforce	Manually	Each activity can be associated with a page	No	Yes

3   Automated Business Process Management (ABPM)

This section corresponds to the design and development step of Design Science Research Methodology (DSRM). We explain each step of the proposal using a real application; therefore, this section also corresponds to the demonstration phase of DSRM. We propose to integrate the activities involved in BPM in a single solution in a way that these activities can be conducted automatically or semi-automatically and maintain a coherent context. In order to do so, we developed a metamodel illustrated by the following Fig. 1.

This metamodel defines the entities of two domains: definition domain (at green and on left) and runtime domain (at red and on right). The entities on the left side (PROCS, TASKS, and FLWDF) are included in the definitions of GENIO and the entities on the right side (workflowprocess and workflowtask) are included in the applications generated by GENIO. The arrows from the left side to the right side (at red) define the relations between runtime and definition domains.

The entity PROCS contains the attributes that define what a process is. The main attributes are CODTABF, CODFORMS, and PROCNAME, that define respectively the main database table associated with the process, the application form that allows to

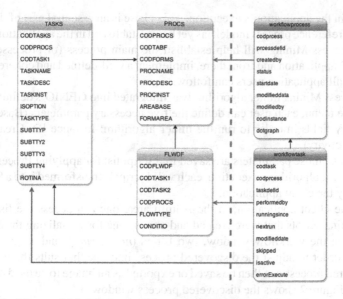

Fig. 1. Metamodel for the integration of ABPM in GENIO (Color figure online)

change that table, and the name of the process. The entity TASKS defines the tasks that are included in a process (PROCS). The main attributes are CODPROCS, TASKNAME, and TASKTYPE that define respectively the task process, name, and type. The entity FLWDF defines the connections between the tasks inside a project. The main attributes are CODPROCS, CODTASK1, and CODTASK2, that define respectively the process, the start task, and the end task.

The entities workflowprocess and workflowtask represent the execution instances of the entities PROCS and TASKS. The main attributes of workflowprocess are therefore related with the execution of processes: createdby, status, startdate, modifieddata, and modifiedby. The same reason can be applied to the workflowtask entity.

Next we detail the phases that are included in our proposal and were integrated into GENIO.

3.1 Phases of the GENIO ABPM

The first phase of our proposal is the process discovery phase (design and modelling activities), then, in process implementation phase we describe how the modelled processes are implemented in the applications generated by GENIO (preparation of execution). Afterwards, we describe the process execution phase and finally the process improvement phase (monitoring and optimization activities).

3.2 Phase 1: Process Discovery

The first phase of GENIO ABPM concerns process discovery by using Process Mining techniques [4]. In this first phase, one can discover what are the workflows being executed within a GENIO client's application by analysing the log of events that have taken place in the application's execution. This phase is an essential part of the GENIO ABPM if no reference process model has yet been established in the application's design. Applying Process Mining will help establish the main process (or processes) behind each GENIO application and from there, implement a well-defined and coherent process from which all application users can follow.

The Process Mining miner algorithm was integrated into GENIO's definition menu. On that same menu, each user can define the five necessary parameters (Base table and the necessary fields in order to run the miner algorithm: Instance ID, Creation Date, Users and Activity).

Afterwards, those parameters are saved in a script list for applying Process Mining. Then, during the algorithms execution, each valid script is transformed into a SQL query to be used by the client application.

Inside the client application, in the Admin area, one can access the list of every Process Mining scripts that were created and choose one for visualizing the discovered workflow. On the workflow window, two filters (*nodes cutoff* and *edges cutoff*) are available in order to adjust the discovered process into one that suits the users needs. The discovered process can then be saved or exported as an image to be used or analysed afterwards. Figure 2 shows the discovered process window.

In the next section we describe the second phase of GENIO BPM cycle - the process implementation phase.

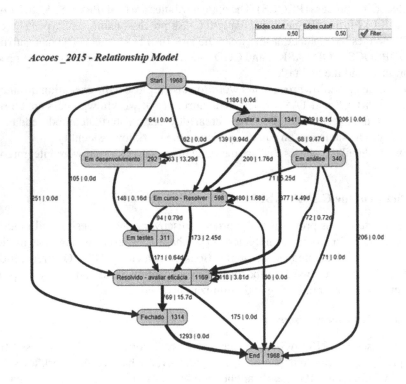

Fig. 2. Process Mining discovered process model

3.3 Phase 2: Process Implementation

In this phase, GENIO uses the discovered process in the first phase to create a workflow process that can be executed directly in GENIO. A workflow engine was implemented in GENIO in order to execute processes that can be defined manually or imported from Process Mining results.

Each implemented workflow process has a base table (INCID in this example) and a Form of that Table associated (Fig. 3). These associations define the main table that is edited by the process activities and the main form that can be used to execute these activities.

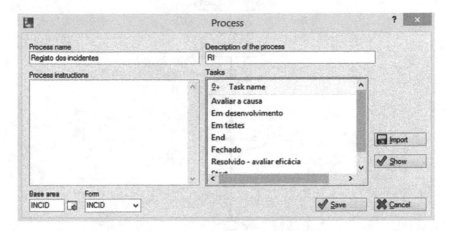

Fig. 3. Form to create the workflow process

To create a workflow process, the client has to indicate the links between activities and the conditions existing between them. The conditions are responsible for moving the workflow process to the next activity (Fig. 4)

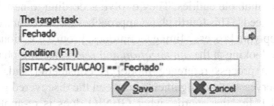

Fig. 4. Form to create links with conditions

3.4 Phase 3: Process Execution

In this phase, the workflow processes will be executed. To access the implemented workflow processes, the "Processes" option was added to the "Administration" menu. When the client clicks in "Processes" the implemented workflow processes are listed.

The links and conditions constructed previously are directly embedded in the generated applications, so when a user uses the applications and changes the state of a variable, through GENIO forms, if that variable is related to a workflow process, then the conditions will be verified and the process will move to the next activity.

In the Form of each workflow process, there is a button to open the visualizer of that process, where one can see in which activity the process has stopped. The green shapes indicate activities that were already executed and the yellow shape indicates the activity where the process stopped (Fig. 5).

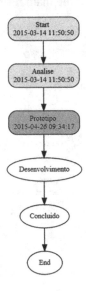

Fig. 5. Workflow process visualizer (Color figure online)

3.5 Phase 4: Process Improvement

Processes are not immutable entities. They evolve according to new business requirements and business needs. This fourth phase approaches the need for a continual process improvement by applying Process Mining techniques. From a traditional BPM life cycle perspective, we are looking at the *optimization* and *reengineering* phases combined.

In this phase, a process reference model is considered and, through process discovery, one observes any misalignments between the discovered process model and the reference model. In other words, what GENIO does is re-applying the process discovery mining algorithm over the new execution instances of the process. However, and for future work, more efficient and proper process optimization techniques can be implemented in GENIO, such as Buijs Evolutionary Tree Miner algorithm [6] that, by taking into consideration the new proposed similarity dimension, pinpoints the similarities between the process reference model and the one discovered by the algorithm. Then, the process manager can decide whether or not to perform process optimizations or reengineering. In the next section, we describe the results of applying the proposed GENIO ABPM approach in a Quidgest internal application.

4 Result Analysis

This section corresponds to the evaluation step of Design Science Research Methodology (DSRM). With the purpose of testing our proposal's applicability, we implemented the GENIO ABPM in Quidgest's CRM application: QUIGENIO. This application records incidents detected by clients or collaborators over a specific Quidgest application that lacks a resolution/response to the problem. After registering the incident, it goes through a set of phases.

The main expectation from performing this test case, besides analysing QUIGENIO's incident record process instances, is the possibility of refinement and improvement of this process.

After applying the ABPM over the incident record process, we conducted a qualitative evaluation of the outcomes through semi-structured interviews with three stakeholders of QUIGENIO application (two technicians, that use the application to solve incidents, and a senior stakeholder, accountable for the research and development at Quidgest and the main accountable for the incident management application). Seven questions were asked with respect to the expected outcomes within the scope of process mining and process execution applications. The questions were as follows with the respective results.

Was it possible to discover any unknown aspect of the process (such as unexpected activities, etc.)?

According to the given answers, and from analysing 2015 data, most of the older employees did not find any unexpected behaviour or unknown aspects within the process. Nevertheless, since the process obeys recent quality criteria inside the organization, few older and most of the newer employees did not completely understand all the aspects and behaviour concerning the process. Furthermore, the application does not have any robust validation in order to ensure the most correct flow for incident resolution, since it allows users not to abide by its own workflow. Therefore, some outliers were discovered, such as data quality errors and repetitive flows.

Observing the outcomes of applying phase one of the GENIO ABPM (process mining), was it trivial to implement the process according to the remaining phases of the cycle?

The low number of activities and being somewhat sequential did not over complicate the process mining application. By also applying the filters, one could discard the least frequent activities and paths. However, in more complex systems with more activities and decision gateways, it might not be trivial to discover the best workflow model. It will always depend on the business, the data quantity and the applied filters. Therefore, in this case from discovering the process to its implementation, there were only minor complications and short effort. This had to do with the facilitated proximity of the data intended for the example workflow, and also with its simplicity. However, increasing complexity also increases the analysis effort and implementation of the results. Therefore, an improvement of interfaces is required to help users understand the objectives of each stage. Furthermore, this cycle also interferes with the client application. It forces him to be available for, together with a process consultant, obtaining the data and analyse the process instances.

Were there any runtime improvements during process execution after applying GENIO ABPM?

Regarding process improvement, it is being developed the ability to parameterize the possibility of blocking the registration action from the incident resolution actions, whenever a user jumps to a non-predicted workflow status. It will be possible to choose whether the workflow allows him to "escape" or not. In the first case, when a non-predicted process status is reached, the process instance simply stops at that point and remains invalid for later analysis. However, being a test case and not being in production for the entire organization, it is not yet predictable to qualify its real impact.

After implementing GENIO ABPM, is there any potential for simplifying the process execution for the users?

Concerning the potential for simplifying process execution, the GENIO ABPM allows a cyclical process analysis. It uses an embedded workflow in the application, linking activities directly to application interfaces. This use of the application and the workflow can be collected through the mining process to identify potential activities within a process that is redundant or have usual paths that are too convoluted. From this information, the process may be represented by the simplified workflow or task number in either the path taken by users participating in the activity.

For example, in the case of QUIGENIO incidents, there is clearly an excess of paths of all activities for all activities, the most worrying being the successive setbacks to the earliest activities of the process end. After an analysis of the use of frequencies, we can design some warnings and follow-up of impediments in order to force the incident to progress to a state of completion. This could even pass for introducing new states to avoid setbacks. With a new version of the process incidents application (with these improvements included), it can guide the user to a correct implementation of the process.

Were there any improvements found in process runtime after the application of GENIO ABPM?

The simplification by reducing underused activities and disposing reverse or exceptional paths will certainly lead to reduced average time of completion with respect to Quidgest incident resolution processes. For example, one can check for empty states in the output of the process mining phase which certainly corresponds to users who, for lacking guidance, lost time trying to understand what to do and gave up in following the reference process. This is clearer by the excessive time average (126 days) transition between this empty state and the state of "resolved". Also, it should be considered the time-consuming transition between the "analysis" and "under development" states, thereby detecting a possible bottleneck in the effective treatment of incidents.

All things considered, the ABPM does, in fact, provide wider and more realistic process awareness through the process mining phase in a real time and automatic manner. It can help new employees to understand the main structural and behavioural aspects of the process. With respect to the process improvement phase, its viability and utility will always be dependable on how the organization intends to implement the process execution in its workflow engine. By employing a closed approach, users can only execute the actions and action paths defined exclusively by the workflow, whereas by applying an open approach, users can still decide, according to internal or external factors, which actions or paths to follow during process execution. Next, we state our main conclusions and themes for future work.

5 Conclusion

Business Process Management applications are getting more attention due to their known advantages, for instance, by applying Process Mining organizations can use all data available in their systems to understand reality, to make decisions and draw new strategic paths. However, an integrated solution that supports all BPM phases (design, modelling, execution, monitoring, optimization and reengineering) is still lacking. In this research, we integrated the BPM phases into a single platform, GENIO. This way we automated most of the phases and simplified the connections between these phases.

This new approach, Automated BPM (ABPM), represents a contribution to the BPM literature and eases the adoption of this kind of techniques. For example, incorporating Process Mining analysis directly into tools that are used by organizations is useful. By doing it this way, users do not need to export the event logs with a specific format that will be imported to an external tool, like ProM or Disco, that they do not know how to use and probably it is not installed in all devices of the organization. By integrating the process mining directly in applications that are already in use, the process of analysing the data is faster and more efficient.

Additionally, our proposal potentiates the BPM advantages since ABPM helps to better understand the processes executed by applications and continuously improves theses processes.

For future work, we intend to apply the ABPM approach in other GENIO applications and collect feedback in order to improve the proposal and its interfaces.

We would like to thank Filipe Almeida and Rodrigo Serafim from Quidgest who helped us to collect and analyse the data.

References

1. Panagacos, T.: The Ultimate Guide to Business Process Management: Everything You Need to Know and How to Apply it to Your Organization. CreateSpace Independent Publishing Platform, Scotts Valley (2012)
2. Ko, R.K.L.: A computer scientist's introductory guide to business process management (BPM). J. Crossroads **15**, 11–18 (2009). ACM
3. Van der Aalst, W.M.P., Hofstede, A.H.M., Weske, M.: Business process management: a survey. In: van der Aalst, W.M.P., Weske, M. (eds.) Business Process Management. LNCS, vol. 2678, pp. 1–12. Springer, Heidelberg (2003)
4. Van Der Aalst, W.M.P., Wijters, T., Maruster, L.: Workflow mining discovering process models from event logs. IEEE Trans. Knowl. Data Eng. **16**, 1128–1142 (2004). IEEE
5. Hevner, A., March, S., Park, J., Ram, S.: Design science in information systems research. J. Mis Q. **28**, 75–105 (2004). Society for Information Management and the Management Information Systems Research Center

6. Buijs, J.C.A.M., La Rosa, M., Reijers, H.A.: Improving business process models using observed behavior. In: Cudre-Mauroux, P., Ceravolo, P., Gašević, D. (eds.) Data-Driven Process Discovery and Analysis. LNBIP, vol. 162, pp. 44–59. Springer, Heidelberg (2013)
7. Van der Aalst, W.M.P., Hofstede, A.K., Weijters, A.J.M.M.: Process equivalence: comparing two process models based on observed behavior. In: Dustdar, S., Fiadeiro, J.L., Sheth, A.P. (eds.) Business Process Management. LNCS, vol. 4102, pp. 129–144. Springer, Heidelberg (2006)
8. Dijkman, R.M., Dumas, M., van Dongen, B.F., Kaarik, R., Mendling, J.: Similarity of business process models: metrics and evaluation. J. Inf. Syst. **36**, 498–516 (2011). Elsevier
9. Van Dongen, B.F., Dijkman, R.M., Mendling, J.: Measuring similarity between business process models. 20th International Conference on Advanced Information Systems Engineering. LNCS, vol. 5074, pp. 450–464. Springer, Heidelberg (2008)
10. Kunze, M., Weidlich, M., Weske, M.: Behavioral similarity - a proper metric. In: Rinderle-Ma, S., Toumani, F., Wolf, K. (eds.) Business Process Management. LNCS, vol. 6896, pp. 166–181. Springer, Heidelberg (2011)
11. Zha, H., Wang, J., Wen, L., Wang, C., Sun, J.: A workflow net similatity based on transition adjacency relations. J. Comput. Ind. **61**, 463–471 (2010). Elsevier
12. Li, C., Reichert, M., Wombacher, A.: The minadept clustering approach for discovering reference process models out of process variants. Int. J. Coop. Inf. Syst. **19**, 159–203 (2010)

A Service-Oriented Living Lab for Continuous Performance Improvement in SMEs

Thang Le Dinh[✉], Manh Chien Vu, Thuong-Cang Phan, and Serge Théophile Nomo

Research and Intervention Laboratory on Business Development in Developing Countries (LARIDEPED), Université Du Québec à Trois-Rivières, C.P 500, Trois-Rivières, QC G9A 5H7, Canada
{thang.ledinh,manh.chien.vu,thuong-cang.phan,serge.nomo}@uqtr.ca

Abstract. The convergence of globalization and digitalization has thoroughly transformed the business environment. Therefore, enterprises need a user-centered and open-innovation ecosystem to promote the value co-creation process in order to perform better than their rivals. This paper presents a service-oriented approach for designing a Living Lab for continuous performance improvement in enterprises, especially small-and-medium-size enterprises (SMEs). The proposed Living Lab is an on-going project for the creation of a living laboratory that will support the upgrading program for SMEs in developing countries. The purpose of this Living Lab is to integrate the co-creation and experimentation of innovative ideas and performance improvements in real-life use cases.

Keywords: Service-Oriented · Living lab · Continuous performance improvement

1 Introduction

The concept of Living Labs was originally used to describe the areas used by students to perform real-world projects [1]. The term "Living Lab" refers to living laboratory that brings experiments out of the traditional controlled environment and into a real-life context [1]. Nowadays, the Living Lab approach is considered as a user-centered and open innovation ecosystem that focuses on engaging stakeholders in research and innovation in order to promote the co-creation process [2].

In a value co-creation network, enterprises propose values by offering products and services to the market; thus, customers continue the value-creation process through the use and evaluation of products and services [2]. Open innovation is a paradigm, which assumes that enterprises can and should utilize both internal and external ideas to create value [3]. An open innovation ecosystem is a specific business ecosystem that promotes open innovation by enabling its members to work cooperatively and competitively with the others in order to co-evolve capabilities, support new products, satisfy customer needs, and incorporate a new round of innovations [4].

The focal point of this research is the Living Lab approach and its application within the context of continuous performance improvement in small-and-medium-sized enterprises (SMEs) in order to integrate their business partners with their improvement effort.

© Springer International Publishing Switzerland 2016
T. Borangiu et al. (Eds.): IESS 2016, LNBIP 247, pp. 299–309, 2016.
DOI: 10.1007/978-3-319-32689-4_23

For this reason, this paper proposes a service-oriented approach for designing a Living Lab for continuous performance improvement. The purpose of this Living Lab is to integrate the co-creation and experimentation of innovative ideas and performance improvements in real-life use cases.

The proposed Living Lab is an on-going project for the creation of a living laboratory that supports the upgrading program for SMEs in developing countries. This project is carried out by the LARIDEPED laboratory (Research and intervention laboratory on business development in developing countries). In order to gain greater economic competitiveness in a global business environment, several developing countries have formulated policies and implemented programs, called upgrading programs, to support SMEs to improve their performance continuously. The objectives of the upgrading programs are to improve productivity and product/service quality, to promote innovation and technological upgrading among local firms and to encourage SMEs co-creating value with their business partners.

This paper is organized as follows. Section 2 describes the theoretical background about continuous performance improvement in SMEs. Section 3 introduces the principles of the service-oriented approach. Section 4 proposes the design of the Living Lab for continuous performance improvement. Section 5 proposes the key activities of the Living Lab. Finally, Sect. 6 provides some conclusions and directions for future work.

2   Theoretical Background

2.1   Living Lab and Applications in SMEs

The concept of Living Lab has emerged from MIT in Boston. Its purpose was to sense, prototype, validate and refine complex solutions in a real-life context [5]. Over the past decade, Living Lab has become an established part of local and regional innovation systems, by using a variety of methods and tools and focusing on a wide array of domains and themes [6]. The Living Lab concept is strongly emerging in Europe as a new method and approach to facilitate innovation in information and communication technologies (ICTs) [7].

There have been many definitions published about Living Lab in the literature. Some authors define Living Lab as a user-centric research methodology for sensing proto-typing, validating and refining complex solutions in multiple and evolving real-life contexts [8–10] Others consider Living Lab as an integrated platform that implements an open innovation model by a successful mixture of ICT-based collaborative environments and open innovation ecosystem [11, 12]. This platform, which advocates user centric product/service development methods and public-private partnership, holds potentially disruptive and long lasting transformational effects on the industry, market, regional economies and societal landscapes [13].

Besides, SMEs play an important role in academic researches and in the socio-economic life of a country. Leaders of SMEs, who are usually owners, make most strategic decisions. Indeed, the decision-making process is more characterized by the owners and is less reliant on a collaborative process [14]. SMEs with limited resources often have to face certain disadvantages in the market and won't compete effectively with large companies [15]; therefore, collaborative competences need to be developed for establishing joint multi-functional working teams in order to share their professional knowledge and to facilitate business process improvements [16]. Furthermore, most SMEs are low to mid-tech in nature, with modest ambitions and low levels of business innovation [17, 18]. It is important to provide SMEs' managers with opportunities to improve their management skills by obtaining feedbacks, requirements and ideas from their business partners and customers [19, 20].

For business founders and SMEs' managers, the Living Lab approach is very attractive in acquiring valuable information about the business environment [7]. SMEs mostly consider Living Lab as a method of innovation that does not require a special and expensive infrastructure [21]. In a Living Lab, SMEs can participate actively in a close relation with business communities, public organizations and research institutions. This participation addresses different issues of economic, legal and ethical matters from various perspectives and maximizes the benefits of innovation in a particular territory. Indeed, the Living Lab model brings new opportunities to both technological and social innovation, viewing them as two sides of the same coin [22]. Even if Living Lab seems like a promising initiative, there is a real challenge to design, implement, and manage the Living Lab to support digital innovation processes [23].

2.2   Continuous Performance Improvement Systems for SMEs

Presently, innovation is regarded as an important competitive weapon for enterprises to penetrate into the market. Innovation is "something new or improved, which is done by the enterprise to significantly add value either directly or indirectly for the enterprise or its customers" [24, 25]. Continuous improvement, which is defined as a collection of activities carried out in order to increase the efficiency of an enterprise, is the main motive for every improvement [26, 27].

Numerous studies have been conducted in order to determine the important success factors of continuous improvement in various business areas such as service quality, operating costs, needs for products and services, information management, product life circle, staff performance assessment, R&D, supply and customer satisfaction [28]. Some researchers assumed that efficiency measurement plays a vital role in the success factor of a change project in the organization in general, and in comprehensive quality management, in particular [28, 29].

In order to promote continuous improvement in an organization, it is a need for corresponding performance improvement objectives against *continuous improvement areas* and for defining *performance factors* to measure results [30]. Thirty-five continuous improvement areas and seventy performance factors were identified from the literature review [30]. The improvement areas concentrate on specific business aspects such as technology, strategies, efficiencies, customers, and environment control. The performance factors usually cover the quality, productivity, investment, cost control, and satisfaction. Several researchers have compared the applications of the proposed continuous improvement areas and the performance factors in theory and in practice. When assessing the relationships among strategy, action and assessment, it is believed that if the enterprise doesn't apply the assessment and measurement system, it shall hardly achieve the profits expected [28, 29, 31]. Moreover, performance measurement is the decisive factor for operating performance, and performance measurement system must be based on success factors [31].

Obviously, there have been many theoretical studies on enterprise performance measurement and assessment. Studies on continuous improvement and performance factors are usually restricted to find the factors that have influence on specific operations of SMEs. For instance, an approach, called Strengthened Business Process Matrix, is used for the continuous improvement on service operations in service SMEs [32]. In general, there is a lack of studies that could cover the whole process of continuous improvement, including diagnostics, measurement, and improvement.

3   Service-Oriented Approach for Designing a Living Lab

In order to design the Living Lab for continuous performance improvement in SMEs, we adopted and enhanced the information-driven approach for designing service-oriented systems [33]. The information-driven approach proposed a set of interrelated concepts representing a service-oriented system, including three levels: services, service systems and value creation networks. This paper proposes the integration of the continuous improving process of a Living Lab and the three levels of a service-oriented system (Fig. 1).

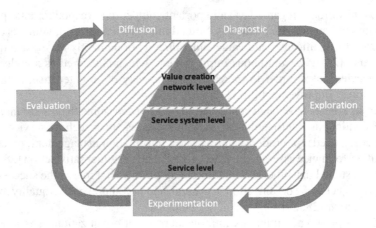

Fig. 1. Service-oriented approach for designing a Living Lab.

The service-oriented approach for designing a Living Lab includes the activities of the continuous improvement process such as Diagnostic, Exploration, Experimentation, Evaluation and Diffusion [34]. Furthermore, the approach consists of three levels [33]: the value creation network level for service proposal, the service system level for service creation, and the service level for service operation (Table 1).

Table 1.   Three levels of the service-oriented approach for designing a Living Lab.

Level	Element	Objectives
Value creation networks	Service proposal	Co-creating business value in a service value creation network by applying effective management practices.
Service system	Service creation	Organizing business services in a service system.
Service	Service operation	Transforming the shared information into organizational knowledge to improve the quality of services.

As mentioned in Table 1, the *value creation network level* depicts particular networks of service systems and shows how values are proposed and co-created among economic entities of the network. The *service system* level describes service systems and clarifies the roles of people, technology, and shared information. The *service level* presents what is provided to stakeholders and how it is provided.

4   Design of a Living Lab

In this section, the design of the Living Lab is presented according the three levels: Value creation network, Service system, and Service levels.

4.1   Value Creation Network Level

The value creation network level aims at modelling services as a chain of value co-creation and exchange in which service systems co-produce common results [33]. A *value creation network* is comprised of a variety of economic entities, which are connected through the proposition, acceptance, and evaluation of value [3]. Service providers propose values in the market based on their competences and capabilities. The value proposition is accepted, rejected, or unnoticed by other service systems in need of resources. Once the value is proposed and the service made available in the market, it is up to other service systems – potential customers – in need of such resources to decide whether to accept the value proposition. Each *economic entity* is a stakeholder of the network, has distinct goals, and assumes a subset of roles in the network. A *value proposition* is a value produced by transferring things or by improving some states of service clients [33].

In the context of a Living Lab for continuous performance improvement, there are economic entities in the value creation network as stakeholders such as Utilizer, Enabler, Provider, and User [8, 35, 36] In our approach, we prefer the term of *Beneficiary* instead of *Utilizer*, which represents enterprises that use the Living Lab to develop or improve their products or services (Fig. 2). *Enabler* creates the general infrastructure and policies to allow the Living Lab to operate. *Provider* promotes continuous performance improvement, including academia as well as emerging technology and service providers. *User* is business partners who hold an important position since they are the driving force for innovation in the Living Lab environment.

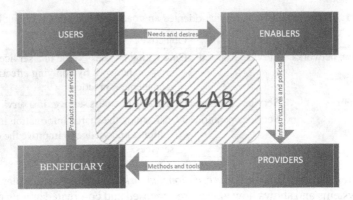

Fig. 2. Stakeholders of a Living Lab.

4.2 Service System Level

The service system level involves the configuration and implementation of business services in a service system to ensure that the service has adequate resources and sufficient technological support. A service system is defined as a value-coproduction configuration of people, technology, other internal and external service systems, and shared information [37].

Concerning people at the service system level, *Enablers* can be public sectors or local governments to drive the development and innovation in the specific region. *Providers* can be academia, emerging technology or service providers. Academia, including academies and research organizations, is key stakeholders in deciding about the efficacy of collaborative approaches [35]. *Users* encompassing the civic sector and end users who are in an important position since they are the driving force for innovation in the validation environment [35]. Concerning technological solutions at the service system level, it is supposed that *Beneficiaries* have been or are going to become digital enterprises, which use emerging systems and tools in the digital age such as enterprise systems, knowledge management and collaboration systems, and business analytics and intelligence. In our approach, there is a focus on promoting open-source systems and software-as-a-service so that SMEs can be able to benefit emerging technologies as large enterprises. Concerning necessary resources at the service system level, there are two categories of services provided by the Living Lab: independent and dependent services. Independent services or autonomous services are those whose realization is independent from the services provided by other economic entities. Dependent services require cooperation with other economic entities for their realization.

4.3 Service Level

The service level concentrates on what is provided to customers and how it is provided. In other words, this level deals with different types of information and knowledge related to the service operation.

The services provided by a Living Lab for continuous performance improvement can be classified based on the life-cycle of a Living Lab [34]. The *diagnostic activity* studies the needs and desires of the *Users*, and analyzes the capacities of the *Beneficiaries* to determine the co-creation process and suggested solution. The *exploration activity* discovers new market opportunities and new use practices of products or services. The *experimentation activity* requires the development of the validation environment (technologically or not) so that the *Users* can experiment with the product or the service in development. The *evaluation activity* allows deepening the understanding of the experiment of the *Users* with the developed product or service in a holistic way. The *diffusion activity* shares the new knowledge and knowing with other stakeholders of the Living Lab and its community.

5 Key Activities of the Service-Oriented Approach

The key activities of the service-oriented approach to design a Living Lab focusing on the activities related directly to continuous performance improvement are the Exploration, Experimentation and Evaluation activities (Fig. 3). We adopted the principles of the *Integrated Performance Measurement System (IPMS)* model [38] to measure the results of the activities of the Living Lab according to its three levels. For each level, there is a need to determine the stakeholders, control measures, environmental positioning, improvement objectives, and internal performance measures [38].

5.1 Exploration Activity

The exploration activity determines critical performance factors before collecting the data about them. The exact definition and the collection of *key performance indicators* (KPIs) will enable the Living Lab to supervise thoroughly the whole continuous improvement process. In this activity, the Living Lab needs to indicate the corresponding data of the defined KPIs. The Living Lab may also compare the indicators in different locations and periods to determine the tendency of each indicator. Moreover, the Living Lab identifies and displays the important indicators for the subsequent analytical process. Information and data are collected through the enterprise's database as well as statistical data and macroeconomic indicators. Measuring instruments and process will be selected as per purpose. After selecting indicators, the Living Lab concentrates on tracking these indicators. The Living Lab selects the measuring instruments for collecting, storing and analyzing related data. Data is tracked on a regular basis within the performance measuring system applied.

After collecting information about the market and enterprise operations with specific indicators, another important task is to store the data in the information system of the Living Lab in a reasonable manner to facilitate the access and processing of business data. Data must be stored immediately after being collected and arranged reasonably. It is important to facilitate the data access through other business software and systems such as spreadsheet, DBMS and reporting systems. Each enterprise can opt to use a tool which is conformable to its size, resources and integrated into the system of the Living

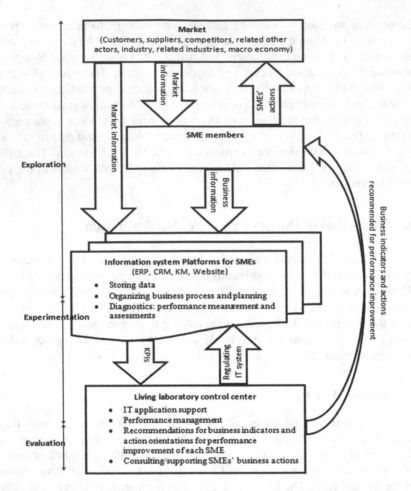

Fig. 3. Key activities of the service-oriented approach.

Lab. *Beneficiaries* can train or hire technological experts as providers to assist them in elaborating software and systems and creating an organizational database in order to meet their operational requirements.

5.2 Experimentation Activity

The experimentation activity is mainly supported and controlled by the Living Lab. *Beneficiaries'* performance is assessed with the indicators collected through enterprise management software such as customer relation management (CRM), supply-chain management (SCM), enterprise resource planning (ERP) and knowledge management (KM). In addition, enterprises as *Beneficiaries* can also use other management software and systems to collect information for their management purpose. Information and data, after being collected by management software, shall be processed at a Living Lab.

A Living Lab can be an innovative ecosystem for *Users* based upon the enterprise-citizen-government relationship. The Living Lab approach can permit *Users* to take an active part in the process of R&D, co-creation and innovation. As for *Users*, the Living Lab influences on the development of services and products to meet the actual needs. Moreover, it also helps in making the improvement process by participating actively in activities of *Beneficiaries*. As for *Beneficiaries*, the Living Lab has the ambition to enable innovation, to rectify and integrate new ideas, and to provide swiftly their services and products for new markets.

5.3   Evaluation Activity

In the evaluation activity, the system highlights the parameters that have a negative impact on the KPIs analyzed, from that the Living Lab system may automatically propose actions to overcome and supervises the positive change of each indicator. Then, for each change in SMEs (information is upgraded by SMEs on their own), the Living Lab may restart the above process. The parameters that have the negative impact on KPIs are compared with before and after the action of producing impact on the operations of SMEs, from more suitable new solutions may be proposed for improving the enterprise's performance.

The focal point of this study is designing and carrying out a Living Lab as an intelligence service system in order to improve SMEs' operating performance through the continuous improvements. This intelligence service system is expected to have some specific advantages such as the followings: (i) the operational data continuously updated in real time; (ii) Information provided by SMEs and related to the main indicators; (iii) Numerous analytical methods used by the Living Lab to maintain a complete control over KPIs. This control supervises indicator development tendency, supervises the negative impacts on the indicators, and forms automatically solutions to overcome and to assess action performance. In general, the Living Lab organizes uniformly all the data about SMEs, thus helping these enterprises take timely measures to improve the indicators.

6   Conclusion

In this paper, we are stepping into a period in which ICTs are playing an integral part in the process of managing and controlling business activities of each enterprise. However, the application of ICTs in SMEs recently was still restricted, especially tools and systems for promoting continuous improvement. The paper proposes a service-oriented approach for designing a Living Lab that supports the continuous performance improvement in SMEs. To achieve this objective, the paper first gives an overview of the SME-related studies and the necessity of applying the Living Lab approach for SMEs. It also presents methods and indicators for SME performance measurement and assessment that could be used in the Living Lab environment. Finally, the paper proposes the design of a Living Lab and its key activities.

This study still has some limitations. It was mainly based on the exploration of previous studies in the literature in order to propose the suitable solution for designing a Living Lab for continuous performance improvement. The paper presents the preliminary results, which have not been fully validated yet. Presently, the implementation of a Living Lab based on an open-source platform and the validation with selected SMEs are carried out by the team. In the future, this Living Lab will be applied and experimented in reality so that the improvement areas and performance factors can be clearly analyzed and validated.

References

1. MIT Living Labs: Products, places, and experiences that respond to a changing world. http://livinglabs.mit.edu
2. Pallot, M.: The Living Lab Approach: A User Centred Open Innovation Ecosystem. Webergence Blog (2009)
3. Vargo, S.L., Maglio, P.P., Akaka, M.A.: On value and value co-creation: a service systems and service logic perspective. Eur. Manage. J. **26**, 145–152 (2008)
4. Chesbrough, H.: Open innovation: a new paradigm for understanding industrial innovation. In: Chesbrough, H., Vanhaverbeke, W., West, J. (eds.) Open Innovation: Researching a New Paradigm, pp. 1–12. Oxford University Press, Oxford (2006)
5. Nystrom, A.-G., Leminen, S.: Living lab - a new form of business network. In: 2011 17th International Conference on Concurrent Enterprising (ICE), pp. 1–10 (2011)
6. Santoro, R.: Interview with the former President of ENOLL, 12 February 2010
7. Veeckman, C., Lievens, B., Schuurman, D., De Moor, S.: The impact of the organizational set-up of Living Labs on the innovation process: a case study between different living lab approaches in flanders. In: ISPIM Conference Proceedings, The International Society for Professional Innovation Management (ISPIM), pp. 1–16 (2012)
8. Eriksson, M., Niitamo, V.-P., Kulkki, S.: State-of-the-art in utilizing Living Labs approach to user-centric ICT innovation-a European approach. Lulea Cent. Distance-Spanning Technol. Lulea Univ. Technol. Swed. Lulea (2005)
9. Bergvall-Kåreborn, B., Eriksson, C.I., Ståhlbröst, A., Svensson, J.: A milieu for innovation–defining living labs. In: 2nd ISPIM Innovation Symposium, New York, pp. 6–9 (2009)
10. Almirall, E., Lee, M., Wareham, J.: Mapping living labs in the landscape of innovation methodologies. Technol. Innov. Manage. Rev. **2**(9), 12–18 (2012)
11. Leminen, S., Westerlund, M., Nyström, A.-G.: Living labs as open-innovation networks. Technol. Innov. Manage. Rev. **2**(9), 6–11 (2012)
12. Schuurman, D., Marez, L.D., Ballon, P.: Open innovation processes in living lab innovation systems: insights from the LeYLab. Technol. Innov. Manag. Rev. **3**(11), 28–36 (2013)
13. Eschenbaecher, J., Turkama, P., Thoben, K.-D.: Choosing the best model of Living Lab collaboration for companies. In: eChallenges, pp. 1–9. IEEE (2010)
14. The Nature of Managerial Work: Prentice Hall College Division. Prentice Hall, Englewood Cliffs (1980)
15. Penrose, E.T.: The Theory of the Growth of the Firm. Basil Blackwell, Oxford (1959)
16. Möller, K.: Role of competences in creating customer value: a value-creation logic approach. Ind. Mark. Manage. **35**, 913–924 (2006)
17. Hirsch-Kreinsen, H., Jacobson, D., Robertson, P.L.: Low-tech industries: innovativeness and development perspectives—a summary of a european research project. Prometheus **24**, 3–21 (2006)

18. Reboud, S., Mazzarol, T., Soutar, G.: Low-tech vs high-tech entrepreneurship: a study in France and Australia. J. Innov. Econ. Manag. **14**, 121–141 (2014)
19. Kilpatrick, S., Crowley, S.: Learning and Training: Enhancing Small Business Success. ERIC (1999)
20. Curtin, P., Stanwick, J., Beddie, F.: Fostering Enterprise: The Innovation and Skills Nexus–Research Readings. ERIC (2011)
21. Lehmann, Valerie, Frangioni, Marina, Dubé, Patrick: Living lab as knowledge system: an actual approach for managing urban service projects? J. Knowl. Manage. **19**, 1087–1107 (2015)
22. Dubé, P., Sarrailh, J., Billebaud, C., Grillet, C., Zingraff, V., Kostecki, I.: Le livre Blanc des Living Labs. In: Umvelt Service Design, p. 133. Montréal (2014)
23. Svensson, J.: Living Lab Principles-Supporting Digital Innovation. Int. Soc. Prof. Innov. Manag. ISPIM. 1–11 (2012)
24. Damanpour, F.: Organizational size and innovation. Organ. Stud. **13**, 375–402 (1992)
25. Business Council of Australia: Innovation Study Commission: Managing the Innovating Enterprise: Australian Companies Competing with the World's Best. Business Library in association with the Business Council of Australia, Melbourne (1993)
26. Michela, J.L., Noori, H., Jha, S.: The dynamics of continuous improvement. Int. J. Qual. Sci. **1**, 19–47 (1996)
27. Harrington, H.J.: Continuous versus breakthrough improvement: finding the right answer. Bus. Process Re-Eng. Manage. J. **1**, 31–49 (1995)
28. Kanji, G.K.: Measurement of business excellence. Total Qual. Manag. **9**, 633–643 (1998)
29. Dixon, J.R., Nanni, A.J., Vollman, T.E.: The New Performance Challenge: Measuring Operations for World Class Competition. Dow Jones-Irwin, Homewood (1990)
30. Chang, H.H.: The influence of continuous improvement and performance factors in total quality organization. Total Qual. Manage. Bus. Excell. **16**, 413–437 (2005)
31. Le Duc, T.: L'impact des connaissances en technologie d'information des dirigeants sur le succès du système d'information des PME: une étude empirique au Vietnam. Clermont-Ferrand 1 (2013)
32. Aarnio, T.: The strengthened business process matrix–a novel approach for guided continuous improvement at service-oriented SMEs. Knowl. Process Manage. **22**, 180–190 (2015)
33. Le Dinh, T., Thi, T.T.: Collaborative business service modelling and improving: an information-driven approach. In: Lee, I. (ed.) Trends in E-Business, E-Services, and E-Commerce: Impact of Technology on Goods, Services, and Business Transactions, pp. 128–147. Business Science Reference, Hershey (2014)
34. Qu'est-ce qu'un Living Lab? Montréal InVivo. http://www.montreal-invivo.com/wp-content/uploads/2014/12/livre-blanc-LL-Umvelt-Final-mai-2014.pdf
35. Sarjanen, S., others: Living Lab-Discovering the Essence (2010)
36. Stahlbrost, A.: Forming future IT the living lab way of user involvement. Luleå Univ. Technol. (2008)
37. Spohrer, J., Maglio, P.P., Bailey, J., Gruhl, D.: Steps toward a science of service systems. IEEE Comput. **40**, 71–77 (2007)
38. Bititci, U.S., Carrie, A.S., Devitt, L.M.: Integrated performance measurement systems: a development guide. Int. J. Oper. Prod. Manage. **17**, 522–534 (1997)

IT-Based Service Engineering

Digital Service Platform for Networked Enterprises Collaboration: A Case Study of the NEMESYS Project

Francesco Bellini[(✉)], Fabrizio D'Ascenzo, Iana Dulskaia, and Marco Savastano

Department of Management, Sapienza University of Rome, Rome, Italy
{francesco.bellini,fabrizio.dascenzo,iana.dulskaia, marco.savastano}@uniroma1.it

Abstract. Enterprises' networks (formal and informal) are an ever-growing economic phenomenon, especially in Europe, characterised by a large number of Small and Medium Enterprises. The new economic opportunities are making possible the creation of new types of organizations where the deployment of information technology into knowledge work will increase organizational productivity and effectiveness. The aim of the paper is to summarise the results of the NEMESYS research project funded under the Lazio Region Structural Funds, where a digital platform has been developed in order to deliver services to enterprise networks independently from the network shape and enabling efficiency and effectiveness of the business activities.

Keywords: Enterprise network · Collaboration tools · Digital services · Business process management

1   Introduction

In the knowledge economy connections and collaborations add significant value. Combination of knowledge from different perspectives can provide new opportunities and respond to challenges in innovative ways [1].

The new economic opportunities are allowing the creation of new types of organizations where the deployment of information technology into knowledge work will increase organizational productivity and effectiveness.

Rapid globalization of business makes enterprises increasingly dependent on their cooperation partners; competition between supply chains and networks of enterprises are growing. Consequently, businesses tend to become more and more information-intensive and networked [2].

The level of dynamic integration capabilities between independent enterprise information and communication technology (ICT) systems is critical for the success of such business networks. Enterprise ICT systems are expected to participate into several, potentially heterogeneous networks simultaneously. They should also react fast to changing partnerships, and use technology-independent tools for managing technical and semantic interoperability [3].

© Springer International Publishing Switzerland 2016
T. Borangiu et al. (Eds.): IESS 2016, LNBIP 247, pp. 313–326, 2016.
DOI: 10.1007/978-3-319-32689-4_24

ICTs can be seen as major enabler for modern enterprise collaborations [4], without appropriate ICT based approaches and infrastructures, cooperative relationships between enterprises would not be possible. By improving the transparency of inter-organisational infrastructures and implementing the advanced organisational approaches, cooperative and flexible solutions can become feasible. These technologies have now become a prerequisite for efficient enterprise collaboration [5].

Information technologies are seen as a great opportunity for networked businesses as they can provide enterprises with the mechanisms that helps to make contacts, check prices, display goods and enter into contracts. Such trends as Web services, IP convergence and on-demand computing still continue to develop. The reliability of the network will become even more important. The business networks are tending to support more and more critical business applications [6].

The dynamic nature of collaborations and the autonomy of enterprises create new challenges for the operational computing environment.

In this scenario, the main goal of this paper is to describe and propose a model through which new digital service platforms enable the collaboration among network enterprises. The authors also aim at contributing to scientific literature by providing a literature review on enterprises networks and the role of information technologies in networked business by providing an example of enterprise networks' digitization process through the analysis of a case study of NEMESYS project.

By using empirical analysis based on a case study, this research analyses NEMESYS project funded by the European Regional Development Fund (ERDF) under Axis I "Research, Innovation and strengthening of the production base."

The aim of the project is to provide solutions to SMEs and enterprise networks by enabling companies to digitized process, sharing information, goods and services with other enterprises, by using cloud computing and process dematerialization methods.

The work is structured as follows. The first part of the study presents a brief literature review in order to build a conceptual framework for analysing the NEMESYS project and consist of: (1) types and main advantages of inter-enterprise collaboration; (2) enterprise digital transformation in a successful network. These theoretical perspectives are integrated in this framework, which are related to the digital service platform.

In the second part of the paper, firstly, the research methodology is presented together with the case description, and secondly, general results were presented. The paper concludes highlighting the main findings, limitations and proposing some further research directions.

2 Theoretical Background

2.1 Identification of the Network Enterprises Types and Models

In the past years, the enterprise network has become an important form of running business. Enterprises now rely on their networks to support mission-critical applications and services, the needs of a business web of suppliers, vendors, partners, customers and employees [7].

The centrality of the enterprise networks for the prosperity of the territories is well known. In recent years, intensive research on inter-organizational networks has developed, but it also developed in various contexts (public, private, associations, media, political, jurisprudential, etc.) [8]. It summarizes the wide variety of approaches used in organizational sciences into three main groups: first group sees the network as a model of relationship between different organizations to achieve common goals [9]; second group defines the network as a series of connections "connections between organizations related to social relationships" [10]; third group sees the network as a set of two or more exchange relationships [11].

This makes clear that only the first meaning implies memberships, boundaries, objectives, and outcomes, something that resembles what used to be called an organization. What remains stable is the pattern of the relationship, but not the economic and social processes neither the structure nor the subjects.

Advantages of Operating in the Network. Beyond the aggregation into districts, is emerging the concept of enterprise network, understood as an aggregation of SMEs around a joint development project or around one or more international enterprise, operating through the provision of all network of their expertise [12].

More and more companies decide to use the Network Agreement as innovative method of doing business, to increase their competitiveness and their ability to innovate. Encourage the aggregation of SMEs in enterprise networks is a way to stimulate organizational development and integration of competences. However, it requires processes, systems and business models that enable efficient and effective business management and that are also integrated with systems and processes of individual companies without changing their identity and operation.

Networking gives businesses many advantages because it makes them act as if they were a single collective subject, driven by economies similar to those that provide benefits to the larger companies but retaining the flexibility and entrepreneurial responsibility widespread [13, 14].

Some authors identify the following main advantages of operating in the form of network include [15–17]: access to a higher quality and volume of financial resources, information, raw materials, legitimacy, etc.; the development of new skills or new products in the collaborative form; the development of new knowledge and new information; the pursuit of processes of specialization or diversification; risk sharing; the reduction of transaction costs; creating incentives for learning and dissemination of information; the value of intangibles such as the tacit knowledge.

The network enterprises, as mentioned above, thus are more like a new collective subject that: manages network processes; controls the "value network"; creates and develops both internal organizational units that operate as quasi-enterprises in order to be economically self-sufficient ("vital nodes"); configures, selects and keeps active the multiple connections between internal organizational units and external companies (bonds or "Network"); presents as a complex of structures: a hierarchical structure, a market information system, logistics system, a communication system, a culture, a political system ("composite structures coexisting"); sets up a system of operating methods and government, between market and hierarchy.

2.2   Type and Topology of Networks Enterprises

A first distinction is between *Informal Networks* and *Formal Networks*, referring respectively to the absence or presence of agreements between undertakings formalized through contracts [18, 19].

A second distinction can consider the possible presence of *one or more companies* of reference. In this context there will be cases (a central network) [20] where there will be only one leader (usually a medium or large company) who holds the key resources (capital, know-how, technology, innovation capacity) and the technical, procedural, commercial, economic conditions to a number of legally independent company. In other cases, companies may also be more of a reference generating system (network with multiple centres of gravity) [21] that revolves around several strategic partners, with complex relations of influence and furniture. They can also form networks without any form of central government (symmetrical networks or horizontal) that are formed generally around one or more objectives/projects shared by the partners constituents, that coordinate and work together to contribute to the achievement of often differentiated common.

An evolution of the symmetrical networks, can lead to systems consisting of a set of autonomous companies, which act in an integrated and organic way, creating, from time to time the most suitable for the business value chain who wishes to pursue ("holonic networks").

A third distinction can be developed with reference to the *main objectives of the network* itself [20], such as information exchange, research, innovation, quality, procurement, production, marketing and internationalization.

With regard to the latter classification developed in accordance with the goals of the prevailing network, they can be divided into two broad categories:

1. **asymmetric networks** (supply chain): also known as **vertical networks or supply chain** [5], in which all the players participate and carry out the functions in the formation and transfer of a product until the final status of utilization: purchase and transformation raw materials in all stages of processing, until the final product, as well as the marketing of the same and after-sales service;
2. **horizontal networks** (sharing) [22]: business networks based on sharing a common goal with differentiated contributions and hierarchical roles: networks of research and innovation (product/service, process); supply networks (co-purchase); networks of production (co-production); marketing networks and marketing (co-market); networks of sub-contracting; networks of the acquisition and/or the provision of goods and services used common.

In the non-hierarchical partnership, the two parties are equal in status, operate as partners (such as engaged in co-development) and where no one dictates the other. In this case, all decisions affecting the partnership are mutually agreed on [5].

2.3   Role of Information Technologies in Network Business

The trends of new technologies have the potential to transform the way to conduct business and simultaneously reduce costs and increase revenue [6].

ICT enables and shape the new economy and becomes an important feature of a business networking [23].

Technological innovation supports the dematerialization process. Economic activities can be reconstructed in order to take advantage of the most valuable assets. A design vision emerges where external actors and new competences are mobilized, old business borders are overcome and actors' roles are reshuffled. This business reconfiguration involves not only products and services but a whole business system. The rules of the game transform, leading to a new infrastructure and new business ideas that influence strategies, actions and networks of actors within the system [24].

Tapscott describes how digital technology influences various sectors [25]. The author highlights that new technologies changes tend at reducing costs, improving overall efficiency, adding value, squeezing out the intermediaries, reducing time and the convergence of computing, communications and content.

During last decade a large number of new collaborative, networked organizations have emerged, as a result of the progress on computer networks and communication systems, but also as a reaction to market turbulence when companies seek complementarities to increase their competitiveness and reduce risks. Advanced and highly integrated supply chains, virtual enterprises, virtual organizations, professional virtual communities, and value constellations, are some examples of this trend. The design and development of invisible, easy to use and affordable ICT infrastructures is a key pre-requisite for the effective large-scale implantation of the collaborative networks paradigm. The ICT infrastructure is usually aimed to play an intermediate role as an enabler of the interoperation among components. In this context, it is intended as the enabler for safe and coordinated interactions among the inter-organizational actors [26–28].

Various studies have shown that ICT could reduce the coordination costs that result from the outsourcing activities and therefore stimulate cooperation between firms [29]. Important IT developments that enable inter-organizational cooperation also include the development of standards for exchanging information [30], the reduction of prices for computational power of processors and the interconnectivity of communication networks, resulting in the Internet.

According to Kerravala [6] the role of the network and the following trends will continue to develop: *Voice, video and data convergence*: full convergence promises to create a competitive advantage for companies by bringing all of their collaborative applications together and delivering truly unified communications. *Web services*: web services will simplify application integration and provide a standardized way for companies to communicate with one another, bringing application integration to mid-size organizations. *Migration to IP*: IP has the necessary openness and flexibility to adapt to current company challenges and will be the delivery mechanism for many new technologies and applications. *On-demand computing*: on-demand computing becomes a new computing model for companies where resources are pooled and allocated as needed by applications and resources. This will help to deliver the true real- time enterprise where information is available to any user, over any device, at any time.

3 Case Study: NEMESYS Project

NEMESYS (Network Enterprise Management EcoSYStem) is a project of industrial research and experimental development approved under the Lazio Region Operational Programme "Regional Competitiveness and Employment" 2007–2013, funded by the European Regional Development Fund (ERDF) under Axis I "Research, Innovation and strengthening of the production base."

The aim of a project is to provide solutions to SMEs and enterprise networks by enabling companies to digitise process, sharing information, goods and services with other enterprises, by using cloud computing and processes/dematerialisation methods for: optimizing processes; facilitating marketing and trade; facilitating the access to information through a "central repository" and promoting the exchange of information between companies.

The industrial research programs provided for NEMESYS in such areas as Intelligent Network Agent (INA), cloud computing, security, BPM (Business Process Management) and others, to define new tools and solutions that will be then combined in an innovative way, following an approach of experimental development, with technologies already available today for example for knowledge & workflow management, business process management and social networking.

The concept at the base of NEMESYS appears from the fact that the networking actors work together to achieve a common goal is now essential for any business that wants to face successfully the challenges of the global market and develop their business in moments of the crisis. This is true particularly for SMEs which account for the majority of the numerical Italian enterprises and that in order to survive in the global market must "internationalize", "critical mass" and combine individual products in strategically integrated solutions that meet the needs of the market.

The NEMESYS project aims to facilitate processes, systems and business models through a platform of advanced accessible services to individual companies and networks of companies.

The NEMESYS platform should satisfy five main requirements:

(1) Help to design, configure and manage the network: able to be used by both networks companies and single enterprise that are interested to seek new synergies on the market. The platform helps individual companies in the research of new partners in technology/financial/commercial and networks areas.

(2) Managing the Network Agreement and the Network's contracts: allow to provide management of the Network agreement and contracts through the formalization of its rules, supporting the activities of planning, control and indicating/monitoring deadlines, events, milestones.

(3) Manage projects: able to manage the project (product/service provide to each customer of a SME or the Network) in collaborative mode using the means most commonly used by individual SMEs, such as task lists, timetables, etc.

(4) Manage documents in collaborative and trusted mode: able to manage the sharing of materials/information at the project, plan, program, enterprise network level (via a System Cooperative Semantic Document Management (CSDM) based on cloud architecture). Individual SMEs use their document management systems/ERP and the

platform will recover, integration and sharing of information in relation to their level of confidentiality and user profiling.

(5) Manage information and operational flow: implements a system of Knowledge Management & Workflow to optimize operations through integrated process management of individual companies (active/passive cycle, marketing, sales, compliance).

Target Clients of NEMESYS Services. The services of NEMESYS can be aggregated for the following types of consumer:

User: The user is allowed to navigate in the NEMESYS platform with utilities obtained previously acquired in the registration process from which the credentials were created. Users can be divided as: user as a physical person (the user registered only with the personal data), user as a company (the user who is registered by entering not only the personal data, but also even the company's one).

Aggregation: all the companies registered at the portal NEMESYS.

3.1 Service Catalogue of NEMESYS Platform

The requirements of each service, the contact points between the different services of NEMESYS and legacy services provided to the customer (networks enterprise or enterprises) were identified.

Two main areas represent the Service Catalogue of NEMESYS platform:

1. Utility services: administration and configuration services of the system (Service Access Management, Service Management organization, certification).
2. Core Services: specifics of business aggregation entity managed by the system: condition of the contract, checklists and compliance regulations, mapping of competencies and responsibilities.

Figure 1 represents the macro application of NEMESYS architecture in which are mapped:

1. Stages of the life cycle of the aggregation: constitution, conduction, extension and dissolution.

2. Areas of aggregation processes:

Area 1: this first area of activity mainly covers all activities related to the organizational structure of the business at a strategic level and includes all aspects of incorporation and the activities conduction for the aggregation.

Area 2: entirely within the conduction of the aggregation, covers the activities of operational management and internal control.

Area 3: given its complexity and criticality for aggregation, opportunity management requires a clear distinction from the rest of the company's activities and can be divided into activities of recognizing opportunities (assessment) and those of development opportunities (development).

Area 4: includes communication and operational marketing.

Services related to the processes of the business (Table 1).

The way of connection between business needs and the catalogue services is delivered through the SaaS platform through Web services and mobile devices.

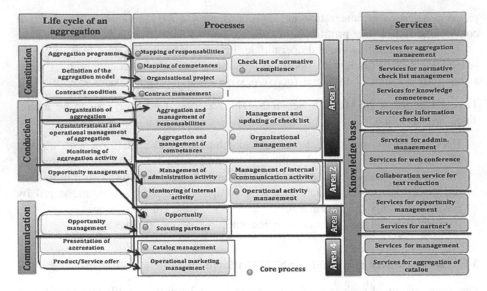

Fig. 1. Macro application architecture of NEMESYS

One of the main problems of the companies' aggregation is the large amount of documents that are not managed in a consistent and integrated manner with the performance of business processes.

The opportunity of dematerialization can be only achieved if the activities and services addressed to them can be inserted smoothly in the performance of the business process in a transparent and optimized manner.

The NEMESYS catalogue services provides services for managing the flow of "business" (non-defined document and its metadata) at the same time "capturing" documents in moments of archival interest (records) and its metadata, for commissioning conservation and the subsequent search and retrieval.

3.2 Method of Analysis

Following the work done so far - in particular, as a result of market analysis carried out, it can be asserted that currently on the market exists a potential demand for the services of the NEMESYS platform (approximately 1.5 million of enterprises).

Italian enterprises which, although diverse, seems to have some common relevant characteristics including – *in primis* - the need of digital services, through which then respond to the information and collaborative needs that can be interesting not only for enterprises, individual or aggregate, but also for individual professionals.

NEMESYS is created to help to find a response to market by providing operational services that potentially can support SMEs and professionals in their dynamic growth and development.

The existence of market sectors that potentially constitutes a fertile area for the implementation of the platform NEMESYS was identified. In particular, crossing

Table 1. General characteristics of services.

Process	First level service	Second level service
ADMINISTRATION	Services internal administration of the platform	Personal data management, Services configuration, Functionality and processes monitoring
ADMINISTRATION	Administration services exposed to NEMESYS customer	Personal data management, services configuration
REGISTRATION	Access management service	Profile creation, Log in and recognition
CONTRACT MANAGEMENT	Service for the management of the contract's aggregation	
MAPPING OF RESOURCES AND SKILLS AND MAP OF RESPONSIBILITY	• Service of the knowledge skills	Service for resource mapping, Service for mapping skills
	• Service of resources and skills mapping	Service for mapping of responsibilities
CHECK LIST DI COMPLIANCE	Service for the management of checklist regulations	Service for the checklist of the establishment of an aggregation and the sector
ADMINISTRATIVE/OPERATIONAL MANAGEMENT	Services for administrative management	Operational services support
OPPORTUNITY MANAGEMENT		Chat, video conference
PRESENTATION OF THE AGGREGATION OF PRODUCTS AND SERVICES OFFER	Service for opportunity management	Certification and Legacy services, Editing of joint documents, Semantic search, Digital signature, Storage.

elements of evaluation such as their need for digital services and service requirement of the platform. The areas most interesting in development of NEMESYS are: (1) Construction sector; (2) Small Office sector (Accountants, Lawyers and Engineers); (3) Consulting Management sector/ICT.

After identified and studied the needs of the market areas of possible implementation of the platform, it is necessary to make a cross-check between the needs of the identified enterprise sector with the market analysis and the practical response of the subjects that populate directly this market. In order to provide such analysis, an experimentation process were conducted during which to a chosen actors the processes and services of the platform were presented in detail in order to receive direct feedback from actors.

The process of experimentation is supported by a methodological framework that allows verifying whether and to what extent the services provided by the portal corresponding concretely to the needs of Italians enterprises and professionals.

Based on these premises a qualitative approach was chosen.

The primary objective of the interview is to enter in the perspective of the studied subject, taking its conceptual categories, and the participants' interpretations about the subject and the motivations of their observations.

For the testing phase of the platform, the focus groups instrument was chosen, a technique, which in recent years has had a particular development in qualitative research and experimentation.

Through the defined methodological approach and provided analysis tools, was put in action the implement of a testing platform and requirements, dividing the implementation in two main parts:

(1) presentation and description of services

(2) execution of experimental tests.

The need to develop ad hoc questionnaire to be submitted to the parties that were included in the selected focus groups accurse from specific objectives to be pursued with the testing phase.

The overall goal is to provide the NEMESYS platform's 'user test', or to record and measure the degree of satisfaction that the subjects reported compared to a designed and studied product for been implemented in the market where they operate.

In particular, the questionnaire are aimed to collect the following information:

Understand the perceived usefulness of the offered services; Verify that the platform services, in terms of single presented service, is perceived as a 'complete'; Check the availability of a user to pay for the presented service/instrument; Investigate the comprehensibility of the offer; Understand if the user is satisfied with the degree of customization of the environment (dashboard).

3.3   Experimentation

The project's experiment was conducted in two phases involving representatives from different companies chosen for the test.

Phase 1. In the first phase of the analysis, in several sessions, representatives of the market categories interested in the analysis were gathered. By organizing focus groups, NEMESYS platform was introduced.

The participants of experiment, in this stage, have gained only theoretical and descriptive information of services and features of the platform by showing to potential users the representations of graphics, images, reports and slides.

Based on these elements, however, the respondents were able to express an initial opinion on the usefulness and functionality that the portal could have. The desired result was the collection of feedback from actual users of the platform, which then was into consideration in order to enhance, implement, correct or modify the elements of the designed computer system.

This phase of experiment was conducted with 4 companies working in the field of ICT consultancy, small office: accountants and lawyers and enterprise network working in construction domain. As the result of the feedback obtained from the participants in this experiment it can be concluded:

1. All services, in general, have been perceived as very useful, especially with a view to standardization of internal processes within enterprises. Users declared to be prepared to use the platform.
2. The integration of collaboration tools (chat, conference call, video-conferencing, joint editing of documents) was considered very useful, in particular, has emphasized a particular interest in collaborative editing.
3. A great potential that the platform could have on the market was recognized, it was also considered as an instrument tends to be more useful for companies and enterprise networks, rather than for individual practitioners.

The focus groups interviewed during the meeting of experimentation gave general feedback of concerns about some elements of the platform, accompanying their answers with some ideas of improvement, for instance, the structure of dashboard was considered as particularly complex, as well as an unclear. It is therefore, suggested to be simplified and to improve usability, in particular, to place a video tutorial on the homepage of the platform, in order to guide the user in its functionality.

Phase 2. In the second round of the platform's testing, the participants had the opportunity to try the demo version. The goal of this stage is to test the various tools of the platform. Not only the quality and effectiveness-efficiency of the platform, was searched through the conducting of experimental tests, but rather, its usability level for users.

Therefore, the main goal of the Phase 2 was the evaluation the quality of the software system and its ability to trigger rapid learning, quick execution of tasks, low error rate, easy to remember basic instructions, high user satisfaction.

The results, in terms of feedback, emerged at this stage is crucial for the construction of the useful guidelines in the planning of a technology roadmap and commercialisation of products and services to be launched on the market.

In this stage of experiment 4 groups of users were involved.

1. *Students of the University of Salerno* were asked to try the platform. This was the only experimental test in which the users were students and not the representatives of small and medium-sized enterprises.

The results of the demo version test, in terms of feedback, are surely considered to be "special" because students are generally more capable of navigating a web platform and on average less prepared to understand the advantages of digital services in the business processes of a company.

The results of the test were very interesting especially because of interest that the audience has shown towards the new platform. Having as a target the students we wanted to give more weight during our investigation to the assessment of the design, verification the ease of use and less weight to the verification of the provided services.

Assessing the overall design: the overall design of the site has been evaluated very positively by the students and described as "innovative" and "captivating", which invites to navigate and to: "find out more..."

Evaluation the ease of use: the site was considered simple to use. There have been suggestions to simplify the use of terms that are too technical or too market.

Suggestions: to give even greater importance to the search engines in all areas of the platform, to use as much as possible open source software to allow, to implement the reserved and dedicated areas.

2. Here the target involved in testing the platform was *representatives of small and medium-sized companies* from different market sectors. Three meetings were held in 3 different cities: Milano, Rome, Palermo.

Being precisely the target of potential future customers of the platform NEMESYS, we wanted to give more weight to analysis of the interest of the users in the provided services and to "willing to pay analysis" and to analysis of the design of the site.

Evaluation of the "Usability" of offered services was judged as: sufficiently guided in use and easy to understand; complete in terms of acknowledgment messages and completion actions.

Evaluation of the actual propensity to "spend" for this type of services: respondents said they were willing to spend in order to purchase these services.

4   Conclusions, Limitations and Future Research

This research has demonstrated how digital service platform can provide solutions to SMEs and enterprise networks by enabling companies to digitized process, sharing information, goods and services with other enterprises, by using cloud computing.

A single-case study was conducted with the representatives of different market areas in order to evaluate the functionality and quality of the software system and its ability to trigger rapid learning, quick execution of tasks, easy to remember basic instructions, high user satisfaction. The results of the feedback obtained from the participated companies have been perceived as very satisfactory and the NEMESYS platform was considered as useful and user-friendly.

Despite the fact that users identified the platform as "satisfactory", in order to function as "All-in-one" platform NEMESYS should be enriched with additional services suggested by participants. The guidelines for the subsequent construction of the technology roadmap and commercial demand can serve, directly from the NEMESYS platform and support: (1) establishment of a start-up (from the assessment of business ideas, to prepare business plans, to support access to financed credit, the establishment of the company including compliance with the law); (2) international-ization of the business (with local market analysis, selection of potential interested companies, business plan and administrative technical support); (3) participation in tenders and competitions.

The main limitation of this study is related to the fact that the NEMESYS platform has only been implemented in the pilot phase of the project. In this respect, only the design and functionality levels were taken into consideration.

It could be very interesting to conduct a research in the future once the platform start to function and to analyse how the inter-organisational relationships develop and change due to a technological support of digital platform.

References

1. Skyrme, D.: Knowledge Networking: Creating the Collaborative Enterprise. Routledge, London (2007)
2. Ricciardi, F., De Marco, M.: The challenge of service oriented performances for chief information officers. In: Snene, M. (ed.) IESS 2012. LNBIP, vol. 103, pp. 258–270. Springer, Heidelberg (2012)
3. Kutvonen, L., Metso, J., Ruokolainen, T.: Inter-enterprise collaboration management in dynamic business networks. In: Meersman, R., Tari, Z. (eds.) On the Move to Meaningful Internet Systems 2005: CoopIS, DOA, and ODBASE. LNCS, vol. 3760, pp. 593–611. Springer, Heidelberg (2005)
4. Za, S., Marzo, F., De Marco, M., Cavallari, M.: Agent based simulation of trust dynamics in dependence networks. In: Nóvoa, H., Drăgoicea, M. (eds.) IESS 2015. LNBIP, vol. 201, pp. 243–252. Springer, Heidelberg (2015)
5. Jagdev, H.S., Thoben, K.-D.: Anatomy of enterprise collaborations. Prod. Plan. Control 12 (5), 437–451 (2001)
6. Kerravala, Z.: As the value of enterprise networks escalates, so does the need for configuration management. The Yankee Group, p. 4 (2004)
7. Dyer, J.H., Harbir, S.: The relational view: cooperative strategy and sources of interorganizational competitive advantage. Acad. Manage. Rev. 23(4), 660–679 (1998)
8. Axelsson, B., Easton, G. (eds.): Industrial Networks: A New View of Reality, vol. 11. Routledge, London (1992)
9. Van de Ven, A.H., Ferry, D.: Measuring and Assessing Organizations. Wiley, New York (1980)
10. Aldrich, H.: Organizations and Environment. Prentice Hall, Englewood Cliffs (1999)
11. Emerson, R.M.: Power-dependence relations. Am. Sociol. Rev. 27, 31–40 (1977)
12. Cagnazzo, L., Tiacci, L., Rossi, V.: Knowledge management system in SMEs within stable enterprise networks. WSEAS Trans. Bus. Econ. 11(1), 155–174 (2014)
13. Parker, H.: Inter-firm collaboration and new product development process. Ind. Manage. Data Syst. 100(6), 255–260 (2000)
14. Lewis, D.J.: Partnership for Profit: Structuring and Managing Strategic Alliances. The Free Press, New York (1990)
15. McLaren, T., Head, M., Yuan, Y.: Supply chain collaboration alternatives: understanding the expected costs and benefits. Internet Res. 12(4), 348–364 (2000)
16. Holton, J.A.: Building trust and collaboration in virtual team. Team perform. Manage. Int. J. 7(3/4), 36–47 (2001)
17. Horvath, L.: Collaboration: the key to value creation in supply chain management. Supply Chain Manage. Int. J. 6(5), 205–207 (2001)
18. Coviello, N., Munro, H.: Network relationships and the internationalisation process of small software firms. Int. Bus. Rev. 6(4), 361–386 (1997)

19. Fuller-Love, N.: Formal and informal networks in small businesses in the media industry. Int. Entrepreneurship Manage. J. **5**(3), 271–284 (2009)

20. Thoben, K.-D., Jagdev, H.S.: Typological issues in enterprise networks. Prod. Plan. Control **12**(5), 421–436 (2001)

21. Kandula, S., Mahajan, R., Verkaik, P., Agarwal, S., Padhye, J., Bahl, P.: Detailed diagnosis in enterprise networks. ACM SIGCOMM Comput. Commun. Rev. **39**(4), 243–254 (2009)

22. Saiz, J.J.A., Bas, O., Alfaro, J.: Performance measurement system for enterprise networks. Int. J. Prod. Perform. Manage. **56**(4), 305–334 (2007)

23. Österle, H., Elgar, F., Rainer, A.: Business Networking: Shaping Collaboration Between Enterprises. Springer, Heidelberg (2001)

24. Resca, A., Za, S., Spagnoletti, P.: Digital platforms as sources for organizational and strategic transformation: a case study of the midblue project. J. Theor. Appl. Electron. Commer. Res. **8**(2), 71–84 (2013)

25. Tapscott, D.: The Digital Economy: Promise and Peril in the Age of Networked Intelligence, vol. 1. McGraw-Hill, New York (1996)

26. Camarinha-Matos, L.M., Afsarmanesh, H.: Virtual enterprise modeling and support infrastructures: applying multi-agent system approaches. In: Luck, M., Mařík, V., Štěpánková, O., Trappl, R. (eds.) ACAI 2001 and EASSS 2001. LNCS (LNAI), vol. 2086, pp. 335–364. Springer, Heidelberg (2001)

27. Bernus, P., Baltrusch, R., Vesterager, J., Tølle, M.: Fast tracking ICT infrastructure requirements and design, based on enterprise reference architecture and matching reference model. In: Camarinha-Matos, L.M. (ed.) IFIP TC5/WG5.5. IFIP — The International Federation for Information Processing, vol. 85, pp. 293–302. Springer, Heidelberg (2002)

28. Camarinha-Matos, L.M.: Infrastructures for virtual organizations-where we are. In: IEEE Conference on ETFA 2003, Emerging Technologies and Factory Automation, Proceedings, vol. 2, pp. 405–414. IEEE Press (2003)

29. Clemons, E.K., Kleindorfer, P.R.: An economic analysis of interorganizational information technology. Decis. Support Syst. **8**(5), 431–446 (1992)

30. Hardwick, M., Spooner, D.L., Rando, T., Morris, K.C.: Sharing manufacturing information in virtual enterprises. Commun. ACM **39**(2), 46–54 (1996)

How Can ITIL and Agile Project Management Coexist?

An Adaptation of the ITIL V.3 Life Cycle in Order to Integrate SCRUM

Bertrand Verlaine[✉], Ivan Jureta, and Stéphane Faulkner

PReCISE Research Center, Department of Business Administration,
University of Namur, Rempart de la Vierge 8, 5000 Namur, Belgium
{bertrand.verlaine,ivan.jureta,stephane.faulkner}@unamur.be

Abstract. A significant proportion of organizations delivering IT services follows and combines some IT management frameworks. At the organizational level, they often act in accordance with ITIL, the most used IT Service Management (ITSM) framework. At the project management level, a growing part of them are willing to work with agile methods. However, ITIL favours the Waterfall life cycle, such as in PRINCE2 or PMBOK, to the detriment of agile methods. Nevertheless, it is also assumed that ITSM best practices have to be adapted to, e.g., the environment, the kind of IT services and the culture of IT organizations. So there is a legitimate issue to raise: How can ITIL v.3 and agile project management coexist in an IT organization?

In this paper, we positively answer to this question by describing *how* to adapt ITIL v.3 when it is associated with SCRUM, the most popular agile method. First, we detail the current ITIL structure when a software implementation project is carried out. Then, we identify and explain which are the ITIL elements to modify in comparison with Waterfall-based project management methodologies. Lastly, we describe and illustrate eight interfaces between ITIL v.3 and SCRUM.

Keywords: It service management · ITIL v.3 · Agile methods · SCRUM

1 Introduction

Organizations delivering IT services often apply an IT Service Management (ITSM) framework. It describes how to manage quality IT services that meet the business needs "through an appropriate mix of people, process and information technology" [1]. In this paper, we refer to ITIL, which is often considered as the most used ITSM framework.

Besides the management of the organizational processes, IT organizations also have to manage their projects. Some of them consist of implementing software. In recent years, these kinds of projects are more and more often managed thanks to agile methods. This means that they respect the *agile manifesto* and its twelve

© Springer International Publishing Switzerland 2016
T. Borangiu et al. (Eds.): IESS 2016, LNBIP 247, pp. 327–342, 2016.
DOI: 10.1007/978-3-319-32689-4_25

principles [2]. Taken as a whole, *agile* corresponds to "the continual readiness of an information systems development method to rapidly or inherently create change, proactively or reactively embrace change, and learn from change while contributing to perceived customer value [...], through its collective components and relationships with its environment" [3]. There are several agile methods: eXtreme Programming (XP) [4], SCRUM [5] and Feature-Driven Development [6], to name a few of them. Each adheres more or less strongly to the agile manifesto and principles. Presently, SCRUM is the most popular agile method in the IT industry [7]; this justifies its use in the scope of this paper.

If we compare agile methods and ITIL v.3 from a conceptual and structural point of view, they could not be more different. Agile methods are seen as loose and very flexible, while ITIL is rather considered as bureaucratic and procedural. However, they share a common objective: both of them aim at providing business value to its customers and users. As first and main principle, the agile manifesto states that its "highest priority is to satisfy the customer through early and continuous delivery of valuable software" [2]; ITIL v.3 "is adopted by organizations to enable them to deliver value for customers through IT services" [8]. However, the way of doing is very dissimilar. The former provides value by quickly implementing what customers and users really want, while the latter provides value by delivering stable IT services respecting the negotiated set of functionalities and the quality levels. The agile manifesto favours informal interactions between the project stakeholders as opposed to a high formalism, which is advocated by ITIL v.3. Therefore, the following research issue is naturally raised.

How can ITIL v.3 and agile project management coexist in an IT organization?

Contributions. In this paper, we analyse the ITIL v.3 best practices by focussing on the relations between them and the structure of software project management methods. We conclude that ITIL favours methods which are based on the Waterfall life cycle or, at least, methods which recommend a full software design before its implementation. Based on four recommendations in order to adapt ITIL v.3 to the principles of the agile manifesto, we discuss the alignment of SCRUM and ITIL v.3. We identify, define and justify eight interfaces between them, as well as the modifications to the ITIL v.3 life cycle in order to enable agile project management. This work aims at helping people wishing to follow the ITIL v.3 best practices associated with SCRUM in their IT organizations.

Organization. First, we present ITIL v.3, its point of view on software project management, and SCRUM (Sect. 2). Then, in Sect. 3, we describe the relations between ITIL v.3 and SCRUM while emphasizing the adaptations to ITIL v.3. Finally, after the related work (Sect. 4), the conclusion and some directions for future research are discussed (Sect. 5).

2 Presentation and Discussion of the Reference Frameworks

In this section, we describe the two main references used, namely ITIL v.3 (Sect. 2.1) and SCRUM (Sect. 2.4). In Sect. 2.2, we describe the relations between the relevant ITIL processes and the project management structure advocated by ITIL. In Sect. 2.3, we make four recommendations in order to adapt ITIL v.3 to an agile project management method.

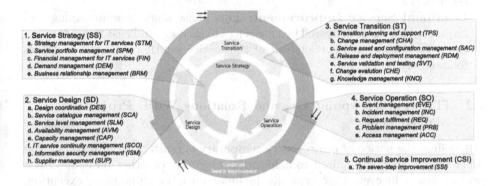

Fig. 1. ITIL v.3 life cycle (based on an official illustration of ITIL [9])

2.1 A Short Description of ITIL V.3

ITIL is a collection of ITSM best practices which requires to focus on the customers and users and, more specifically, on the value that they get by using IT services [10]. A recent empirical study [11] demonstrates that ITIL strongly helps companies delivering IT services to improve their processes and to increase their benefits. ITIL[1] v.3 is structured into five phases, each being composed of processes. An ITIL process is defined as "a structured set of activities designed to accomplish a specific objective. A process takes one or more defined inputs and turns them into defined outputs" [9]. These five ITIL v.3 phases along with their processes are depicted in Fig. 1 and described below.

- **Service Strategy:** This phase aims at guiding the whole IT service creation and delivery strategy through an effective management of its life cycle. Topics covered are mainly the creation and management of the IT strategy, the analysis and the development of the markets (including the internal customers), the feasibility analysis related to the conception of IT services and the financial management [9].

---

[1] The third version of ITIL was released in 2007 and revised in 2011. In this paper, each time we mention ITIL v.3, we refer to its last version.

- **Service Design:** This phase provides the guidance for the conception of
  services and their future management [1]. The conception lies in defining
  how the organization assets will be transformed to bring value to customers
  through the use of the future IT services. This phase also defines how to
  improve the existing IT services.
- **Service Transition:** This phase explains how to organize the implementation of the designed services and how to manage the changes applied in
  existing services [12].
- **Service Operation:** This phase focuses on the delivery and support of IT
  services [13].
- **Continual Service Improvement:** This phase aims at maintaining and
  improving the value delivered by IT services to its users and customers through
  the measurement and the analysis of the service solutions and the processes
  followed [14].

2.2   ITIL V.3 Viewpoint On, and Relations With, Project Management

ITIL defines the notion of project as "a temporary organization, with people and
other assets, that is required to achieve an objective or other outcome. Each
project has a lifecycle that typically includes initiation, planning, execution,
and closure" [12, p. 324]. This definition is very similar to the ones proposed
in the PMBOK [15] or in other related references (e.g., [16,17]). The notion of
Project Management Office (PMO) is another important notion in the scope of
this work. From the ITIL point of view, the purpose of the PMO is "to define and
maintain the service provider's project management standards and to provide
overall resources and management of IT projects" [1, p. 254]. Actually, it is
a combination of two processes, namely, *Design coordination* and *Transition
planning and support*. The former focuses on the creation of the service design
package while the latter focuses on the effective implementation of IT services
and of their modifications. A quick look to the PMBOK indicates that this notion
is similarly understood: a PMO is "a management structure that standardizes
the project-related governance processes and facilitates the sharing of resources,
methodologies, tools, and techniques" [15, p. 10].

Concerning the project management, ITIL suggests to combine its best practices with a methodology such as PRINCE2 or PMBOK [12, p. 324]. Although
ITIL aims at managing the whole life cycle of an IT service, the projects leading
to the effective creation or modifications of IT services are not directly managed through the ITIL processes. This is consistent with the project notion; the
PMBOK explains that "a project is a temporary endeavor undertaken to *create*
a unique product, service[2] or result" [15]. Actually, ITIL supports this creation
by, e.g., providing information, but it not *directly* manages projects. In the ITIL
Service Design book [1, Sect. 3.11.3], the project management in an iterative,

---

[2] The notion of service in the PMBOK is different from the notion of service in ITIL v.3,
but this discussion is out of the scope of the paper.

incremental and/or adaptive life cycle is briefly discussed. The Rapid Application Development (RAD)[3] [18] and XP [4] methods are mentioned. However, there is no explanation concerning the way for combining one of these two methods with ITIL. The structure of the ITIL v.3 processes, as illustrated by the left side of Fig. 2, does not fit with agile methods. Indeed, this structure corresponds to a Waterfall life cycle, also called "conventional development" in the ITIL literature: the requirements are elicited, then the system-to-be is specified, which leads to its implementation and, lastly, to its testing and deployment. This is illustrated by Fig. 2 and discussed hereafter. The legend of Fig. 2 is available in Table 1, and is also applicable to Figs. 3 and 4.

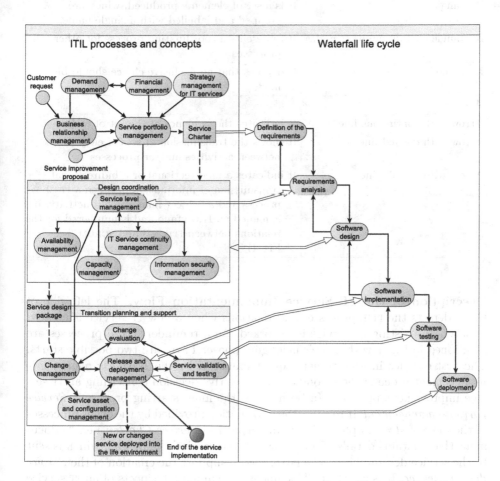

Fig. 2. Relations between the ITIL v.3 processes and the Waterfall life cycle

---

[3] RAD is not always considered as fully agile, but this discussion is out of the scope of the paper.

Table 1. Legend applicable to Figs. 2, 3 and 4

Form	Description
Nodes	
Light circle	It is a trigger of the flowchart
Dark circle	It depicts the end of the flowchart
Rectangle with rounded edges	It is a set of tasks to be performed, which corresponds to the rectangle label; this is a process in ITIL v.3, otherwise this is an activity in the scope of project management
Rectangle	It is a set of elements produced, which are grouped and labelled with a single name
Rectangle containing other nodes	It represents a coordinating process for other ITIL processes
Diamond	It denotes that an exclusive choice should be made.
Arrows	
Arrow with continuous line	It indicates the sequence of the set of tasks
Arrow with dashed line	It shows the transmission of sets of elements between activities and/or processes
Arrow with double line	It indicates a unidirectional or a bidirectional transmission of information between a ITSM process and a project management activity. It is named an **Interface** and is numbered for the relations between ITIL v.3 and SCRUM (see Fig. 4)

Description of the IT Service Implementation Flow. The left side of Fig. 2 depicts the ITIL processes and relations when a new IT service is created or when an existing IT service is reworked. As a reminder, these processes are mentioned in Fig. 1 within their belonging phase. There are two possible starts. The first one lies in a customer request managed by the *Business relationship management* process; the second one is a positive decision concerning an IT service improvement proposal. In both cases, the main starting process is *Service portfolio management*. It receives the information provided by the other processes of the *Service strategy* phase. Its main output is a *Service Charter*, i.e., "a document that contains details of a new or changed service" [9, p. 452], which is sent to the service design phase. The latter has to support the creation of the *Service design package*. It is a (set of) "document(s) defining all aspects of an IT service and its requirements through each stage of its lifecycle[, which] is produced for each new IT service, major change or IT service retirement" [1, p. 418]. At the organizational level, the design tasks are coordinated by *Design coordination*. The other processes are used to provide information about the expected service level and the four quality properties; these information exchanges are managed by *Service level management*.

Once created, the *Service design package* is transferred to *Change management* for its implementation, which is coordinated by *Transition planning and support*. The workflow is as follows. First, the *Service design package* is transformed into several requests for change, which is "a formal proposal for a change to be made [on a configuration item, which contains the] details of the proposed change" [1, p. 415]. Once authorized, they are grouped under a service release and, then, they are effectively implemented. *Service validation and testing* is in charge of validating the deployment of the service release. This leads to the *Service operation* phase, which is out of the scope of this paper.

The right side of Fig. 2 depicts the Waterfall model [19, 20], which is the main project life cycle model behind the structure of PRINCE2 and of PMBoK: these methods recommend to design first the software and, then, to implement it. That is, if the software specifications are sufficiently detailed after an in-depth requirements analysis, it will be coded such as. In this context, we consider the software engineering as a linear process with possible steps backward. The first steps focus on the requirements engineering and their specifications (see the right side of Fig. 2). Then, the specified software is coded and tested. The last step is the software deployment. One should move to the next step only when the previous step is achieved, although a step back is always possible in order to improve or to remake a previous output. However, returning to a former step often involves additional costs and delay. The lack of contact with the stakeholders is also a drawback often underlined when using this software engineering model.

In Fig. 2, the arrows with a double line illustrate the relations between the ITIL processes and the steps of the project management workflow. The first information transfer occurs when the *service charter* is communicated to the step *Definition of the requirements*, so that the software engineers can elicit the requirements and design the future software during, respectively, the steps *Requirements analysis* and *Software design*. This specification work is facilitated and supervised by the processes of the service design phase, coordinated by the *Design coordination* process. The next step, *Software implementation*, lies in the coding of the designed software by respecting the service release previously defined. This leads to its test through the step *Software testing* and, lastly, to its deployment through the step *Software deployment*.

2.3   ITIL Associated with an Agile Project Management Method: Recommendations

To be considered as agile, a project management method has to respect the agile manifesto [2] and have to be incremental, iterative and adaptable [21]. Based on the observations made in Sect. 2.2, we make four recommendations in order to associate ITIL with an agile project management method. Note that ITIL v.3 adaptations are allowed if we respect its main principles and ideas. Indeed, the ITIL content is not prescriptive, in the sense that IT organizations are encouraged to adopt the main ITSM principles and "to adapt [the best practices] to work in their specific environments in ways that meet their needs" [12, Sect. 1].

1. The *Service design package* has to be created incrementally along with the software implementation and testing.
2. The software development team should be able to modify the *Service design package*, and thus the requests for change, even when the implementation has already begun.
3. The phases *Service design* and *Service transition* have to be conducted in parallel.
4. Service managers have to progressively release their IT services, on the same pace that the underlying software implementation is carried out.

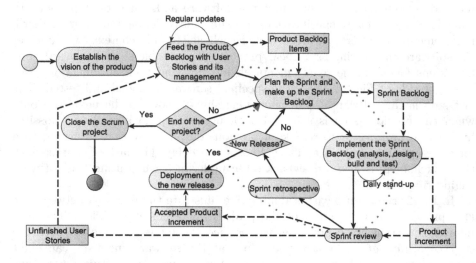

Fig. 3. The SCRUM process framework (based on [5,22,23])

2.4   An Introduction to SCRUM

SCRUM is an agile process framework for managing software development projects. It consists of roles, events, rules and artefacts [24]. Its main objectives are the transparency, the inspection and the adaptation during the software implementation [5,24]. Figure 3 illustrates the SCRUM framework and its steps, which are described hereafter[4].

When a SCRUM project starts, the vision of the product, which corresponds to the future software to be created, is determined. The client and the SCRUM team have to write down how the future product is going to support the client's organization strategy. This is the essence of the business value that will be got from the product use. In particular, this includes the definition of the targeted users and

---

[4] For more details about SCRUM, the reader can refer to [5,22].

customers of the product, the main use situations addressed by the product, the business model, its "must-have" characteristics, its desired qualities and a comparison with the possible competing products [22]. Note that the SCRUM team is composed of (i) the product owner—s/he is in charge of the product backlog management—(ii) the SCRUM master—s/he is responsible for ensuring that the SCRUM team correctly follows the SCRUM philosophy and its rules, without any hierarchical relation—and (iii) the development team—the latter is composed of professionals who carry out the work leading to the product implementation[5]. All SCRUM teams have to be self-organized and cross-functional.

The second SCRUM step is the feeding of the product backlog, which is a prioritized list of requirements. It is managed by the product owner. It is continually updated even after the start of the product development, hence the fact that SCRUM is an adaptive software project management method. Product backlog updates come from the customer or from the Sprint review (see further for a description of this SCRUM event). These updates include modifications, additions and removals of product backlog items.

Once the product backlog is defined and prioritized, a first Sprint may be organized. The dotted line in Fig. 3 represents its life cycle. This SCRUM iteration is a fixed period of time (about four weeks) during which a subset of the product backlog, called the Sprint backlog, is analyzed, designed, implemented and tested. A Sprint begins with its planning and ends with the Sprint review and, after that, the Sprint retrospective. The Sprint review is an inspection of the product increment created during the Sprint. This inspection is achieved by the customer and the product owner with the help of the development team. The second meeting, i.e., the Sprint retrospective, is held by the SCRUM team to inspect and to improve their way of working for the next Sprints.

After the Sprint review and the Sprint retrospective, the customer and the product owner decide if the product increment is deployed as a new product release, and thus made immediately usable. Then, the customer has to determine if the current version of the product meets his expectations, or if an additional Sprint is needed in order to integrate some more backlog items to the product and/or in order to improve it. The closing of the SCRUM project corresponds to, i.a., the creation of the documentation.

3 Coexistence of ITIL and SCRUM: Alignment and Description of the Interfaces

In this section, we describe the alignment between SCRUM and ITIL v.3 as well as all the interfaces between them through which information exchanges occur. In Table 2, we sum up these interfaces, which are numbered in Fig. 4. In this picture, we illustrate how to combine ITIL v.3 with SCRUM. The left part of Fig. 4 contains some differences compared to the left part of Fig. 2 illustrating

---

[5] In the scope of this paper, we consider that the development team includes the SCRUM master.

the structure of ITIL v.3. These differences, detailed hereafter, are due to the recommendations made in Sect. 2.3. The right side of Fig. 4 is exactly the same than Fig. 3 illustrating the SCRUM method.

At the beginning, there is not difference compared to the traditional life cycle of ITIL v.3 detailed in Sects. 2.1 and 2.2: the *Service strategy* phase is covered as usual. Afterwards, there is a key difference in comparison with the traditional structure of ITIL v.3 (cf. Fig. 2). There is no more a direct relation with the phase *Service design* before the start of the software implementation projects. In other words, the *Service charter* is sufficient to start a SCRUM project. The *Service charter* document is used to establish the vision of the product in SCRUM (see **Interface** 1 in Fig. 4 and its summary in Table 2). Of course, it is also transferred to the next ITIL phase and, more precisely, to *Service level management*. This difference is explained by the fact that the service design will be progressively achieved along with the carrying out of Sprints[6].

Then, the product backlog has to be created and fed based on the *Service charter* and on the communication between the product owner and the identified stakeholders. For utility and quality considerations, information provided by *Service level management* should be used (e.g., service improvement opportunities, service quality plans, reports on operational level agreements and underpinning contracts, and so on [1, p. 121]). This is captured by **Interface** 2, which is referenced by its number in Fig. 4 and in Table 2. After the next SCRUM step, i.e., the Sprint planning, the first Sprint starts.

During a Sprint, the Sprint backlog is implemented; this includes the analysis, the design, the coding and the testing of the objective(s) introduced in the Sprint backlog. There are several information exchanges with ITIL processes during a Sprint. The first main concerns *Design coordination* (cf. **Interface** 3). Indeed, for analysis and design tasks achieved during the Sprints, this ITIL process coordinates the transfer of knowledge about the design of a service—or of a service modification—in order to reach the adequate service level. The second main information exchange involves *Change management* (cf. **Interface** 4). Indeed, the designed changes made during a Sprint have to be assessed and authorized by the Change Advisory Board (CAB), which is "a group of people that support the assessment, prioritization, authorization and scheduling of changes" [12, p. 306]. In the context of our work, the scheduling of changes is automatically determined: the authorized changes are carried out during the current or the next Sprints. Similarly, it is not relevant to prioritize changes achieved during projects seeing that it is an ITIL artefact applied for operational changes.

A second key difference is the removal of the ***direct*** relation between *Service level management* and *Change management*, i.e., between the ITIL phases *Service design* and *Service transition*. In the common ITIL structure, the phase *Service design* ends with the completion of the *Service design package*, which is

---

[6] If other types of configuration items than software, activities or processes have to be modified, and thus specified in a *Service design package*, a parallel project should be carried out or it could be included in the agile project. This possibility is left for future work (see Sect. 5).

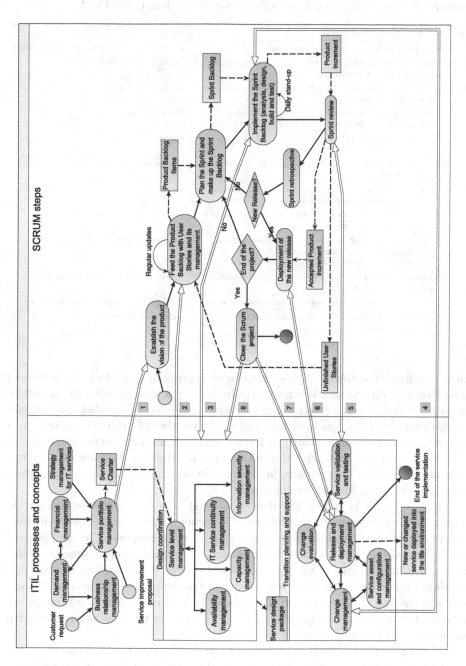

Fig. 4. Alignment of, and interfaces between, ITIL v.3 and SCRUM

Table 2. Description of the interfaces between ITIL v.3 and SCRUM; the numbers (#) correspond to the digits used to identify the interfaces depicted in Fig. 4

#	*From*: Information transferred	*To*
1	*Service portfolio management*: Service charter	*Establishment of the vision of the product*
2	*Service level management*: Service quality plan & Service improvement opportunities	*Product backlog management*
3	*Design coordination*: Service portfolio updates & Revised enterprise architecture	*Sprint*
	Sprint: Documentation obtained from the analysis and design tasks & Identified constraints	*Design coordination*
4	*Change management*: Authorized and rejected RFCs & Changes to services and infrastructure	*Sprint*
	Sprint: Software modifications to assess & Sprint planning and updates	*Change management*
5	*Service validation and testing*: Configuration baseline of the testing environments & Analysis of tests results	*Sprint review*
	Sprint review: User stories considered during the Sprint & Software modifications achieved	*Service validation and testing*
6	*Release and deployment management*: Deployment plan, Service notification, Tested environments and facilities & Updates for the release and deployment activities	*Deployment of the new release*
	Deployment of the new release: Reviewed and accepted product increment	*Release and deployment management*
7	*Scrum project closing*: Final version of the product created	*Release and deployment management*
8	*Scrum project closing*: Functional, technical and user documentation created	*Design coordination*

then transferred to the *Change management* process in order to be transformed into *Requests for change*. When associating ITIL v.3 with SCRUM, the activities of *Service design* and *Service transition* are conducted in parallel. The *service design package* is thus gradually created as the number of Sprints increases. As a reminder, one of the agile principles favors "working software over comprehensive documentation" [2], but this does not mean that there is no more documentation produced [24]. This remains indispensable for, e.g., the IT service operation management or its further modifications [13].

Once a Sprint is ended, the next SCRUM step is the *Sprint review* during which the development team, the product owner and the stakeholders inspect the newly created product increment. This step is supported by the process *Service validation and testing* (cf. **Interface** 6). In particular, it provides automated testing solutions to support the *Sprint review*. If the product increment is validated for release, it is deployed thanks to the support of the process *Release and deployment management* (cf. **Interface** 5). It is important to automate the deployment of software seeing that this activity proves to be more frequent with an agile project management method.

After the *Sprint retrospective* and, if so decided, after the deployment of the product increment, a new Sprint can be planned. Note that, along with the Sprints execution, the product backlog is regularly updated, always with the support of the process *Service level management* (cf. **Interface** 2).

Once the last version of the product fulfils the stakeholders' expectations about the software-related utility and warranty provided, the SCRUM project may end by its final deployment (cf. **Interface** 7). During this last SCRUM step, the *Service design package* is finalized according to the operational conventions prescribed by ITIL (cf. **Interface** 8). The objective is to make accessible the IT service description, including the documentation created during the Sprints, in a single and comprehensive source of information. It is indispensable for further support and maintenance activities carried out during the operation activities structured around the ITIL phase *Service operation.*

4 Related Work

Several research works deal with ITSM frameworks and agile principles in order to integrate the latter into the ITSM processes and environments (e.g., [25,26]). These works are quite far away from the topic tackled, seeing that we study the consequences of associating an ITSM framework with an agile project management method.

In [27], there is a description of how to manage projects and services in an agile way. To do so, they explain how to combine three frameworks: ITIL v.3 edited in 2007, PRINCE2 and DSDM Atern (Dynamic Systems Development Method). The latter is an agile project method for delivering software. This book does not directly describe the relations between ITIL and an agile project management framework, seeing that PRINCE2 is used as an intermediary between them.

In [28], Pollard et al. argue for a deeper focus on ITSM issues, including the consequences of new project management methods, such as agile methods, on the common ITSM structure and operations. They underline the need for solutions taking into account both highly structured ITSM frameworks and agile frameworks, which provide minimal guidelines according to the authors. In the same line, [29] is a claim for combining ITSM frameworks with agile methods in order to improve the business and IT alignment (BIA). However, the author does not explain how. He focuses on the technological issue in BIA through an agile service provisioning system based on the principles of the service-oriented paradigm.

In [30], the authors describe how to apply SCRUM in the IT support, which is one of the components of an ITSM. This work covers the operational processes of ITIL v.2 and discusses the use of SCRUM during the maintenance and incident management, and when a small modification to an existing service has to be carried out.

Another related paper contains a large discussion about ITIL v.3 edited in 2007 and software implementation methodologies [31]. A part of the discussion is about agile software implementation methodologies. They stay at a very high level without describing practically how to integrate ITIL v.3 with an agile method. Nevertheless, the observations made in this paper are similar to our four recommendations (see Sect. 2.3).

Lastly, [32] reports an experiment about the use of XP combined to ITIL v.2, and concludes that agile methods share more similarities with ITIL than often believed.

5   Conclusion and Future Work

How can ITIL v.3 and agile project management coexist in an IT organization?
By tackling this research issue, we argue for an adaptation of the most used ITSM
framework, ITIL v.3, in order to facilitate its coexistence with an agile project
management method, SCRUM. Although ITIL and agile methods share the same
main objective, i.e., providing business value to customers and users, the way of
doing is very different. This is explained by their respective structure. Basically,
ITIL favours the complete design and specifications of an IT service before starting
its implementation. Unlike ITIL v.3, agile methods favour a parallelism of the
design, specifications, implementation and testing activities, which are indeed
carried out at each SCRUM iteration, i.e., at each Sprint. The main contribution
of this paper is the identification and the description of eight interfaces, i.e.,
information exchange channels, between ITIL v.3 and SCRUM, which can be put
into action thanks to some described adaptations in the structure of the ITIL v.3
life cycle.

This paper also opens the way for several future works. Applying SCRUM
is only possible for the management of *software* implementation project and
not for other kinds of projects, such as the installation of hardware. Studying
the structure of ITIL v.3 in order to organize both agile and traditional project
management is relevant. Indeed, many IT organizations face both software and
hardware projects, sometimes mixed.

Another future work is the generalisation of the ITIL adaptations for other
agile project management methods. In this context, the integration of this work
with the alignment between ITIL v.3 and the service implementation life cycle
proposed by the same authors in [33] is an interesting research direction. The
objective would be to map the life cycle of the ITSM procedural structure of
an IT organization, of the service implementation life cycle in a service-oriented
system, and of the agile management of software implementation projects.

A last future work is the execution of a case study in one or several IT
organizations working with ITIL v.3 and willing to conduct their software implementation projects with SCRUM. Based on this work, the theoretical propositions
made in this paper would be improved thanks to the comments provided and
the observations made. Note that this could be a good opportunity to conduct a
validation of the SCRUM method seeing that, taken as a whole, the agile research
lacks of empirical validation [34,35].

References

1. Hunnebeck, L., Rudd, C., Lacy, S., Hanna, A.: ITIL V3.0 - Service Design, 2nd
   edn. TSO (The Stationery Office), London (2011)
2. Beck, K., Beedle, M., Bennekum, A.V., Cockburn, A., Cunningham, W., Fowler,
   M., Grenning, J., Highsmith, J., Hunt, A., Jeffries, R., et al.: Manifesto for agile
   software development (2001). http://www.agilemanifesto.org/
3. Conboy, K.: Agility from first principles: reconstructing the concept of agility in
   information systems development. Inf. Syst. Res. **20**(3), 329–354 (2009)

4. Beck, K., Andres, C.: Extreme Programming Explained: Embrace Change, 2nd edn. Addison-Wesley, Boston (2004)
5. Schwaber, K., Sutherland, J.: The SCRUM Guide. http://www.scrumguides.org/docs/scrumguide/v1/scrum-guide-us.pdf
6. Palmer, S., Felsing, J.: A Practical Guide to Feature-Driven Development. Prentice Hall, Upper Saddle River (2001)
7. Rubin, K.S.: Essential Scrum: A Practical Guide to the Most Popular Agile Process. The Addison-Wesley Signature Series. Addison-Wesley Professional, Boston (2012)
8. Addy, R.: Effective IT Service Management: To ITIL and Beyond. Springer, Heidelberg (2007)
9. Cannon, D., Wheeldon, D., Lacy, S., Hanna, A.: ITIL V3.0 - Service Strategy, 2nd edn. TSO (The Stationery Office), London (2011)
10. Hochstein, A., Zarnekow, R., Brenner, W.: ITIL as common practice reference model for it service management: formal assessment and implications for practice. In: IEEE International Conference on e-Technology, e-Commerce, and e-Services (EEE 2005), pp. 704–710. IEEE Computer Society (2005)
11. Marrone, M., Kolbe, L.: ITIL and the creation of benefits: an empirical study on benefits, challenges and processes. In: Proceedings of the 18th European Conference on Information Systems (ECIS), P. 66 (2010)
12. Rance, S., Rudd, C., Lacy, S., Hanna, A.: ITIL V3.0 - Service Transition. TSO (The Stationery Office), London (2011)
13. Steinberg, R., Rudd, C., Lacy, S., Hanna, A.: ITIL V3.0 - Service Operation, 2nd edn. TSO (The Stationery Office), London (2011)
14. Lloyd, V., Wheeldon, D., Lacy, S., Hanna, A.: ITIL V3.0 - Continual Service Improvement, 2nd edn. TSO (The Stationery Office), London (2011)
15. PMI Standards Committee: A Guide to the Project Management Body of Knowledge (PMBOK®R GUIDE). 5th edn. Project Management Institute (2013)
16. Jurison, J.: Software project management: the manager's view. Commun. AIS 2(3), 2–57 (1999)
17. Royce, W.: Software Project Management: A Unified Framework. Addison-Wesley Professional, Reading (1998)
18. Martin, J.: Rapid Application Development. Macmillan Publishing Company, New York (1991)
19. Benington, H.D.: Production of large computer programs. Ann. Hist. Comput. 5(4), 350–361 (1983)
20. Royce, W.W.: Managing the development of large software systems: concepts and techniques. In: Proceedings of the 9th International Conference on Software Engineering (ICSE), pp. 328–339. ACM Press, New York (1987)
21. Cohn, M.: Succeeding with Agile: Software Development Using Scrum. The Addison-Wesley Signature Series. Addison-Wesley Professional, Boston (2010)
22. Pichler, R.: Agile Product Management with Scrum: Creating Products that Customers Love, 2nd edn. Addison-Wesley Professional, Boston (2010)
23. Schwaber, K.: Scrum development process. In: Sutherland, J., Casanave, C., Miller, J., Patel, P., Hollowell, G. (eds.) Business Object Design and Implementation, pp. 117–134. Springer, London (1997)
24. Schwaber, K., Beedle, M.: Agile Software Development with Scrum, 1st edn. Prentice Hall PTR, Upper Saddle River (2001)

25. Göbel, H., Cronholm, S., Seigerroth, U.: Towards an agile method for itsm self-assessment: a design science research approach. In: Proceedings of the International Conference on Management, Leadership and Governance (ICMLG 2013), pp. 135–142. Academic Conferences and Publishing International (ACPI), Sonning Common (2013)

26. Komarek, A., Sobeslav, V., Pavlik, J.: Enterprise ICT transformation to agile environment. In: Núñez, M., Nguyen, N.T., Camacho, D., Trawiński, B. (eds.) Computational Collective Intelligence. LNCS, pp. 326–335. Springer, Switzerland (2015)

27. Office of Government Commerce (OGC): Agile project and service management: delivering IT services using ITIL, PRINCE2 and DSDM Atern. The Stationery Office, London (2010)

28. Pollard, C.E., Gupta, D., Satzinger, J.W.: Integrating SDLC and ITSM to 'servitize' systems development. In Nickerson, R.C., Sharda, R., eds.: Proceedings of the 15th Americas Conference on Information Systems (AMCIS 2009), Association for Information Systems, pp. 3306–3314 (2009)

29. Chen, H.: Towards service engineering: Service orientation and business-it alignment. In: Proceedings of the 41st Hawaii International International Conference on Systems Science (HICSS-41 2008), p. 114. IEEE Computer Society (2008)

30. Shalaby, M., El-Kassas, S.: Applying scrum framework in the IT service support domain. J. Convergence 3(1), 21–28 (2012)

31. Hacker, W.: Intersection of software methodologies and ITIL v3. In: Proceedings of the IASTED International Conference on Software Engineering, pp. 232–236. ACTA Press (2008)

32. Hoover, C.: ITIL vs. agile programming: Is the agile programming discipline compatible with the ITIL framework?. In: Proceedings of the 32nd International Computer Measurement Group Conference, Computer Measurement Group, pp. 613–620 (2006)

33. Verlaine, B., Jureta, I., Faulkner, S.: Towards the alignment of a detailed service-oriented design and development methodology with ITIL v.3. In: Nóvoa, H., Drăgoicea, M. (eds.) IESS 2015. LNBIP, vol. 201, pp. 123–138. Springer, Heidelberg (2015)

34. Dingsøyr, T., Nerur, S.P., Balijepally, V., Moe, N.B.: A decade of agile methodologies: towards explaining agile software development. J. Syst. Softw. 85(6), 1213–1221 (2012)

35. Dybå, T., Dingsøyr, T.: Empirical studies of agile software development: a systematic review. Inf. Softw. Technol. 50(9–10), 833–859 (2008)

SStream: An Infrastructure for Streaming Multimedia Content Efficiently and Securely in a Heterogeneous Environment

Claudiu Olteanu[1]([✉]), Mihai Bucicoiu[1], and Marius Popa[2]

[1] Faculty of Automatic Control and Computers,
University Politehnica of Bucharest, Bucharest, Romania
vasilica.olteanu@cti.pub.ro, mihai.bucicoiu@cs.pub.ro
[2] Teamnet, Bucharest, Romania
marius.popa@teamnet.ro

Abstract. The rapid evolution of Internet had a big impact on how digital media is being shared and distributed. Nowadays, copyright violation is a major concern, as security issues still exist in video content traffic. Moreover, a heterogeneous environment often increases the need for retransmission of content, so, the bandwidth consumption is larger and creates congestion at the network level and higher energy consumption. In this paper, we try to tackle these problems and introduce SStream, a solution which can be used to deliver multimedia content in an efficient and secured manner. Our solution is based on a new and innovative encryption scheme, Attribute-Based Encryption. SStream protects the digital content by avoiding piracy and enforcing access control. We evaluated our solution and show that the added security layer does not impact the quality of the content.

Keywords: Video-streaming · HTTP adaptive streaming · Cryptography · Attribute-based encryption · Content delivery network · Software development approach

1 Introduction

Video streaming services account for a large share of Internet traffic [1]. According to the last year Total Audience Report, online video streaming viewers was growing at an impressive 60 % rate per month pace in December 2014, whereas TV had declined roughly 4 % [2]. A huge percentage of it is based on mobile or tablets clients [3]. The rapidly growth and interconnectivity of the Internet and gadgets had required the introduction of new protocols for faster and better video streaming. Moreover, the security aspects are important as intellectual property must be protected.

Our scope is to introduce a new solution for video streaming based on an open source project which uses HTTP-Based Adaptive Streaming. The advantage of this approach is not only that it has a lower cost, but it also ensures

© Springer International Publishing Switzerland 2016
T. Borangiu et al. (Eds.): IESS 2016, LNBIP 247, pp. 343–354, 2016.
DOI: 10.1007/978-3-319-32689-4_26

content protection while filtering access based on user attributes. Our proposal is beneficial for existing video streaming platforms as well as other digital content distributors who are focused on security issues when user privileges are involved.

In media distribution there are three entities: *the consumer, the distributor,* and *the producer. The consumer* receives the video content, decodes it and renders it to the end user. The job of *the producer* is to create and encode the content using a chosen protocol. *The distributor* takes the content from the producer and delivers it to the client. The most important role in terms of security is on the producer and consumer side. Both parties need to agree on encrypting the digital content in a safe and efficient way in order to assure its protection.

Digital Rights Management (DRM) systems have become top priorities for the Publishing and Entertaining Industries [4]. DRM systems manage and control the access and utilization of digital assets and their scope is to protect the intellectual property. Until today, several DRM systems have been proposed, based on different cryptographic schemes [5]. However, the current security issues of video streaming traffic require further investigation. The biggest disadvantage of the encryption schemes deployed today is that the access is controlled based on whether *the consumer's* key can decrypt or not the content.

In this paper, we present SStream, a DRM-like system based on a newly encryption scheme, Attribute-Based Encryption (ABE) [6]. The access to a video content can be built on user's attributes and not on the access to a certain key. Attribute-Based Encryption is a public key encryption algorithm that allows users to encrypt and decrypt messages based on their attributes.

We've also wanted our solution to be available to multiple devices such as phones and tablets, thus the media content will be delivered using an HTTP-Based Adaptive Streaming protocol, MPEG-DASH [7]. We found that the overhead brought by ABE is insignificant and it can be easily integrated and used to filter the access to the shared content.

The structure of this paper is as follows: in Sect. 2 we describe the technologies used, along with their advantages. Next, in Sect. 3 an overview of the SStream is presented while, Sect. 4 details on how we've implemented it. In Sect. 5 the experimental setup is presented and the obtained results. Section 6 presents similar work, while Sect. 7 concludes this paper.

2   Background

The concept of streaming means deliveries of continuous content from a server to a client where the packages are almost instantaneous consumed. One important aspect of streaming is that, preferably, the server transmission rate should match the client consumption rate. This is not trivial as this usually fluctuates, e.g., the client moves from a 4G connection to a Wi-Fi. Another important aspect of video streaming is the quality experience, if there are frequent stalls of the video or long startup delays, the overall experience of the client will suffer.

The Dynamic Adaptive Streaming over HTTP (MPEG-DASH) is an international, standardized, efficient solution for HTTP-based streaming of MPEG media. It uses the existing codecs, formats, protocols, signaling and content protection to offer backward-compatibility for the existing proprietary technologies.

Typically, the video/audio source is cut into many short segments, encoded to the desired delivery format and finally hosted on an HTTP Web server. A client requests the chunks from the Web server in a linear fashion and downloads them using plain HTTP progressive download. As the chunks are downloaded to the client, the client plays back the sequence of chunks in linear order. Because the chunks are carefully encoded without any gaps or overlaps between them, the chunks playback as a seamless video. Providing multiple encoded bit rates of the same media source also allows clients to dynamically switch between bit rates depending on network conditions and CPU consumption.

In terms of security, MPEG-DASH offers built-in support for content protection using the Common Encryption Scheme (CENC) [8]. It specifies standard encryption and key mapping methods. These can be utilized by one or more DRM systems to enable decryption of the same file. DRM systems usually imply techniques like encryption, watermarking, public/private keys, hashing, fingerprinting, digital certificates or others. We used this property of MPEG-DASH and created our own DRM system based on the Attribute-Based Encryption (ABE) scheme as detailed in the *Implementation* section.

Standard encryption is inefficient when selectively sharing data with many people since the data needs to be re-encrypted using every users public key. Firstly introduced by Amit Sahai and Brent Waters, the *ABE* scheme is a type of public key encryption [6]. It can generate keys based on a list of attributes and the decryption is possible only if the attributes set of the user matches those from the content. Currently, two different ABE schemes are proposed: (1) *Ciphertext-Policy ABE* where users have attributes and they receive a key from an authority for their set of attributes [9]. The ciphertext contains a policy which is a boolean predicate over the attribute space. The users can utilize their keys to decrypt the ciphertext only if their set of attributes satisfies the policy. (2) *Key-Policy ABE* where the attributes are assigned to a ciphertext when it is created and the policies are assigned to the users by the authority which creates the key [10].

In our solution we make use of the Ciphertext-Policy ABE implementation due to its binding of the attributes to the user. In order to protect the video content and to serve it to the end-users with high availability and high performance, the video chunks, and their encryption keys are delivered using a Content Delivery Network (CDN) system.

3 SStream Architecure

In this section, we present a high-level overview of *SStream*, a scalable and efficient adaptive streaming system which can be used to securely deliver multimedia content in a heterogeneous environment. First, we define the requirements of such systems:

- (*R1*) access to the media content should be allowed only for specific users. For example, only the Premium users should be allowed access to HD sports videos.

- (*R2*) media content should be distributed by a Content Delivery Network (CDN). The CDN should not have access to the content.
- (*R3*) videos keys should be safely distributed also through the CDN while preserving the privacy of the media content.
- (*R4*) be backward compatible.

SStream (Secured Stream) is an attribute based solution for video streaming which uses MPEG-DASH protocol for content encoding.

SStream adds an extra encryption layer using the *ABE* scheme over an existing solution which uses *Advanced Encryption Standard (AES)* for video content encryption [11]. The ABE encryption is applied only to the AES key and the overhead brought is insignificant compared to its benefits. Adding a short overhead to the encryption/decryption process, we managed to filter the access to the video content using users' attributes and to safely store and deliver the content through the CDN.

In order to see if *SStream* is a reliable solution, we tested its applicability, scalability, and performances on video streaming security. Since we added an extra layer of security using the ABE scheme, the major focus was to see how big is the overhead brought by that layer.

3.1   Security Overview

In this section, we detail on how our system protects the media content. Figure 1 depicts the high-level process. First, the video content was encrypted using AES. We chose to extend a solution based on the AES encryption because it is a symmetric-key algorithm which has high speed and low Random Access Memory requirements. Second, the video key is protected using ABE. In this way, only the users with some specific attributes can obtain the AES key to decrypt the video content.

In this paper, we will not focus on the AES algorithm because it is a well-known algorithm and we will concentrate on Attribute-Based Encryption applicability. As said before this will add an extra layer of security.

On the server side, in order to create the video key we need *a set of attributes* and the *ABE Master key*. The two are used to derive the *ABE Video Key (Step 1 in* Fig. 1*)*. The next step is to encrypt the video content with AES (*2*), generating an *AES Video Key*. Both the *ABE Video Key* and the *AES Video Key* are used as input for the *ABE Encryption (3)* step. The video key generation ends with the *key publication (4)*.

In order to obtain the user key, we derive *(5)* the *ABE Master key* and *a list of attributes* which describes the user.

To decrypt the video content, first we need to obtain the *AES Video key*. This is easily retrieved using the *ABE Decryption* process *(6)*. For the decryption process, we use as input the published *encrypted video key* and the *ABE private key* of the user. Note that this process can take place only if the user holds a proper private key with the same attributes as those used when encrypting the video.

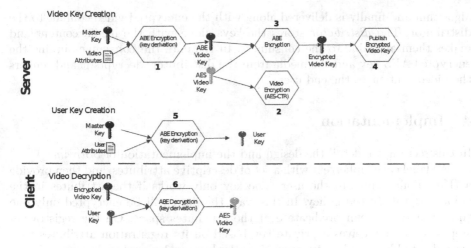

Fig. 1. Security mechanism overview

By adding the ABE security layer, we managed to handle the first three requirements presented in the beginning of the section. The access to a video content is filtered using the registration attributes of a user (*R1*) and the content is safely distributed and hosted by the CDN(*R2, R3*).

3.2 Content Delivery Overview

Next we outline the infrastructure used to distribute the video content. The job of each entity involved in the process is illustrated in Fig. 2.

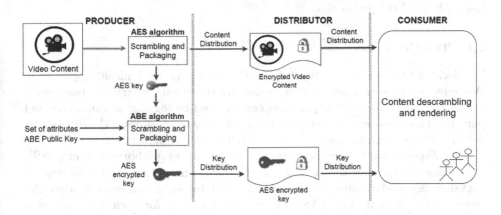

Fig. 2. Architecture of the system

The video content is taken by the *producer*, encoded and encrypted with AES. Next, the resulted AES key is encrypted with the Attribute-Based Encryption algorithm and finally is delivered along with the encrypted video content to the distributor. The *distributor* stores the keys along with the media content and makes them available to the consumers. In the end, the *consumer* obtains the encrypted AES key and the media from the distributor, decrypts it and renders the video content to the end user.

4   Implementation

In this section, we detail the design and the implementation of *SStream*.

We label each ciphertext with a set of descriptive attributes, and then provide a (Key, Policy) pair to the user. The key only works if the attributes in the ciphertext satisfy the policy. In this way, the data will be encrypted only one time using a boolean predicate over the attributes space. On the registration step, each user receives a private key based on its registration attributes that are validated by an administrator. Next the key can be used to decrypt only the content which was encrypted with a set of attributes that are satisfied by the user's attributes.

SStream follows the structure of similar streaming solutions: a consumer(C), a distributor(D) and the producer(P). *The consumer(C)* is represented by an Android application which uses a DASH player to decode and to render the video content. The player dynamically adapts the frame rate, the resolution and the bit rate depending on network conditions and CPU power. *The distributor(D)* uses an *HTTP Web Server* and hosts the encoded media content along with the encryption keys. Finally, the hosted content is delivered to the clients on their demand. *The producer(P)'s* job is to encode the media content using the MPEG-DASH standard and to publish the encoded chunks on the CDN. Before the publication, it encrypts the video chunks using AES protocol and the AES key with the ABE protocol.

4.1   The Consumer

We decided to do our prototype of the Consumer as an Android application. We opted for this as usually smartphones are those with restrictive bandwidth capabilities. The Android application can be used to register to the server and play the video content. It contains three important modules: (1) *Registration Service*, (2) *Decryption Module* and (3) *MPEG-DASH player*.

The *Registration Service* interacts with our Trusted Authority Server (TAS). It initiates a request with the TAS to collect the encryption keys. The request contains user's attributes which are validated by an administrator after the account was created. The TAS generates unique keys for each user. The service receives as input a public ABE key (the one used to encrypt the content), a master ABE key and a list of attributes. Using this three entities, it generates a private ABE key and it sends it along with the ABE public key to the consumer. The two are securely saved and can be used to decrypt and obtain the AES key of a video.

The connection between the TAS and the Registration Service is protected by an HTTPS channel and the whole process is illustrated in Fig. 3.

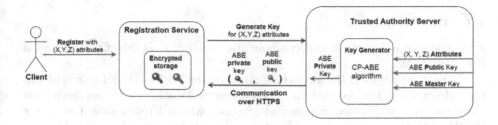

Fig. 3. Registration step

The *Decryption Module* uses the API provided by the Ciphertext-Policy Attribute-Based Encryption library [12](the same library is used by the key generator service from Trusted Authority Server) to decrypt the AES key using the ABE keys obtained on the registration step.

In order to display the video content we chose to extend a *JavaScript player (Dash.js)* which decodes the MPEG-DASH segments encrypted with AES [13]. We modified the source code and added a hook which calls our decryption module to obtain the AES key. Further, the library follows its normal flow.

Both modules are represented in Fig. 4.

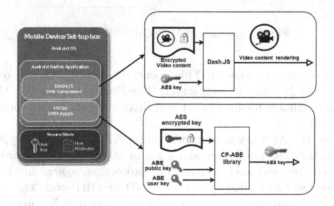

Fig. 4. Overview of consumer's architecture

4.2 The Distributor

For content distribution, we chose to install and configure an Apache Tomcat server. The server stores the encrypted AES keys and the encrypted video content received from the producer. Next it acts like a *distributor* which delivers the content on client demand.

Even though in our prototype the CDN was represented by an Apache server, in real world, the distributor can be replaced with other content distributors like *Youtube, Hulu,* etc...

4.3 The Producer

The producer is based on two components: an *MPEG-DASH Encoder* and a *Security Module.*

The *Encoder* ciphers the media content using the MPEG-DASH standard and the publication of the encoded chunks on a specific location. It breaks down each video file into small video chunks and creates a Media Presentation Descriptor (MPD) [14]. MPD is a file format used to provide information for a DASH client in order to be able to download the media segments from an HTTP server. The media segments can be encoded in different bit rates. This allows the DASH clients to dynamically switch between bit rates depending on network conditions (Fig. 5).

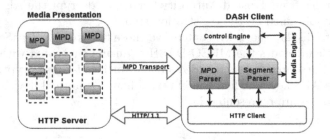

Fig. 5. Overview of MPEG-DASH protocol

Each video chunk and the MPD file is encrypted using AES by our *Security Module* and published on the web server. The clients will use the MPD file to lookup for the available media content and finally, depending on their privileges they will play the video.

At its turn, the AES key is encrypted using ABE. For the encryption of the content, ABE uses the public key and a set of attributes. There are two types of rules that can be used to enforce content protection: *logical* and *composition.* The first ones use the logical operators (AND or OR) while the second ones follow the form X out of (A, B, C, D) and means that if X equals 2, the user should have minimum 2 of the A, B, C or D attributes.

Both rules can contain other attributes groups as elements. The properties are based on attributes and can be either simple (has the "X" attribute. Example: "has a premium account") or arithmetical (has the "X" attribute > 18. Example: "AGE > 18"). The application can compute a very large set of properties rules. As a proof of concept we decided to use only three properties: age, country and account type (premium or regular) and the rule was always "*The user is from X country, has a Y account type and his age is greater than Z.*".

5   Evaluation

In order to evaluate our solution, we focused on the overhead brought by the layer of ABE encryption on two of the entities: the consumer and the producer. After the ABE encryption, the encrypted AES key has the same size. Therefore, the distribution layer was not affected by our changes, i.e. the size of the content is not altered by our solution.

Since we use the ABE to encrypt the AES key (256 bits), we look at the overhead when we introduce a large number of attributes with different types of attributes groups. We believe that a comparison with other encryption algorithms is not relevant since there is no other similar algorithm which solves the privileges problems using a list of properties assigned to a user and incorporated in the encryption keys. We demonstrate that we can benefit from content filtering using user's attributes adding a small overhead to the fast AES encryption algorithm. We show that the benefits of ABE are higher than the cost.

For the producer, all the tests and the benchmarks have been run on a workstation with a 4th Generation Intel Core i7-4700MQ Processor, 2.40 GHz frequency and 6 MB of L2 cache, 8 GB of DDR3 RAM memory at 1600 MHz. The OS used is Linux Mint with a 3.11.0-12-generic kernel version. On the other side, the environment for the consumer was represented by a Nexus 5 device with a 2.26 GHz quad-core Snapdragon 800 processor, 2 GB of RAM, 16 GB of internal storage and Android 6.01 operating system.

On the producer side, we run a number of tests where we measured the encryption time of the same 256 bits file for 10, 100, 200, 500 and 1000 attributes groups:

1. simple logical attributes groups: contains simple properties like *"(BIG and GREEN)"*
2. compositional attributes groups: has the form "2 of (A, B, C, D, E)" with A, B, C, D, E as simple properties. E.g. *"(2 of (PROGRAMMER, TESTER, STUDENT, TEACHER, GRADUATED))"*
3. simple logical attributes groups, with logical properties: For example *"(AGE < 20 and Height > 1.80)"*.

In Fig. 6 we can observe that as the predicate boolean difficulty increases, the encryption time is getting bigger. On the consumer side, we did the same tests and we measured the decryption time of the encrypted AES 256 key. Therefore, we had an ABE private key of the consumer based on three attributes and the AES key encrypted with a policy of 10, 100, 200, 500 and 1000 attributes groups (based on that three attributes). Similar with the encryption results, the decryption time is directly proportional with the predicate boolean difficulty, see Fig. 7.

Considering the fact that in our implementation of *SStream* we need to assign to the user only three kinds of attributes (Country, Age, Account Type), the overhead brought by the ABE algorithm is insignificant ($\approx$250 ms on consumer, $\approx$20 ms on producer). Note that the producer does not have time constraints as it can prepare the content ahead.

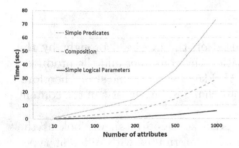

Fig. 6. ABE encryption time of AES 256 key

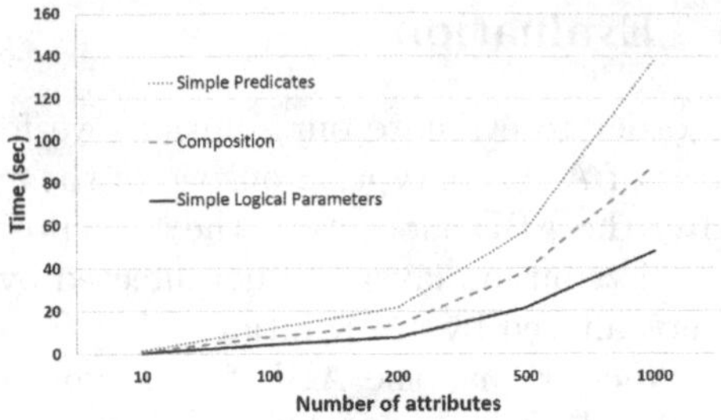

Fig. 7. ABE decryption time of AES 256 key

Moreover, in a real video streaming system, 10 attributes are more than enough to filter the access of the users using policies based on simple predicates. Even with this number, the overhead is small ($\approx$485 ms on client side, $\approx$90 ms on server side) and can be overlooked.

6   Related Work

In this section, we discuss similar solutions built on HTTP-Based Adaptive Streaming.

HTTP Live Streaming is an adaptive streaming communications protocol that can be used to distribute both live files and video-on-demand. The protocol was introduced by Apple and is compatible with Apple TV and iOS devices. For other platforms than iOS and Mac, it requires a special plugin such as Flash and Quicktime [15].

The protocol breaks down the streams into several video chunks encoded with MPEG2-TS, transcoded for different bit rates and delivers them to the client. The client is responsible for requesting the appropriate video chunks based on its available bandwidth. In contrast, *SStream* can be used on any device with any modern operating system. Also, it has support for other metrics than the bandwidth (i.e. the CPU usage).

Microsoft Smooth Streaming, known as IIS Smooth Streaming, was created by Microsoft team as an extension of Internet Information Services 7.0. It uses the MPEG-4 Part 14 (ISO/IEC 14496-12) file format for storage and transport [16].

With Smooth Streaming the file chunks are created virtually upon client request, but the actual video is stored on disk as a single full-length file per encoded bit rate. Same as HLS, Smooth Streaming is a proprietary implementation and its features can be used only if you pay a fair amount of money. In comparison, our solution breaks down the video into several chunks which can be stored on different servers, increasing the performance and the high availability of the system.

The main reason we chose MPEG-DASH over the others adaptive streaming communications protocols was because it is an open standard. Also, it can be integrated on the client side without the need of a specific plugin. Moreover, the protocol has native support for metrics which can be used to improve the quality of the client's experience.

7   Conclusions

In this paper, we introduced *SStream*, a video streaming solution that allow media distribution in a secure way.

The ABE protocol can be efficiently used to gain access to the digital content only for users with some specific attributes. In this way, we can easily select which user can see the content and which not. The main advantage is that in our DRM system we can encrypt the video content only once, using a set of attributes. We don't need to re-encrypt the media using the private key of each user. Therefore, we save time and space while we distribute our content safely.

Since the ABE algorithm is used only to encrypt the AES key, we demonstrated in the *Evaluation* section that the overhead is insignificant. We can benefit from content filtering using user's attributes adding a small overhead to the fast AES encryption algorithm. By adding the ABE security layer, we managed to handle some of the problems encountered by the media streaming providers. Firstly, we restricted the access to the media content using the registration attributes of a user (*R1*). Secondly, the media content and the videos keys can be hosted and distributed through untrusted CDNs (*R2, R3*).

Moreover, using the MPEG-DASH protocol *SStream* is an interoperable and scalable system which offers backward compatibility with most of the browsers, TVs, tablets and smartphones (*R4*).

Acknowledgments. We would also like to mention that the research for this paper was done within the MITSU (next generation MultImedia efficienT, Scalable and robUst Delivery) project financed through the Celtic-Plus - EUREKA Programme. The main objective of MITSU is to study and develop the next generation of multimedia streaming systems to be used over wireless networks [17].

References

1. Kafka, P.: re/code Tech News: Streaming Video Now Accounts for 70 Percent of Broadband Usage, December 2014. http://recode.net/2015/12/07/streaming-video-now-accounts-for-70-percent-of-broadband-usage/
2. The Total Audience Report. http://www.nielsen.com/content/dam/corporate/us/en/reports-downloads/201420Reports/total-audience-report-december-2014.pdf
3. Total Audience Report: Q2 - Media usage on device (2015). http://www.nielsen.com/us/en/insights/reports/2015/the-total-audience-report-q2-2015.html
4. Arnab, A., Hutchison, A.: Digital rights management - an overview of current challenges and solution (2004)
5. Fazio, N.: On cryptographic techniques for digital rights management (2006)
6. Sahai, A., Waters, B., Goyal, V., Pandey, O.: Attribute-based encryption for fine-grained access control of encrypted data

7. ISO, IEC 23009–1(2011) Observation of strains: Information technology - Dynamic Adaptive Streaming over HTTP (DASH)
8. W3C: ISO Common Encryption EME Stream Format and Initialization Data. https://w3c.github.io/encrypted-media/cenc-format.html
9. Waters, B., Bethencourt, J., Sahai, A.: Ciphertext-policy attribute-based encryption. In: Proceedings of the 2007 IEEE Symposium on Security and Privacy, SP 2007, pp. 321–334 (2007)
10. Attrapadung, N., Libert, B., de Panafieu, E.: Expressive key-policy attribute-based encryption with constant-size ciphertexts. In: Catalano, D., Fazio, N., Gennaro, R., Nicolosi, A. (eds.) PKC 2011. LNCS, vol. 6571, pp. 90–108. Springer, Heidelberg (2011)
11. Schaad, J.: RFC 3565 - Advanced Encryption Standard (AES) Key Wrap Algorithm (2003)
12. Bethencourt, J., Sahai, A., Waters, B.: Ciphertext-policy attribute-based encryption library. http://acsc.cs.utexas.edu/cpabe/
13. Dash Industry Forum: Dash.js player. https://github.com/Dash-Industry-Forum/dash.js/wiki
14. ISO, IEC 23009–1: 2014: Information technology - Dynamic adaptive streaming over HTTP (DASH), Part 1: Media presentation description and segment formats
15. May, E.W., Pantos, R.: HTTP Live Streaming (2015)
16. Microsoft: Smooth Streaming Protocol Specification (2012)
17. MultImedia efficienT Scalable and robUst Delivery. http://mitsu-project.eu/

Integration of Hazard Management Services

Anca Daniela Ionita[1]([✉]), Cristina-Teodora Eftimie[1], Grace Lewis[2],
and Marin Litoiu[3]

[1] University Politehnica of Bucharest,
Spl. Independentei 313, 060042 Bucharest, Romania
anca.ionita@upb.ro, cristina.eftimie@stud.acs.upb.ro
[2] Carnegie Mellon Software Engineering Institute,
4500 Fifth Ave., Pittsburgh, PA, USA
glewis@sei.cmu.edu
[3] York University, 4700 Keele Street, Toronto, ON, Canada
mlitoiu@yorku.ca

Abstract. Software migration to services is composed of three important parts: source code characterization, target code modeling, and transformation of legacy artifacts to develop services. Moreover, if the same target code model is defined as a common migration target for several existing applications with similar functionality, it is also possible to support interoperation and integration, in addition to migration to software services. This method for software migration may be applied in hazard management, where the availability of systems to manage particular environmental or social hazards may be insufficient when chain reactions and correlated events have to be treated simultaneously. Existing applications for monitoring hazards and emergency response may be migrated towards service-oriented systems, capable to orchestrate decision making and response actions. The target model proposed in this paper is a process template for integrating services irrespective of the hazard type, with the possibility to reuse the realizations of visualization and notification activities. The example implemented in our study was based on process binding to services specific for water and air pollution management.

Keywords: Migration to services · Process modeling · Modeling and design of IT-enabled service systems · Hazard management

1 Introduction

Legacy software represents a valuable asset for any organization, but it has to evolve in order to fit in today's ecosystems dominated by services, in which Cloud Computing and Service-Oriented Architecture (SOA) complement and leverage each other. Redevelopment from scratch for creating a service-oriented system is a lengthy and costly approach that is prohibited for many businesses. A potentially faster and easier solution with reduced risks is to integrate the legacy applications into new environments via wrapping and adaptation, but there would still be old software that has to be maintained. Another solution, which is potentially slower but better in the long term, is to migrate the legacy code to a new system, but reuse its assets [1].

© Springer International Publishing Switzerland 2016
T. Borangiu et al. (Eds.): IESS 2016, LNBIP 247, pp. 355–364, 2016.
DOI: 10.1007/978-3-319-32689-4_27

We investigated the case of modernizing a set of similar applications by migrating them to conform to common models representing their business, architectural, process or enterprise aspects. This is the situation of systems managing various natural, technological or environmental degradation hazards [2]. Currently, there are many systems for early warning and alert, more or less based on Information Technology (IT); a report of United Nations Environment Programme (UNEP) includes more than a hundred examples, classified by type of event, source and geographic coverage [3]. The United Nations Office for Disaster Risk Reduction (UNISDR) discusses national platforms and international frameworks aiming to implement the Hyogo Framework for Action for building resilience to hazard consequences [4].

The idea proposed in this paper is that various hazard management systems may be migrated to service-orientation based on a common process template, which is further configured by means of sub-processes and concrete services specific to various types of hazards, means of collecting data, methods for decision making and notification distribution. This may represent a step forward for creating systems that are able to interoperate if multiple hazards occur at the same time, e.g. a hurricane that produces floods, and then water pollution and biological hazards.

After discussing the general context of migrating to services in Sect. 2, the paper is focused on the modeling phase of the software migration target for a general hazard management process in Sect. 3. Its mapping to REST services is exemplified for water and air pollution in Chapter 4, by using Drools for defining business rules, and by performing simulations with real data made public by national and regional authorities.

2 Migrating to Software Services

In this chapter we discuss how to make the migration decision and how to realize it.

Decision. To make the decision of migrating or not, a list of options has to be put together, considering Return of Investment (ROI), payback, and alignment with the strategic objectives of the organization. There are three essential analyses that have to be performed for this purpose (see Fig. 1):

- *Technical analysis* – determines the readiness of the legacy software for migration, which is often referred to as *serviceability* or *cloudability*. This requires determining the degree of distribution of the legacy architecture, the usage of services, and the existence of Internet clients and their number. The use of metrics for complexity, coupling, and cohesion is common.
- *Business analysis* – defines business goals and drivers, user priorities, costs, and it identifies risks. Several criteria considered are licensing, availability of services associated to the software product, changes in business process, and impact on organizational structure (new roles or departments).
- *Analysis of options* – estimates the potential benefits of various strategies for migrating to services, compared to the option of not migrating [5].

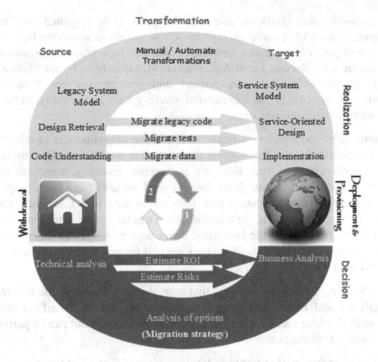

Fig. 1. Decision and realization aspects for migration to services

The decision of migration to Cloud and SOA should be accompanied by a well-motivated strategy. Generally, a direct transition in the "Cold Turkey" style is not recommended, because it may introduce risks and discontinuities to the business, and the costs may be difficult to support. Incremental approaches, often called "Chicken Little" approaches, are preferred because they establish a plan for gradually migrating parts of the legacy code towards services [6]. When creating a strategy for evolving towards service provisioning, the following options should be considered:

- wrap the entire application without changing its structure and transform it into a service;
- decompose it into reusable services offered to other service-oriented platforms;
- migrate the entire system to SOA;
- adopt a mixed architectural style, e.g. migrate part of the legacy code to SOA or modernize the application by using third-party services;
- deploy the entire system on an Infrastructure as a Service (IaaS) cloud provider;
- restructure and deploy part of the legacy application in the Cloud (or in multiple clouds);
- integrate available Software as a Service (SaaS) products into the legacy software.

The strategy also decides the software migration life cycle and the timing and dependencies between basic activities, such as decomposing the legacy system into parts, adding specific architectural elements, designing for non-functional properties such as scalability and elasticity, selecting the parts to be migrated, and selecting technologies. At the end of a migration phase it is necessary to sunset the legacy system making sure to preserve a fallback version, to abandon legacy processes, and to clean up data. Beforehand, Service Level Agreements (SLAs) have to be established for the new services, in addition to deployment and provisioning for launching the service-oriented system. In an incremental strategy this is normally executed via multiple withdrawal/launching steps.

Realization. After the decision is made, the software migration has to effectively be realized. The foundation for this stage is the horseshoe model, initially introduced for reengineering, in which its three sides are architecture recovery, transformation, and architecture-based development. Since then, several variants have been proposed for reverse engineering, transformation and forward engineering. Each side can have several levels of abstraction and the transformation can take place at multiple levels [7]. Generally, the three sides of the horseshoe cover aspects related to the source of the migration, its target, and the transformations applied for getting from the source to the target (see Fig. 1).

Migration Source. The legacy software that represents the source of the migration has to be analyzed and modeled. Program understanding can be based on static and dynamic analysis using various reverse engineering techniques and can be performed at multiple levels of abstraction:

- *code level*: separation of reusable code; slicing; identification of functional and data dependencies;
- *design level*: design pattern detection; architecture reconstruction; feature location;
- *business level*: business process modeling; discovery of business knowledge (rules, concepts, patterns).

Migration Target. The service-oriented system represents the software migration target obtained via forward engineering techniques. Classical development models can be used, but there are also specific elements at each level of abstraction:

- *modeling level*: service identification based on candidates discovered from the legacy software; reuse of third-party services; selection of service candidates with feasible implementation; modeling of "to-be" business processes;
- *design level*: introduction of architectural elements for Cloud (virtualization infrastructure; multitenant architecture; NoSQL databases; data replication; components for billing, monitoring, security) and/or SOA implementations (service registry, discovery, composition, monitoring and management);
- *implementation level*: implementation of services (e.g. based on SOAP or REST); use of SOA tool suites; adoption of proprietary environments for the Cloud.

Transformations. Transformations are a part of any maintenance approach and can be applied at three levels of abstraction: *code* (stripping, restructuring), *design* (component-to-service transformation) and *business models* (service provisioning adoption, pricing models adjustment). Migration to SOA and Cloud requires two other types of transformations:

- *composition model* – for SOA (e.g. modification of business processes for service orchestration);
- *deployment model* – for Cloud (e.g. addition of a load-balancing component for deployment into an IaaS platform).

An important trend in transformations is automation based on Model-Driven Engineering (MDE), using standards for discovering knowledge or for modeling service-oriented architecture and cloud environments [9]. MDE is used for *horizontal transformations* (between similar source and target levels of abstraction) and for *vertical transformations* – both for reverse and forward engineering.

In addition to code migration, automatic transformations are also useful for migrating existing relational databases to document-oriented data stores that support terabytes of data and distribution on thousands of commodity servers. In addition, migrating tests for core and third-party services is also useful and potentially challenging. Table 1 summarizes the challenges discussed above for migration decision, as well as for the three elements of realization: source, target and transformation.

Table 1. Summary of software migration challenges

Source challenges	Transformation challenges
- Complexity and scale - Monolithic code - Missing interfaces - Too many dependencies - Incompatible data types	- Restructuring databases - Building correct transformations - Assessing if transformations maintain essential functions and data - Performing time-consuming manual transformations
Decision challenges	Target challenges
- Estimating the global cost of migration - Estimating ROI - Assessing transformation time - Identifying new roles for managing services - Changing business models - Pricing for all parties involved - Dealing with employee resistance to change	- Dealing with federations of infrastructures - Testing involving third-parties - Versioning services - Defining the appropriate granularity of services - Avoiding vendor lock-in for Cloud services - Maintaining the coherence of the target system in an incremental migration - Determining the right thresholds for scaling up and down predicting QoS failures - Selecting the Cloud platform for data storage, taking into account the amount of data processed, and random access patterns - Defining architectures for distributed clouds - Dealing with admission control in multiple geographical location - Scaling out to public Cloud providers

3   Software Migration Target Model for Hazard Management

This chapter is only focused on one of the three realization elements discussed above: the migration target modeling. Our study was performed for a specific application domain — hazard management. In this context, we propose a process template that is general enough for any hazard management system and may be transformed into an executable process by binding its activities to abstract and then concrete services [10]. A preliminary theoretical study had the aim to identify typical activities, information flows and architectural modules in existing systems. For instance, disaster monitoring, decide & act and warning dissemination were identified as important steps in the information flow of early warning systems [11]. Other desirable features are: problem analysis, scope assessment, population and institutional notification [12]. The procedures for hazard and emergency management are generally well defined and involve many actors with clearly specified responsibilities and hierarchical relationships.

However, the aim of our analysis was to extract the essential activities that would characterize a generic service process [13], within the context of hazard management systems, and would define an orchestration template for the service-oriented system that represents the migration target.

Figure 2 shows the proposed process model represented in BPMN (Business Process Modeling Notation), composed of four basic activities: two of them specific to the type of hazard – *Monitoring* and *Decision Support* – and the other two general – *Visualization* and *Notification*. The realization of these activities has a high diversity; for example, *Notification* may consist of an informative message, an early warning or an alert, depending on the severity of the situation and the time left for performing preventive, mitigation or response actions.

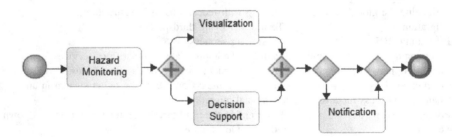

Fig. 2. Process template for hazard management

Increased complexity may require the definition of a sub-process (later exposed as a web service), as the example from Fig. 3, which corresponds to *Hazard Monitoring*. An important way to monitor physical quantities, relevant as inputs for *Visualization* and *Decision Support*, is to use sensor networks and integrate data collected by them on a regular basis. The example considered here is a sub-process for integrating data from sensor observations and transforming them for interoperation purposes, based on SOS (Sensor Observation Service), a standard of the correspondent web service interface adopted by OGC (Open Geospatial Consortium) [14].

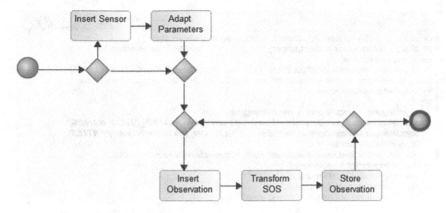

Fig. 3. Sub-process example for hazard monitoring

4 Example of Integrated Services

The process template presented above was used for integrating services for two particular hazards — air and water pollution — based on the experience of two research projects: prediction and decision support in case of accidental pollution of rivers [15] and early warning against radioactive clouds potentially induced by nuclear facilities [16]. Water and air quality are an important topic of research for improving prevention and control in various areas of the globe [17, 18].

For both cases we adapted services corresponding to the generic process activities (see Fig. 4) and we implemented and executed the resulting concrete processes on Activiti BPM Platform. For *Hazard Monitoring* we applied the sub-process described in Fig. 3. The Sensor Observation Service was realized with the Sensor Web infrastructure available from 52°North [19]. A REST client was created for querying sensor properties with SOS and sensor descriptions conforming to SensorML (Sensor Modeling Language) [20]. Three web services were bound to *Insert Sensor, Insert Observation,* and *Store Observation* activities.

The decisions were managed in terms of business rules specified in Drools, as a series of *if-then* statements [21], with the suite offered by JBoss Enterprise BRMS (Business Rules Management System). The language allows to make a clear separation between the reasoning itself and the data it is applied to. Two web services were implemented for our example, for identifying water and air pollution respectively. Their aim was to determine if there is a low, medium or high pollution, according to configurable thresholds, and to decide whether it is necessary to send alerts regarding the polluted area, characterized in terms of latitude and longitude and visualized using Google Maps API. The color codes were: red for high pollution levels and yellow for medium ones. A pop-up allows the visualization of geographical coordinates when pressing the right mouse button.

Water Pollution Services. The water pollution example was configured for a risk area in the proximity of Popesti-Leordeni and not far from the Romanian capital city, with a

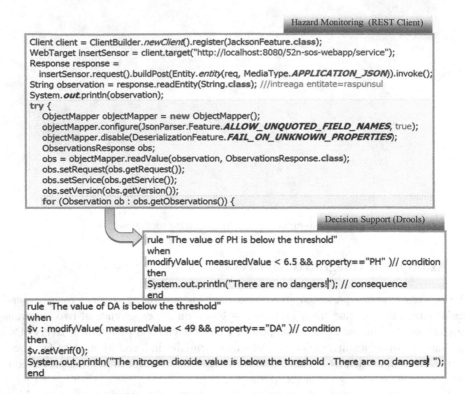

Fig. 4. Example of process activities implementation

population of almost 2 million inhabitants. The observations monitored in this case were related to six quality attributes: pH, turbidity, conductivity, color, nitrites and bacteria. The values used in our simulations were originated from the water analysis reports made public by a company that provides public water supply and sewerage services in Bucharest [22]. We only considered the properties that conform to WaterML, a standard model adopted by OGC for water observations data, including water quality [23].

Air Pollution Services. A specific decision service was defined for identifying air pollution also. The quality attributes considered for monitoring in this case were: sulfur dioxide, nitrogen dioxide, ozone, carbon monoxide, suspension powders with diameter less than 2.5 μm and suspension powders with diameter less than 10 μm. The simulations were performed with public data supplied by the National Network for Monitoring Air Quality [24] and collected from more than 150 automated and mobile stations.

5   Conclusion

The realization of migration to software services is confronted by many challenges regarding its three important aspects: the legacy software representing the source, the target service-oriented system, and the required transformations. They are influenced by the legacy code complexity and preparedness for migration, as well as by the required scalability, elasticity and maintainability of the new system.

This paper proposes a process template capable of integrating services for multiple types of hazards, which may be used for modeling the software transformation target of existing early warning and alert systems, such as water and air pollution management, implemented for our example. We applied this template by implementing specific REST services for monitoring: (i) water characteristics on a river segment in the proximity of a potential source of pollution, and (ii) the concentration of the main pollutants used in estimating the air quality index. The simulations were performed with public data from national and regional authorities. The decision activity was realized based on specific rules defined in respect with multiple threshold values.

Future work should be focused on migrating more complex algorithms for decision support, currently used in legacy hazard management systems, including predictions such as: atmospheric dispersion of radioactive emissions and cloud propagation based on weather conditions, as well as pollutant propagation downstream the source where it was flushed into the river, based on hydrodynamic equations. More flexibility in the process execution may also be attained by defining a mechanism for late binding of services, based on location, risk probability and impact, as well as other factors that need to be investigated.

Acknowledgments. The work of Anca Daniela Ionita was supported by the Partnerships in Priority Areas Program - PN II, MEN-UEFISCDI, under the projects 47/2012 and 298/2014.

References

1. Ionita, A.D., Litoiu, M., Lewis, G. (eds.): Migrating Legacy Applications: Challenges in Service Oriented Architecture and Cloud Computing Environments. IGI Global, Hershey (2013)
2. Working Background Text on Terminology for Disaster Risk Reduction. The United Nations Office for Disaster Risk Reduction (2015)
3. Early Warning Systems: A State of the Art Analysis and Future Directions. Division of Early Warning and Assessment (DEWA). United Nations Environment Programme (UNEP), Nairobi (2012)
4. UNISDR Annual Report 2014. The United Nations Office for Disaster Risk Reduction, Geneva (2014)
5. Lewis, G., Morris, E., Simanta, S., Smith, D.: SMART: Analyzing the Reuse Potential of Legacy Components in a Service-Oriented Architecture Environment. Technical Note CMU/SEI-2008-TN-008 (2008)
6. Brodie, M.L., Stonebraker, M.: Migrating Legacy Systems: Gateways, Interfaces & The Incremental Approach. Morgan Kaufmann Publishers, San Francisco (1995)
7. Kazman, R., Woods, S., Carrière, J.: Requirements for integrating software architecture and reengineering models: CORUM II. In: Proceedings of the Firth Working Conference on Reverse Engineering (WCRE), pp. 154–163. IEEE Computer Society Press (1998)
8. Razavian, M., Lago, P.: A frame of reference for soa migration. In: Di Nitto, E., Yahyapour, R. (eds.) ServiceWave 2010. LNCS, vol. 6481, pp. 150–162. Springer, Heidelberg (2010)

9. Wagner, C.: Model-Driven Software Migration: A Methodology: Reengineering, Recovery and Modernization of Legacy Systems. Springer, Heidelberg (2014)
10. Ionita, A.D., Catapano, A., Giuroiu, S., Florea, M.: Service oriented system for business cooperation. In: Proceedings of the 2nd International Workshop on Systems Development in SOA Environments, SDSOA 2008, pp. 13–18. ACM, New York (2008)
11. Wächter, J., Babeyko, A., Fleischer, J., Häner, R., Hammitzsch, M., Kloth, A., Lendholt, M.: Development of tsunami early warning systems and future challenges. Nat. Hazards Earth Syst. Sci. **12**, 1923–1935 (2012)
12. Hristidis, V., Chen, S.-C., Li, T., Luis, S., Deng, Y.: Survey of data management and analysis in disaster situations. J. Syst. Softw. **83**, 1701–1714 (2010)
13. Borangiu, T., Oltean, V.E., Dragoicea, M., e Cunha, J.F., Iacob, I.: Some aspects concerning a generic service process model building. In: Snene, M., Leonard, M. (eds.) IESS 2014. LNBIP, vol. 169, pp. 1–16. Springer, Heidelberg (2014)
14. Ciolofan, S.N., Mocanu, M., Ionita, A.D.: Cyberinfrastructure architecture to support decision taking in natural resources management. In: Dumitrache, I., Florea, A.M., Pop, F. (eds.) Proceedings of the 19th International Conference on Control Systems and Computer Science (CSCS), Bucharest, pp. 617–623. IEEE (2013)
15. Vacariu, L., Hangan, A., Mocanu, M.: Pollution detection on the CyberWater platform. Environ. Eng. Manage. J. **14**(9), 2043–2050 (2015)
16. Gheorghe, A.V., Vamanu, D.V.: Disaster risk and vulnerability management from awareness to practice. In: Gheorghe, A.V. (ed.) Integrated Risk and Vulnerability Management Assisted by Decision Support Systems, pp. 1–320. Springer, Netherlands (2015)
17. Ismail, Z.: Evaluating trends of water quality index of selected Kelang river tributaries. Environ. Eng. Manage. J. **13**, 61–72 (2014)
18. Stefan, S., Barladeanu, R., Andrei, S., Zagar, L.: Study of air pollution in Bucharest, Romania during 2005–2007. Environ. Eng. Manage. J. **14**(4), 809–818 (2015)
19. Martínez, A.P.: Implementation and documentation of Sensor Web Enablement at KNMI. Internship Report, Royal Netherlands Meteorological Institute, De Bilt (2011)
20. OGC® SensorML: Model and XML Encoding Standard, Version 2.0.0. Open Geospatial Consortium (2014)
21. Ary, J.: Instant Drools Starter. Packt Publishing, Birmingham (2014)
22. Apa Nova Bucuresti, Water analysis reports. http://www.apanovabucuresti.ro/en/water-analysis-reports
23. OGC® WaterML 2.0: Part 1- Timeseries, Version 2.0.1, Open Geospatial Consortium (2014)
24. National Network for Monitoring Air Quality. http://www.calitateaer.ro/

Servitization in Sustainable Manufacturing: Models and Information Technologies

Service Oriented Mechanisms for Smart Resource Allocation in Private Manufacturing Clouds

Octavian Morariu, Theodor Borangiu, Cristina Morariu,
and Silviu Răileanu[✉]

Department of Automation and Industrial Informatics, Research Centre in CIM
and Robotics - CIMR, University Politehnica of Bucharest, 313,
Splaiul Independentei sector 6, Bucharest, Romania
{octavian.morariu,theodor.borangiu,
silviu.raileanu}@cimr.pub.ro

Abstract. Cloud manufacturing (CMfg) represents an evolution of networked and service-oriented manufacturing models, focusing on the new opportunities in networked manufacturing enabled by the emergence of cloud computing platforms. The paper reports results obtained in developing service-oriented mechanisms that optimize resource allocation in a private cloud implemented with IBM CloudBurst 2.1 for manufacturing enterprises. A predictive mechanism is described that augments the generic threshold-based implementation by recognizing repetitive patterns in application usage. Then, a queued resource allocation bus architecture extended with computation of alternative schedules is proposed; this is a service oriented mechanism assuring adaptability of the private CMfg system to workload fluctuations; the implementation is on IBM CloudBurst 2.1 and uses a genetic algorithm for smart resource allocation. A multilayer QoS monitoring architecture, designed for the cloud, is reported.

Keywords: CMfg · Private cloud · Predictive capacity provisioning · QoS · Service oriented resource allocation · Service choreography · Queued bus architecture

1 Introduction

Cloud manufacturing (CMfg) represents an evolution of networked and service-oriented manufacturing models, with specific focus on the new opportunities in networked manufacturing (NM) enabled by the emergence of cloud computing platforms [1]. While the concept itself refers to the most important issues related to cloud adoption, it does not cover the redundancy requirements specific to MES workloads. Other cloud based services for the manufacturing industry like product design, product scheduling, batch planning, real time manufacturing control, testing, management, and all other stages of the product life cycle are described in [2]. Manufacturing enterprises have started to adopt cloud computing, especially in the upper side of the software stack: the enterprise resource planning (ERP), supply chain management (SCM) and customer resource management (CRM) areas. Another important research direction is

© Springer International Publishing Switzerland 2016
T. Borangiu et al. (Eds.): IESS 2016, LNBIP 247, pp. 367–383, 2016.
DOI: 10.1007/978-3-319-32689-4_28

represented by the study of resource virtualization techniques and the resource sharing in manufacturing systems [3, 4].

A structured approach to cloud adoption and MES virtualization is considered by manufacturing companies that are organized using the 5-level ISA-95 model, focusing especially on level 3 (the Manufacturing Execution level on which mixed production planning, product scheduling and resource allocation prepare the execution of production processes controlled on ISA-95 levels 0, 1 and 2), where private clouds can offer support for a virtualized MES.

The communication pattern between MES and the physical workloads in shop floor is, from SOA perspective, service choreography with point to point message exchange in real time. When considering migration to cloud environments, these characteristics of MES specific workloads can be assured by private cloud implementation with workload virtualization.

In this context, MES virtualization involves migration of all MES workloads that were traditionally executed on physical machines to the data centre, specifically to the private cloud infrastructure as virtual workloads. The idea is to run all the control software in a virtualized environment and keep only the physical resources with their dedicated real time controllers on the shop floor. This separation between hardware resources and software that controls them provides a new level of flexibility and agility to the manufacturing solution [5, 6].

The innovations in virtualization technologies together with real time monitoring capabilities implemented by cloud providers allow development of cloud based elastic systems. Elasticity is defined as the capability of a system to automatically increase and decrease its capacity based on real time load without the intervention of the system administrator. System elasticity has been studied as part of self-optimization problems in autonomic computing area [7] focusing on the system design, which has a great impact on elasticity.

Commercial cloud providers offer various techniques to support elasticity for customer applications. Amazon E2C cloud offers a service called Elastic Load Balancing that abstracts the complexity of managing, maintaining, and scaling load balancers [8]; this service is designed to automatically add and remove capacity as needed, without any manual intervention. In private cloud implementations like IBM CloudBurst 2.1 scalability is implemented based on predefined thresholds [9]. The thresholds can be defined in low level metrics like CPU usage, memory usage or disk usage; this is implemented by IBM Tivoli Monitor that uses a Linux based OS agent to collect real time metrics and monitor predefined thresholds. When a threshold is reached a new workload instance can be provisioned or de-provisioned based on the predefined workflow. The workflow is executed by IBM Tivoli Provisioning Manager [10] and interacts with the underlying virtualization technology, VMware VCenter.

One characteristic common to the implementations discussed above is that these are reactive in nature. In other words the decision to scale up and down is taken based on some predefined rules that are evaluated against real time metrics. This approach is flexible and works well for generic applications. However, for real life applications with a more specific purpose, like the MES ones, an advanced predictive scalability model based on repetitive usage patterns can assure better resource utilization.

Section 2 of this paper presents such an approach for a private CMfg implemented with IBM CloudBurst 2.1 that augments the threshold mechanism, with information based on the historical repetitive usage patterns. Section 3 proposes a queued resource allocation bus architecture extended with computation of alternative schedules. Section 4 describes a service oriented mechanism for assuring adaptability of a typical private CMfg system to workload fluctuations that is capable of intelligent resource allocation; the implementation is on IBM CloudBurst 2.1. A genetic algorithm for smart resource allocation is proposed. Section 5 presents a multilayer QoS monitoring architecture implemented on top of IBM CloudBurst 2.1 private cloud solution and integrated with IBM TSAM product stack.

2 Predictive Capacity Provisioning Mechanism

An important factor to consider in private CMfg systems is the time taken to provision an additional resource. This typically includes the provisioning of the workload in a virtualized environment, the start-up of the workload, dynamic configuration of services and load balancing and start-up of the application. This provisioning time cannot be ignored when planning capacity requirements and elasticity, because it is significant even for simple applications. In practice, the provisioning time introduces the need to set thresholds at a lower level than actually dictated by the capacity requirements, in order to allow time for the new instance to become active before the capacity is exceeded by the user load. This approach has many disadvantages. One of the most obvious is that it introduces the risk of false positives that lead to poor resource utilization by unnecessary provisioning of additional resources. When using simple thresholds along with a small granularity of the application scalability the effects are amplified. We propose a predictive mechanism that augments the generic threshold based implementation by recognizing repetitive pattern in application usage.

The capacity supported by one instance is an intrinsic property of an application. For example the amount of concurrent users for one instance can be determined by load testing. The results obtained with load tests serve as baselines for determining the initial thresholds for the deployment and configuring the dynamic scalability of the applications.

To augment this we propose a daily and weekly usage pattern model that would predict the future required capacity and would act before the threshold is reached, allowing setting higher levels for thresholds and so avoid false positive triggers.

The implementation described in this paper is targeted at IBM CloudBurst 2.1 on System x, but the concept does apply to any API based cloud platform, either public or private. To encapsulate the predictive algorithm we introduce the Elastic Scalability Module (ESM) that augments the CloudBurst 2.1 threshold mechanism. The architecture of the Elastic Scalability Module proposed for IBM CloudBurst 2.1 is illustrated in Fig. 1. The ESM works by collecting real time usage metrics provided by IBM TUM; it has two operational phases: the learning phase and the driving phase. In the learning phase, the ESM stores in the metrics provided by IBM TUM per day for each day of the week in a relational database together with the threshold trigger events generated by TUM. This is done several times until a pattern is established. The ESM determines a pattern for a day of the week by comparing the metric variati-on against an average of previously recorded metrics for the same day of the week. If the difference for each hourly average is smaller than a preconfigured threshold, the pattern is considered valid.

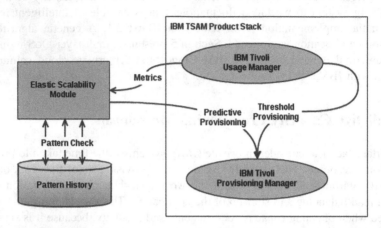

Fig. 1. Architecture of ESM for IBM Cloud Burst 2.1 implementing the MES CMfg

The algorithm for the learning phase is presented below:

Algorithm 1 Validate Pattern

function validatePattern(hourOfDay, currentLoad) is
* saveInDatabase(hourOfDay, currentLoad)*
* if hourOfDay=0 then*
*   weekPatternFound = true*
*   for i=0 to 23 do*
*   avg = computeAvgDayWeekHour(i, 10)*
*   if abs(avg/currentLoad) > patternThreshold then*
*   weekPatternFound = false*
*   endif*
* endif*
* if weekPatternFound = true then*
*   swithToDrivingPhase()*
*   setHigherThresholds()*
* endif*
end function

Once the pattern is validated, the ESM begins to function in the driving phase, by sending predictive provisioning instructions to the IBM Tivoli Provisioning Manager (TPM), eventually replacing the trigger based behaviour of Tivoli Usage Manager (TUM). Also at this point, the thresholds are set to higher values, to avoid false positives. Even in the driving phase the current usage load is validated against the pattern stored in the database and if the pattern validation fails, the ESM will transition back to learning phase and will set relaxed values for the thresholds. This behaviour helps in exceptional scenarios like special days of the year when rush orders are received and must be planned or a situation in which the system load is unexpected. In this case, the system would fall back on threshold based provisioning and de-provisioning.

Algorithm 2 Predictive Set Capacity

function predictiveSetCapacity(dayOfWeek, hourOfDay) is
  loadDayPattern(dayOfWeek)
  nextProvisioningTime = hourOfDay + provisioningDelay
  estimatedCapacity = getPatternCapacity(nextProvisioningTime)
  instances = (currentCapacity - estimatedCapacity)/instanceCapacity
  if (instances > safeCapacityThresholdProv) then
    provision(instances)
  endif
  if (instances < safeCapacityThresholdDeprov) then
    deprovision(abs(instances))
  endif
end function

The predictive provisioning algorithm is invoked each hour and based on the provisioning delay it computes the next provisioning time. The next provisioning time re-presents the time when a new machine would be active, if the decision to provision it is taken now. Based on the daily pattern, the estimated capacity is retrieved. The difference between the current provisioned capacity and the estimated capacity divided by the instance capacity represents the number of instances that need to be provisioned or de-provisioned, depending if the difference is positive or negative. The result is compared with a safe capacity threshold and the decision is made to provision or de-provision additional instances. ESM considers the average provisioning time in the *provisioningDelay* constant. The overall goal followed by the ESM algorithm is to keep the capacity as close as possible to the average user load using historical usage patterns.

3 Queued Resource Allocation Bus Architecture

Private cloud computing involves several initial steps to setup the system. The first step consists in resource enrolment and discovery, grouping the resources in resource pools and abstraction of physical resources. The next logical step is the creation of a service catalogue which allows publishing of resource pools and available workloads. Based on this service catalogue, cloud customers can request resources and configure the required workloads for their business requirements. The final step is represented by the actual operational model for consuming the available cloud resources and published workloads. However, due to the limited nature of resources in private clouds, the actual resource allocation is implemented through a request approval process.

Microsoft is using System Center 2012 SP1 Service Manager and Orchestrator to offer a self-service interface access to the service catalogue; this is a request based process triggering an administrator approval for required resources. The administrator has a set of built-in tools that allows a quick decision or even auto approval for requested resources based on pre-defined policies. IBM uses Tivoli Service Automation Manager (TSAM) software stack to manage the resources in the private cloud offerings. As part of the Tivoli stack the Tivoli Service Request Manager (TSRM) allows customers to create tickets that are triggering an internal approval workflow. TSRM implements an initial ticket validation that prevents customers to create requests if the system does not have the required capacity for provisioning in the in the required interval.

The solution presented in the paper is adding two key abilities for decision support compared to the implementations above. The first is the ability to offer alternative schedules for customers in case the resources are not available at the required time, instead of a simple deny of the request either automatically or assisted-manual by the system administrators. The second is the ability to use federated resources for request fulfilment, in the scenario where two or more private clouds are interconnected.

The proposed resource allocation architecture is presented in Fig. 2.

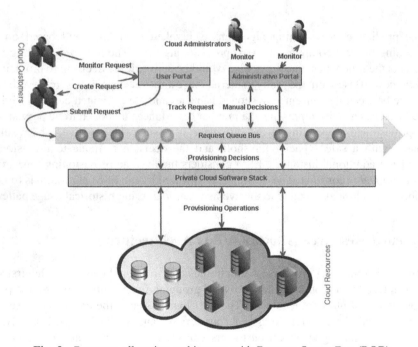

Fig. 2. Resource allocation architecture with Request Queue Bus (RQB)

The proposed solution consists in a Request Queue Bus (RQB) where the requests are submitted by the customers using a user portal. The requests are considered stand-alone entities that are queued for processing rather than assigned directly for an immediate decision. The user portal allows creation of requests, based on the services catalogue offered by the underlying private cloud software stack, without performing a prior validation in regards to the available capacity in the time interval required. To offer a superior user experience the requests are created in a "shopping cart" fashion, allowing the customer to add multiple workloads and associated resources in a single request. The request object data structure contains references to the service catalogue items selected together with the associated amounts. At the same time the request data structure contains the initial time interval for which the respective resources should be provisioned. The user portal assembles the request object and submits it in the resource allocation queue, see Fig. 2. The user portal also allows customers to track requests created and provide further responses on the options for request fulfilment provided by the system.

The administrative portal is used by cloud administrators and serves two major roles. The first one is to allow creation of request fulfilment policies. These policies contain a matching rule for requests and a link to the corresponding decision process. If the rule is evaluated to true for a request, then the corresponding request fulfilment policy is applied and the decision process is triggered. The decision process can be a SOA BPEL process, representing a multi-level approval process or the invocation of a specialized module that computes alternatives for request fulfilment. The expected scenario is that when the resources can be allocated in the requested interval, the approval process is invoked, and when there is not enough capacity for provisioning the requested resources the alternatives are computed and presented to the cloud customer in the request object. The request lifecycle is detailed in Fig. 3.

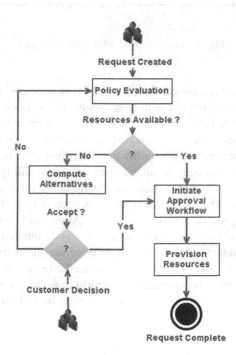

Fig. 3. The request lifecycle

The cycle starts when the request is created by the customer, containing the requested resources along with the initial timeframe. If the resources are available, an approval workflow is initiated. If approved either manually or automatically, the resources are provisioned or a resource reservation is created, depending on the support of the underlying cloud infrastructure. If the resources are not available in the timeframe requested, the alternatives are computed and presented to the customer (Fig. 4). If the customer accepts one of the alternatives proposed, the approval workflow is initiated and the normal flow for provisioning is started. If not, the request remains in the request queue and policies are reapplied.

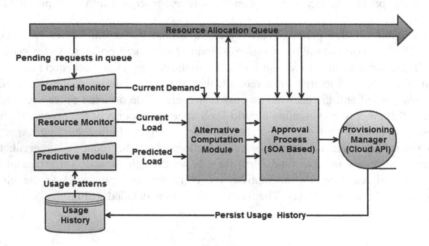

Fig. 4. Interactive scheduler architecture

The alternative schedules are computed based on two factors: timeframe requested and possibility to fulfil the request with burst resources, or in other words, resources provided by interconnected private clouds; both factors are provided by the customer in the initial request. When a request is created the timeframe is entered in the form of StartTime and EndTime, and the possibility of using burst resources is a logical value.

The algorithm that computes the alternatives starts by shifting the timeframe with preconfigured intervals in both directions on the timeline; for each shift the resource availability is computed. The closest alternatives, in regards to the timeframe, are added to the set of options presented to the customer. Along with these alternatives, the availability for the initially requested timeframe is computed when using burst resources from interconnected private clouds. If there are alternatives found with burst resources in the initial requested timeframe, these are added to the set of options. Once the set of alternative options is generated, the algorithm evaluates the feasibility of each option against a set of constrains obtained in real time from 3 other modules:

- *Demand Monitor* – implements a cyclic behaviour and checks the requests currently present in the allocation queue. The resources being requested are summed up on each component (CPU, memory, storage). These vectors represent the current demand for the system.
- *Resource Monitor* – is responsible for monitoring in real time the status of the cloud resources. The output of this module represents the current available capacity of the cloud system on two components: local capacity and burst capacity. This can be seen as real time system load.
- *Predictive Module* – provides predictive load information based on usage patterns stored in a persistent storage. Most private cloud implementations have a specific purpose and thus there are usually diurnal or weekly usage patterns. This information is useful when evaluating the alternative schedule options.

The algorithm for computing and evaluating the alternative scheduling for requests is:

Algorithm 3 Compute Alternatives

ComputeAlternatives(Request)
  currentDemand = getCurrentDemand()
  currentLoad = getCurrentLoad()
  usagePattern = getPreditedPattern()
  For each time interval +-
    alternativeStartTime = StartTime +- interval
    alternativeEndTime = EndTime +- interval
    if (allowBurst) then checkIfBurstPossible()
    altOpt= createAlternative(
                        alternativeStartTime,
                        alternativeEndTime,
                        burstStatus)
    scoreDemand = evaluateAltDemand(altOpt,currentDemand)
    scoreLoad = evaluateAltLoad(altOpt,currentLoad)
    scorePattern = evaluateAltPattern(altOpt,usagePattern)
    globalScore = computeScore(scoreDemand, scoreLoad, scorePattern)
    if (globalScore within thresholds) then
                include alternative in the final list
    else
                disregard alternative option
  EndFor
  Return alternatives option list
  End

The algorithm itself can be considered a highly simplified version of the "yield management" class of algorithms. A survey of the advanced algorithms in "yield management" class used in industry can be found in [11]. We argue that the resource allocation problem in private cloud can be expressed and resolved with this class of algorithms, due to the similar nature of resource allocations especially when resources are limited and shared between concurrent customers. Another class of meta-heuristic algorithms that would be suited to compute valid alternatives are genetic algorithms [12] on private cloud resource allocations.

Once the alternatives are computed, the requester can accept one, in which case the request will be completed, or reject them in which case the request will be re-evaluated against the new conditions of the cloud; cloud conditions, in terms of provisioned capacity can change during this process, so a re-evaluation of the request is important, mainly in scenarios where dynamic matching rules are used for policy matching.

4 Adaptive Resource Allocation in Private Manufacturing Clouds

In order to improve predictability of resource utilization in private cloud systems, the private cloud resource management layer needs to implement an adaptive behaviour to automatically adjust the resource allocation for cloud applications according to the real time capacity requirements. Modern applications are more and more aware of the fact that the underlying platform is virtualized and so resources might be allocated and de-allocated in an adaptive fashion in regards to the current load and capacity. Active monitoring of cloud applications at multiple layers (MES, web, J2EE, database) and recording multiple factors (CPU, memory, I/O, networking) can provide relevant information that represents complex triggers for the cloud adaptive behaviour and smart resource allocations. A similar approach for assuring platform adaptability for such applications is to extend them in order to explicitly trigger resource allocation changes depending on specific application requirements. The general idea is that the more information is provided to the private cloud system by both monitoring tools and application specific triggers, the more accurate the adaptive behaviour will be, and so better resource utilization and better SLA's can be achieved.

This chapter presents a service oriented mechanism for assuring adaptability of a CMfg private cloud system to workload fluctuations that is capable of intelligent resource allocation in both terms of amount and co-locations based on virtualization optimization. The real time monitoring information is gathered with a multi-agent monitoring system capable of multi-layer and multi-factor monitoring. The smart resource allocation is achieved with a distributed genetic algorithm that considers the workload characteristics in conjunction with physical optimum allocation and the current load. The pilot implementation is presented in the context of IBM Cloud Burst 2.1 private cloud implementation with a study on DayTrader J2EE benchmark appli-cation in load test scenarios. The results illustrate how the private cloud can show an adaptive behaviour in regards to the workload variations.

4.1 Workload Classification and Types of Triggers for Adaptive Allocation

Characteristics such as: virtualization overhead on CPU, memory and IO performance have created the need for a scheduling algorithm that would consider the requirements of workload scheduling and virtualization optimization (memory over-commit, uniform distribution of IOPS), in order to provide best performance possible. Table 1 describes the workload types based on operating system, CPU profile and IO profile.

Table 1. Workload profiles

OS	CPU Profile	IO Profile
Windows	High	Low
Windows	Low	High
Linux	High	Low
Linux	Low	High

For example, a MES workload can run parallel processing applications which have a CPU intensive profile (e.g. mixed batch planning and product scheduling) or run a high end relational database system, which has an IO intensive profile (e.g., inventory, Supply Chain Management). Similarly the operating system used can differ according to each customer. In real life implementations the applications are typically designed in three layers: UI layer, business layer and database layer. When running such applications in cloud environments, the mapping with virtual machines is at the UI/Business layers, where clustering is configured at the application server layer and at the database backend. Out of these, the application server workloads are the ones that drive the application capacity most of the time. The application server workloads show a high CPU profile, while the database workloads have a high IO Profile. However, these characteristics depend greatly on the application implementation and so a baseline should be established before a workload profile can be established.

The events affecting the adaptive resource allocation process can be triggered from two main sources: the monitoring layer and the application itself. The monitoring layer considered in this paper is part of our previous work described in [13]; the solution uses a multi agent system to gather real time data at multiple layers in the cloud application stack: hypervisor layer, OS layer, application layer and can be extended with custom monitoring data. The data generated by the monitoring solution sends multi-factor data (CPU, Memory, IO, Network) in a repository in a continuum stream. This allows a central monitoring agent to trigger events based on a set of rules, either on a single metric or on complex multi-factor conditions. Table 2 presents types of event triggers that can be defined to invoke the adaptive resource allocation process.

The event can be triggered either by simple threshold based conditions, e.g., when CPU usage on a given VM is higher than a value or by pre-defined rules. A rule definition is essentially an XML file with a simple scheme that supports nested definitions of rules consisting of operands, comparators and logic operators. A rule has a name, a comparator and two operands. The comparators can be HIGHER or LOWER and the operands can be a metric or a constant. Example of such a rule is presented below:

Table 2. Event triggers

Metric	Definition	Type
CPU (OS Layer)	Threshold	Simple
Memory (OS Layer)	Threshold	Simple
Disk IO (OS Layer)	Threshold	Simple
Network (OS Layer)	Threshold	Simple
Combined (OS Layer)	Rule	Complex
CPU (App Layer)	Rule	Simple
Memory (App Layer)	Rule	Simple
Disk IO (App Layer)	Rule	Simple
Network (App Layer)	Rule	Simple
Application Defined	Rule	Simple
Combined (App Layer)	Rule	Complex

```
<rule name="high_cpu_mem">
    <operator>AND</operator>
    <rule name="high_cpu">
        <comparator>HIGHER</comparator>
        <operand>cpu_os_prc</operand>
        <operand>50</operand>
    <rule>
    <rule name="high_mem">
        <comparator>HIGHER</comparator>
        <operand>cpu_mem_prc</operand>
        <operand>70</operand>
    <rule>
</rule>
```

The association between the rules and the events triggered is stored in a XML file in the Adaptive Rules repository. An example of such an association is presented in the outline below:

```
<association>
    <event>trigger_horizonal_add</event>
    <rule>high_cpu_mem</rule>
</association>
```

4.2 Adaptive Provisioning Mechanism for Optimal Resource Allocation

The architecture of the adaptive provisioning mechanism designed for optimal resource allocation is shown in Fig. 5.

The mechanism consists in a comprehensive multi agent monitoring solution that is capable to gather real time metrics from both operating system layer and application layer, a multi-factor monitor that triggers reconfiguration events based on administrator

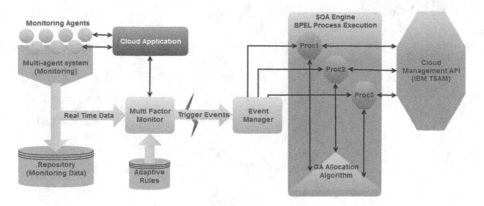

Fig. 5. Adaptive provisioning mechanism architecture

defined rules, a business process that manages the life cycle of the cloud project and a genetic algorithm for optimal resource allocation in the private cloud.

The adaptive provisioning mechanism illustrated in Fig. 5 aims to scale up and down the resources required by the application, being aware of three important questions: "when to scale?", "what to scale?" and "how to scale?" The solution is implemented as a BPEL process (Fig. 6) and runs on top a SOA engine. The overall flow is:

- **Step1:** A new project is created in the cloud management system. The monitoring agent instantiates a new process instance, which will be running for the entire life cycle of the cloud project;
- **Step2:** The BPEL process is initialized and starts to listen for adaptive scaling events triggered by the Event Manager based on thresholds or rules;
- **Step3:** The multi-factor monitoring agent matches on a threshold trigger or a predefined rule and triggers an event;
- **Step4:** The event is sent to the BPEL process that computes the scale up/down requirements based on the event received;
- **Step5:** The genetic algorithm is invoked to determine the optimal resource allocation/de-allocation based on the current status of the cloud;
- **Step6:** The process continues until the project is finished.

In this architecture the Event Manager has the responsibility to match the event triggered with the corresponding BPEL process and to sequence the events that might be triggered for the same process in short amounts of time. This aspect has been proved to be very important in: (a) reducing the impact of resource allocation overhead and resource configuration on the decision making process, and (b) eliminating duplicate events that can be generated from a local monitoring perspective.

The business process is exposed as a web service end point called SmartAllocationServiceEndPoint (Fig. 6 left). The process starts with a receiveInput activity that parses the payload containing the project identifier, the organization and the event actions. The values from the payload are assigned to the process variables in Assign_Parameters activity. At this point the process starts to listen for events in a

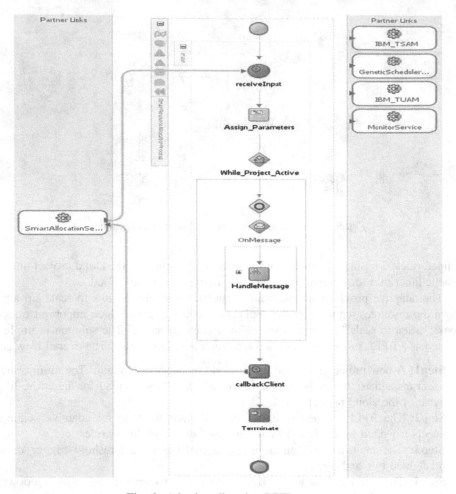

Fig. 6. Adaptive allocation BPEL process

while loop; this behaviour will continue for the entire life cycle of the project. When an event is received, the OnMessage activity will be triggered and the event is processed by the HandleMessage block. The callbackClient informs the caller, in this case the agent invoking the web service end point, of the process completion. The Terminate activity finalizes the process in the BPEL execution engine.

The next activity invokes the web service exposed by the multi-agent monitoring solution to fetch the current load. The current allocation, the current load and the event generated are used to compute the changes (scale up or down decision). Once all this information is gathered and structured, the genetic algorithm (GA) is invoked to compute the best allocation pattern for the event. Once the decision on what and how to provision is in place, the InvokeCloudAPI activity invokes the cloud API to perform the resource allocation changes. In our pilot implementation the cloud API is offered by IBM Tivoli Service Automation Manager as a set of REST web services.

4.3 Genetic Algorithm for Smart Resource Allocation

The workload scheduling is a NP-Complete problem, so the solutions generated would be sub-optimal. There are several hard conditions that need to be respected in order for a schedule to be accepted as a viable solution such as resource allocation levels and cloud capacity, and several soft conditions that are meant to exploit the virtualization features and minimize performance overhead of concurrent workloads.

As these conditions are sometimes conflicting a genetic algorithm would be able to generate only sub-optimal solutions for the scheduling problem. The genetic algorithm starts with a randomly generated population of solutions and by applying operations as selection, crossover and mutation on individuals create new generations evaluating the fitness of each individual of the population in the process. When the fitness level in the population reaches a satisfying value, a set of solutions are obtained. In the design of the GA prototype, there are six objects as shown in Fig. 7.

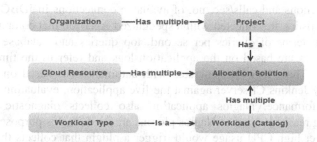

Fig. 7. Data Objects class diagram

The new schedule is generated by randomly assigning a new alternative set of resources (CPU cores and virtual disks) for the selected Workload instance. The Genetic Algorithm has the following structure:

Step1: generateInitialPopulation()
Step2: while(best individual fitness < min_fitness){
Step3:   do_crossover(best 65% individuals)
Step4:   calculate_fitness(offsprings)
Step5:   remove_worst(worst 35% individuals)
Step6:   calculate_best_individual_fitness }

5   Closed Loop QoS Monitoring in Private Clouds. Conclusions

This conclusion section presents a multilayer QoS monitoring architecture implement-ted on top of IBM CloudBurst 2.1 private manufacturing cloud solution designed and integrated with IBM TSAM product stack.

The solution developed uses several open-source tools to assure a closed loop QoS monitoring solution: Jenkins CI, Munin, Nagios and Jira. The solution uses a set of monitoring jobs executed by the Jenkins server; these jobs are implemented as ANT tasks and executed at repeating time intervals. The general role of the monitoring job is to collect QoS data from each layer in the application stack: Tivoli, Hypervisor, J2EE/JMX/MBeans, DB, application logs and HTTP access logs. Each job creates one or more artefacts, which are typically simple text files containing metrics for the time interval since the last execution of the job. These artefacts are pushed to a shared network location where they are processed by Munin. Nagios is used for event monitoring on these metrics, implemented using thresholds on each metric. If a threshold is reached, Nagios invokes the Jira plugin to create a tracking ticket.

A set of metrics are collected in this implementation at various layers. From Tivoli Stack: CPU, RAM Usage, Disk I/O rate, Network I/O; from VMware hypervisor: workload uptime, CPU quota usage, memory quota usage, virtual disk usage. At OS layer, the metrics collected are: CPU usage per process and per kernel/user, memory usage per process, disk I/O per device, network traffic/interface. J2EE layer metrics are collected using JMX access to runtime MBeans and include the average no. of EJB container transactions and calls/sec, no. of available connections in JDBC pools.

Database statistics are collected with a specialized ANT job that computes average usage reports in terms of queries per second, top queries and database locks. The application metrics are based on the application logs and refer to the time taken for page transitions. These logs are generated with automatic tests based on WebDriver and executed by Jenkins CI server against the live application, evaluating directly the application performance. Nagios application also collects diagnostic data upon thresholds being reached. A set of Nagios plugins are used for this purpose, e.g., J2EE application server high CPU usage would trigger a plugin that collects thread-dumps from Java process usage by sending a SIGQUIT message. Thread-dumps are automatically attached to the Jira issue created, together with application server log files.

This approach helps system administrators to detect the problems in an early stage and prevent further system QoS degradation. The availability of real time artefacts also supports root cause analysis for one off events.

Acknowledgements. This work is partially supported by the IBM FA2016 Project: Big Data, Analytics and Cloud for Digital Transformation on Manufacturing – DTM.

References

1. Li, B.H., Zhang, L., Wang, S., Tao, F., Chai, X.D.: Cloud manufacturing: a new service-oriented networked manufacturing model. CIM Syst. **16**(1), 1–7 (2010)
2. Xun, X.: From cloud computing to cloud manufacturing. Robot. Comput. Integr. Manuf. **28**(1), 75–86 (2012)
3. Morariu, O., Borangiu, T., Răileanu, S.: vMES: virtualization aware manufacturing execution system. Comput. Ind. **67**, 27–37 (2015)
4. Morariu, O., Borangiu, T., Răileanu, S.: Redundancy mechanisms for virtualized MES workloads in private cloud. In: Borangiu, T., Thomas, A., Trentesaux, D. (eds.) Service Orientation in Holonic and Multi-agent Manufacturing. SCI, vol. 594, pp. 147–155. Springer, Heidelberg (2015)

5. Zhang, L., Luo, Y.L., Tao, F., Ren, L., Guo, H.: Key technologies for the construction of manufacturing cloud. CIM Syst. **16**(11), 2510–2520 (2010)
6. Cheng, Y., Tao, F., Zhang, L., Zhang, X., Xi, G.H., Zhao, D.: Study on the utility model and utility equilibrium of resource service transaction in cloud manufacturing. In: Proceedings of Industrial Engineering and Engineering Management (IEEM), pp. 2298–2302 (2010)
7. Azbayar, D., Chase, J., Babu, S.: Reflective control for an elastic cloud application: an automated experiment workbench. In: Proceedings of HotCloud 2009, pp. 234–241 (2009)
8. Best Practices in Evaluating Elastic Load Balancing, Amazon E2C (2013). http://aws.amazon.com/articles/1636185810492479
9. Lemos, A., Moleiro, R., Ottaviano, P., Rada, F., Widomski, M., Braswell, B.: IBM CloudBurst on System x, IBM RedBooks (2012)
10. Olivieri, A., Pintus, A., Santucci, C.: IBM Tivoli Provisioning Manager V7.1.1: IBM RedBooks, Form Number SG24-7773-00 (2009)
11. McAfee, R.P., Velde, V.: Dynamic pricing with constant demand elasticity. Prod. Oper. Manag. **17**(4), 432–438 (2008)
12. Morariu, O., Morariu, C., Borangiu, Th.: A genetic algorithm for workload scheduling in cloud based e-learning. In: Proceedings of the 2nd International Workshop on Cloud Computing Platforms. ACM
13. Morariu, O., Morariu, C., Borangiu, T.: Transparent real time monitoring for multi-tenant J2EE applications. J. Control Eng. Appl. Inf. **15**(4), 37–46 (2013)

Modeling a Manager's Work as a Service Activity

Yuval Cohen[1(✉)], Shai Rozenes[1], and Maurizio Faccio[2]

[1] Department of Industrial Engineering, Tel-Aviv Afeka Academic
College of Engineering, Mivtsa-Kadesh 38, 69988 Tel-Aviv, Israel
{yuvalc,rozenes}@afeka.ac.il
[2] Department of Industrial Engineering and Management,
University of Padova, Padova, Italy
maurizio.faccio@unipd.it

Abstract. Planning of manager's workload is an elusive and challenging issue that has no exact quantitative tools. This paper develops for the first time (to the best of our knowledge) an analytical model that shows how a manager's activity and its associated workload can be analyzed as a provision of various services. The model is essentially a queuing model of tasks with arrivals, waiting time, and services (with a single server). The model is first analyzed in the most general way, finding the mean values of waiting times and queue length. While the proposed model is for one manager, it is based on very general assumptions and would fit most practical environments. Then, a simpler model for determining the optimal span of control for a manager is developed and illustrated using a numerical example.

Keywords: Manager load · Span of control · Queuing · Server · Workload

1 Introduction

Quantitative planning of a manager's workload is an elusive and challenging issue [1, 2]. Moreover, to the best of our knowledge, this paper presents for the first time an analytical tool for estimating a manager's workload. This paper uses queuing theory and models to analyze the work load of a manager, and recommend an efficient control span.

This is a novel approach since organizational hierarchy and structure were determined in a different way that is often more art than science. One reason for this is the variety of different managerial roles and managerial styles which make the managerial work to be considered as composed of non-standard tasks. This variety of managerial roles was summarized and categorized by Mintzberg [3] as shown in Table 1.

While managerial task durations may have a variety of distributions, the single manager is still working as a single server with a general distribution of workload of accumulated managerial tasks which characterizes a single server queuing system. One of the most prevalent objectives for the use of queuing models is estimating the load on various servers and the resultant waiting time and line length. While typical servers usually face an end customer (examples may range from call center operators to

© Springer International Publishing Switzerland 2016
T. Borangiu et al. (Eds.): IESS 2016, LNBIP 247, pp. 384–391, 2016.
DOI: 10.1007/978-3-319-32689-4_29

Table 1. Henry Mintzberg's 10 managerial roles

Category	Roles
Interpersonal	Figurehead
	Leader
	Liaison
Informational	Monitor
	Disseminator
	Spokesperson
Decisional	Entrepreneur
	Disturbance Handler
	Resource Allocator
	Negotiator

cashiers and hotel front-desk clerks and from bank tellers to flight stewardesses) some extensions propose special use of queuing for special purposes.

An important such model is the classical Ashcroft [4] machine interference model. This model is used to determine the workforce of operators that serve several machines simultaneously. Thirty years later Bunday and Scraton [5] proved that, for queues with independent service times, machine interference model gives the same result for models that have the same three parameters: (1) mean arrival rate, (2) mean service duration, and (3) the same number of servers.

A more recent review of the subject is given in Haque and Armstong [6]. Queuing theory has a pivotal role in assessing the workload in call centers [7] and recently queuing theory has been used for determining workforce in public service [8, 9]. However there has not been any trial to model the load of a manager as a server of a queue of jobs arriving at his/her desk.

2 The Proposed General Model

A manager has three hierarchical levels of interface: with subordinates, with peers, and with higher-up managers. This interface is also the core of categorizing tasks:

(1) Tasks that are related to upper management requirements and plans,
(2) Tasks that are related to the interface with other units of the organization, and
(3) Tasks that are related to subordinates.

In most systems this could be described as the three arrival processes that coalesce into one queue as depicted in Fig. 1.

In this figure, λ_i is the mean arrival rate of task type i and E[Si] is mean service time of task type i.

Prioritizing these tasks is key to efficient and effective management. Typically the importance of tasks to the manager is related to the hierarchy: the higher the source, the higher the importance. However, urgency of tasks is often opposite to the managerial hierarchy: the most urgent tasks are often related to the subordinates, the next urgency

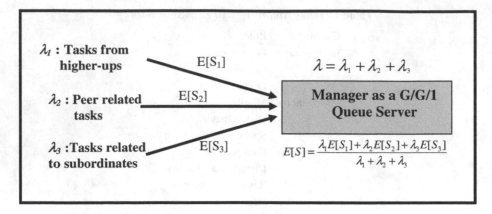

Fig. 1. The manager as a queuing system

is typically the interface with other peers, and least urgent are the ones related to higher management. Sequencing the work could be done on the basis of multiplying importance level by urgency, but more important task should get more time devoted to them (according to their importance and nature).

2.1 General Description of the Model

It is clear from the discussion that the manager could be modeled as a single server in a queueing system. If we assume that arrival rate is smaller than service rate, the most general system to model the manager (using Kandall notation) is: G/G/1.

For G/G/1 no assumption need to be made regarding the arrival pattern or the service times. To continue the discussion the following notations are presented.

Notations.

- i – Index for the type of task
- λ_i – Mean arrival rate of tasks type i
- λ – Total arrival rate
- $E[Si] = \mu_i$ – Mean service rate of tasks type
- ρ – Utilization of the manager
- σ_a – Standard deviation of arrival intervals
- σ_s – Standard deviation of service times
- P_O – Probability of idle time
- W_q – Mean waiting time
- W – Mean time duration in the system
- L_q – Mean number of waiting entities in line
- L – Mean number in system
- t – requires random amount of managerial attention (t)
- NS – Number of subordinates
- Y – Overall demand for managerial attention

2.2   Mathematical Description of the G/G/1 Model

Since there is one server, the manager, his average utilization is easy to predict once the mean rate of each task stream (λ_i) is known, and the corresponding mean service time (μ_i) is known [10]. The average utilization is given in Eq. 1.

$$0 \le \rho = \sum_{i=1}^{3} \left(\frac{\lambda_i}{\mu_i} \right) \le 1 \tag{1}$$

Also, the utilization represents the percent of time the server is busy. Therefore, the percent of server idle-time is [11]:

$$0 \le P_0 = 1 - \rho \le 1 \tag{2}$$

The waiting time could be estimated using Kingman's formula approximation [10]:

$$W_q \approx \left(\frac{\rho}{1-\rho} \right) \left(\frac{\left(\sigma_a \sum_{i=1}^{3} \lambda_i \right)^2 + \left(\sigma_s \sum_{i=1}^{3} \mu_i \right)^2}{2} \right) \left(\frac{\sum_{i=1}^{3} \lambda_i \cdot \mu_i}{\sum_{i=1}^{3} \lambda_i} \right) \tag{3}$$

From Little's law we have:

$$L_q \approx \lambda W_q = \left(\frac{\rho}{1-\rho} \right) \left(\frac{\left(\sigma_a \sum_{i=1}^{3} \lambda_i \right)^2 + \left(\sigma_s \sum_{i=1}^{3} \mu_i \right)^2}{2} \right) \left(\sum_{i=1}^{3} \lambda_i \cdot \mu_i \right) \tag{4}$$

Also, having one server, the mean number of tasks in service is simply ρ. Thus, Little's law yields:

$$L = L_q + \rho \approx \left(\sum_{i=1}^{3} \lambda \right) \cdot W_q + \sum_{i=1}^{3} \left(\frac{\lambda_i}{\mu_i} \right) \tag{5}$$

Note that the task arrival rate (of subordinates' tasks) increases with the number of subordinates. Thus, we must limit the number of subordinates to meet maximal utilization of $\rho < 0.9$. This maximal utilization should be observed even in peak hours.

$$W = \frac{L}{\lambda} = W_q + \frac{\rho}{\lambda} = W_q + \frac{\sum_{i=1}^{3} \left(\frac{\lambda_i}{\mu_i} \right)}{\sum_{i=1}^{3} \lambda_i} \tag{6}$$

The tendency to give priority to certain jobs could be developed into a queuing model with priorities. However, this is left for future research. The workload on the manager depends both on the tasks arrival rate and the required time.

Assuming a subordinate generates an independent task arrival process with rate of λ_i and that the task execution durations has a certain distribution with mean $1/\mu$, and standard deviation σ, the cumulative workload is a complex Poisson process having a mean of:

$$Mean(Work\_load) = \frac{\left(\sum_i \lambda_i\right)}{\mu} \tag{7}$$

$$Var(Work\_load) = \left(\sum_i \lambda_i\right)\left(\sigma^2 + \left(\frac{1}{\mu}\right)^2\right) \tag{8}$$

$$\sigma_{(Work\_load)} = \sqrt{\left(\sum_i \lambda_i\right)\left(\sigma^2 + \left(\frac{1}{\mu}\right)^2\right)} = \sqrt{\left(\sum_i \lambda_i\right)} \cdot \sqrt{\left(\sigma^2 + \left(\frac{1}{\mu}\right)^2\right)} \tag{9}$$

Thus, a unit time should allow most of the work to be completed even in the peak hours, so determining the number of standard deviations above the average could be determined using Chebyshev's inequality [12]:

$$\Pr(|X - \mu| \geq k\sigma) \leq \frac{1}{k^2} \tag{10}$$

$$Mean(Work\_load) + k\sigma_{(Work\_load)} < 1(time\_unit) \tag{11}$$

For example taking 3 standard deviations above the mean ensures about 89 % that the workload per time unit would be met. Therefore, the maximal workload ($\Sigma\lambda i$) that still meet Eq. 11, will be chosen by this approach. For $k = 3$ this yields:

$$\frac{\left(\sum_i \lambda_i\right)}{\mu} + 3\sqrt{\left(\sum_i \lambda_i\right)} \cdot \sqrt{\left(\sigma^2 + \left(\frac{1}{\mu}\right)^2\right)} < 1(time\_unit) \tag{12}$$

Equation (12) could be the basis of an upper bound for the manager's load.

3   The Case of a Simple Foreman

In this section, the managerial span of control of a simple foreman of an assembly line is modeled as a service model. The foreman gives managerial and relief service to all the subordinates under his/her control, and the duration of all other tasks are negligible. Span of control is a function of the attention allocation.

A foreman or a leader can focus his/her attention at most 100 % of the time. If the attention is uniformly allocated among the NS (Number of subordinates) in each section, the attention allocated to each station is $1/NS$ of the time.

Attention allocation to stations could be spread uniformly, or in Pareto manner, or in other patterns and forms, but it would always be a decreasing function of the number of stations in a section (NS).

On the other hand, the performance of a line-section depends on the attention spread. So increase of attention would increase performance but with a decreasing marginal addition.

We assume the events that require management attention are independent. This assumption leads to an exponential distribution of time intervals between these events, and consequently to a Poisson arrival process. Since each station contributes a rate of λ events per time unit, the event rate of a line-section is $(NS)\lambda$.

Since each event requires random amount of managerial attention (t), it is imperative to consider its duration distribution ($F(t)$). Assuming independent and identically distributed (i.i.d.) event durations, the overall demand for managerial attention (Y) for a specific foreman is a compound Poisson distribution with the following mean and variance.

$$E[Y] = \lambda(NS)(E[t]) \tag{13}$$

$$\text{Var}[Y] = (\lambda(NS))(E[t^2]) = (\lambda(NS))\left(Var[t] + (E[t])^2\right) \tag{14}$$

The lack of managerial attention may cause defects and serious problems. It is therefore, reasonable to assume that the section length must permit managerial attention most of the time.

Taking the cycle-time (C) the as the time unit, it is desirable that:

$$E[Y] + k\sqrt{Var[Y]} < C \tag{15}$$

or using (13) and (14):

$$\lambda(NS)(E[t]) + k\sqrt{(\lambda(NS))\left(Var[t] + (E[t])^2\right)} < C \tag{16}$$

So, inequality (16) gives an upper bound on the section's length (NS) for any combination of estimated event rate (events which require managerial intervention), and the mean and variance of the managerial intervention duration.

The following numerical example illustrates this point: Consider an assembly line with cycle-time (C) of one minute, where each operator in a station generates a managerial time-consuming event every 100 cycles on the average, foreman's mean intervention duration of 0.5 min. with a large variation of 0.25.

Summarizing the parameter values we have: $\lambda = 0.01$ per cycle, and $C = 1$, $E[t] = 0.5$ and $Var[t] = 0.25$, in minutes.

Requiring three standard deviations above the mean, inequality (16) could be written as:

$$0.01(NS)(0.5) + 3\sqrt{(0.01(NS))\left(0.25 + (0.5)^2\right)} < 1 \tag{17}$$

Multiplying both sides of (17) by 200 and some manipulation yields:

$$(NS) + 6\sqrt{50(NS)} - 200 < 0 \tag{18}$$

Designating $U = \sqrt{NS}$ inequality (18) turns into quadratic expression:

$$U^2 + 6\sqrt{50}(U) - 200 < 0 \tag{19}$$

Which results in $U < 4.28$ or $NS < 18.33$

Thus, the number of subordinate workers under a single manager should be under 18. This is reasonable if we realize that each worker on average needs the manager once every 1:40 h (100 min.) for about half a minute. Thus, having 18 workers is possible without having to stop the line too often.

4 Conclusion

In this paper, we developed for the first time an analytical method to estimate a manager's workload. The manager was modeled as a server of managerial tasks.

The manager's tasks were categorized and a G/G/1 queuing model was applied with some general results for mean utilization, waiting time, and queue length. A clear bound on the total load of the manager was developed.

A special model was developed for finding the maximal span of control for an assembly line foreman. In the future this model should be validated using simulation and real empirical data.

References

1. Wong, C.A., Elliott-Miller, P., Laschinger, H., Cuddihy, M., Meyer, R.M., Keatings, M., Burnett, C., Szudy, N.: Examining the relationships between span of control and manager job and unit performance outcomes. J. Nurs. Manage. **23**, 156–168 (2015)
2. Nasrallah, W.F., Ouba, C.J., Yassine, A.A., Srour, I.M.: Modeling the span of control of leaders with different skill sets. Comput. Math. Organ. Theory **21**(3), 296–317 (2015)
3. Mintzberg, H.: Mintzberg on Management. Free Press, New-York (2007)
4. Ashcroft, H.: The productivity of several machines under the care of one operator. J. R. Stat. Soc. B **12**(1), 145–151 (1950)
5. Bunday, B.D., Scraton, R.E.: The G/M/r machine interference model. Eur. J. Oper. Res. **4**, 399–402 (1980)

6. Haque, L., Armstrong, M.J.: A survey of the machine interference problem. Eur. J. Oper. Res. **179**, 469–482 (2007)
7. Gong, J., Li, M.: Queuing time decision model with the consideration on call center customer abandonment behavior. J. Netw. **9**(9), 2441–2447 (2014)
8. Ernst, A.T., Jiang, H., Krishnamoorthy, M., Sier, D.: Staff scheduling and rostering: a review of applications, methods and models. Eur. J. Oper. Res. **153**(1), 3–27 (2004)
9. Dawndra, J., McLaughlin, M., Gebbens, C., Terhorst, L.: Utilizing a scope and span of control tool to measure workload and determine supporting resources for nurse manager. J. Nurs. Adm. **45**(5), 243–249 (2015)
10. Bhat, U.N.: The general queue G/G/1 and approximations. In: Bhat, U.N. (ed.) An Introduction to Queueing Theory, 2nd edn, pp. 169–183. Birkhauser, Boston (2015)
11. Gross, D., John, F., Shortle, J., Thompson, M., Harris, C.M.: Fundamentals of Queueing Theory, 4th edn. Wiley-Interscience, Haboken (2008)
12. Haviv, M.: Queues: A Course in Queueing Theory. Springer, New York (2015)

Servicizing as a Tool for Increasing the Sustainability of Product Life Cycles

Adi Wolfson$^{(\boxtimes)}$ and Dorith Tavor

Green Processes Center, Sami Shamoon College of Engineering,
Bialik 56, 84100 Beer-Sheva, Israel
adiw@sce.ac.il

Abstract. The design and delivery of services have changed tremendously over the last decade. Yet the conceptualization of services should place a greater emphasis on the social and environmental aspects of value design, and services should also be incorporated as an essential part in the production and delivery of products. The addition of clean services (CleanServs) to the various stages of the product's life cycle can reduce both resource use and pollution emission. Moreover, servicizing the product's life cycle can also add various environmental and social values, and thereby increasing the sustainability of the final solution. Finally, the potential of servicizing to increase the sustainability of the physical resources based life cycle of goods was illustrated by the example of the life cycle of printed book.

Keywords: Sustainability · Services · Servicizing · Life cycle

1 Introduction

In terms of goods or services, the life cycle of every product encompasses myriad physical or tangible resources and non-physical or intangible resources [1, 2]. During the product's life cycle, some of these resources are directly incorporated in the final product while the rest are discharged or emitted to the surroundings.

Resource managements, in general, and natural resource management, in particular, which relates to the right and efficient allocation of resources to every step of a process, is a key element in any process management [3, 4]. With this regard, product life cycle management, which is generally defined as a strategic business approach for the effective management and use of corporate capital [5, 6], is gaining high acceptance as a tool for resource managements [7, 8]. Yet, the coordination and balance of resources use in a process has also numerous effects on many external circles, and on social, economic and environmental demands. In fact it affects the ability of nature to provide ecosystem services. Thus, managing the process life cycle in more sustainable fashion is one of the main challenges of industry nowadays [9].

The ultimate value of the product, which is determined by the integration of all these resources, can be defined based on a calculation that combines its monetary value, e.g., its price or its contribution to gross domestic product (GDP), its social value, e.g., based on issues of equity and social justice, and its environmental value, e.g., the impact of the product on ecosystems. The product's actual value, however, is

T. Borangiu et al. (Eds.): IESS 2016, LNBIP 247, pp. 392–402, 2016.
DOI: 10.1007/978-3-319-32689-4_30

represented by the sum of these three values weighted against the sustainability value of the production process or the life cycle of the product.

Sustainability is a measure of the stresses imposed by manmade activities on the social and the natural environments and the ability of ecosystems to withstand these stresses while renewing their resources and ensuring that the next generation can also supply its needs [10–12]. Sustainability measures comprise environmental, social and economic aspects that should be integrated in a way that generates added value and that follows triple bottom line principles [13]. From a more practical perspective, sustainability entails adopting habits defined by greater environmental and social consciousness to achieve sustainable development, i.e., "development that meets the needs of the present without compromising the ability of future generations to meet their own needs". [14]. Sustainable development, therefore, depends on balancing social, economic, and environmental needs when making decisions about the physical resources based life cycle of a product.

The first stage in the life cycle of a product in terms of the physical resources used in its production is initiated by the extraction of the raw materials that are employed in the second stage of manufacturing (Fig. 1). The following stage of delivery transfers the value from the supplier to the consumer, who exploits the product's value until the product's final stage in its life cycle, "end-of-life", when the product is either discarded as waste or recovered for reuse or recycling. Note that each stage in a product's life cycle not only consumes physical resources, e.g., materials and energy, it also discharges materials and energy to the environment. Moreover, when these discharges harm the social and/or natural environments, they can be defined as pollution.

Alterations in the physical resources based life cycle of a product can affect its value from the social, economic and environmental perspectives, the last of which is defined by the extent to which resources are used rationally and the amount of pollution

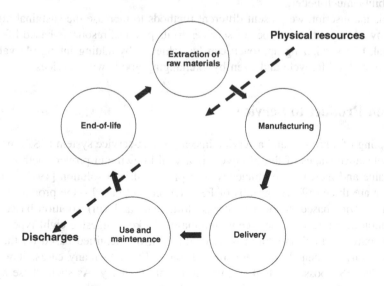

Fig. 1. Generic physical resources based life cycle.

discharged to the environment during the product's life cycle. In addition to the physical resources consumed during its life cycle, however, a product's environmental value must also consider other measures, such as the extents to which its life cycle is guided by the preservation of biodiversity and a respect for animal rights. For example, even if the utilization of materials and energy entailed in the life cycle of a coat produced with real sheep's wool is much higher than that of a synthetic wool coat, the ultimate environmental value of the former product must also consider how the sheep are raised and how the wool is produced. Finally, all the stages of the physical resources based life cycle should also take into account social issues such as human rights, equity and social justice. Thus, a product life cycle that entails violations of the social rights of the workers is unsustainable.

The utilization of physical resources and the efficiency with which these resources are used during the manufacturing process have strong impacts on the sustainability of the final product. Thus, enhancement of a product's value by increasing the sustainability of its life cycle via the rational use of resources, which leads both to less intense resource use and lower pollution emissions, is straightforward. A less intuitive approach to increasing value, however, involves changing the arrangement of the product's non-physical resources and adding supporting and supplementary services to its life cycle, i.e., servicizing the life cycle, which can also increase its sustainability [15, 16]. In addition, because service involves the co-creation of values, i.e., using a constellation of integrated resources and capabilities, servicizing the life cycle can change the rules that define the tasks of both supplier and consumer, in the process transforming the former into a provider who supplies the platform for the exchange and engaging the customer to assume an active role in the provision of the service or product. Moreover, while the production and delivery of goods is usually perceived as a linear value-chain [17], service co-creation is often viewed as a non-linear process [18], and as such, the notion of service co-creation can reflect the complexity of sustainability much better.

In this manuscript, we present different methods to increase the sustainability of a product by adding different types of services to its physical resources based life cycle. In general, this servicizing approach can be achieved by adding intangible values to each stage of the life cycle and even by exchanging goods with services.

2   From Product to Service

The coupling of a product and a service into a product-service system (PSS) in the use and maintenance stages of the life cycle is a well-known and proven method to gain added value and increase the efficiency of a product-driven solution [19–22]. In general, there are three different groups of PSS: (i) product-based – the product is dominant, (ii) service-based – the service is dominant, and (iii) solution-based – the combination of product and service is dominant. Tukker suggested eight types of PSS between 'pure product' and 'pure service' that can be identified based on their economic and environmental characteristics (Table 1 [21]). In many cases, it was also reported that PSS possesses higher environmental efficiency. As such, these systems were also termed eco-efficient services, a term that emphasizes the role of the service in effecting a more eco-efficient solution [23, 24]. Eco-efficiency, a term coined in 1992 by the World Business Council for Sustainable Development, refers to the extent to which processes are based on the use of fewer resources and the generation of less waste and pollution [25].

Table 1. PSS types [21].

PSS type	Explanation	Example
Product-oriented service		
Product-related service	The provider delivers to the customer a product together with the services that are needed during the product use-phase	Car or house maintenance services
Advice and consultancy	The provider delivers to the customer a product together with services related to the use of the product	Services that assist in the operation of domestic electric devices
Use-oriented services		
Product lease	The provider delivers to the customer a service that includes a product owned by the provider and used solely and for a limited time by the customer together with supportive and complementary services.	Car lease
Product renting or sharing	The provider delivers to the customer a service that includes a product owned by the provider and used by the customer for a certain time or used sequentially with other customers together with supportive and complementary services	Apartment rental by using the Airbnb website
Product pooling	The provider delivers to the customer a service that includes a product owned by one customer and used by other customers for a certain time, together with supportive and complementary services	Car pooling
Result-oriented services		
Activity Management/outsourcing	The provider delivers to the customer a solution comprising services and products and the customer does not buy the product but only the result of the product	Public transportation

(Continued)

Table 1. (*Continued*)

PSS type	Explanation	Example
Pay per service	The provider delivers to the customer a solution comprising services and products and the customer does not buy the product but only the result of the product according to the level of use	Pay per view of movie
Functional result	The provider delivers to the customer a solution that comprises services and products and how the solution is delivered is at the provider's sole discretion.	Carbon labeling [26, 27].

As previously mentioned, the addition of supporting and complementary services not just to the use stage of the product's life cycle but also to all the other stages can increase the sustainability of goods. We recently proposed a new framework for sustainable service innovation termed clean services, or CleanServs [26–28], which helps promote the realization of more sustainable solutions. CleanServs are services that are competitive with, if not superior to, their conventional tangible or intangible counterparts, that reduce the use of natural resources, and that cut or eliminate emissions and wastes while increasing the responsibilities of both provider and customer. In general, five types of CleanServs were offered in descending order from most to least sustainable: Prevention, reduction, replacement, efficiency and offset (Table 2).

Table 2. Various types of CleanServs [26].

CleanServ type	Explanation	Example
Prevention	Exchanging a good with a 'pure service' that yields the same solution	Paying with Bitcoin instead of conventional cash, i.e., coins or bills
Reduction	Addition of a service to a good that increases the intensity of its use and thus cut its production	Using laundromat services instead of buying private laundry machine.
Replacement	Providing an alternative solution by coupling a service with another good	Using public transportation instead of private cars
Efficiency	Addition of a service to a good's life cycle to increase the efficiency of the final solution	Using *Waze* or *Moovit* applications to increase the efficiency of transport
Offset	Addition of a complementary service to compensate resource utilization during the production or delivery of a good	Bottle recycling service

The CleanServ opportunity with the most sustainability potential is the replacement of the entire life cycle of a pure product with pure service, thus eliminating the need for further production or delivery of the good. Yet the exchange of physical resources with non-physical means is not a trivial matter. Indeed, the production and delivery of a service usually also require physical resources. Therefore, when considering an option based on the prevention type CleanServ, the physical resources based life cycle of both solutions, i.e., the good and the service, must also be compared based on other environmental values and on social and economic values, and not merely from the perspective of physical resources. For example, using a massage service instead of purchasing a one's own massage chair may initially be perceived as more economical and effective. However, in addition to the high costs incurred via payments for a series of massage treatments, there are other, equally important considerations: the need to coordinate the times for massage appointments instead of using the massage chair in the comfort of one's home, and transportation to and from the massage business also requires resources while emitting air pollution and greenhouse gases to the environment.

Any exploration of the opportunities that exist to exchange a particular good with a service or group of services must also take into account both the quality of the good and its quantity. This notion is particularly important today, as cultures around the world increasingly emulate the consumption-driven culture of the West, where people seem to almost worship consumerism, and they typically purchase many more goods than they actually need or use. The ultimate and perhaps inevitable result of this global embrace of the consumer culture has been the rampant production of products with very short life-times but that can be used again and again, as the resources consumed throughout their life cycles are not exploited to their full potentials. In this scenario, the addition of a reduction type CleanServ to a good can lead to more intense use of that good and, consequently, more a rational use of the resources involved in its life cycle. Indeed, this type of CleanServ is applicable mainly to the use stage of a product's life cycle, and as such, it refers to the product-oriented service type of PSS, i.e., product-related service and advice and consultancy, and the use-oriented service type of PSS, e.g., leasing, renting, sharing or pooling, for example, a bike rental service (Table 1).

Though many goods are neither efficiently used nor necessary, we still need them to perform a variety of actions. However, many of our purchases are driven by the quest for a solution. This means that in many cases, we can replace one good with another or that good can be replaced with a result-oriented service type of PSS, i.e., activity management, pay per service or functional result. In this replacement type of CleanServ, not only is the use stage of the life cycle changed, but also all the other stages are affected, since the original good has been replaced with another. Therefore, the final solution should be evaluated to verify that it is indeed more sustainable than the good that it replaced. For example, using *YouTube* or *ITunes* to watch and listen to online content or to download movies or music instead of buying or renting a CD will lead to a reduction in the use of the resources that were previously consumed by CD production, packaging and storage as well as those used in the delivery of the CD.

The efficiency of each stage of the life cycle can be enhanced by both the rational use of the physical resources associated with each stage and a reduction in the overall pollution discharged to the surroundings. Improvements in efficiency can be realized by using clean technologies (CleanTech) or efficiency type CleanServs. The focus of this type of CleanServ is not on the good itself, on the number of goods or on its replacement by another good, but rather, it emphasizes the addition of supplementary services that can streamline the life cycle with respect to resource utilization. A highly relevant example of a efficiency type CleanServ is a service that facilitates smart traffic navigation and in so doing, it saves fuel and decreases air pollution.

Finally, the resources that were utilized in the production of a good can be partially offset by the addition of a service dedicated to the reuse or recycling of the product as a viable alternative to its disposal in a landfill. Alternatively, a service that invests in planting trees or in developing clean energies can offset the amounts of greenhouse gases that were emitted during the production and delivery of a good, i.e., an offset type of CleanServ.

Figure 2 illustrates the possible combinations of product and service along the continuum of 'pure-product' to 'pure-service' [27].

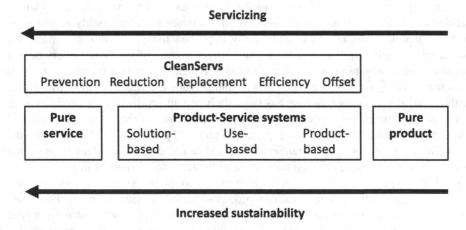

Fig. 2. Servicizing – from product to service [27].

3 Example

The potential of servicizing to increase the sustainability of the physical resources based life cycle of goods can be evaluated using as an example the production of a dedicated guidebook, for example, a travel book for tourists. The main activities in each stage of the life cycle (Fig. 1) of a printed book and the inputs into and outputs from the cycle are listed in Table 3 [28].

3.1 Prevention

The purchase of a guidebook can be prevented by using a consultation service run by an expert or by hiring a tourist guide for a guided tour. In this case, the service will likely not only provide a more professional and up-to-date solution, it will also lead to

Table 3. Life cycle inventory of a printed book [28].

Stage	Extraction of raw materials	Manu-facture	Delivery	Use	End of life	Total
Activities	Paper and ink production	Book printing	Packing, distribution, storage	Personal transportation, book reading	Disposal	–
Material input (kg)	113	21	1	15	0	151
Water consumption (L)	3174	26	55	500	0	3754
Energy (MJ)	1653	724	122	1305	0	3794
Air emission (g)	99	64	5	55	0	222
Water emission (g)	562	87	57	523	0	1229
Solid waste (kg)	4	75	0	16	0	94

a reduction in use of all the resources that are exploited during the book's life cycle. Yet besides the relatively higher monetary investment entailed in paying for the service, a book offers a more flexible option, and it can be used several times by the same user. Furthermore, though using the above-mentioned services requires many fewer resources, as it eliminates all the stages of the book's life cycle, the use of the service still requires transportation for the provider as well as the physical facilities used by the provider, e.g., an office equipped with a computer and whatever else is needed by the consultant. But because these same resources are used repeatedly to provide service on a regular basis (e.g., daily), the relative amounts of resources used in any single transaction (i.e., service provision) are very low. In addition, the same provision of service can be used simultaneously by several customers (i.e., groups of tourists), and therefore, the level of resource use per person is further decreased. Finally, included among the prevention type of CleanServs are educational services that, although they do not prevent the production of a product per say, they can effect more conscious consumption habits.

3.2 Reduction

Services also exist that can significantly reduce the number of books produced and still supply the customers with the same solution, i.e., a guidebook. One example of a reduction type of CleanServ is a book borrowing service (e.g., a library) that loans books, thereby eliminating the need to purchase and own them. Consider, for example, a scenario in which one book is used by 12 customers per year: with the exception of the resources consumed during the book's use stage (i.e., transportation to the book store or to the library), those associated with all the other life cycle stages of the book are divided by 12, thus significantly reducing the amounts of resources used per service instance. Although the resources used in library operation should also be added to this evaluation, because these resources are split between hundreds or thousands of books, they account for only negligible amounts of resources per single service instance. Alternatively, a second-hand book store is another CleanServ of the reduction type, but it typically involves fewer uses per book when compared to the library service. In addition, book sharing service can also be used to reduce the production of books.

3.3 Replacement

New technologies, and especially information technologies and the Internet, have not only expanded the opportunities to provide services, they have also drastically changed how we produce and deliver those services. When paired with the myriad software applications available today, electronic devices now allow the e-version of a book to be downloaded instead of buying a hard copy. As such, the e-book has changed both the total amount of resources of the life cycle as well as the types of materials used, e.g., metals and plastic instead of paper and ink. Nevertheless, because each electronic device is typically used with multiple books as well as for other purposes, the amount of resources per service use is much lower than that used over the life cycle of a printed book. The inventory of input and output resources associated with the life cycle of an e-book is summarized in Table 4. It can be seen that in all the stages of the life cycle, e-books use and emit fewer resources.

Table 4. Life cycle inventory of a printed e-book [28].

Stage	Extraction of raw materials	Manu-facture	Delivery	Use	End of life	Total
Activities	Metal and plastic production	E-reader produc-tion	Packing, distribution, storage	Personal transportation, e-reader use	Disposal	–
Material input (kg)	3	21	1	17	0	42
Water consumption (L)	28	1	13	6	0	48
Energy (MJ)	47	214	28	453	1	742
Air emission (g)	3	8	2	37	0	50
Water emission (g)	26	123	16	297	0	463
Solid waste (kg)	0	3	1	72	1	77

3.4 Efficiency

Efficiency type CleanServs are services that reduce resource utilization and pollution emission by streamlining the various stages of the life cycle. Different services, from life cycle assessment to research into new methods, tools and technologies, can be employed to this end. For example, the development of stiffer, lower weight paper or the creation of a service that promotes a more effective delivery process, e.g., a smart distribution application that can help drivers reduce the amounts of gasoline they need to run their deliveries, are efficiency type CleanServs. In addition, services can also be designed and implemented to improve the resource balance at the book's end-of-life or disposal stage by managing the resources more efficiently to maximize their potential. For example, garbage separation and sorting services can promote increased books reuse or recycling rates. While in a book recycling service, used books or printed papers can be returned to the book life cycle or be used to produce carton materials for packing, respectively, on a smaller scale, books can also be reused when their original owners pass them on to other readers or donate them to a library or to a second-hand book shop. Finally, some of the resources used in the manufacture of books can be returned to the larger resource pool via decomposition and resource recovery, i.e., decomposition of the organic matter used to produce books can yield compost that, in turn, can be used to improve the soil and to fertilize plants. However, note that poorly controlled or uncontrolled decomposition processes can lead to increases in the amounts of pollution discharged to the soil and to water sources.

3.5 Offset

Resource use can be offset by implementing different services, such as paper recycling or book reuse as mentioned above, and carbon can be offset by planting trees that will absorb the carbon dioxide emitted during the book's life cycle. Alternatively, the greenhouse gasses that were emitted during the whole life cycle of the book can be traded with other processes whose carbon emissions were cut.

4   Conclusions

The physical resource based life cycle of a product summarizes the transfer of input and output resources in the various stages of the production and delivery of a product from "cradle-to-grave" and preferably from "cradle-to-cradle". The addition of CleanServs to the different stages of the product life cycle can promote more efficient resource management. This approach can increase the sustainability of the product and offer PSS frameworks that yield more sustainable solutions than those of just a decade ago.

References

1. Klepper, S.: Entry, Exit, Growth, and Innovation over the Product Life Cycle. The American Economic Rev. 562–583 (1996)
2. Stark, J.: Product Lifecycle Management. Springer, London (2011)
3. Berkes, F.: Common Property Resources: Ecology and Community-Based Sustainable Development. Belhaven Press, London (1989)
4. Mahoney, J.T., Pandian, J.R.: The resource-based view within the conversation of strategic management. strategic management J. **13**(5), 363–380 (1992)
5. Amann K.: Product Lifecycle Management: Empowering the Future of Business, CIM Data, Inc. (2002)

6. Sudarsan, R., Fenves, S.J., Sriram, R.D., Wang, F.: A product information modeling framework for product lifecycle management. Comput. Aided Des. **37**(13), 1399–1411 (2005)
7. Immonen, A., Saaksvuori, A.: Product Lifecycle Management. Springer, Heidelberg (2013)
8. Terzi, S., Bouras, A., Dutta, D., Garetti, M., Kiritsis, D.: Product lifecycle management-from its history to its new role. Int. J. Product Lifecycle Manage. **4**(4), 360–389 (2010)
9. Westkämper, E.: Life cycle management and assessment: approaches and visions towards sustainable manufacturing. CIRP Ann. Manuf. Technol. **49**(2), 501–526 (2000)
10. Clark, W.C., Dickson, N.M.: Sustainability science: the emerging research program. Proc. Natl. Acad. Sci. **100**(14), 8059–8061 (2003)
11. Turner, R.K.: Sustainable Environmental Economics and Management: Principles and Practice. Belhaven Press, London (1993)
12. Adams, W.M.: Green Development: Environment and Sustainability in the Third World, Routledge (2003)
13. Glac, K.: Triple Bottom Line. Wiley Encyclopedia of Management. Wiley, New-York (2015)
14. World Commission on Environment and Development. Our Common Future, p. 27. Oxford University Press, Oxford (1987)
15. Rothenberg, S.: Sustainability through servicizing. MIT Sloan Manage. Rev. 48(2) (2012)
16. Chen, Y.Y., Ye, L.Z.: Environmental effect of manufacturing industry servicizing. J. Commercial Res. **8**, 20 (2009)
17. Porter, M.E., Millar, V.E.: How information gives you competitive advantage.. Harvard Business Rev. **63**(4), 149–160 (1985)
18. Normann, R., Ramirez, R.: Designing interactive strategy. Harvard Business Rev. **71**(4), 65–77 (1993)
19. Mont, O.K.: Clarifying the concept of product–service system. J. Cleaner Production **10**(3), 237–245 (2002)
20. Baines, T.S., Lightfoot, H.W., Evans, S., Neely, A., Greenough, R., Peppard, J., Wilson, H.: State-of-the-art in product-service systems. Proc. Inst. Mech. Eng. Part B J. Eng. Manuf. **221**(10), 1543–1552 (2007)
21. Tukker, A.: Eight types of product–service system: eight ways to sustainability? Bus. Strategy Environ. **13**(4), 246–260 (2004)
22. Morelli, N.: Developing new product-service systems (PSS): methodologies and operational tools. J. of Cleaner Production **14**(17), 1495–1501 (2006)
23. Hockerts, K.: Innovation of eco-efficient services: increasing the efficiency of products and services. Greener Mark. Global Perspect. Greening Mark. Pract. **95**(108), 95–108 (1999)
24. Brezet, J.C., Bijma, A.S., Ehrenfeld, J., Silvester, S.: The Design of Eco-Efficient Services. Delft University of Technology, Design for Sustainability Program, Delft 2001))
25. World Business Council for Sustainable Development. Eco-Efficiency: Creating More with Less, Geneva (2000)
26. Wolfson, A., Tavor, D., Mark, S.: Editorial column—from cleantech to cleanserv. Serv. Sci. **5**(3), 193–196 (2013)
27. Wolfson, A., Tavor, D., Mark, S.: CleanServs: clean services for a more sustainable world. Sustain. Acc. Manage. Policy J. **5**(4), 405–424 (2014)
28. Kozak, G.: Printed scholarly books and e-book reading devices: a comparative life cycle assessment of two book options, University of Michigan (2003). http://css.snre.umich.edu/css_doc/CSS03-04.pdf

Service Architecture for CSP Based Planning for Holonic Manufacturing Execution Systems

Gabriela Varvara[✉]

Department of Automatic Control and Applied Informatics,
Technical University "Gheorghe Asachi" Iasi, Iasi, Romania
gvarvara@ac.tuiasi.ro

Abstract. In the last period substantial effort was dedicated to solve resource allocation, planning and coordination problems for loosely coupled multi-agent systems through combinatorial techniques, especially Distributed Constraint Satisfaction Problem (DisCSP). Some preoccupations were directed to the extension and adaptation of these results to manufacturing planning/scheduling problems. This work will exploit the DisCSP techniques that could be used to manufacturing execution systems based on holonic organization in order to integrate a DisCSP planning mechanism and then reformulate the agent-holon model and the inter-holon connections from a service perspective.

Keywords: Distributed constraint satisfaction problem · Multi-agent planning · Holonic manufacturing execution systems · Service oriented design

1 Introduction

Modern manufacturing systems, distributed by their nature, have to face the challenges of post globalization period defined by frequent changes of the manufacturing scenarios that results in dynamic adjustments while guaranteeing scalability and optimal use of resources. From this perspective, aspects regarding distributed planning/scheduling combined with dynamic coordination at the execution level are continuously reevaluated to identify decentralized agile solutions able to ensure autonomous, safe and secure operation. At shop floor level, the versatile connection between holonic organization and multi-agent computing results in Holonic Manufacturing Execution Systems (HMES), a new paradigm that already proved to be a powerful tool to enhance decentralization and autonomous behavior. Despite all the recent advances concerning planning/scheduling techniques, some problems already persist and require specialized central entities. For instance, the planning process made by an Order Holon (OH) for two products that will be executed simultaneously could cause allocation problems for shared resource holons (RH). Classical techniques based on bidding processes, especially Contract Net Protocol (CNP) could not find a solution in absence of a central synchronization mechanism inserted at staff holon (SH) level [1, 2].

Recent research on combinatorial problems solution through Constraint Satisfaction Problem (CSP), its distributed algorithm (DisCSP), could bring benefits on

T. Borangiu et al. (Eds.): IESS 2016, LNBIP 247, pp. 403–416, 2016.
DOI: 10.1007/978-3-319-32689-4_31

manufacturing systems planning/scheduling or resource allocation at the shop-floor execution level [1, 3–5]. The CSP solution is obtained at the end of a search process made into a constraint network whose nodes are agents of a multi-agent system (MAS). Each agent holds and controls one variable and its assignment inside a predefined domain of values. The final solution represents a set of agents' variable assignments that satisfy all the problem constrains.

The DisCSP extends CSP solution in order to accommodate to the requirements of physical distributed problems and becomes, from one step to another, more than simple extensions of the centralized algorithm [6–8]. At the first development stage, the solution was centralized, CSP based, and obtained by a leader agent selected from all the MAS agents [9]. Thereafter, new algorithms were developed in order to ensure a complete decentralization and the agent autonomy. On the other hand, the distributed methods could assign the agent variables in two different ways, an asynchronous one were a single agent is allowed to make assignments at a time and a synchronous one with concurrent processes at agent level, which exploits the parallelism of distributed systems. Both assignment approaches have been used to solve multi-agent planning problems. Their representatives as The Asynchronous Forward Checking (AFC) algorithm or the Asynchronous Back-tracking algorithm (ABT) have been already used to solve simple planning problems. A robotic system with parallel execution of robots' actions [3], a shared resources alloca-tion problem involving two product holons with concurrent planning activities [1] are DisCSP best practice examples. For all of these situations the DisCSP approach proved its completeness by founding a solution were BDI (belief-desire-intention) agent mechanism and CNP negotiation failed in resource allocation.

Despite this, the direct use of the DisCSP algorithms for realistic more complex planning problems is not possible due to their major drawbacks regarding the use of a unique agent variable, the assumption that only binary inter-agent constraints are possible, the order the agents made their assignments and the time evolution of the system state. Interesting research papers as [10, 11] focus on adapting and extension of classical algorithms in order to overcome the above mentioned limits. They allow an increased number of variables for each agent of the constraint network to cover planning aspects regarding both public and private agent actions, a significant decreasing of the variables domain and a "goal-achieving" heuristics for ordering the agents execution.

In order to apply the DisCSP methodology to HMES planning, the next step proposed by this work is to connect the MAS constraint network to holonic organization of MES. The PROSA based holon architecture has to be adapted in order to accommodate to DisCSP mechanisms and the basic holon roles redefined. Moreover, MAS communi-cation aspects during plan elaboration have to be local and global integrated in holon interfaces in a reliable, safe and secure, service-oriented manner. Accordingly, after this short introductory paragraph, the second one identifies the model of the DisCSP planning agent for two known basic algorithms (AFC for synchronous and ABT for asynchronous agent assignments) and a new general planning methodology defined by [10, 11] adapted to the reality of HMES ("Planning First"). The third paragraph integrates DisCSP MAS at different holonic level and explains holarchy formation according to planning constrains at different organization levels. The last paragraph is devoted to service identification from communication paths during DisCSP planning in HMES. Some final remarks are presented at the end of the paper.

2 The DisCSP Agent Architecture

This paragraph is devoted to architectural details regarding the operation and communication of agents from MAS during the distributed constraints solving for a planning process. The first two presented algorithms namely ABT and AFC can be directly used for simple resource/plan actions allocation problems, while the third algorithm named "Planning first" represents an enhancement of AFC algorithm, to include complex planning scenarios with agent local and global actions, scheduling aspects in an optimized procedure. The analysis concerns the identification of the execution flow at agent level, emphasizing on the communication paths among the agents of the constraint network. It is based on the use of the following notations:

- $A_1, A_2, \ldots, A_{i-1}, A_i, A_{i+1}, \ldots A_n$ represent the agents of the constraint network ordered by priority such that A_i is the successor of A_{i-1} and the predecessor of A_{i+1}
- $v_1, v_2, \ldots, v_{i-1}, v_i, v_{i+1}, \ldots v_n$ are the variables manipulated by the agents such that v_i is hold by A_i
- $D_1, D_2, \ldots, D_{i-1}, D_i, D_{i+1}, \ldots D_n$ are the variable domains such that v_i has the domain $D_i = \{val_{i,1}, \ldots val_{i,ik}\}$ where $ik = size(D_i)$
- For A_i it is defined the Current Partial Assignment (CPA) as being the state of the assignments made by the agents with higher priority, namely the set $\{(v_1, val_{1,p}), \ldots (v_{i-1}, val_{i-1,q})\}$, where $p \leq size(D_1)$ and $q \leq size(D_{i-1})$
- The AgentView – is the agent memory location for storing the CPA and other algorithm specific data.

2.1 The Asynchronous Backtracking (ABT) Algorithm

As presented in [6, 9], this is the first complete asynchronous search algorithm for solving DisCSP. Agents, subject to a total order, execute autonomously their local consistent assignments in order to satisfy the global problem constraints. On the basis of known higher priority agents (predecessors) assignments, the current agent A_i tries to find a value v_i for its variable x_i to comply with the constraints. If the assignment is possible, it sends the selected value to its successors. If the agent can't find an appropriate value it reports to the higher neighbor the received previous assignment as being nogood. The ABT algorithm can compute the solution or detect that no solution exists in a finite time only if agents are subject to a static total order. Thus, the acyclic graph provided by ABT considers two types of agents [9]: those from which the link departs as being value-sending agents and those to which the link arrives as being constraint evaluating agents. The local information about the global search, in the form of the most updated values believed to be assigned by all the predecessors, is stored in the agent AgentView. A NogoodStore keeps all the nogoods as justification of value removal.

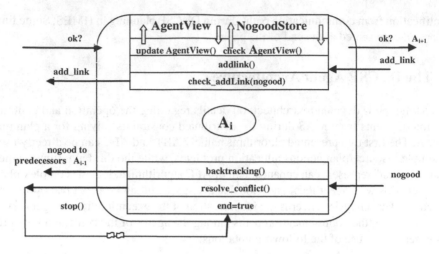

Fig. 1. The procedures execution at the ABT agent level

At agent level are manipulated the following messages:

- *ok?* to inform the successors about the agent assignment
- *nogood* to inform the predecessor about a new nogood
- *add_link* to request a predecessor to setup a link
- *stop* will be broadcasted to all the other agents if the current agent generates an empty nogood resulting in an insolvable DisCSP problem.

The messages received by the agent A_i will trigger the following procedures as detailed by [9] and represented in Fig. 1:

- The check_AgentView() procedure checks if a current assignment is consistent with the values received from the predecessors and stored in the AgentView. If a consistent assignment is found the agent notifies all its successors about it in a form of an *ok?* message.
- The backtracking() procedure solves the received nogoods and derives new nogoods or consistent value sent as an *ok?* message.
- The resolve_conflict() procedure will be called every time a *nogood* message is received and its associated nogood inconsistent assignments are the same with variables assignments found in the AgentView. Then it will call the Check_addLink() procedure to update the AgentView with assignments from nogood made by other agents not directed linked with A_i. This is followed by a request for a new link sent to agents owing these variables.
- The procedure CheckAgentView() is called in order to find a new consistent value after an older inconsistent one was removed.
- The link setup request from a received *add_link* message is treated by *addlink()* procedure. It adds the sender as being one of the agent successors. As result, the agent sends it an assignment as an ok? message if this value is different from that received in *add_link* message.

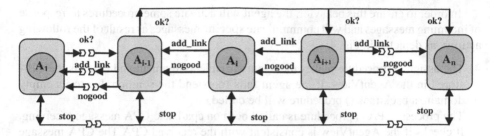

Fig. 2. The ABT inter-agent communication paths

An extended representation of these messages at MAS level will define the communication paths as represented in Fig. 2:

2.2 The Asynchronous Forward Checking Algorithm

This algorithm is the most used representative of the classical DisCSP with synchronous search. As presented in [9], the AFC agents communicate according to their following distinctive features, as represented in Fig. 3:

– The agent assignments are allowed only in the moments it holds the CPA named "token", as a privilege of taking operational decisions to extend it. The token will be passed to one agent to another according to their precedence order.
– The agent in possession of the "token" will try to extend the CPA. If it succeeds the extended CPA will be sent to its successor and the CPA copies to successors that have no assignments in the CPA. If it fails to make an assignment consistent to problem constraints, a back_CPA (AgentView) message will be send to its predecessor.
– The agent receiving the CPA copy will perform a forward check and remove from its domain the values unassigned and not consistent with the CPA. If its domain becomes empty, it will send a not-OK message to inform the agents with no assignments in CPA about its non consistency. The next step, the agent owning the original CPA will send a back_CPA (AgentView) message.

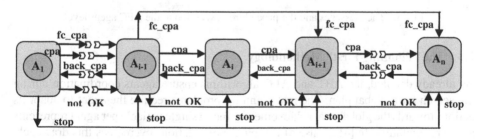

Fig. 3. The AFC inter-agent communication paths

In order to ensure this behavior, the agent will activate some procedures as response of incoming messages and will communicate specific messages as result of the following actions, as depicted in Fig. 4:

- The assign () procedure makes the agent variable assignment and extends the CPA stored in the AgentView. If the agent fails to extend the solution due to its empty domain, a backtrack () procedure will be called.
- The process_CPA () procedure is called both on cpa/back_CPA message receiving. It checks if the AgentView is consistent with the received CPA The CPA message of the last agent is the problem solution, while a back-CPA from the first agent will stop the procedure and broadcast a stop message.
- The process_fc_CPA() procedure will start as result of receiving a fc_cpa(CPA) message in order to check if the unassigned values of the active agent are consistent with the received CPA.
- The backtracking () procedure allows agents to reconsider an entire path of assignments.
- The not_OK (CPA) procedure updates the AgentView with the received inconsistent CPA.

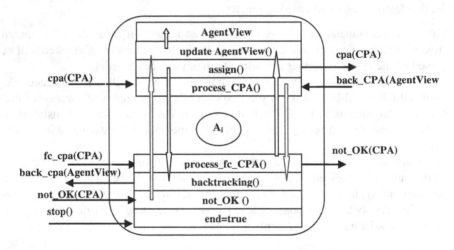

Fig. 4. The messages and the procedures execution at the AFC agent level

2.3 The "Planning First" Methodology

As already detailed, the ABT and AFC algorithms ensure agents coordination during the search for a global plan. The real planning problems require the agent to adapt its actions towards the global goal achievement. Since a single variable per agent represents a severe limitation. In [4] the use of n-tuple representations overcomes this drawback, but this does not allow a complete separation in treating the variables including different preconditions, or possible relationships of causality between them. In [10, 11] the authors proposed an enhanced AFC algorithm and an associated methodology, named "Planning First" to be used for general planning purposes in networks with loosely coupled agents as represented by the HMES with extended RHs autonomy. The algorithm allows local planning at agent level and agents coordination for both planning and execution activities. Moreover, the proposed methodology includes a goal-achieving heuristics for the order of agents' assignment to optimize the search process. It offers a coherent global solution that overcomes also other drawbacks of classical algorithms, namely: the intra-agent constraints are of unary type and the inter-agent constraints are only of binary type, the complexity of the problem associated with a large amount of messages among the agents, the necessity of total ordering of the agents associated to the efficiency dependence of this ordering process.

The algorithm introduces two types of agent actions: private used to achieve local intern plans, and public required for the execution of the system plan. The global plan is obtained through the DisCSP coordination of the agents, while the local plan is established by a local planner and ensures that the agent can execute the sequence of its public actions. In order to obtain this quite general planning behavior, four action directions are proposed by [11]:

The Agent Holds Three Variables. Each agent holds two ordered sequences of public actions (ActVar) and associated times to start these actions (TimeVar), and set of requirements (ReqVar) addressed to other agents in order to ensure the preconditions of local actions. This improvement will cut entire paths from the search tree by choosing only the assignments of ActVar actions directed to the achievement of the global goal.

The Local Planning. Agent starts with planning before any assignments of one of its variables. It comprises the following sequence of actions:

- The identification of a local plan that satisfies all the private goals. It contains local actions and no more than δ public actions and does not consider the preconditions provided by other agents. It takes into account only the agent capacity to meet the requirements addressed by other agents.
- The ActVar are assigned with the actions of the above relaxed plan in their appearance order. The ActVar domain is optimized through the essential actions that appear in any instance of the global plan. A local plan that does not contain essential actions will be dropped and then it results a decreasing of the ActVar values domain.
- The TimeVar are instantiated with values consistent with the assigned actions and then
- The ReqVar values are assigned. This involves the creation of action landmarks for the actions requested to be executed by the neighbor agents from the constraint network.

If TempVar/ReqVar domains become empty during the search process, the current ActVar assignment is added to the forbidden plans. The agent will start the search for a new plan different from the previous. If it fails to find a new plan it will perform a backtrack.

The Enhancement of the DisCSP Heuristics. The classical algorithms assume a predefined order for agent assignments. The "Planning First" methodology proposes a dynamic ordering that comply with two principles:

- "The most constraint" that imply the descending ordering of agents by the number of their gathered action landmarks. An agent with a great number of action landmarks is most likely to be unable to find a feasible plan and to make backtrack.
- "Goal-achieving" accomplished by the local planning through the order of assignments. Starting the process with ActVar will direct the search to the agent goal achievement. Furthermore, the ReqVar assignment will follow the principle "least constraint first" by ordering the unassigned agents in ascending order of their action landmarks.

Adapting the DisCSP Solver Algorithm. The DisCSP AFC classical algorithm has to be adjusted in order to allow dynamic generation of variable domains and then of constraints, to include local planners with consistent requirements and precise actions' execution moments. The proposed solution [11] is to use a back-jumping mechanism as a backtracking technique. This implies that each variable keeps the track to the deepest variable conflicting with it and backtracks to it when no consistent value can be found. The agent from the constraint network has a distinctive operation mode as depicted in the next figure:

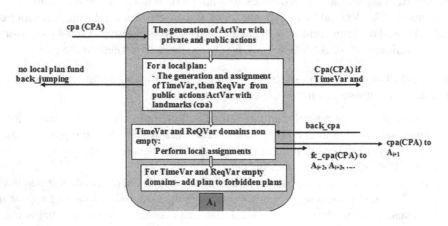

Fig. 5. The communication and the execution model at the "Planning First" agent level

3   The DisCSP Based Planning for HMES

As already known, HMES are distributed by their nature and assume dynamic formation of holarchies associated with horizontal and vertical communications flows. Their planning problems are solved through centralized, semi-centralized and decentralized methods and involve mainly the Product Holon (PH) and Resource Holon (RH) of the basic PROSA architecture. A constant research effort is directed to the transfer of the decision activities to the execution level while preserving the system performance. Hence, a RH with an enhanced autonomy has to perform coherent planning/scheduling and execution activities. Referring to distributed planning/execution activities, a key point remains the coordination at all the decision levels. HMES solve this problem at higher integration Order Holon (OH) level or at the intermediate PH level through centralized bidding mechanisms, CNP being the most used protocol. As already mentioned, the drawback of these mechanisms is their lack of completeness. They could fail in identifying concurrent plans that use shared resources or with limited availability. Moreover some of the potential contractors could decide not to negotiate. To overcome this problem, a third centralized component should be added to relax the bidding conditions. On the other hand, the distributed planning is accomplished by MAS with belief-desire-intensions (BDI) AI mechanisms at agent level. It assumes the existence of a library with alternative plans, the planning process meaning the selection of a suitable plan to achieve the system goal under current circumstances. In this light, the possibility of decentralized planning of HMES through DisCSP techniques represents a new promising research area. This new type of coordination algorithms comes firstly with the completeness characteristic and a few important features, namely:

- The outcome plan is unique for a given constraint network, the agent priorities being settled static or dynamic.
- The planning process implies the participation of all the agents, none of them being able to refuse the collaboration. As a consequence, when an agent fails, the process must be restarted or the algorithms should be adapted to include a recovery process.
- The resource allocation and scheduling processes can run simultaneously through an abstract time added as an explicit working variable.
- At the end of the procedure, each agent stores in the AgentView its perspective of the partial assignments made by all its predecessors (agents with higher priorities).

The case studies presented in [1, 3] emphasize some aspects regarding the hierarchical level in the HMES holarchy the DisCSP planning could be added. This approach can be extended to define the following possible levels of DisCSP integration:

- The complete decentralization associated with a heterarchical organization and decisions at RH level. The agents of the constraint network are included in the RH processing component. The PH is free from making planning activities. Its role is to provide the working configuration for a given product: RHs and associated priorities for static assignment, manufacturing goal constraints, specific public actions associated to each RH and their domains, actions timing sequence, atoms (parts, locations, actions, propositions) affected by/affecting the agents actions and their domains.
- The centralized planning at PH level enables centralized keeping of the information regarding DisCSP network formation and starting. The planning process is independent of the RH processes as the MAS reside in the processing part of PH. At this level it is possible to have PHs holarchies that imply the access of two or more PHs on critical resources (shared/limited access). The agents' variables from the constraint networks will be the actions needed to produce all the products managed by the already referred PHs. Their priority is related to the execution priority of different plans and, inside a particular plan, of the associated actions. Due to its completeness, a DisCSP RH allocation solution will be found even when conflicts arise among PHs accessing the same shared RH.

- The centralized planning at OH level could use a DisCSP based planning in order to solve conflicts among different manufacturing orders requiring the same product to be made for multiple orders in the same time.

From other perspective, the HMES allows the decomposition of the manufacturing problem in sub-problems that could be solved concurrently by DisCSP MAS. For large scale systems were cluster decomposition is obvious the method is applicable and offers scalable solutions as presented in [5] for a similar scheduling problem. A DisCSP constraint network could be defined for each cluster represented as a holarchy, and different appropriate algorithms could be used for each MAS in a concurrent manner. The clusters are correlated in the way that a higher priority cluster solves the problem at its level obtaining a solution named *consistent partial state* and sends it to the lower priority neighbor cluster. Then both clusters will obtain a new solution and so on until the system solution is found. Each cluster receives a partial solution from its predecessor and tries to extend the solution with assignments of its own variables that conform to the local constraints.

4   SOA for HMES DisCSP Planning

From service perspective, as presented in [12–14] the integration of the DisCSP planning mechanisms in HMES means the reformulation of the inter-agent, MAS and inter-holon specific communication paths. Consequently, aspects referring interoperability, re-configurability, maintenance addressed by service based communication have to be added and adapted to new operational mechanisms. The agents that solve the DisCSP planning problem could be superimposed over holonic system agents or not. If this was happened, the problem of encapsulation is essential as RHs differ as structure and are distributed. The planning system servitization in a SOA based formulation of HMES should be captured in a product-service system capable of ensuring reliable, safe and secure operation [15]. This process will start with the identification of reusable resources and their necessary interface communication in the form of a request/response protocol type. Then the requestors and the providers should be specified along with a discovery mechanism and the structure of the exchanged messages.

This paragraph initiates this process by identifying of the communication flows inside HMES with DisCSP planning, taking into account different operation setups. The planning problem is considered to be solved inside the HMES holarchies at different levels. The DisCSP MAS will be integrated as a single entity if the integration is made at PH and OH decision level.

At RH planning level each agent from the constraint network must be integrated in the holon architecture. Consequently, each RH will participate in planning process. Thereby, the RH associated agent will extend its functionality with the procedures depicted in Figs. 1, 3 and 5. Accordingly, the inter-agent message exchanges as represented in Fig. 2 or Fig. 4 become the service oriented communication paths depicted in the next diagram:

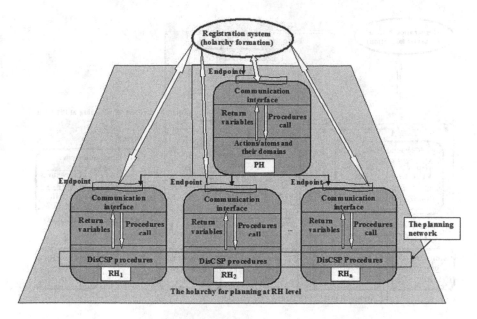

Fig. 6. Service communication path for planning at the RH level

The diagram highlights two types of exchanging messages: the agent from the higher priority RH will request from PH, or other third entity, information about actions/atoms and their domains, and problem constraints. Each agent will receive from specified predecessors cpa, fc_cpa and not_OK or equivalent messages and from its successor a back_cpa message type. All the input/output messages are mediated by the holons communication interfaces through service endpoints. A registry system is necessary to integrate new holons in the holarchy (Fig. 6).

Following the same principle, the DisCSP planning network could be integrated at PH or OH level, as represented in the next figures. In Fig. 7, the MAS agents of the planning network are distributed among PHs processing parts. On the other hand, every PH develops its own holarchy in order to make the resource allocation for product manufacturing. Hence, different PHs coordinate their allocation problems in such a way that shared resource problem becomes a global planning constraint and can be solved by product holons collaboration.

In a similar way, the planning process could be moved upward, at OH level as depicted in the Fig. 8. This architecture could solve conflicts among OHs that share downward PHs and further RHs.

The clustering problem presented in the above paragraph assumes that, at the top level, the system holarchy has a MAS planning system. Besides this, the holarchies resulting from system decomposition act themselves as being agents in a constraint network as depicted in Fig. 9. This horizontal planning decomposition assumes that each holarchy solves its own constraint problem but it is subject to variable assignment generated by the predecessor holarchy. Thus, the solution found by the upstream holarchy is sent to the downstream one in the form of a consistent partial state message.

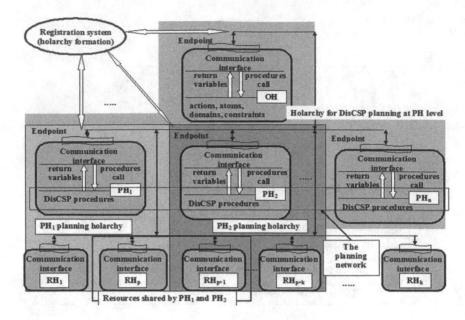

Fig. 7. Service communication path for centralized planning at PH level

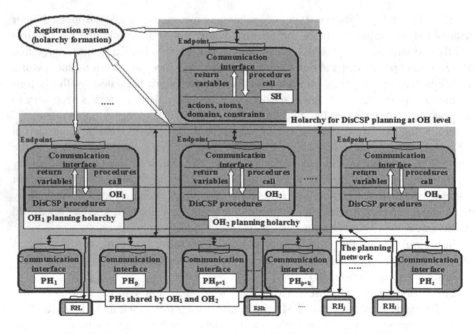

Fig. 8. Service communication path for centralized planning at OH level

Then both holarchies work together to find their own solutions affected by the assignments made on the common variables by each of them.

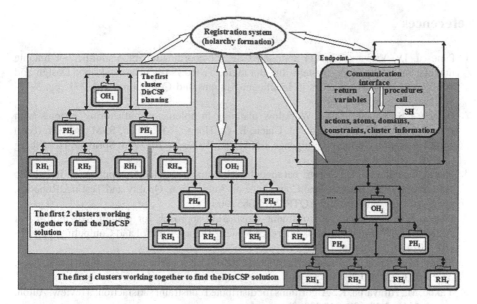

Fig. 9. DisCSP planning for cluster holarchies

The process will extend and, finally, all the holarchies work together to find a final solution. The exchanged messages refer the partial state and the common variable assignments. A third part is necessary to establish the constraint partition with all the required information about each sub-problem to be solved.

5 Conclusions

The focus of this work consists in sketching the main distributed CSP algorithms suitable to be integrated in HMES. On this basis, the architecture of PROSA holons was adapted to integrate the DisCSP MAS at different type of holon and decision level inside the holarchies. The inferred architecture was reformulated to ensure data encapsulation, portability and secure communication, in a way that could improve the efficiency of the manufacturing systems, especially of the execution ones. Thus, exchanged messages and service mechanisms were identified in order to further develop service oriented architectures.

Behind the reported results stands the idea that CSP could be an alternative way of thinking and designing the planning process for manufacturing purposes. It should be integrated in the already developed HMES in such a way its algorithmic benefit not to be surpassed by an inherent complexity or message traffic congestion. Of course, the distribution must be considered, but in a fair balance with the efficiency at the system level.

Further work will be directed to the architecture details and implementation aspects associated to robotic systems.

References

1. Pănescu, D., Varvara, G.: On applying CSP for coordination of a multi-robot holonic manufacturing execution System. In: Borangiu, T. (ed.) Advances in Robot Design and Intelligent Control. Advances in Intelligent Systems and Computing, vol. 371, pp. 3–12. Springer, Switzerland (2015)
2. Hsiech, F.S., Chiang, C.Y.: Workflow planning in holonic manufacturing systems with extended contract net protocol. In: Chien, B.-C., Hong, T.-P., Chen, S.-M., Ali, M. (eds.) Next-Generation Applied Intelligence. LNAI, vol. 5579, pp. 701–716. Springer, Heidelberg (2009)
3. Pascal, C., Pănescu, D.: A petri net model for constraint satisfaction application in holonic systems. In: IEEE International Conference on Automation, Quality and Testing, Robotics, pp. 1–6 (2014). doi:10.1109/AQTR.2014.6857900
4. Pănescu, D., Pascal, C.: A constraint satisfaction approach for planning of multi-robot systems. In: 18th International Conference System Theory, Control and Computing, pp.157–162 (2014)
5. Salido, M.A., Giret, A.: Feasible distributed CSP models for scheduling problems. Eng. Appl. AI 21, 723–732 (2008)
6. Yakoo, M., Hirayama, K.: Algorithms for distributed constraint satisfaction: a review. Auton. Agent. MAS 3(2), 198–212 (2000)
7. Faltings, B., Yokoo, M.: Introduction: Special Issue on Distributed Constraint Satisfaction. Artificial Intelligence, vol. 161, pp. 1–5 (2005)
8. Leitao, R.A., EnenBreck, F., Barthes, J.-P.A.: Distributed constraint optimization problems: review and perspectives. Expert Syst. Appl. 41, 5139–5157 (2014)
9. Wahbi, M.: Algorithms and Ordering Heuristics for Distributed Constraint Satisfaction Problem. Wiley-ISTE, NewYork (2013). ISBN 978-1-84821-594-8
10. Brafman, R.I., Domshlak, C.: From one to many: planning for loosely coupled multi-agent systems. Technical report. Association for the Advancement of Artificial Intelligence AAAI (2008)
11. Nissim, R., Brafman, R.I., Domshlak, C.: A general, fully distributed multi-agent planning algorithm. In: van der Hoek, W., Kaminka, G.A., Lesperance, Y., Luck, M., Sen, S. (eds.) The 9th International Conference of Autonomous Agents and Multi-Agent Systems, AAMAS 2010, Toronto, Canada, pp. 1–8 (2010)
12. Varvara, G.: Service-oriented agent-based systems for manufacturing. Technical report. The 14th IFAC Symposium INCOM Bucharest, May 23–25 (2012)
13. Pănescu, D., Varvara, G., Pascal, C.: Planning and coordination mechanisms in service oriented manufacturing. Technical report. The international INSEED Seminar, Bucharest, May 21–25 (2012)
14. Barbosa, J., Leitao, P.: Enhancing service-oriented holonic multi-agent systems with self-organization. In: International Conference on Industrial Engineering and Systems Management 2011, Metz, France, pp. 1373–1381 (2011)
15. Garcia-Dominguez, A., Marcos-Barcena, M., Medina-Bulo, I., Prades-Martel, L.: Towards an integrated SOA-based architecture for interoperable and responsive manufacturing systems. In: Brunone, B., Giustolisi, O., et al. (eds.) Proceedings of MESIC 2013, Procedia Engineering, vol. 63, pp. 123–132 (2013)

Product-Service Systems

Designing Product Service Systems in the Context of Social Internet of Things

Pazanee Carpanen[1(✉)], Lia Patrício[1], and Bernardo Ribeiro[2]

[1] FEUP – Faculdade de Engenharia da Universidade do Porto, Rua Dr. Roberto Frias,
4200-465 Porto, Portugal
{mesg1301159,lpatric}@fe.up.pt
[2] CEIIA – Centro para a Excelência e Inovação na Indústria Automóvel,
Rua Eng. Frederico Ulrich 2650 (Tecmaia), 4470-605 Maia, Portugal
bernardo.ribeiro@ceiia.com

Abstract. Technology has taken its toll on human life and is present everywhere. Within the context of smart cities projects, there is a need to see how social relationship can be translated to objects and a new paradigm - the Social Internet of Things tries to address this transition. This research aims to develop a new approach for the product service systems design in the context of the social internet of things, with a case study of the development of a new smart social bike service. The research uses the design thinking approach to integrate concept of product service system into the multi-level service design. New service concepts are proposed and an architecture is designed for the operationalization of the service based on the Social Internet of Things paradigm. This research aims to show how service design methods can be applied in the context of product service systems and social internet of things.

Keywords: Product service systems · Service design · Smart services · Social Internet of Things

1 Introduction

Services are increasingly important as the service sector grows in economies and as manufacturing companies add services to their offerings to become more competitive in the market, moving from products to product-service systems. This trend, together with technology evolution, raise new challenges to service design, as it requires the orchestration of product, service and technology components to develop integrated solutions to customers. Service design is a systematic process based on a human centred approach [1] and is crucial to service innovation [2]. Service design is a rapidly evolving interdisciplinary field that synthesizes service science and design thinking, representing a human-centered, creative, iterative approach to the creation of new services [3] that incorporates multiple contributions from service marketing, operations, and information technology, all integrated through design-based methods and tools [4]. Indeed, advances in technology has changed the way services and products are designed.

© Springer International Publishing Switzerland 2016
T. Borangiu et al. (Eds.): IESS 2016, LNBIP 247, pp. 419–431, 2016.
DOI: 10.1007/978-3-319-32689-4_32

Service delivery and experience has been revolutionised through technology advances [2]. There are more opportunities for better quality and personalised services as well as deeper customer relationship due to the rise of information technology such as Internet of Things, social networks, mobile technologies and cloud computing. These technologies enable omnipresent customer communication, storage and analysis of big data [5]. Big Data can be characterized by huge volume, high velocity of real-time information and generation, and a wide variety of data sources and types [6]. The evolution of cutting-edge technologies has helped companies to improve service offerings as they look to service as a differentiating factor that promote growth [2].

Information Technology has also created new opportunities to innovate product service systems. These product service system solutions are now more complex, including hardware, sensors, data storage, microprocessors, software, and connectivity, they are more than just an object comprising of mechanical and electrical parts. An amalgam of ubiquitous wireless connectivity, advancement in processing power and device miniaturization has been the pillar for the so called 'smart, connected products' [7].

One advancement in technology has been the Internet of Things. The internet of things is defined as the 'interconnection of sensing and actuating devices providing the ability to share information across platforms through a unified framework, developing a common operating picture for enabling innovative applications. This is achieved by seamless ubiquitous sensing, data analytics and information representation with Cloud computing as the unifying framework' [8]. This raises the concern of properly addressing services that will function under the IOT so as to adapt well to the market.

This paper contributes to address these challenges by showing how a service design and technology approaches can be integrated to design new product service systems in the context of the social internet of things. The research objectives therefore relate to the integration of Product Service System concept in the service design process. The research aims to create a smart service in the context of the Social Internet of Things Paradigm by integrating concept from Product Service System and Service Design. The research questions identified are:

1. How to integrate the concept of PSS in the design of a new services under the 'Social Internet of Things Paradigm'?
2. How to design an architecture to support such new Product Service System?

To this end, the following section covers extent research on smart services and Social Internet of things, product service system, and service design, analyzing their contributions and gaps to address the research questions. Then, the case study of the design of a smart social bike system, showing how the combination of service design and product-service systems approaches can be useful for the creation of integrated product service system solutions in the context of the social internet of things. Finally, managerial and research implications are discussed, identifying opportunities for future research.

2   Literature Review

2.1   Smart Services

Smart services can be defined as a service conveyed through the use of intelligent prod-ucts that possess some kind of awareness and connectivity [9]. Such services include pre-emptive services, such as remote monitoring of intelligent machines [10], self-serv-ices, such as information services made available for the customer through Internet access via car electronics [11], or highly interactive services, such as collaborative remote repair of machines or remote surgeries with collaborating physicians at distant locations [12]. An intelligent product are those that 'contain information technology (IT) in the form of microchips, software, and sensors and provide companies with the means to collect, process, and produce information to serve customers and provide solutions in many domains' [13]. It has been argued that smart services help boost business to business and business to consumer settings such as mechanical engineering, health care, information and communication technology (ICT), automotive, and household appli-ances [14]. Others argued that the application of smart services foresee a consequent increase in efficiency for the providers and users in terms of cost reductions, increased flexibility, increased access and time savings [9]. Biehl, Prater and McIntyre 2004, argue that to gain customer acceptance and usage of new innovative services is a big challenge despite the rapid emergence of smart services [10]. Keh and Pang 2010 argue that customers perceive technology-mediated services as risky [15]. 'As these perceptions influence customers buying decisions, smart service providers need to overcome these obstacles to raise user acceptance of smart service innovations' [16]. They further point out that 'some smart services are delivered object-to-object with no human contribution whatsoever, others involve customers and employees as integral participants' [16]. 'The defining characteristic of smart services is the delivery to or through intelligent products or connected objects.' 'Smart services form a heterogeneous group of services that exhibit different levels of customer interactivity involved in the service delivery' [16].

As such, to embrace the smart service concept, the technical aspect is not the main issue as technologies are pretty well developed. The issues lies in getting the required support of senior management to utilize the new perspective unfolding. With the rise of competition and commoditization taking its toll on production lines, manufacturers have adopted a new business infusion to maximise benefit from service activities. This leads to going beyond the traditional life cycles of product and looking into usage of the product by the customers [9]. Indeed, the research on smart services helps answering the research questions. There is a mismatch in understanding how technologies changes the perspective of how business will be done from the management point of view.

2.2   Product Service Systems

Mont defines the product service systems as "a marketable set of products and services capable of jointly fulfilling a user's need" [17]. Companies using a product service system gain competitive advantage by modifying the traditional usage of their product by adding a service element to it. Moreover, increasing profitability by proposing alternative scenario of usage is another aim of PSS as it seeks to create a balance between economic, social and environmental issues [18]. PSS comprise of the following elements:

1. the product
2. the service
3. relationships

Manzini and Vezzoli argued that 'the PSS is a strategic design intended to integrate a system of products, services and communication based on new forms of organization, role reconfiguration, customers and other stakeholders' [19]. "Strategic design for sustainability" stands for the ability to create new stakeholder configurations and develop an integrated system of products, services and communication that is coherent with the medium-long-term perspective of sustainability [18]. According to Morelli, a PSS is a social construction whose foundation are goals, expected results and problem-solving criteria that stimulate the involvement of different partners. Such participation creates a value co-production process whose efficiency depends on a shared vision of possible and desirable scenarios [20]. Nicolas et al. 2007 proposed a method for designing PSS based on the Functional Analysis and Agent-Based Value Design. This method aims to help designers detail values and costs required to meet functions [21]. Indeed, research gives a useful insight on current way of designing PSS and also shows that there is a gap in designing a PSS using the service design perspective and the research aim to address it.

2.3 Social Internet of Things

Currently there is a new concept being studied, Social internet of things (SIoT), whereby objects established social relationships with each other's. The idea came from creating a service that allows similar devices to share best practices to solve problems among friends given proper authorization. The aims of such relationship is defined as follows [22]:

1. Structure IOT to guarantee network accessibility so that efficient service discovery can be carried out while ensuring scalability.
2. Create trust to leverage level of interaction between things that are friends.

Atzori et al. 2011 argue that the benefits of SIOT for humans are they become visible, find resources/old friends, obtain context information, and get filtered information and discover new resources. On the other hand, the benefits for objects are publish information/services, find information/services, and get environment characteristics. They came up with an architecture consisting of three layers. The base layer consists of the database for storage and management of data such as human and objects behaviors. It also comprise of the ontologies, the semantic engines and the communications. The component layer includes functional tools such as profiling, ID management, owner control, relationship management, service discovery, service composition, and trustworthiness management. The application layer is the link to the objects, humans, and services through the use of interfaces.

Indeed, the survey shows that most research on Social Internet of Things have mostly focused on the technical and technological aspects of such paradigm and there is a need to look how to design a smart service using such paradigm as a supporting tool. This research aim to bridge this gap.

2.4 Conclusion and Research Contribution

With the rapid advent of technology and the fast growth of portable devices with strong communicating capabilities, the idea behind the Internet of Things is taking form. Indeed, Smart services are gradually growing and adapting to the concept of Internet of things. Both smart services and product service system has the aim to provide something which is sustainable and efficient to the society. Also, the Social Internet of Things being a new paradigm, there is a lack of research on its applicability. To this end, this research aim to reduce the gaps identify by designing a product service system under the context of the Social Internet of Things which eventually leads to a creation of a smart service.

3 Methodology

The research used a design science research methodology [23] nested in the design thinking approach. The research approach proposed uses five steps with different techniques along the steps. The steps follows the iterative process of inspiration, ideation, reflection and implementation [4] and extend the multi-level service design approach [24] to include a technique from product service system namely Actor Network Mapping [25]. While designing a product service system, there was a need to show the different value that is offered to the stakeholders involved in the project. Figure 1 shows the steps used in the research approach as well as the techniques used in each steps. As a first step, the problem and/or goal is defined. Step two deals with understanding the customer experience. Techniques such as interviews, question-naire, stakeholder map and benchmarking are used to gather rich set of data to under-stand the context. Then, tools such as Customer Journey and Customer Experience Modelling [26] are used to draw the customer experience of the given context. Step three involve the conceptualisation of the service offering using tools such as Customer Value Constellation, Service System Architecture, Service System Navi-gation, Service Experience Blueprint and Actor Network Mapping. Step four involve the design of the system architecture that will support the new service and uses tools such as Social Internet of Things Architecture [22], Scenario, Use Cases, KAOS [27] and Mockups. The last step involve in defining the business model.

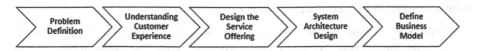

Fig. 1. Steps of the approach

3.1 Case Study

To validate the steps proposed above, a case study of a bike sharing service is used. Yin 2005 argue that unit of analysis is primordial in the case of a case study methodology [28]. In the present case, the unit of analysis is CEIIA (Centro para a Excelência e Inovação na Indústria Automóvel), an innovative and engineering centre based in Portugal, that wish to implement such service on their mobility platform. A study was first performed on the current bike sharing systems to understand the different elements; people, processes and technology that constitutes such systems. A preliminary insight was obtained about its users and stakeholders. The stakeholders for smart social bike were identified, as they will be the ones responsible to make the system operable. The stakeholder map is given in Fig. 2. Stakeholder analysis gives an insight on who is involved in such type of project and what kind of support they eventually bring in.

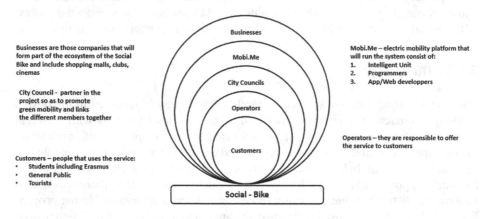

Fig. 2. Stakeholder map

3.2 Data Collection

Interviews, observation and questionnaires are tools that are used to gather useful information about the current context of bike sharing system and it helps to validate the initial idea as well. Through the qualitative and quantitative study, the market segment is identified and assumptions and constraints for the new project are defined. By identifying the market segments, you are in a position to tailor-made services for each need of the different segments. Within the context of the project, understanding the experience of bike sharing users and operators of these systems is very important to understand problems faced, the level of satisfaction and their needs. Six operators of bike sharing system were contacted. The data collection was made as follows:

1. Preliminary investigation on social media to get a first insight on the feeling of people using the current bike sharing system were undertaken. The different bike sharing systems were searched on Facebook in order to get a view from the customers. Nowadays, social media is being used as a channel to reach customers since more

people are active on the social media. It is interesting to see how current bike operators uses such channel.

2. Interview of operators of bike sharing system to get insights on how they manage the system, what problems, and challenges they faced. In this case, the sample will be selective as in Portugal, the Municipality usually operates the scheme.

3. Interview the users of bike sharing to gather data on their level of satisfaction. It is important to get a face to face interaction with the users as it provide not only qualified data and also allow the interviewee to observe the body language of the user. Here, the sample was random because different people from different background use the bike. The questions were designed into two sections where the first section concentrate on gathering data on the current system and the second section, selling the new concept indirectly.

4. Observations were undertaken on the day of the interviews to grasp how the people behave while using the bike sharing. This helps in understanding the activities involved and identifying solutions to given problems.

5. Using an online questionnaire to try and reach the different users of bike sharing system. The survey was published on social media including bike sharing groups. Also, it was sent to university students with the aim of getting maximum information. Questionnaire brings in quantitative data that helps in designing the service system architecture in the later stages of the research.

4   Smart Social Bike Case Study

4.1   Understanding the Customer Experience

The data gathered was analysed and a better insight was obtained about the current experience of users of bike sharing system. The problem encountered was identified as well as the customer segments. Also, the new concept that was proposed got a positive response. A benchmarking of the different bike sharing was undertaken to assess the different components and technological advances possess. This is done so as smart social bike can be conceived in a way that brings competitive advantage in the market. For smart social bike, the Customer Experience Requirement's are derived from the service requirements which address the issues raised during the data collection phase. The CER identified as more important after analyzing the Customer Experience Modelling were availability, convenience, and reliable, fulfilling, range of service.

4.2   Designing the Service Offering

The design of the new service use the three steps of the Multi-Level Service Design: service concept, service system and service encounter [24]. The tool used for designing the service concept is the customer value constellation (CVC). The service concept of current bike sharing systems was drawn based on the previous studies undertaken. Then to satisfy the needs of the customers, to address the issues raised and with the concept of smart social bike, a new service concept is developed for the smart social bike and is presented in Fig. 3.

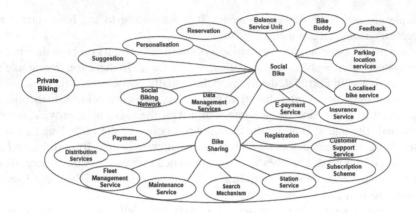

Fig. 3. CVC for smart social bike

The new services will allow users to personalise their riding experience and keep in touch with their peer on a social biking network. Reservation of bike is possible and distribution of bike among station are made easy with the parking location services. Also, private users can connect to the ecosystem and uses the service available.

The next step was to design the service system using two tools namely the service system architecture (SSA) and the service system navigation (SSN). The SSA for smart social bike shows the main activities in the new service and which service interface is responsible for its execution (Fig. 4). While with the use of Personas, SSN goes into a higher level of detail showing the journey of the customer using a scenario where he enquires about the system, register and uses the service.

Activity	Information Search	Register to system	Payment	Generate membership card	Set Preference	Use Bike
Customer	☐		☐		☐	☐
Employees	☐	☐	☐			
Station						☐
Physical Store	☐	☐	☐			
Card				☐		☐
Smartphone	☐	☐	☐	☐		☐
Web Portal	☐	☐	☐	☐		
Black Box						☐
Maintenance						
Backend System	☐	☐	☐	☐	☐	☐

Fig. 4. Service System Architecture for the smart social bike

Figure 5 shows the Service Experience Blueprint for the activity using the bike, assuming that the user will use the e-card. The user logins on the mobile app and chooses the option card. He scans the card at the station and unlocks the bike. Then he connects his smartphone with the bike. The black box on the bike synchronises with the smartphone and reads the preferences of the user. During the ride, the black box will only capture information as set by the user and sends the appropriate notification. Note that, the system will track the positioning of the bike. The failure might arise during synchronisation due to network problem. The analysis of the riding behaviour might take some time due to the influx of information to process according the need of the user.

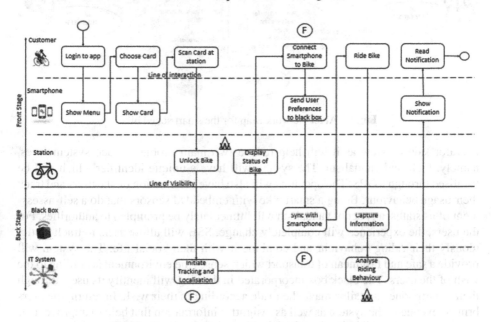

Fig. 5. Service experience blueprint for using the bike

Extending the Multi-level Service Design steps, Actor Network Mapping (Fig. 6) which depicts the networks of actors and components in a system [25] is used to show the different value given to and through to the stakeholders previously identified.

Figure 6 depicts the actor network map for the Smart Social Bike. The actors for SSB are the users, municipality, businesses, operators and Mobi.Me. To be able to implement SSB, the municipality need to provide the appropriate structure such as defining the places that will serve as stations, and making sure that the infrastructure that the system will need are available such as internet, power supply and lighting. On the other hand, SSB provides a platform to help municipalities in Urban Planning. Traditional bike sharing system do allow urban planning but is only limited to the determination of station positioning. SSB goes a bit further as it will allow municipalities to see zones of interest to users through the use of heat maps. Also, an electric bike allows the reduction of carbon foot print of a city and help reducing congestion and traffic thereby decreasing parking costs. Indeed, SSB will help improve the business on the

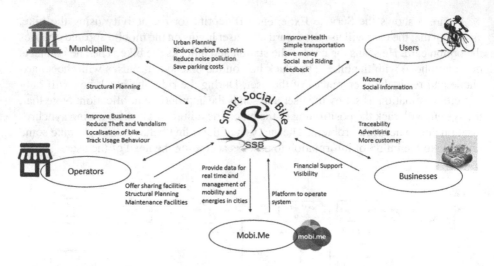

Fig. 6. Actor Network Map for the smart social bike

operator side of view as it will help reduce two main problems such system faces, namely, theft and vandalism. The system will have a unique identifier which will be localised through a GPS. The operators will also have information on the users and track their usage behaviour. Being a smart bike with embedded sensors that do a self-assessment of its status, any act of vandalism will immediately be prompted to authorities. For the users, the experience will completely change. SSB will allow users to track meticulously their riding behaviour and combine it with their social life. The system will provide a safe and fast mean of transport which senses the environment according to the wish of the users. The black box incorporated in the bike will identify its users through their smartphone and tailor-made their ride according to their wish. In return, the users brings revenue to the system as well as insightful information that help to improve their experience.

4.3   Smart Social Bike System Architecture Design

The architecture diagram (Fig. 7) is designed based on the SIOT architecture [22]. The three main actors that interact with the system using either a laptop or a mobile device are the users, operators and administrator which are connected to the data warehouse provider in the service cloud. The web service-based component which provides the bike sharing system consists of 6 main components which are connected by interface component.

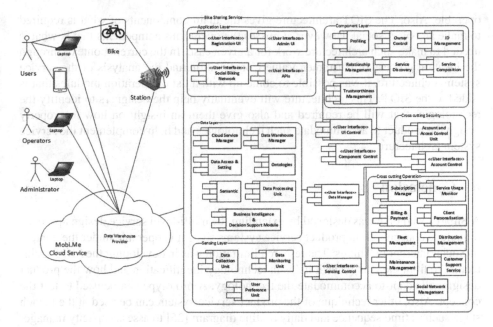

Fig. 7. Smart social bike System Architecture

5 Discussion

The aim of this research was to see the applicability of service design in designing a product service system in the context of social internet of things. The current approach to design product service system does not use a service design perspective while the acceptance of technologies in smart services faces an issue from the managerial perspective. Indeed, the Social Internet of Things being a new paradigm, as such there is no applicability of the concept. This research proposes a set of steps that uses several concepts to address the gap. Understanding the customer experience as a first step allow the collection of a rich set of information that helps in the design of a service offering of value that uses sufficient advances in technology that solve customer needs. The Multi-level Service Design was used in order to design the service in a systematic way. New services were ideated through the Customer Value Constellation, the Service System Architecture and Service System Navigation were drawn in order to understand which actors, service interface and technologies are responsible during the different activities of the customer journey. After that, the service encounters are illustrated through the use of service blueprinting which shows the potential point of failure and helps in the design of service recovery. These visual techniques helps see where and how technologies interfere to solve problems. Indeed, there was a need to go beyond the touchpoints to show what value is being given to the different stakeholders during a particular activity. The actor network mapping helps to bridge this gap by showing what is offered to the different stakeholders during the usage of the service. This process also helps in the identification of requirements that is important to make the system operable. Also, The SIOT architecture gives the main components of what is required to make an object social. However, it misses the operations components that is what is needed to make such architecture work for a given case. In the current context, through the ideation process of Customer Value Constellation and the analysis of the service system architecture, it was possible to come up with a list of operation modules that is added to the SIOT. This architecture will eventually help the designers to identify the technologies that will be required and also give them an insight on how to properly design the product to accommodate such technologies and help complement the service system architecture.

6   Conclusion

A Smart social bike was designed by extending the multi-level service design approach to include concepts from product service systems so as it is operable under the context of Social Internet of Things. The research limitation was in developing the SIOT architecture to fit in the context as it helps in technology identification and how the product design will adapt to accommodate the technology. A prototype can be used to test the concept. Also, other technique of the product service system can be used at the launch stage such as time sequence and daily routine diagram [25] to assess capacity management. This helps the operator offer new services at off peak time. Indeed, the business model can be improved to better fit the context.

References

1. Evenson, S., Dubberly, H.: Designing for service: creating an experience advantage. Introduction Serv. Eng. 403–413 (2010)
2. Ostrom, A.L., Parasuraman, A., Bowen, D.E., Patrício, L., Voss, C.A.: Service research priorities in a rapidly changing context. J. Serv. Res. 18, 127–159 (2015)
3. Blomkvist, J., Holmlid, S.: Service prototyping according to service design practitioners. Proceedings of ServDes (2010)
4. Patrício, L., Fisk, R.P.: Creating new services. In: Fisk, R.P., Russell-Bennett, R., Harris, L.C. (eds.) Serving Customers: Global Services Marketing Perspectives, pp. 185–207. Tilde University Press, Melbourne (2013)
5. Rust, R.T., Huang, M.-H.: The service revolution and the transformation of marketing science. Mark. Sci. 33, 206–221 (2014)
6. McAfee, A., Brynjolfsson, E., Davenport, T.H., Patil, D., Barton, D.: Big data. Manage. Revolution. Harvard Bus Rev. 90, 61–67 (2012)
7. Porter, M.E., Heppelmann, J.E.: How smart, connected products are transforming competition. Harvard Bus. Rev. 92, 11–64 (2014)
8. Gubbi, J., Buyya, R., Marusic, S., Palaniswami, M.: Internet of Things (IoT): a vision, architectural elements, and future directions. Future Gener. Comput. Syst. 29, 1645–1660 (2013)
9. Allmendinger, G., Lombreglia, R.: Four strategies for the age of smart services. Harvard Bus. Rev. 83, 131–145 (2005)
10. Biehl, M., Prater, E., McIntyre, J.R.: Remote repair, diagnostics, and maintenance. Commun. ACM 47, 100–106 (2004)

11. Lenfle, S., Midler, C.: The launch of innovative product-related services. Lessons Automot. Telematics. Res. Policy **38**, 156–169 (2009)
12. Sila, S.: Long-distance Surgery. Glob. Telephony **9**, 12–14 (2001)
13. Rijsdijk, S.A., Hultink, E.J., Diamantopoulos, A.: Product intelligence: its conceptualization, measurement and impact on consumer satisfaction. J. Acad. Mark. Sci. **35**, 340–356 (2007)
14. Fano, A., Gershman, A.: The future of business services in the age of ubiquitous computing. Commun. ACM **45**, 83–87 (2002)
15. Keh, H.T., Pang, J.: Customer reactions to service separation. J. Mark. **74**, 55–71 (2010)
16. Wünderlich, N.V., Wangenheim, F.V., Bitner, M.J.: High tech and high touch a framework for understanding user attitudes and behaviors related to smart interactive services. J. Serv. Res. **16**, 3–20 (2013)
17. Mont, O.: Clarifying the concept of product–service system. J. Clean. Prod. **10**, 237–245 (2002)
18. Beuren, F.H., Gomes Ferreira, M.G., Cauchick Miguel, P.A.: Product-service systems: a literature review on integrated products and services. J. Clean. Prod. **47**, 222–231 (2013)
19. Manzini, E., Vezzoli, C.: A strategic design approach to develop sustainable product service systems: examples taken from the 'environmentally friendly innovation' Italian prize. J. Clean. Prod. **11**, 851–857 (2003)
20. Morelli, N.: Developing new product service systems (PSS): methodologies and operational tools. J. Clean. Prod. **14**, 1495–1501 (2006)
21. Nicolas, M., Tomohiko, S., Peggy, Z., Daniel, B.: A model for designing product-service systems using functional analysis and agent based model. Guidelines for a Decision Support Method Adapted to NPD Processes, pp. 282–292 (2007)
22. Atzori, L., Iera, A., Morabito, G.: Making things socialize in the internet—does it help our lives? In: Kaleidoscope 2011: The Fully Networked Human? - Innovations for Future Networks and Services (K-2011), Proceedings of ITU, pp. 1–8. IEEE (2011)
23. Hevner, A.R., March, S.T., Park, J., Ram, S.: Design science in information systems research. Mis Q. **28**, 75–105 (2004)
24. Patrício, L., Fisk, R.P., Cunha, J.F.E., Constantine, L.: Multilevel service design: from customer value constellation to service experience blueprinting. J. Serv. Res. **14**(2), 180–200 (2011)
25. Morelli, N., Tollestrup, C.: New representation techniques for designing in a systemic perspective. Nordes (2009)
26. Teixeira, J., Patrício, L., Nunes, N.J., Nóbrega, L., Fisk, R.P., Constantine, L.: Customer experience modeling: from customer experience to service design. J. Serv. Manage. **23**, 362–376 (2012)
27. Pohl, K.: Requirements Engineering: Fundamentals, Principles, and Techniques, 1st Edition edn. Springer, Heidelberg (2010)
28. Yin, R.K.: Case Study Research: Design and Methods. Sage Publications, Thousand Oaks (2008)

An Event-Driven Service-Oriented Architecture for Performing Actions on Business Organization Items

Vasilica-Georgiana Puiu and Adrian Alexandrescu[✉]

Faculty of Automatic Control and Computer Engineering, "Gheorghe Asachi" Technical University of Iasi, 27 Prof. Dr. Doc. Dimitrie Mangeron, Iasi, Romania
georgianapuiu@ymail.com, aalexandrescu@cs.tuiasi.ro

Abstract. In order to improve the client experience but also to increase revenue, there are single-point access websites which offer services belonging to multiple business organizations, and which employ ad services to entice the potential clients by presenting related products.

This paper presents a generic business model that uses an event-driven service-oriented architecture for performing actions on organization items (e.g., reserving a room at a hotel or a table at a restaurant, making a doctor's appointment, or purchasing a product). The system can be viewed as an aggregator of organizations to which businesses can adhere and offer their services to potential clients. There is also proposed a novel method that uses service composition in order to allow scheduling algorithms to be efficiently implemented. Due to its modularization, flexibility and extensibility, the proposed model is an effective tool for enhancing the user experience by offering the clients easy access to items from different business organizations and by making suggestions for other related organization items depending on the user's actions and preferences.

Keywords: Event-driven · Service-oriented architecture · SOA · Business model · After-sales service

1 Introduction

Nowadays, more and more people have constant access to online resources. There are many services that offer the possibility of performing common tasks and activities over the Internet (e.g., shopping, paying bills, planning trips, ordering food, or making reservations to hotels and restaurants), thus significantly reducing the time it would otherwise take to perform those actions.

People need quick access to a variety of services like making appointments, paying bills or purchasing items. Because one of the most important aspects of everyday life is time management, an online user must be able to perform the aforementioned actions in a timely manner. This means making with ease appointments and reservations to the desired places (e.g., hotels, restaurants, hospitals or medical clinics) while having an overall pleasant user experience. In order to both improve the user's overall impression and to help increase the revenue of business organizations, benefitting from a service

© Springer International Publishing Switzerland 2016
T. Borangiu et al. (Eds.): IESS 2016, LNBIP 247, pp. 432–443, 2016.
DOI: 10.1007/978-3-319-32689-4_33

must also come with an after-sales offer which will suggest to the user other available and related services.

For example, if someone wants to plan a wedding, that person usually makes a reservation at a selected restaurant for a specific date. After the appointment is made, the restaurant or the website used to make the reservation can suggest a flower arrangement firm, a music band or even a hotel where out of town guests can stay. This is the after-sales aspect of using the *wedding restaurant reservation* service, which can be implemented for any action (reserving, ordering or paying) that a user or client performs.

This paper suggests a multi-purpose and generic solution for handling reservations and appointments which can be easily extended to making online purchases. The proposed system uses an event-driven service-oriented architecture which businesses can employ to increase the user experience by providing the user other services of interest. This is achieved by considering the characteristics of the services that are provided by the organizations which use the proposed business model.

When a client wants to use the system, a custom request is built based on the user's preferences and a suitable response is provided; this is usually a confirmation that the request was successfully processed. Afterwards, the user receives recommendations for other related services.

Depending on the action type (reservation or appointment), the user must provide details about an item (room, table, seat, doctor's service) for which the action is made, an organization where the item is located (hotel, restaurant, cinema/concert/sport game, medical clinic), a time interval in which over the item is made the action (booking period, concert/film date, doctor visit date), the number of persons for which the action is made (a single, double room, concert/film individual seat, individual doctor visit or maybe for mother and child) and the preferences regarding the item (TV, breakfast, air conditioning, parking lot).

Based on all these characteristics the system is able to reserve the most suitable item from a selection of organizations and it is also able to recommend the user other connected services from businesses that adhere to this system.

This paper is organized as follows. The Related Work section shows some related systems which are compared to the proposed method. The Problem Statement section takes a look at a few typical appointment and reservation scenarios and clearly defines the concepts that are used throughout the paper (i.e., action, organization and item). Next the proposed generic system is described; taking into account the system characteristics, this section presents a general overview of the system architecture along with motivations for the design choices that were made, followed by a short presentation of the final product, which includes a typical usage scenario. A few novel improvements for the proposed system are shown in the next section and, finally, the last section takes an overall look at the proposed system and offers ideas of extending and improving the considered service-oriented architecture.

2   Related Work

There are many papers related to web services and service-oriented architectures that focus on the fine details of the proposed solutions which implement the two concepts. SOA is "defined and explained" [1] in many articles because it is based on solid principles [2] and it has easily and early started to be the best choice of web design and development [3, 4]. The focus of the system presented in the current paper is more on the business approach and the chosen backend solution of using a SOA is just a means to an end.

A less used technique is to have an event-driven architecture applied in the web services domain. Such an example is presented in [5, 6] where the authors propose a web service framework which is meant to lead to an event-driven web. The approach described there is based more on subscribing to web topics, whereas our proposed solution uses generic action-taken events which are interpreted by the modules that are registered to the event management module (e.g., the registration module).

In [7], two solutions are provided in order to emphasize how an event-driven approach leaded to loosely coupled domains and systems, "to a more flexible and agile architecture".

The current paper also refers to concepts like recommendation systems [8] and after-sales services [9], but only as to show the capabilities of the proposed system and possible improvements and application of the presented event-driven service-oriented architecture.

3   Problem Statement

There is an increasing need for making appointments and reservations in a quick and efficient manner by means of a user-friendly single-access point. In order to provide a solution for this wide area problem, the study started from basic examples. The general analysis of a hotel room reservation, a concert seat reservation and a medical clinic appointment has emphasized the common and different attributes.

When somebody wants to reserve a hotel room, beside the fact that he should choose a hotel and a room, he should provide the booking period, the number of persons and, in order to make the stay pleasant, an amount of preferences such as TV, Wi-Fi, air conditioning, etc. The concert seat reservation is a similarly example. The one who makes the reservation must choose a concert, a seat, the period is given by the concert organizer, the number of persons is obviously one and, to make his experience memorable, some preferred facilities (e.g., air conditioning, parking lot, snacks). The last example shows how much this case can be extended. When making a medical clinic appointment, one would choose a medical clinic, a doctor, a period for the visit, a number of persons that, in some real cases, can be greater than one, and some facilities such as air conditioning, heating system, TV, parking lot, etc.

After these exemplifications, it is easy to deduct the standard and the distinct characteristics. So, whenever someone wants a room reservation or an appointment, it is clear that he must provide information about his **action** (to reserve or to make an appointment), about the **organization**, the place where that action can be made (either a hotel, a concert, a medical clinic), the **item** that he wants to occupy (a room, a seat, a doctor's service), the **period**, the **number of persons** involved in that action and certain preferred facilities that will guarantee a satisfying experience. Because the **preferences** differ from an organization to another, from a person to another one, they represent the flexible side of the input data. This part is composed of elements from a list of facilities: Wi-Fi, TV, telephone, radio, air conditioning, heating, sound proofing, bathroom, Minibar, parking lot, children's play area, etc.

Taking into account the aforementioned characteristics, this paper presents a solution focused on the possibility of creating a custom request and receiving a suitable response (or suggest) regardless of the reservation/appointment type. Custom, in this context, means that the request it is formed by a fixed part and a flexible, user created part. Even so, the input data remains simple due to the general but clear perspective and is formed by an action, an organization, an item, a time interval, a number of persons and a list of preferences.

To make clear the representation of each fixed parameter, three practical examples are considered:

- In a hotel room reservation, the action is reservation, the organization is hotel, the item is room, the time interval is the booked period, and the number of persons is the number of people for whom the reservation is made.
- In a concert seat reservation, the action is reservation, the organization is concert, the item is seat, and the time interval is the period of the concert, the number of persons is the number of people for whom the reservation is made.
- In a medical clinic appointment, the action is appointment, the organization is medical clinic, the item is doctor, and the time interval is the period in which the meeting is scheduled, the number of persons is the number of people for whom the appointment is made, by default 1.

Another aspect considered in this paper is a recommendation component, which makes suggestions, usually, when a client makes an action (e.g., reservation, appointment or purchase). For example, when a client reserves a room at a hotel, based on that reservation and past actions, the system must be able to suggest a nearby restaurant with a specific style of food.

The recommendation must be made either manually, by an organization manager, or automatically, by using a recommendation algorithm. Details regarding this aspect are discussed in the Improvement of the Proposed System section of this paper.

4 Proposed Generic System

4.1 General Context and Overview

Social web has a significant role of how the humanity is perceiving and understanding the Internet. Everyone is nowadays realizing that time is very important and wants to start using it as wisely as possible, to plan it in a comfortable and easy way.

These two facts are related and the Internet can now provide solutions for some of our everyday problems.

The proposed system is a generic online solution that allows users to make reservations at hotels for rooms, reservations at restaurants for tables, appointments at medical clinics for a specialist consult, etc. The common elements of these use-cases, as discussed in the Problem Statement section of this paper, are: actions, organizations, items, period, number of persons and preferences. All these form a custom request which the proposed system interprets and takes the appropriate action.

The system responds to every custom request with the status of the wanted action. In case that it is not achievable (e.g., maybe the specified room is not available in that period), the system provides suggestions based on the initial requirements, i.e., displays other available rooms in the period mentioned with the same characteristics.

Therefore, *the goal of the system is to allow users to make actions on the items of organizations by specifying a period, the number of persons and other preferences, and, in return, to also receive recommendations for complementary items from other organizations*.

For example, when someone wants to reserve a room at a hotel, the system makes the reservation, if it is not possible it suggests alternatives, and then it recommends a reservation for a table at a restaurant nearby.

There are two types of users in the online system: business organizations and clients. A business organization provides a service or offers a product to potential clients. The term client is used very loosely and it refers to the user that makes the reservation or appointment. This can imply a money exchange between the client and the business organization, but not necessarily.

From a business organization's point of view, if it wants to allow clients to make actions on its items, then the organization needs to be part of the system. This implies creating an account and configuring the available items (number or persons/item, periods and available preferences). A client has the possibility of choosing from all the businesses in the system when deciding to make an action on an organization item.

Basically, the proposed system is an aggregator of businesses and it offers clients a central point for making reservations, appointments and even purchases. Having many businesses in the same system is advantageous because a client of one business can benefit from the services of other businesses by means of the recommendations.

4.2 System Architecture

The design choice for the system architecture is based on the fact that it is an online solution which needs a high degree of flexibility and extensibility. This is why the chosen solution is an event-driven service-oriented architecture.

A Service-Oriented Architecture (SOA) is grounded on the "separation of concerns" [10], a software engineering theory that allows the logic to be divided into smaller related pieces which form a functionality or a concern. Services are highly flexible, customizable, extensible, loosely coupled, reusable, stateless, share a formal contract, and, a very important aspect, services abstract the underlying logic so they can be used generically. Using an event-driven architecture allows the system to be developed in a manner that increases responsiveness and extensibility. Event-driven systems are a very good solution in dynamic and asynchronous environments [11].

The proposed solution guarantees an answer to the user's request with the status of the action made and, asynchronously, recommendations of related items, so each possibility is taken in consideration and the workflow becomes complex. In order to prevent any bottleneck, an event-driven approach is proper. The flexibility is increased and the maintenance and testing become easier. Another advantage is bound to after-sales services because any future improvements are going to be easily integrated. Towards a user friendly interface, the system uses a single account type: the organization can be a client of another organization, and a client can manage, if he desires, one or more businesses.

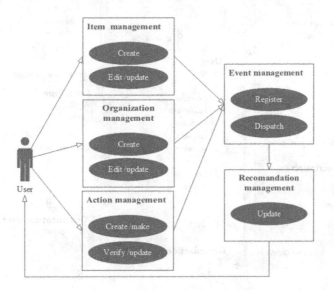

Fig. 1. Use-case diagram representing the actions that the user can take and the basic interaction between the modules of the proposed system

The main modules are user/account management, organization management, item management and reservation management. Figure 1 shows the main actions a user can take and the basic interaction between the modules. A user must have an account in order to have access to all the services. From this point on, he can administrate organizations by registering them and their characteristics (the items). A logged in user can search items for making actions, see the item details, start the process of making a new action (e.g., reservation) and verify the status of previous requests.

4.3 Implementation of the Proposed System

Database Structure. The database design delivers the data model used by the proposed solution. The main tables map the modules representing the User, Organization, Item, Action, Event and Recommendation; these and the relationship between the tables are shown in Fig. 2.

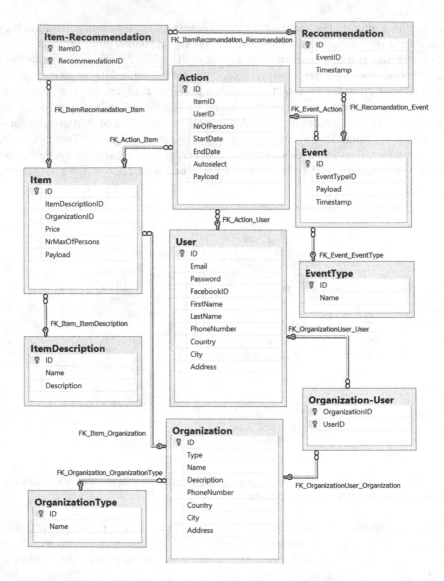

Fig. 2. Entity–relationship diagram for the database used by the proposed system

The **User** table contains the personal information like first name, last name, e-mail address and the full address, and the **Organization** table holds the name, description, address and phone number of each business. To store records in an effective way, the organization types (hotel, restaurant, medical clinic), are separated in a different table, **OrganizationType** that contains an id and a name. In order to connect the user to the organizations that he created, an extra table **Organization-User** is needed.

The **Item** table has a complex structure because it contains not only particular but also general data. In order to reuse the generic fragment, this information is stored in the **ItemDescription** table that has an id, a name (e.g., twin room, single room), and a basic, common description (e.g., TV, air conditioning). The Item table is then constructed from an ItemDescription id, the organization id from where it belongs, the price, the maximum number of persons (e.g., the room capacity, the number of persons at a table) and the specific characteristics for that item (e.g., sea view, non-smoking) and represents the preferences available to the user.

The **Action** table reflects an important module. It contains information about the user that has made the action (user id), the item upon the action was made (item id), the number of persons for which the action is made, the period represented by the start and the end date, the user preferences. In order to offer the client, the best available items for this selection, an auto-select option is given. When the user chooses this, the system will return the item whose characteristics best match this action's user preference. If not, the user will receive a list of several items that pair with the input data.

The **Event** table depends on an auxiliary table **EventType** that specify the type of the event occurred (item created/updated, action created/updated) through a foreign key, a timestamp that marks the moment when the event happened and the characteristics specific to that event.

The **Recommendation** table is connected to events and items because items recommendation is made when an event arises. This logic is represented in the database through foreign keys and an additional table **Item-Recommendation**. Recommendation table is formed by an id, and event id and a timestamp. Here is made the link between the recommendations and events. Further, the recommendations are linked to the items using the Item-Recommendation table. This one contains a recommendation and an item foreign key.

Application Modules. The proposed solution is light and simple due to the separation of concerns in modules such as User, Organization, Item, Action, Event and Recommendation. Each one covers functionality that is reusable, replaceable and increasable.

They intercommunicate through web services so a module is in charge only to make a request and wait a response, independently of the processing needed to provide that answer. Every module, except Event and Recommendation, exposes basic CRUD (i.e., Create, Read, Update and Delete) operations through the web services interface. These two are distinct because they implement the observer pattern. The Recommendation module is the observer and the Event is the observable module. The observer registers first and must send recommendations (update) each time an event it is dispatched. Based on the information given by the event occurred, the solution decides what it is suitable to suggest next to the user. An interaction example between the user and the modules is presented in Fig. 3. There is presented a typical scenario where a user makes a reservation at a hotel and then receives recommendations.

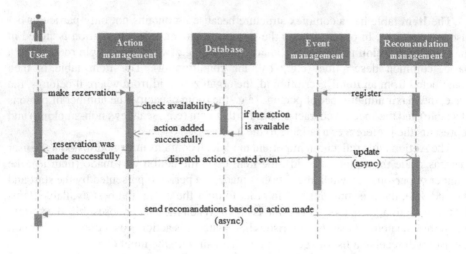

Fig. 3. Sequence diagram representing a user making a reservation using the proposed system

4.4 Practical Example

As a practical example, this paper presents a hotel room reservation scenario, choosing a single room that has the wanted characteristics and receiving recommendations about the near restaurants. The selection flow is shown in Fig. 4.

First of all, the user fills in the details regarding the location, the period and the organization type (that is hotel in this case). A list of hotels with the wanted address that are available in the mentioned time interval is then given.

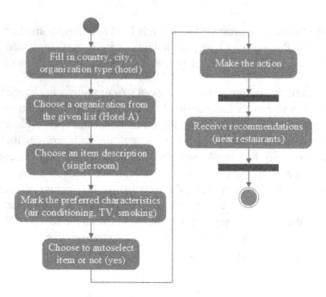

Fig. 4. Activity diagram representing the selection of the preferences when a user makes an action

The user chooses a hotel, an item description (single in this case). After that, a list of facilities (air conditioning, non-smoking, mini-bar) is given. The user marks the one that he prefers and decides if he wants to be able to select the item (room) from the filtered items list or to let the solution provide the best room that matches the required details.

When the action is made, based on the input data, an event is created and dispatched. Because the Recommendation module is an observer, when an event (the observable entity) is dispatched, the solution sends asynchronous suggestions back to the user through a SMTP server.

5   Improvement of the Proposed System

The proposed system has the disadvantage of keeping most of the organization item details in a characteristics field (i.e., payload) in the Item database table. This is because of the abstraction required in order to have a generic system. For example, when reserving a hotel room, the item is the room and the payload contains the room characteristics: non-smoking, with TV, air-conditioning, sea-view, etc. These characteristics are not available when reserving a seat at cinema or when making a doctor's appointment.

In the current state, the proposed system does not take into account the preferences selected by the user, only the period and the number of persons. A simple solution is to let the user who manages the organization to manually change the action items (e.g., manually change the room which was assigned by the system to a certain user). Another solution is to have a scheduling algorithm that has knowledge of each business type and which knows how to interpret the specific characteristics.

The novel proposed method of solving the abstraction problem is to have another layer between the user and the generic system. Figure 5 shows the interaction between the components of this new model. Basically, between the web server and the proposed generic solution there is a Concrete Layer which contains web services for every business type. Those web services translate between a concrete request and an abstract request.

For example, the client wants to reserve a non-smoking with air conditioning single room at hotel Holiday for February 13th, 2016. The request if sent from the Web Server to the Hotel Web Services which interprets it and sends to the Generic SOA a request containing the organization type (hotel), the organization id (id of hotel Holiday), the number of persons (1 person), the period (February 13th, 2016) and the specific characteristics (which contain the information that the room is non-smoking and it must have air conditioning).

This approach is very useful if the scheduling algorithm is a genetic algorithm and the fitness function, which calculates the quality of a candidate solution, is obtained from web services in the Concrete Layer corresponding to the business organization type.

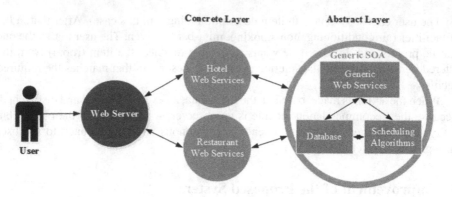

Fig. 5. Proposed improvement of the system presented in this paper

6   Conclusions

Planning our time is very important nowadays and this process is usually made online. For that, this paper proposes a single-point access for making reservations to hotels, restaurants and various events (sports games, concerts), and appointments to hospitals, medical clinics, dentists. Using a multi-purpose platform and providing a minimum input data, the time management and scheduling is much easier.

This paper presents a generic business model that uses an event-driven service-oriented architecture for performing actions on organization items (e.g., reserving a room at a hotel or a table at a restaurant, making a doctor's appointment, or purchasing a product). The system can be viewed as an aggregator of organizations to which businesses can adhere and offer their services to potential clients. It is an effective tool for enhancing the user experience by offering the clients easy access to items from different business organizations and by making suggestions for other related organization items depending on the user's actions and preferences.

The novelty of this paper is the fact that the proposed solution puts together different types of businesses (e.g., hotels, restaurants, cinemas) and it uses the same database structure to store all the organization information. Therefore, the system is very flexible and it also allows for different module and algorithms to be added in order to improve the overall user experience. For example, the recommendation module which can easily use an intelligent suggestion making algorithm because it has access to all the information regarding the users, businesses and the actions that were made.

Another novel aspect is the proposed improvement which removes the drawback of having a generic system by adding an extra layer with concrete implementations. This is particularly helpful in interpreting the preferences set by the users; those interpretations can be used to have a more effective recommendation algorithm.

References

1. Erl, T.: SOA Principles of Service Design. Prentice Hall PTR, Upper Saddle River (2007)
2. Event-driven services in SOA. Design an event-driven and service-oriented platform with Mule. http://www.javaworld.com/article/2072262/soa/event-driven-services-in-soa.html
3. What Is Service-Oriented Architecture. http://webservices.xml.com/pub/a/ws/2003/09/30/soa.html
4. SOA Advisor: The principles of service-orientation. http://searchsoa.techtarget.com/feature/SOA-Advisor-The-principles-of-service-orientation
5. Erl, T.: Service-Oriented Architecture (SOA): Concepts, Technology, and Design. Prentice Hall PTR, Upper Saddle River (2005)
6. Daigneau, R.: Service Design Patterns: Fundamental Design Solutions for SOAP/WSDL and RESTful Web Services. Addison-Wesley Professional, Upper Saddle River (2011)
7. Li, L., Chou, W.: REST-Event: a rest web service framework for building event-driven web. Int. J. Advances in Networks Serv. **4**, 292–301 (2011)
8. Architecting Event-Driven SOA: A Primer. http://www.oracle.com/technetwork/articles/oraclesoa-eventarch-097519.html
9. Event-Driven SOA: Events Meet Services. http://www.oracle.com/technetwork/articles/soa/schmutz-soa-eda-405955.html
10. Mahboob, T., Akhtar, F., Asif, M., Siddique, N., Khanum, M.: A survey and analysis on recommendation system algorithms. Int. J. Comput. Sci. Issues **12**(3), 162–168 (2015)
11. Saccani, N., Johansson, P., Perona, M.: Configuring the after-sales service supply chain: a multiple case study. Int. J. Prod. Econ. **110**(1), 52–69 (2007)

Improving After-Sales Services Using Mobile Agents in a Service-Oriented Architecture

Adrian Alexandrescu[✉], Cristian Nicolae Buţincu, and Mitică Craus

Faculty of Automatic Control and Computer Engineering, "Gheorghe Asachi" Technical University of Iasi, 27 Prof. Dr. Doc. Dimitrie Mangeron, Iasi, Romania
{aalexandrescu,cbutincu,craus}@cs.tuiasi.ro

Abstract. Nowadays, businesses have one main goal: to make profit. But this cannot be done at the expense of the customer, and, in order to keep the customer happy and to make him purchase more products, businesses offer after-sale services and promotions. This paper proposes a system that allows online businesses to benefit from each other's customer base, without breaching the user privacy, by monitoring purchases and recommending to the customer products and services from other businesses in the system. This is achieved using a service-oriented architecture that employs mobile agents in order to increase the system flexibility, extensibility and security. The considered approach allows dynamical changes to the system's structure and also module updates, largely due to the autonomy of the mobile agents. Therefore, the proposed system is an effective method of increasing business revenue and improving the customer experience, while also offering the possibility of implementing other marketing techniques in a high-level privacy and security environment.

Keywords: Business model · Service-oriented architecture · Mobile agents · After-sales service · Recommendation system

1 Introduction

In its simplest form, a typical business model is "businesses provide services to clients and clients mean money". Therefore, the more clients the businesses have, the more money they make.

There are a few techniques and concepts that are used in marketing in order to determine an existing customer to purchase another product or service, which is more or less related to his initial purchase.

After-sales services refer to offering a customer some sort of support and service after he purchased a product. Usually this implies free technical support, extended warranty, or creating a rapport with the customer by asking for feedback regarding his purchase or even calling at one point to exchange pleasantries and to present the latest products that might interest him.

Another, less common, concept is *affiliate marketing*, in which products are promoted by independent individuals and, in turn, those individuals receive a percentage from each sale made. This approach can have a negative connotation because people

© Springer International Publishing Switzerland 2016
T. Borangiu et al. (Eds.): IESS 2016, LNBIP 247, pp. 444–456, 2016.
DOI: 10.1007/978-3-319-32689-4_34

who purchased at one point a product from a website will periodically receive emails with offers for products from other websites in the same affiliate network. The problem is that those products are sometimes over-priced for what they are worth.

This paper presents a solution to increase product sales by offering customers recommendations for other products from different online businesses. This is in some regard similar to the affiliate marketing approach, but no one receives a percentage from the sales and therefore only the most relevant offers are sent to the customers. Also, the proposed solution can be considered an after-sales service because it focuses on making recommendations to clients for products that complement their initial purchase. For example, after a customer purchases a washing machine from a business, he can receive a recommendation to purchase washing detergent from another website.

The proposed solution is a mobile-agent platform built on a service-oriented architecture at which existing online businesses can register in order to have their products recommended to clients of other websites. Basically, when a customer purchases a product from an online business which is registered on the mobile-agent system, the information regarding the purchase is sent by a mobile agent and the system decides when and what recommendation will the customer receive.

Although this paper presents several suggestions of implementing a recommendation module, such a module is not the focus of the research presented here. This paper describes the mobile-agent system used by online businesses which obtain the input data needed by the recommendation module, and which processes the output of that module accordingly. Also, throughout the paper, the term *online business* is used to refer to a website selling products and services when explaining the problem statement and when presenting some practical examples of the proposed solution, while the term *business organization* is used when describing the system; both terms represent roughly the same concept, but the latter has a broader meaning and does not pertain exclusively to websites.

This paper is organized as follows. The Problem Statement section focuses on the presentation of the considered business problem and defines the characteristics of environment used throughout the paper. In Sect. 3 is discussed the related work concerning mobile agents and service oriented architectures used to solve business problems. Next is described the proposed system including the platform architecture, a description of the basic system model and its implementation. Section 5 presents a novel advanced system model and a discussion on the proposed system's effectiveness. Finally, the Conclusions and Future Work section takes an overall look at the proposed models and presents ideas to further expand the research from this paper.

2   Problem Statement

One of the main problems that any business has is how to find customers and, most importantly, how to determine those customers to make more purchases (returning customers) and to recommend other potential clients to buy products and/or services from that business.

There are several marketing techniques as discussed in the Introduction section of this paper, but the most widely used implies offering after-sales services.

When purchasing a product, the customer can receive a recommendation for another product or service, and, similarly, when purchasing a service, another service or even a product can be recommended to the client. For example, when a customer purchases a vacation to the seaside, the system can recommend a snorkeling equipment and a car rental service from two different businesses.

Therefore, the considered system must have certain features and restrictions.

Online businesses must be able to be part of the system seamlessly and without much modification to the existing software. Also, the system must be able to have nodes (businesses) added or removed without any impact on the existing modules and algorithms.

The system must be extensible: different modules added to the central node; e.g., a module that monitors all the purchases and the recommendations that were made, or a module that performs an analysis based on user feedback.

An important restriction is that the businesses, which are nodes in the system, must not be able to tamper with the communication between the central node which has the recommendation module and the other nodes. Of course a certain degree of trust is expected especially as to the validity of a purchase, but there are ways to detect if a node offers fake data which are discussed later in this paper.

Probably the most important two caveats that must be made are:

- The businesses must be willing to share their purchase data with a third-party (the system) in order to benefit from their eventual increase in the number of customers and purchases;
- The users must allow third parties to access their information (at least email address and the purchases that they made). This is not necessarily a significant problem because, nowadays, online businesses already have that clause in their terms and conditions and without accepting those terms the purchase cannot be made.

3   Related Work

There are multiple articles related to after-sales services but they mostly focus strictly from a marketing and economic point of view. These research papers refer to studies regarding after-sales supply chains [1] or to the importance of the after the sale interaction with the customer in order to increase a business' profits [2] and to solutions for applying an after-sales model in different situations [3]. This is also the case with the research presented in the current paper, but here the after-sales strategies are applied in combination with the affiliate marketing technique, because the after-sales service that is offered does not necessarily come from the same business, but from another business in the proposed system.

In terms of after-sales services in a service-oriented architecture there is very little research, although there are papers on applying marketing and consumer behavior techniques in an online environment [4], and research concerning the applications of service-oriented architectures in product service systems [5] and in service co-production [6]. These papers have only tangential link with the research presented in the current paper.

Regarding the applications of mobile agents in sales, the book Intelligent Systems for Manufacturing: Multi-agent Systems and Virtual Organizations [7] contains various designs of multi-agent systems in manufacturing. The difference compared to the research presented in the current paper is that the latter uses a less complex agent system, i.e., the mobility of the agent is limited and is mostly use to hide the computation logic from the online business.

As opposed to existing research, we propose a novel method of aggregating business customers and offering them products from other business in the system. The mobile-agent component and the service-oriented architecture are straight-forward and are kept fairly simple in order to increase extensibility by offering the possibility to easily add new modules to the system.

4 Proposed Method

4.1 General Overview

Taking into account the discussion in the Introduction and Problem Statement sections of this paper, two main goals of the proposed system can be distinguished:

- Improve the customer's experience by offering him products that he might be interested in, from businesses where he purchased before or from other businesses, while keeping these offers in check (the offers must not be made too often) in order not to alienate him.
- Allow the businesses to expand their customer base and to also share their customers with other businesses in the system, thus, increasing their revenue, but all this must be done while having the customer's privacy in mind.

In order to understand how the proposed solution works, next are presented the three basic steps (communication situations) needed to be performed by an online business to be part of the system:

1. Register itself in the system (one time only),
2. Every time a purchase is made, allow the system (or part of the system) to access the transaction information (i.e., details about the purchased product and details about the user that made the purchase),
3. When needed, allow the system limited or filtered access to some of the products and services that are being offered by the online business.

Any online business which implements all the aforementioned steps is part of the proposed system and can seamlessly opt-out if it chooses to do so. In this way the system can dynamically change by having nodes added and removed at runtime without any impact on the performance.

Regarding the customers, each business has its own customer base, i.e., even though a customer can receive an offer from another business in the system, that business does not have access to the client's personal and behavioral (purchase-wise) details from the first business. The system has some knowledge of all the customers from each business but it does not share that information and instead it is used to make recommendations tailored to the customer's needs. All this implies some security concerns which are discussed in a subsequent section of this paper.

4.2 Platform Architecture

In order to facilitate the integration of online businesses in the system, the proposed method uses a *service-oriented architecture*. By using this approach, a business organization can just call a registration service to be part of the system via a web API. The decision of using an architecture which is based on web services was made because the proposed solution is addressed to online businesses and it is easier for those organizations to implement the communication with the system because they already have a web business logic in place and are already familiar with accessing and processing URIs. Also, the system benefits from the advantages of web services and SOA [8], like:

- Interoperability: the system logic and the businesses' logic do not need to be written using the same programming languages,
- Loose Coupling: there is no need for a permanent direct connection between an organization and the system; the communication between the two is done as needed,
- Standardized Protocol: each communication situation is clearly defined and each organization must comply with those standards,
- Flexibility: the system logic can change at runtime without affecting in any way the business organizations,
- Simplicity: the requests and responses contain only the relevant data in XML or JSON format (e.g., the product information).

One of the most important aspects of the system is its ease-of-use. A business must make as few changes as possible to be part of the system and most, if not all, of the communication with the system must be a black-box. For these reasons, the considered approach uses *mobile agents* which hold the communication information (system hostname, credentials, and encryption and communication protocols) and can contain data processing modules pertinent to the system.

A mobile agent is essentially a piece of software that can move from one network node to another and can perform certain tasks. An important particularity of a mobile agent is that it can suspend the task execution on a node and resume its state on another node of the system [9, 10]. Another concept used in this paper is the *agent platform*, which is the environment in which the mobile agent performs its tasks.

As a result of taking into consideration the aforementioned aspects, the proposed solution architecture is a mobile-agent platform which uses web services in order to handle the inter-node communication.

This paper proposes two system models: a basic model, in which the mobility of the agent limited and the final decision is taken by the central node, and an advanced model, in which the agents move between system nodes and have most of the decision logic.

4.3 Basic System Model

The proposed system, in its simplest form, is composed of a Central System Node (CSN) and multiple Business Organization Nodes (BONs); there is one node for each Business Organization (BO) that adhered to the system. Each BON communicates with the CSN by means of a mobile agent (MA). As shown in Fig. 1, there are three communication situations between entities: BO with CSN, BON with CSN and BON with the customer.

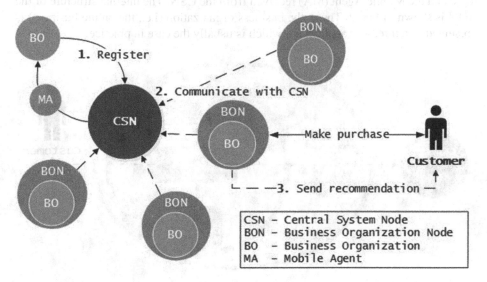

Fig. 1. The proposed basic system model and the communication between the system nodes

The Communication Between a Business Organization and the System. The communication between the BO and the CSN occurs only initially, when the business organization registers itself in the system. The organization calls a registration web service from the Central System Node and sends information like: business name, website, email address, a list of categories of the products and services, and other pertinent data. Using the received information, the CSN creates and configures a mobile agent which is then sent to the business organization. After this point, the organization communicates directly only with the mobile agent, which holds all the details needed to contact the CSN.

The Mobile Agent, the Business Organization Node and the Central System Node. The role of a *Mobile Agent* is to monitor the purchases that are made at the business organization where it is located and to obtain the product information required by other mobile agents in the system. The mobile agent is basically an application which acts as an intermediary or facade between the business organization and the system. It contains the logic needed to contact the CSN and data filtering methods which process the information received from the business organization. The MA has also the capability to evolve and adapt to changes, e.g., if the CSN address changes. This is particularly useful in regards to scalability, if the CSN is composed of a cluster of nodes; in this case, the MA can contain a module with a load balancing logic which defers the recommendation processing (or any other processing) to the most appropriate system node. Changes to the MA structure and behavior can be triggered by the CSN, but an advanced MA can decide to move to another system node to perform the processing and return once that is finished.

The *Business Organization Node* represents a business organization which is part of the system and contains the mobile agent application used for communicating with the rest of the system. In Fig. 1 the BON is composed of the Business Organization (BO) logic and the Mobile Agent (MA) received from the CSN. The internal structure of the BON is shown in Fig. 2. There, the business organization (i.e., the online business) is presented as a three-tier application, which is usually the case in practice.

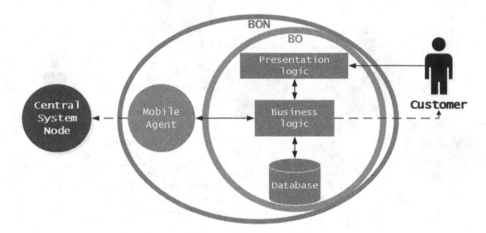

Fig. 2. Internal structure of the Business Organization Node

A critical part of the system is the *Central System Node*, which manages the Business Organization Nodes, creates and manages the Mobile Agents and makes the product and service recommendations based on the information received from the MAs. When it is notified that a purchase was made, it sends that data to the recommendation module, which then makes a request for product details from the business organizations depending on specific criteria. Those requests are satisfied by each mobile agent and are aggregated by the CSN, which, finally, makes its recommendation. In practice, the central node is not necessarily a single computer, but rather a cluster of computers or even a computational cloud; this is because the CSN requires enough resources to properly handle the communication with the other nodes and to process the received information in a timely fashion.

The Communication Between the Mobile Agent and the Business Organization. Each time a customer makes a purchase, the business logic module of the BO notifies the mobile agent by sending the customer information and the purchase details. Depending on how the mobile agent is configured, it can filter certain data for reasons of speed and security. For example, if the recommendation system does not require specific user details or no user details at all, this information can be omitted when the mobile agent sends the data to the central node. The mobile agent data filter configuration is initially performed by the CSN when the MA is created depending on the requirements of the recommendation system.

The proposed system, in its basic form, does not require private user information (e.g., username, email, address, phone number). Also, the recommendation can be sent only by the business logic module of the BO, as presented in Fig. 2. This is the second communication situation between the MA and the BO. After the MA receives the recommendation info (i.e., details about the product or service that is being offered) from the CSN, it forwards that information to the BO which, in turn, will send it to the customer. Between the MA and the BO there is a bidirectional channel which can be permanent in order to reduce the communication overhead.

In the proposed basic system model, the Central System Node requires product information from the businesses in the system in order to make a recommendation. Therefore, the MA must obtain that information from the BO, so the third communication situation implies receiving certain product data. The mobile agent must be able to obtain data from the business organization based on specified criteria.

The Communication Between the Mobile Agent and the Central System Node. A key aspect of this communication is that the MA is the one who contacts the CSN. The communication is of the type request-response, because the MA can be under a firewall or even in a sub-network and, in this case, the CSN cannot connect to the MA without a security opening or a port-forwarding rule in the router. Also, the CSN address can change so it this case the security settings made by the BO would need updating, therefore the system would lack transparency.

The MA contacts the CSN in the following communication situations:

- Notify that the business organization is an active part of the system, and it is not currently offline or removed from the system,
- Notify that one or more purchases were made,
- Check if there is a recommendation for one or more customers of the business organization where the MA resides,
- Check if there are updates for the MA regarding the CSN address, the mobile agent logic or if a new module is to be added to the MA,
- Check if there are requests for product details that need to be obtained from the business organization,
- Send product details for a previously made request.

An important behavior is that the mobile agent does not always send the data to the CSN immediately after a purchase is made. It can be configured to wait for multiple purchases and then to send all the accumulated data or even part of the data (which the MA deems important) to the CSN. More about this and the modules that can be added to the MA is discussed in the *Advanced system model* section of this paper.

4.4 Implementation

The proposed system has two main components: the Mobile Agent (MA), which handles the communication between the Business Organization (BO) and the system, and the Central System Node (CSN), which mainly coordinates the activity of the mobile agents.

The Mobile Agent component has three modules:

– *Business Communication Module* – handles the communication with the business organization,
– *System Communication Module* – handles the communication with the central system node,
– *Data Processing Module* – uses the two previously mentioned modules and also takes limited decisions based on an initial configuration.

The communication scenarios between the modules and the CSN and the BO are shown in Fig. 3.

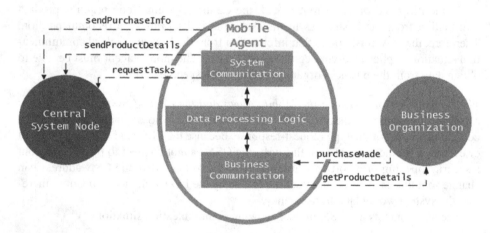

Fig. 3. Mobile Agent communication with the Central System Node and the Business Organization

When a business organization becomes part of the system it must implement a communication API with the Mobile Agent component, which can be configured in one of three modes:

– *Web Service Mode* – the MA-BO communication is done by calling web services: this means that the MA has to implement a *getProductDetails* service and the business organization a *purchaseMade* service,
– *Shared Memory Mode* – the MA-BO communication is done by both processes accessing the same memory segment using a specified protocol,
– *Direct Access Mode* – the BO allows the MA to make direct queries to the database; this requires additional configuration of the MA by specifying the database, tables and columns that need to be accessed in order to obtain the product details and by adding triggers for when purchases are made.

The communication between the CSN and the MA is done by means of web services. The CSN has the *sendPurchaseInfo* web service method which is called by the MA when a purchase is made; the information being sent contains the product details, the user details and the timestamp. At regular time intervals, the MA calls the *requestTasks* method which does three things: signals the CSN that the BON is active (heartbeat design pattern), gets recommendations if available and gets product details requests if required. Another web service method is *sendProductDetails*, which is called when the MA obtained from the BO the product details for the request which was previously performed by the CSN.

Besides the aforementioned communication module, the Central System Node has also a recommendation module whose functionality is presented in Fig. 4. How the product or service suggestion is determined by the Recommendation Module is beyond the scope of this paper, but the proposed system has the means to obtain all the data required by the module and also the means to send the recommendation to the customer.

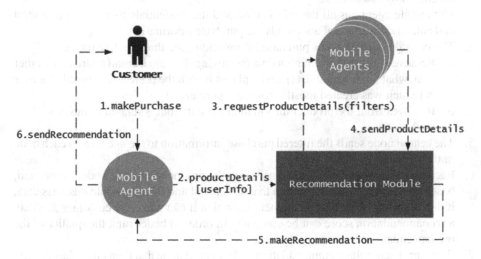

Fig. 4. Recommendation module functionality

5 Advanced System Model

5.1 General Overview

The advanced system model is a variation of the basic model but instead of having a central point for determining the best recommendation, each mobile agent has its own recommendation module, which determines a local suggestion. A usage example when using this approach is presented in the next subsection of this paper.

Another particularity of this system is the possibility of migrating a mobile agent from a Business Organization Node to a Central System Node if the BON does not have the required computational capabilities. This implies extra logic that needs to be implemented at both the BON and the CSN.

In terms of presenting the implementation details of the advanced system model, this paper outlines only the main ideas and system characteristics; all the communication and decision implications will be further researched and published in another paper.

5.2   Use-Case Scenario

The following is an extensive example of what happens when a customer purchases a product from an online business which is a node in the proposed system. Some of the steps can be skipped depending on the desired complexity and distributivity of the system; the presented situation considers that each mobile agent is capable of making recommendations (each agent has the recommendation module).

1. Customer X purchases a product P from online business A.
2. Business A notifies the mobile agent which resides there that product P was purchased by customer X.
3. The mobile agent has all the information and the credentials to contact the central node and it does this and also sends the purchase information.
4. The central node filters the purchase information (i.e., the sensitive data):
   a. Removes the user information data (removing the name, email address and other somewhat confidential data), and replaces it with the preferences profile for user X (which was created mostly from past purchases).
   b. Removes from the product information the data that is related to business A (if any).
5. The central node sends the filtered purchase information to the agent from each node in the system.
6. Each agent has somewhat limited access to the products from the node it is on, and, based on the purchase information that it received and the accessible business data, it decides what is the best recommendation that it can make for customer X. Also, a recommendation score can be computed in order to better rank the quality of the recommendation).
7. Each agent sends the recommendation to the central node that then takes the decision as to which recommendation (or top percentage of recommendations) is to be made to customer X.
8. The central node sends the recommendation to customer X, and/or that data is sent to the agent on node A, which in turn will give the recommendation to the online business to do as it pleases (it can show the recommendation on the website when the customer logs in, or it can send an email directly to the user).

5.3   System Effectiveness, Reliability, Updates and Security Concerns

The initial communication between a business organization and the system, when the organization registers itself in the system, is done over HTTPS and the immediate response that comes from the Central System Node is only and acknowledgement that the request is valid and will be processed. In order to be sure of the authenticity of the business organization, the received email address must have the same domain as the website (the website name is used to uniquely identify an organization in the system) the mobile agent can be sent via email; this is also a good approach in case the communication fails when sending the response or in case the creation and configuration of the mobile agent takes too long for various reasons.

Regarding scalability, the Central System Node can be replaced by a cluster of computers or a computational cloud. Also, if a Business Organization Node is not able to perform computations due to resource limitations, the Mobile Agent can move the computation in the Central System Node.

When there are updates to be made to the system, the Central System Node can send updates to the mobile agent or it can trigger a replacement of the mobile agent without affecting the system's stability.

A very important issue is user privacy. The customer must be able to opt-out from receiving recommendations from the system and to decide how much private information he shares. For example, knowing the user age and gender would help the recommendation module make a better suggestion, but some customers would feel reluctant revealing this information.

The proposed basic system model makes a recommendation each time a purchase is made. This is a problem if there are businesses that sell many products and services (e.g., a general-goods online store) and other businesses that sell daily few products (e.g., an online car dealership). In this case, the products from business that sell less will be recommended more. The solution is to make the number of recommendations for a businesses' products be directly proportionate with the number of products sold by that business. Also, the user can be involved by offering feedback on purchases and on the quality-of-service of the online businesses.

Also, there can be implemented solutions for preventing notifications of fake purchases and, maybe a few solutions for monetization, e.g., the system owner and businesses can receive a percentage for every purchase made as a result of a recommendation.

6   Conclusions and Future Work

Increasing profit is the goal of any business and the easiest way to achieve this is to increase the customer base and also to improve customer care. The solution proposed in this paper is an effective method for improving after-sales services which also allows online businesses to share their clients, their product list and their purchase info.

This is a novel strategy which is based on a combination of traditional after-sales strategies with the affiliate marketing technique. The system uses mobile agents deployed in a service-oriented architecture in order to offer flexibility and, most importantly, to better handle the discussed security concerns and limitations. There are two system models described depending on the desired architecture complexity: a basic system model, in which the central node makes the most important decisions, and an advanced model, in which each mobile agent is more than a simple forwarding proxy because it can make local decisions, therefore reducing the computation performed at the central node, by using the business organization's resources.

The presented practical example for using the proposed approach implies the existence of a recommendation system and has the advantage that a business organization can present their products to customers from other organizations in the system, while keeping the customer information and purchasing preferences hidden from the businesses. In this way, if an organization decides not to be part of the system or to sabotage the other organizations, it cannot have access to any information regarding the other businesses and their customers.

As stated throughout the paper, the logic behind the recommendation system is not the scope of the presented research, but it is described the method by which the input data for the recommendation system is obtained from the business organizations and also the way the recommendation reaches the customer.

For future work, it is interesting to integrate in the system and test existing recommendation algorithms, also to research new techniques and to implement a tool for comparing recommendation algorithms.

Due to the system's extensibility another research point is to see what modules can be added to the system (particularly to the mobile agents) in order to improve the system's functionality (e.g., benchmark, logging, load balancing logic), to increase the business' profits (e.g., offer package deals with products and services from different businesses) and to improve the customer experience (e.g., offer free products and services from different businesses, obtain feedback from the user regarding the received recommendations).

References

1. Saccani, N., Johansson, P., Perona, M.: Configuring the after-sales service supply chain: a multiple case study. Int. J. Prod. Econ. **110**(1), 52–69 (2007)
2. Knecht, T., Leszinski, R., Weber, F.A.: Making profits after the sale. McKinsey Q. **4**, 79–86 (1993)
3. Legnani, E., Cavalieri, S., Ierace, S.: A framework for the configuration of after-sales service processes. Prod. Plan. Control **20**(2), 113–124 (2009)
4. Koufaris, M.: Applying the technology acceptance model and flow theory to online consumer behavior. Inf. Syst. Res. **13**(2), 205–223 (2002)
5. Huang, G.Q., Qu, T., Zhong, R.Y., Li, Z., Yang, H.D., Zhang, Y.F., Chen, Q.X., Jiang, P.Y., Chen, X.: Establishing production service system and information collaboration platform for mold and die products. Int. J. Adv. Manuf. Technol. **52**(9–12), 1149–1160 (2011)
6. Ordanini, A., Pasini, P.: Service co-production and value co-creation: the case for a service-oriented architecture (SOA). Eur. Manag. J. **26**(5), 289–297 (2008)
7. Camarinha-Matos, L.M., Afsarmanesh, H. (eds.): Intelligent Systems for Manufacturing: Multi-agent Systems and Virtual Organizations. IFIP, vol. 1. Springer, New York (1998)
8. Albreshne, A., Fuhrer, P., Pasquier-Dorthe, J.: Web Services Technologies: State of the Art: Definitions, Standards, Case Study. Working paper, Department of Informatics, University of Fribourg (2009)
9. Milojicic, D.: Mobile agent applications. IEEE Concurr. **7**(3), 80–90 (1999)
10. Jansen, W., Karygiannis, T.: Mobile Agent Security. National Institute of Standards and Technology, Gaithersburg (1998)

Designing and Configuring the Value Creation Network for Servitization

Barbara Resta[✉], Paolo Gaiardelli, Sergio Cavalieri,
and Stefano Dotti

Department of Management, Information and Production Engineering,
CELS - Research Group on Industrial Engineering,
Logistics and Service Operations, viale Marconi 5, 24044 Dalmine, BG, Italy
{barbara.resta,paolo.gaiardelli,sergio.cavalieri,
stefano.dotti}@unibg.it

Abstract. Despite the numerous benefits that the implementation of a servitization strategy can bring to manufacturing companies, several challenges have to be faced. Among others, changes in competences, resources, organisational structure and value network relationships are required in order to create, capture and deliver new value. In such a context, this paper investigates how the servitization level of a product-service offering impacts on a product-service provider as well as on its value-creation network. A theoretical conceptual model, derived from literature, is developed and then expanded into an explanatory conceptual framework through a case-based methodology. Evidence from the empirical investigation is then discussed and summarised into twelve propositions. Finally, contribution to both theory and practice, as well as some directions for future research, is pointed out.

Keywords: Product-Service system (PSS) · Servitization · PS provider · Value network · Competences · Resources

1 Introduction

The current situation faced by manufacturing firms is characterised by a fierce global competition and the saturation and commoditisation of their core product markets [1], with consequent negative effects on sales and margins [2]. In addition, customer needs and expectations are becoming more complex and comprehensive, often based on what a product does for the user, not on the product itself [3], and on expectation of benefits. These two factors have pushed companies to move beyond manufacturing towards the service arena [4]. This transformation, also called as "servitization of manufacturing" [5], began in the early 1990s [6], when most manufacturers started to offer services to varying degrees. As summarised by Mathieu [7] and further refined by other authors [8], benefits deriving from a service transformation may be grouped into four categories: financial, strategic, marketing and environmental.

However, many manufacturing firms have struggled to succeed in the service realm, heavily investing in extending their service business, without obtaining the expected correspondingly higher returns [9], as empirically investigated by Neely [4].

© Springer International Publishing Switzerland 2016
T. Borangiu et al. (Eds.): IESS 2016, LNBIP 247, pp. 457–470, 2016.
DOI: 10.1007/978-3-319-32689-4_35

Even if further empirical research is needed to examine the impact of a firm's service transition strategy on its value and profitability, it is clear that this evolutionary journey is fraught with difficulties and involves several challenges [10] in all areas of a company's business model [11]. Modifications are needed not only internally, but also externally, downstream towards customers, and upstream towards suppliers and partners.

Based on this discussion, the general purpose of this paper is to understand how manufacturing firms can successfully provide Product-Service (PS) offerings to the customers. In particular, it is of interest to understand what are the different dimensions that need to be considered to analyse a PS offerings and what value they assume in accordance with different levels of servitization. Moreover, the paper aims at investigating how these different dimensions impact on the business model of a manufacturing company that provide such offerings, in particular on its resources, competences, organisational features and network relationships.

The paper is structured as follows. In Sect. 2 the theoretical background and the research questions are presented. Section 3 is devoted to the description of the conceptual model, while Sect. 4 outlines the research design process. Section 5 discusses the empirical results from the case studies. Finally, Sect. 6 concludes the paper with a summary of the research contribution, managerial implications, and suggestions for future research.

2 Theoretical Background and Research Questions

In recent years, the servitization phenomenon has been put under the magnifying glass by both scholars and practitioners, as demonstrated by a noticeable growth in managerial and scientific studies. However, despite the presence of considerable and extensive research activities, there is little agreement among scholars. The fragmented and disaggregated nature of the field is reflected in the existence of separate silos of knowledge, characterised by different terminologies, definitions, objective of investigations, theories and methodologies, from engineering to sociological disciplines and from a traditional customer-centric to a sustainable network-based stakeholder approach [12]. It has contributed to the existence of a number of gaps in the understanding of the field [13]. In spite of different genesis, motivation, cultural and methodological approach, there is consensus in the scientific community that this evolutionary process requires at its foundation a thorough change of what Bettis and Prahalad [14] termed a business paradigm or dominant logic. The ten functional premises at the basis of the SDL perspective [15] are expressions of the profound change of the worldview from a technocratic to a customer-centric culture, in which managers have to conceptualise the business and carry out all the strategic and tactical decisions.

Moving towards an innovative dominant logic requires the surmounting of a hill, to create a shift of the mindset that pervades the overall organization and the value network in which a company operates [4]. As such, servitisation is not merely related to the introduction of new services in the company's portfolio or the proposal of integrated solutions. It is the gradual and consistent evolution of the entire business model of a manufacturing firm [16], including its value proposition, its position and role in the value creation network, its capabilities and organisational structure and its relations with the customers [17]. In this context, a Product Service System (PSS) can be defined as a servitised business model.

If abruptly and uncritically embraced, a change of paradigm could determine a traumatic response in an organization paving the way for what Gebauer et al. [9] termed as service paradox. As summed up in Fig. 1, to reach a new equilibrium, a consistent and robust strategic roadmap needs to be followed by the formulation of business models that should incrementally drive the progression from a transactional product-oriented vision of the market towards relational result-oriented solutions [18].

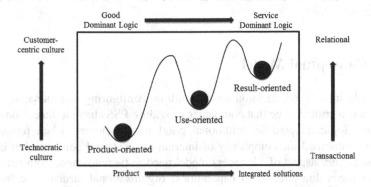

Fig. 1. The serivitzation evolution towards the achievement of a new equilibrium

Several gaps in the research still exist, hindering a comprehensive understanding of the servitisation domain. In particular, despite the widespread uptake of servitisation, questions remain regarding the nature of evolution trajectories. There is no predefined transition process that solves all the servitisation challenges, and therefore not all situations warrant the same approach to change. Rather, different combinations of trajectories to reach the new equilibrium positions can be developed by a company in response to particular market requests.

Moreover, scant attention has been dedicated to understanding the difficulties that companies have to tackle when they embark on a servitisation journey. The debate about factors that can either speed up or delay the surmounting of the hill, either facilitating or hindering the jump from a trajectory to another, is still at an early stage. In particular, the investigation on barriers and enablers has focused mainly on the analysis of a single business model, neglecting both a corporate and a value network perspective.

Finally, the new equilibrium reached with a servitisation evolution can be characterised considering both the new business models to adopt and the change of paradigm. To understand how this evolution occurs, it is fundamental to recognize what evolves: the way a manufacturing firm creates value. When characterising the new equilibrium reached with a servitisation evolution, the majority of existing studies conceptualizes servitised offerings as a single strategic response. In practice, on the contrary, there might be different types of product-service systems and the commitment–performance linkage for each service strategy could be mediated by different business model configurations. On these premises, the research activities presented in the reminder of this paper aim at shedding light on the following research question: "How does the servitization level of a PS offering impact on a PS provider?". In particular:

- **RQ1:** How does the servitization level of a PS offering impact on the organisational configuration of a PS provider?
- **RQ2:** How does the servitization level of a PS offering impact on the resources and competences required in its management and provision?
- **RQ3:** How does the servitization level of a PS offering impact on the value network of a PS provider?

3   The Conceptual Model

As previously introduced, decision about building, configuring and managing the new equilibrium is a critical issue that companies providing PSSs have to face. Compared to the business logic adopted by traditional good manufacturers, when products and services are combined the complexity of internal and external configuration increases [19]. Almost every aspect of a business model need to be renovated, from strategy and position in the value stream, to capabilities, organisational structure, cultures and mind-set [20]. In particular, new human resources and skills could be required [21], and new departments could be created to facilitate the development of customer-centred services [22], with an impact on relationships between the business functions within the company and, in general, on the organisational structure [23]. Moreover, since the development of a PSS often requires resources and capabilities which may be new to the company [24] a collaboration with other partners and suppliers could be required [25], where all but core-competences can be outsourced [8]. This shift from a supply-chain concept to a value-creation network logic [15] is characterised by various intensities and realities along with a "collaborative continuum" [7]. The consequential PSS value-creation network comprises not only the partners necessary for the production of the physical products, but also the actors responsible for delivering service components [26]. Thus, it is fundamental investigating how different types of PS offerings impact on the business model of a manufacturing company that provide such offerings, in particular on its resources, competences, organisational features and network relationships.

In theory building research, no matter how inductive the approach, a prior view of the general constructs or categories and their relationships is needed [27]. As suggested by Miles and Huberman [28], this can be done through the construction of a conceptual model that underlies the research. Such a model explains the main aspects that have to be studied and the presumed relationships amongst them. Compared to conceptual frameworks, a conceptual model is used to represent or describe a phenomenon, but not to explain it [29].

In such a context, the conceptual model that underlines this research (Fig. 2) was built on the Osterwalder's business model canvas [30], combined with results from the systematic literature review.

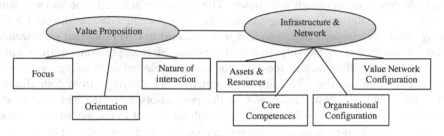

Fig. 2. The research conceptual model

The constructs and the variables considered in this research are described as follows:

Value Proposition. It corresponds to the bundle of products and services offered and represents the substantial value to the customer for which he/she is willing to pay. It can be described using four variables [31]:

– Orientation, in terms of ownership, use and decision-making power (product-, use- and result-oriented);
– Focus, concerning the objective of the service (product vs. processes);
– Nature of the interaction between the Customer and the PS provider (transaction-based vs. relationship-based).

Infrastructure and Network. It defines how products and services can be produced and delivered to clients in order to create value. It can be represented through the following variables [32, 33]:

– Assets (Tangible, Intangible and Human assets), describing the resources involved in the production of value;
– Source of Core Competences, related to company's collective knowledge about how to coordinate skills, resources and capabilities in order to support its competitive advantage;
– Functional Configuration, representing activities, processes and internal relationships among business functions;
– Value Network Configuration, describing inter-organisational interactions of a company with the other actors of the value-creation network.

4 Research Design

Since this study focuses on a how-type question about a contemporary phenomenon not yet thoroughly researched, a case-based approach seemed to be the most appropriate methodology [34].

4.1   Level of Analysis and Sample Selection

Since the paper aims at investigating the impact of different PS offerings, characterised by different levels of servitization, on selected business model elements of a company, a multiple-case study approach was chosen. The cases were selected in accordance with a theoretical (analytical) sampling to illuminate and extend relationships and logic among constructs. In particular, the cases were selected to cover different servitization levels. Additionally, to partially isolate the effects of strategic context from other potentially confounding factors, the case studies were selected from a single industrial macro-sector: automotive. The sample consisted of 13 offerings from four distinct companies (Table 1). Nine cases refer to the product-oriented area and four to the use-oriented category. Even if result-oriented solutions exist in the automotive sector, they are not provided by manufacturing companies and are not included in the research design.

Table 1. Description of cases

Case study	Product offering	Service offering	Orientation	Focus	Nature of interaction
Truco	Light, medium, heavy and special vehicles	Repair Services	PO	PD	TR
		Teleservices	PO	PD	RL
		Repair&Maintenance contracts	PO	PD	RL
		Road Assistance	PO	PD	RL
		Training	PO	PR	RL
		Fleet management	PO	PR	RL
Tenco	Commercial vehicles and transport solutions	Repair Services	PO	PD	TR
		Repair&Maintenance contracts	PO	PD	RL
		Fleet management	PO	PR	RL
		Contract hire	UO	PR	RL
Carco	Automobiles	Leasing	UO	PR	RL
		Long term renting	UO	PR	RL
Elmoby	Premium cars, buses and trucks	Electric Mobility	UO	PR	RL
Orientation - PO: Product-Oriented; UO: Used-Oriented; RO: Result-Oriented					
Focus - PD: Product-Based; PR: Process-Based					
Nature of interaction - TR: Transaction; RL: Relationship					

4.2   Data Collection, Analysis and Coding

Data were collected through semi-structured interviews with managers belonging to sales, after-sales services, marketing, spare part logistics, network development, customer centre and financial services functions. Questions to be followed in carrying out the data collection were developed from the conceptual model and included in the case study protocol. Although the initial set of interviews was agreed during the first planning meeting, the list of informants was expanded through interviewees' referrals. The diversity of informants provided a more complete picture of the phenomenon being studied and helped ensure construct validity. Moreover, having multiple researchers gathering information from multiple respondents helped to mitigate potential sources of bias. Finally, direct observations and extensive reviews of archival data, such as company documentation, annual reports and corporate website, were used for triangulation, to check the internal consistency of data.

Data analysis had two main components: within and across case analysis. Within case analysis for each case helps to examine the static view of the PSS, while the analysis across cases serves for understanding the relationships between the constructs (transformational/systemic approach). First, after each visit, the interviews were taped and then transcribed. Then, a draft the case study report was written, primarily from one researcher's field notes and then reviewed by the other interviewer, also inserting follow-up questions to clarify and extend content. Finally, the summary was sent to the informants for their corroboration and discussed during a follow-up meeting. Once all the data was collected, coding and within case analysis started. To minimise researchers' biases during the data analysis, for each case, researchers coded the data independently on the selected PSS elements, then compared the coding as a validity check for the coding. Then, for each case, the researchers jointly assessed the relationships between the elements. The coding process for each case did not progress until the involved researchers reached agreement on the constructs and their relationships.

Based on the conceptualization and the findings from this study, 12 propositions were elaborated as described in the next subsections.

5   Main Findings

5.1   The Evolution of the Competencies and Their Allocation

A manufacturer that moves into the service realm needs to develop or acquire new competences, depending on the type(s) of offerings introduced in its product portfolio. In particular, as demonstrated by all the case studies, product-based services require technical competences on the product and on its components. Since OEMs already have an intimate understanding of the product they have designed and developed, they are well placed to provide services to inspect, maintain and upgrade a vehicle during its operational life. Given that the involved capabilities for such offerings are close to the traditional core competences of a PS provider, product-based services are managed and delivered directly by the company or through its assistance network. On the contrary, the introduction of offerings characterised by a focus on how the customer uses the product involves two different categories of capability. On the one hand, it is necessary to understand customer's activities and processes involved in owning and using the product, through the development of consultancy competences. For instance, in the Tenco case, consultancy capabilities are developed internally, through proper training programs delivered to the sales force to become "transport consultants". On the other hand, specific competences related to each specific service are required to complement PS provider's core competences on product. Since the desired capabilities are not strictly adjacent to PS provider's traditional competences, in most of the cases, they are brought by external partners. For offerings that are characterised by a shift in product ownership, financial and risk management competences become essential. Moreover, even if the financial partner is an independent firm, it belongs to the same corporate group and it is considered as an internal business unit. Summarising:

- **P1:** Offerings focused on the product are related to traditional technical competences on the product and are delivered directly by the PS provider, generally with the support of its assistance network.
- **P2:** The shift of the PS offering focus from product to process requires consultancy capabilities and involves the transformation of salesmen into consultants who are able to understand customer's activities and processes.
- **P3:** The shift of the PS offering focus from product to process entails an increasing need of specific competences related to the provided services and the involvement of external partners.
- **P4:** A change of product ownership requires the development of financial competences.

5.2 The PS Provider's Evolution

As a heritage of the past, After-Sales is the organisational unit responsible for firm's technical support activities, with a central role in providing and managing product-focused offerings. In all the case companies, the After-Sales function is at the same hierarchical level as product functions and it is not considered a cost- but a profit-centre, with its own identity and responsibility on profits and losses. Moreover, After-Sales not only controls technical support activities, but also manages the processes related to the spare parts business (pricing, logistics and delivery).

However, traditional after-sales services (as repair and maintenance, inspection and diagnosis, extended warranties, etc.) are only one type of the services that a manufacturing company can potentially offer to its customers since the entire life cycle of a product has many pockets of value. Similarly, the After-Sales function is only one of the functions involved in the service provision. Even maintaining a strong importance, it must not be perceived as isolated from other organisational functions. In particular, the Sales function plays a fundamental role in the service realm. Traditionally, the Sales function refers to the organisational unit in charge to sell (directly or through a dealer network) firm's traditional product offering. With the introduction of new services, the Sales function holds both product and service responsibilities, and the salesmen become the first customer-provider interface also for the service domain. In order to push the sales force to promote and sell services to the customers, all the case companies provide bonus schemes, where a portion of the available incentives are related to the number of service contracts sold. Also the Marketing function (or Business Development) has an important role in promoting new offerings to the market

(Elmoby), as well as in understanding market's needs and segmenting customers, with the support of operational information and data from the After-Sales function (Truco and Tenco).

Nevertheless, every function works independently, with informal coordination activities. However, as the extent of the Value Proposition shifts from unbundled to bundled offerings, the need of formal synchronisation increases through cross-functional information and communications flows and shared databases containing customers' data. Therefore, Sales, After-Sales and Marketing function should work closely together, ideally in a symbiotic relationship.

The autonomy and independence of the service business builds momentum, but it must not lose the critical points of contact with the product business. First of all, service activities provide access to operational information of products, which can be used to improve the development and the quality of following product generation. As shown in the Truco case study, the Engineering department can benefit from feedback data on product quality, collected by the After-Sales and Marketing functions, through the assistance network and telematics instruments, installed on the vehicle for providing new services.

When financial services that impact on product ownership are introduced a new function is established, generally managed by an external company belonging to the same corporate group.

A process-focused offering requires competences related to each specific service, that in most of the cases are brought by external partners. Consequently, service provision activities do not involve only the After-Sales function and other internal entities, but takes also into account the possible roles of various third-parties actors in the PS value network. The "virtual" sum of the different functions and partners involved in service design, provision and management represents the Service Organisation. As a virtual enterprise, the involved actors bring complementary core competencies without the creation of a new legal entity, where the PS provider hold the focal position and acts a system integrator. In summary:

- **P5:** The internal Service Organisation involves After-Sales, Sales and Marketing functions.
- **P6:** The introduction of new services that requires innovative technical product features entails the involvement of the Engineering department in the product design phase.
- **P7:** A change of product ownership requires the establishment of an ad hoc function.
- **P8:** The shift of extent from unbundled to bundled solutions entails a higher coordination between the involved units.

5.3   The PS Value Network's Evolution

Service partners are external sources of complementary competences and are part of the service organisation, both for the service and PS provision network. As demonstrated by all the case companies, the assistance and sale network is the principal actor in the

PS provision network for product-focused services, as external reflection of the internal Sales and After-Sales functions. It can be composed by wholly owned or private capital dealers and workshops, or both. There is a high level of vertical control of the PS provider over the network through the requirement of standards enclosed in legal contracts. In addition, strategic objectives are defined centrally by the PS provider and then adapted to the network through the definition of proper KPIs and the related target values. The fulfilment of the assigned objectives is linked to a reward schemes, based essentially on technical aspect of the service provision process and its quality. However, as demonstrated by the Elmoby case, the assistance and sale network can have a mediator role, being the main customer-interface, where the customers can turn not only for technical issues related to the product, but also to create the first contact with the partner responsible for installing the charging station at home. Moreover, a product supplier can also become a PS provision network actor, especially for critical components in case a new technology is in the introduction phase.

With a shift of the offering focus from product to customer's activities and processes, the assistance network loses its role as partner of the PS provision network, while the sale network maintain its front role. However, this aspect is not reflected internally since the After-Sales function still plays a coordination and integration role. As a matter of fact, new partners (competing in industries different from the automotive sector) are involved in the PS offering management and provision, and they are centrally coordinated by the PS provider After-Sales function. The partners act both as service suppliers for the PS provider and as direct service providers for the customers. While for the sale and assistance network the PS provider wields a high vertical control, the service suppliers (that can act also as service providers) are tied to the focal company through partnership relations.

Moreover, the Carco case shows that there can be different tires of partners: the financial company (service partner), in turns, has a partnership with an insurance company to provide the customer with financial and insurance services.

For services that require new technical product features for their provision, there could be the necessity to involve external technical partners, that are in direct relation with the Engineering department.

Finally, the higher is the degree of Service Extent, the higher is number of partners involved and the higher is the need of coordination mechanisms and tools (ICT tools and shared databases), where the After-sales function plays a central role as system integrator. Therefore:

- **P9:** The shift of the PS offering focus from product to process entails the establishment of partnership relations with external companies.
- **P10a:** The involved partners are managed by the After-sale function of the PS provider. For services that requires innovative technical product features developed through an external company, the partner is managed by the Engineering department.
- **P11:** The After-sale function of the PS provider acts as a system integrator for mixed bundled and bundled offerings.

5.4 The Resource's Evolution

The evolution of resources is led by a change in the PS Offering Focus. Indeed, for product-focused offerings, the resources required for the provision and management are both tangible (such as tools, spare parts, and their supply chain) and intangible (predominantly product knowledge and information). As the focus of the offering changes from product to process, more intangible -information and knowledge- and human resources are needed. This aspect derives from the characteristics of pure services claimed by literature, where the relevance of human capital for services production and management, the critical role of customers and the importance of information are highlighted as service distinctive features.

Firstly, the important role played by the human factor in managing and delivery services is associated with substantial investment in human resources and their training, especially underlined by the Tenco case study. Moreover, the creation of employee commitment to service business may find beneficial to redirect their reward policy accordingly. The investigated companies have structured reward systems for the assistance network, based on technical aspects of the service. Truco and Carco have introduced also bonuses related to customer satisfaction. Other incentives that refer to the service area are given to the sales force in accordance with the number of service contracts sold. At the moment, no company has shown an horizontal reward system that cuts across the functional silos and linked or a compensation based on customer satisfaction (except for the Truco's assistance network), or on corporate/business cluster outcomes instead.

Secondly, the importance of knowledge and information resources is reflected into the nature of service technologies and ICT tools, that is a recurring theme in all the case studies. Indeed, service technologies are typically described as knowledge technologies, with high capacity for information processing within the technical core. For example, for telematics and fleet management solutions, the companies' (Truco and Tenco) desire is to better utilise vehicles' technological possibilities and proper information technology applications. Thus, ICT tools are a critical enabler and supporting elements for servitization. In particular, they enable intra- and inter-firm communication flows and the creation of databases where companies can save information, creating a stock of knowledge. Thus:

- **P12:** The shift from a focus on the product to a focus on the process entails an increasing importance of intangible (information and knowledge) and human resources.

6 Conclusion

Traditional manufacturers have moved into the service realm to maintain their positions in increasingly competitive markets, with a consequent evolution of their business models from a "pure product" orientation towards an integrated PSS. Despite some successful stories do exist, many manufacturing firms have struggled to survive in the service domain. As a matter of fact, tackling a servititization journey involves several challenges for a manufacturing company.

In this context, the overall purpose of this paper was to understand how manufacturing firms can successfully provide PS offerings to the customers, investigating how the characteristics of such offerings impact on the business model of a PS provider, especially on its resources, competences, organisational features and network relationships. In order to shed light on this aspect, an empirical investigation based on a multiple case study methodology has been conducted, leading to a more comprehensive understanding. In particular, when moving from product-based to servitized offerings, the required competences move from technical to consultancy- and customer's business-related. Moreover, the importance of intangible (information and knowledge) and human resources increases, as well as the need of establishing partnerships with external companies coming from different value chains. Finally, the establishment of a separate business unit that acts as a system integrator towards both internal functions (in particular Sales and Marketing) and external partners is a fundamental step in the PS provider servitization path. The developed model and the final propositions help managers to support service activities, easily analysing and re-engineering the network structure of a PSS business model.

Some directions for future research can be pointed out to overcome the limitations of this work. When Result-oriented PSSs provided by OEMs become available in the automotive sector, additional case studies should be conducted in this category, that represents the highest servitization level of an offering. Then, the developed propositions should be tested through statistical methodologies in order to assess their reliability, validity and statistical significance. Moreover, the empirical enquiry can be replied in different industries to create a base for inter-sector generalizability and to analyse commonalities and differences between diverse sectors. Another important area of research concerns the impact of servitization on the customer-PS provider interface and on the economic, environmental and social value created. Finally, what are the factors that support (or hinder) the servitization of manufacturing companies is an issue that deserves further investigation.

Acknowledgements. The research leading to these results has received funding from the European Community's Seventh Framework Programme (FP7/2007–2013) under grant agreement no PIRSES-GA-2010-269322.

References

1. Matthyssens, P., Vandenbempt, K.: Service addition as business market strategy: identification of transition trajectories. J. Serv. Manag. **21**(5), 693–714 (2010)
2. Cohen, M.A., Agrawal, N., Agrawal, V.: Winning in the aftermarket. Harv. Bus. Rev. **84**(5), 129–138 (2006)
3. Sawhney, M., Balasubramanian, S., Krishnan, V.: Creating growth with services. MIT Sloan Manag. Rev. **45**(2), 34–43 (2004)
4. Neely, A.: Exploring the financial consequences of the servitization of manufacturing. Oper. Manag. Res. **1**(2), 103–118 (2008)

5. Vandermerwe, S., Rada, J.: Servitization of business: adding value by adding services. Eur. Manag. J. **6**(4), 314–324 (1988)
6. Davies, A., Brady, T., Hobday, M.: Charting a path towards integrated solutions. MIT Sloan Manag. Rev. **47**(3), 39–48 (2006)
7. Mathieu, V.: Product services: from a service supporting the product to a service supporting the client. J. Bus. Ind. Mark. **16**(1), 39–58 (2001)
8. Baines, T.S., Lightfoot, H.W., Benedettini, O., Kay, J.M.: The servitization of manufacturing: a review of literature and reflection on future challenges. Int. J. Tech. Manag. **20**(5), 547–567 (2009)
9. Gebauer, H., Fleisch, E., Friedli, T.: Overcoming the service paradox in manufacturing companies. Eur. Manag. J. **23**(1), 14–26 (2005)
10. Martinez, V., Bastl, M., Kingston, J., Evans, S.: Challenges in transforming manufacturing organisations into product-service providers. J. Manuf. Tech. Manag. **21**(4), 449–469 (2010)
11. Kindström, D.: Towards a service-based business model - key aspects for future competitive advantage. Eur. Manag. J. **28**(6), 479–490 (2010)
12. Gummesson, E.: Extending the service-dominant logic: from customer centricity to balanced centricity. J. Acad. Mark. Sci. **36**(1), 15–17 (2008)
13. Velamuri, V.K., Neyer, A.K., Möslein, K.M.: Hybrid value creation: a systematic review of an evolving research area. J. Betriebswirtschaft **61**, 3–35 (2011)
14. Bettis, R.A., Prahalad, C.K.: The dominant logic: retrospective and extension. Strat. Manag. J. **16**(1), 5–14 (1995)
15. Vargo, S.L., Lusch, R.F.: Evolving to a new dominant logic for marketing. J. Mark. **68**(1), 1–17 (2004)
16. Zott, C., Amit, R., Massa, L.: The business model: recent developments and future research. J. Manag. **37**(4), 1019–1042 (2011)
17. Baines, T., Lightfoot, H.: Servitization of the manufacturing firm: exploring the operations practices and technologies that deliver advanced services. Int. J. Oper. Prod. Manag. **34**(1), 2–35 (2013)
18. Tukker, A.: Eight types of product-service system: eight ways to sustainability? Experiences from suspronet. Bus. Strat. Env. **13**(4), 246–260 (2004)
19. Becker, J., Beverungen, D.F., Knackstedt, R.: The challenge of conceptual modeling for product-service systems: status-quo and perspectives for reference models and modeling languages. Inf. Sys. e-Bus. Manag. **8**(1), 33–66 (2010)
20. Oliva, R., Kallenberg, R.: Managing the transition from product to services. Int. J. Serv. Ind. Manag. **14**(2), 160–172 (2003)
21. Gebauer, H., Friedli, T.: Behavioural implications of the transition process from products to services. J. Bus. Ind. Mark. **20**(2), 70–80 (2005)
22. Galbraith, J.: Organizing to deliver solutions. Organ. Dyn. **31**(2), 194–206 (2002)
23. Neu, W., Brown, S.: Manufacturers forming successful complex business services. Int. J. Serv. Ind. Manag. **19**(2), 232–251 (2008)
24. Davies, A.: Moving base into high-value integrated solutions: a value stream approach. Ind. Corp. Chang. **13**(5), 727–756 (2004)
25. Pawar, K.S., Beltagui, A., Riedel, J.C.K.H.: The PSO triangle: designing product, service and organisation to create value. Int. J. Operat. Prod. Manag. **29**(5), 468–493 (2009)
26. Schweitzer, E., Mannweiler, C., Aurich, J.C.: Continuous improvement of industrial product-service systems. In: Roy, R., Shehab, E. (eds.) Proceedings of the 1st CIRP Industrial Product-Service Systems Conference, pp. 16–23. Cranfield University Press, UK (2009)
27. Voss, C., Tsikriktsis, N., Frolich, M.: Case research in operations management. Int. J. Operat. Prod. Manag. **22**(2), 195–219 (2002)

28. Miles, M., Huberman, A.: Qualitative Data Analysis: an Expanded Sourcebook. SAGE Publications, Beverly Hills (1994)
29. Meredith, J.: Theory building through conceptual methods. Int. J. Operat. Prod. Manag. **13** (5), 3–11 (1993)
30. Osterwalder, A., Pigneur, Y.: Business Model Generation– A Handbook for Visionaries. Game Changers and Challengers. John Wiley and Sons Inc, Hoboken, New Jersey (2010)
31. Gaiardelli, P., Resta, B., Martinez, V., Pinto, R., Albores, P.: A classification model for product-service offerings. J. Clean. Prod. **66**, 507–519 (2014)
32. Gaiardelli, P., Resta, B., Songini, L., Pezzotta, G.: Aligning the servitization level of a company with its organizational configuration. In: Frick, J., Laugen, B.T. (eds.) Proceedings of APMS International Conference. University of Stavanger, Norway (2011)
33. Resta, B., Gaiardelli P., Pezzotta, G., Songini, L.: Configure the service network managing inter-firm relationships. In: Holweg, M., Srai, J. (eds) Proceedings of 18th EurOMA Conference: Exploring Interfaces. University of Cambridge, Institute for Manufacturing, UK (2011)
34. Yin, R.: Case Study Research: Design and Methods. SAGE Publications, Beverly Hills (1994)

Business Software Services
and Data-Driven Service Design

Generic Data Synchronization Algorithm in Distributed Systems

Dragoş Dumitrescu and Mihai Carabaş(✉)

Faculty of Automatic Control and Computers, Computer Science Department,
University Politehnica of Bucharest, Bucureşti, Romania
dragos.dumitrescu92@stud.acs.upb.ro, mihai.carabas@cs.pub.ro

Abstract. The increasing number of mobile users raises serious challenges upon middle-tier synchronization techniques and algorithms. The dynamics of backend systems, as well as those of frontend devices translates into an ever-growing demand for service standardization and flexibility. The current paper describes a flexible, scalable, platform-independent system relying on a distributed backend to provide data synchronization services in a multi-user system. The paper describes the desired architectural model used for this approach, continues with the description of the algorithm used by the backend subsystems and briefly describes an exemplary implementation of the aforementioned design.

Keywords: Rule-based processing · Data synchronization services · Distributed systems · Business software services

1 Introduction

Data synchronization is the process of maintaining a consistent state across multiple systems. Many of the major software development companies have devised their own data synchronization frameworks and technologies that are already offering benefits such as a high throughput, online/offline capabilities, peer-to-peer collaboration, and replication servers.

In this paper, an approach towards data synchronization in terms of a service-based software architecture will be presented. Service-based architectures have long been considered powerful tools for enhancing scalability and increasing system-wide performances [1].

The model we are proposing relies on loose coupling between its members, yet in the meantime provides configurability and closeness to human reasoning.

The context of data synchronization depicted throughout this paper is comprised mainly of the topic of structured data synchronization, namely database synchronization. Current solutions to this ends are suffering from strong coupling between clients and servers, vendor dependence of synchronization platform and lack of flexibility as will be underlined in Sect. 2 of the current paper.

© Springer International Publishing Switzerland 2016
T. Borangiu et al. (Eds.): IESS 2016, LNBIP 247, pp. 473–484, 2016.
DOI: 10.1007/978-3-319-32689-4_36

In order to surpass the aforementioned drawbacks, the objectives of the current paper will be presented, in terms of providing solutions and solving the tradeoffs between efficiency, level of abstraction, configurability, reliability.

The primary purpose of this paper is to present a highly flexible, loosely-coupled architecture for synchronizing data in business scenarios. Even though out of the scope of the current paper, the matter of security should be taken into account by implementers of the proposed architecture.

The proposed solution resides in a rule-based system, providing flexibility – as the most notable aspect in the current paper, scalability, high abstraction level, vendor independence.

The approach proposed throughout this paper provides the end-user with a broad spectrum of controls for managing complex business systems while in the meantime not requiring explicit programming skills. The drive is towards generalizing a complex service-oriented architecture for business systems, while keeping the effort of configuration at bay.

All the message passing interfaces are defined using web standards, implemented on top of well-known technologies and frameworks, while entity management is abstracted in an object-oriented format, distinguishable and implemented across multiple platforms.

The proposed system is a middle-tier – service level – application developed for offering data consistency in a multi-user environment while keeping the components loosely coupled and not interfering in the business logic definition and implementation process.

Another desiderate for the current system is the provision of stateless service discovery throughout the system, while using rule-based deliberation on service provider assignment in a parameterized context (where the parameters can be, but are not restricted to: type of user, type of device, GSM operator etc.).

This paper is structured as follows: Sect. 2 describes existing solutions to data synchronization as well as to rule-based management systems; in Sect. 3 we describe the terms and notations to be used throughout this paper; Sect. 4 focuses on the system's architecture; in Sect. 5, an overview of the communication protocol is described; Sect. 6 covers some ideas regarding the proof-of-concept implementation, while Sect. 7 presents the conclusions and the possibilities for further development of the current work.

2   Related Work

Data synchronization is process of establishing consistency among multiple data sources in a networked system. Examples include file synchronization, database synchronization, version control systems etc. [2].

Nowadays, the problem of data synchronization is becoming more and more of a challenge since the massive development of mobile computing. The restrictions one must follow when designing a synchronization framework are dictated not only by the rules of the business but also by performance and energy concerns.

Throughout this section, current approaches towards data synchronization, as well as insights into production systems will be presented.

The concept of database synchronization is not a novel one. Tools have been developed and have grown into mature, full-featured solutions. Close to the needs of decentralized synchronization between multiple platforms is Microsoft Sync Framework. It is a data store and transport independent, online and offline unified framework that allows integrating and synchronizing multiple clients on some common schemas [2]. Its main drawback consists on the fact that it requires a common schema on the client-side and on the server side and provides few levers to allow customized control over data flows inside the distributed architecture it tackles.

A major database vendor, Oracle, also provides a tool for synchronizing mobile devices to a central store, the Oracle Mobile Server. As the main drawbacks, note that it it only offers support for an Oracle central database and provides a highly centralized architecture, where the synchronization services must be placed on a single server to the ends of providing consistent data among multiple devices [3].

Vendor-dependence is also an issue with the Couchbase Sync Gateway, which provides synchronization between a Couchbase Lite database on the client side and a Couchbase NoSQL database on the server side.

The thesis of Hammarberg and Gustafsson [4] presents some insights into the basics of data synchronization, while also providing an integrated synchronization solution with an existing system. Another architecture taken into account for the design and development of the proposed approach can be found in [5]. Among others the authors stresses on the necessity of optimizing the quantity of data transferred through the network and provide a solution to schema and vendor independence with their approach.

The novelty in the approach proposed throughout this paper is inspired by Liu et al. [6] who propose a scalable solution for dataset synchronization for multiple connected devices. Another approach that was inspirational to the scope of this paper is that of Winstein and Balakrishnan [7] who propose, among others, a state synchronization algorithm in mobile devices and prove their concept implementing a different approach towards SSH. Seminal to the proposed algorithm is the idea of propagating changes from the client towards the server, and not the entire state of the application at a given point.

While the patent of Liu et al.[6] focuses on simple rule-based routing and execution of production rules, the contents of this paper argue for an extended measure, in the sense that administrator-defined rules will provide control of data-flow as well as logic control of the replication of data.

The subject of the current paper is closely related to that of data replication. In that respect, we follow guidelines offered by Oracle [8], Couchbase [9] and Microsoft [10]. An important asset in this concern is that of conflict resolution, a topic approached by all the synchronization methods above. Our approach, however, relies on leveraging the full control of conflict resolution to the administrator of the data flow process, offering fine-grained resolution for the possible conflicts.

As the approach proposed in this paper for data synchronization relies on the use of production rules, we stress that the idea of employing these kinds of systems [5] in the field of business processing is not novel. Currently, multiple such solutions exist [12, 13]. The main contribution of this paper resides in the usage of rule-based reasoning for the purpose of data synchronization in a distributed system. Efforts to standardize such systems have been made; JSR-94 (Java Specification Request) [14] is an example of such attempt for the Java Language.

In the proof-of-concept implementation depicted in Sect. 6, we employ *Drools* [13], an implementation of JSR-94, which provides a powerful rule-based API as an extension to the Java programming language.

3   Background

Data synchronization is usually found in a number of applications ranging from enterprise resource planners, to version control systems, distributed file systems, mirroring and file synchronization.

In the following section, the terms and notations used throughout this paper will be defined. The terms *synchronization* and *data synchronization* will be used interchangeably.

An important aspect while designing a proper algorithm for synchronizing data objects between multiple sites is that changes may occur at multiple points in the system at the same time.

Throughout this paper, *clients* will be defined as entities in the distributed system, their existence being justified by their capacity to authenticate into the system and to receive and send messages via some standard protocol.

The term *agent* refers to a special kind of *client* which is used to provide consistency between the various data sources that might push changes to a *client A* and provides a notification method towards its serviced *client A*. We might be thinking about an agent as an aggregator for all messages concerning *client A*. At the agent-level, we will be also talking about change *conflict mitigation* or *revision control*.

The term *service provider* refers to a *client* capable of providing a service described by a *contract*. A *contract* is a software interface described in an *IDL (Interface Description Language)*. Multiple service providers may offer the same services. The *backend* is responsible for solving the exact client to ask for a request.

A *client* might implement one or more contracts and may provide services inside distributed systems.

The term *generic data-message* or *message* is defined as a string describing a desired action. Each message contains a *type,* a *source* and, optionally, a *destination*.

The process of finding the proper destination for a given message will be called *message routing*. A client performing the task of routing generic messages will be called a *message router*. Usually, all the backend system clients have the capability of routing messages between system workstations.

A *rule* is the fundamental building-block in the proposed architecture. The *rule-base* provides a description of the system's behavior at any given moment in time. Thus, the *client* uses a *rule-base*, an inference engine and a *knowledge base* to assimilate the messages it receives and either to make the appropriate changes to its own state or to route the message to another host.

4 Architecture

In the following section, the main high-level components of the current distributed architecture will be presented. To begin with, the desiderates regarding the current system's functioning are to be discussed.

The main functionalities to be provided by the proposed system can be classified are: online/offline data synchronization unified distributed services, routing capabilities, message passing.

All functionalities are primarily based upon the implementation of a message passing protocol with standard message description. Therefore, the provision of a functional system (as designed in the following chapters) relies on the proper design and implementation of a message distribution system and of a proper routing scheme.

The proposed design offers a generic message interface consisting of a series of fields. Upon receipt on a backend node, the message is analyzed and inserted in a rule engine. The rule-engine evaluates the message and acts accordingly calling various services to solve the message, filter it, map it and reroute the resulted message/messages to the corresponding nodes.

Interactions between clients and the synchronization system will be performed in the following scenarios:

- When the client application performs a significant state change, a dataset signaling message is passed to its corresponding agent
- When the client application needs to call a service, a service request message is passed to its corresponding agent
- When the agent receives a dataset changed event from a different agent that concerns a given client, a message is passed from the recipient agent to the given client

The proposed system must be platform independent and also language-independent. Even though our exemplary implementation is made in Java, this should not be an obstacle for the development of similar modules in any other language.

One of the key requirements of the proposed design resides in a high throughput and a very fast message manipulation engine. Therefore, the routing algorithm, as well as any other rule-based reasoning must function as close to optimal as possible.

In the following sub-section, system architecture is presented, focusing on the components and on the relations between them.

4.1 System Architecture

In Fig. 1, the main components of the proposed system are introduced. The architecture presented in the below figure corresponds solely to the process of dataset synchronization. Note that each arrow corresponds to some data flow. For clarity of the dataset synchronization architecture, Fig. 1 omits some other components that make up the system. One of them is the *Name Resolver*, a component that acts as a mapper from clients to their corresponding agents. It is the duty of the name resolver to aid the client to discovering its corresponding agent.

The term *Dataset signaling* is defined as a message comprising information on the changes that have occurred in the client-side dataset. The depicted *Agent Communication Bus* is used for illustration purposes only to depict inter-agent communication as well as agent to rule-base communication.

The rule-base is a dedicated component that is used to propagate the centrally defined business rules that are to be executed by each agent's rule engine.

In the following paragraphs we present architecture of the stateless service layer proposed within the system. Figure 2 depicts the main components of the architecture and the interfaces between them from this point of view.

In the below figure, note that the terms *Service Request / Service Redirect* specify that the traffic between clients and agents is reduced to queries to identify a certain type of service (i.e. a Service definition) and the response the Agent provides to the querying entity. A service provider advertises the service it implements and communicates its capability to the database. Whenever a client requests a service, its corresponding agent takes all the existing service providers from the database and decides, based on its assigned rules (as depicted in Fig. 1) the provider that the respective client is bound to use.

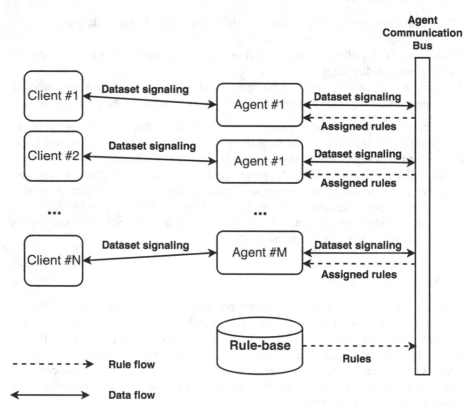

Fig. 1. High-level view of the system architecture

In Fig. 2, an extra step has been omitted for the clarity of the schema. After the resolution of the actual service provider for the requested service, the communication between the client and the service provider is performed without agent intermission.

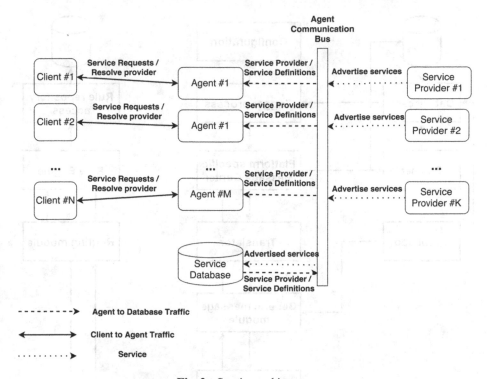

Fig. 2. Service architecture

4.2 Client-Side Architecture

One of the most important aspects of our design is the *client*. A proper implementation and design at this level is the key factor to a successful deployment. In this chapter, we are describing the client side architecture design of a generic client, exposing the intrinsic modules that compose the subsystem. In Fig. 3 the data flow between the components that make up a client subsystem is presented.

The client app can access either the data access layer to alter the current state of the application, or the generic message module by issuing *SEND* and *RECEIVE* commands upon the generic message queue. Upon sending a message the routing module is responsible for finding the right destination for the submitted message based on the rules it knows about and finding the right resolution for the data message and thus virtually filtering the message in either a data or a user level message.

The most important aspect in this design resides in the generality of the message and in the performance of the routing module. Upon receiving a message, it is pushed forward to the data access layer in order to ensure data patching. Patching data means translating a message into a storage operation and thus assuring the data consistency. Increments of data will be used in order to patch the client's known records and update the client's internal state.

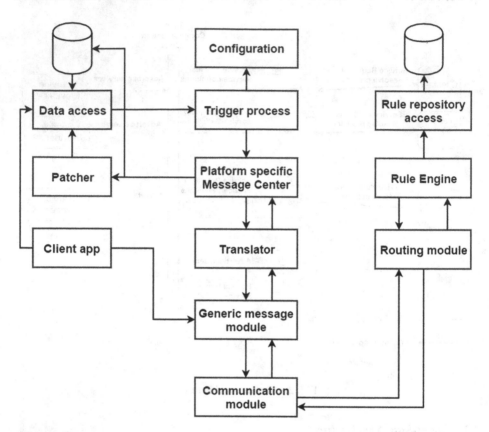

Fig. 3. Detailed description of the client side architecture. The arrows depict data flow between the components of the system

5   Design of the Communication Protocol

The actual functioning of the proposed system strongly relies upon the distribution and the application of sets of rules. In that respect, we argue that the flexibility that can be attained using this approach surpasses some of its disadvantages.

Usage of the proposed approach implies that every *message* that enters the system is regarded as an *event*. Furthermore, its underlying data context resides in all accessible facts in the system.

In this chapter we will be going in the details of the workflows supported by the proposed system and describe the main algorithms to be used for the *ECA* (Event Condition Action) inference engine as well as for the incremental data synchronization algorithm.

We define a Client-Agent mapping as a correspondence between a user-assigned *client* and an *agent* client. There can be multiple correspondences between Clients and Agents. A mapping can be defined statically or dynamically (upon first entry of the user in the system).

After the client discovers its agents, it needs to establish a communication channel to the remote side (the agent) and then perform the rest of the message passing. The structure of the first two steps could be described as follows:

1. Client asks the *Name Resolver* who his agent is
2. Name Resolver responds
3. The Client asks the Agent to start a connection
4. The Agent accepts or not the request

The next step after the connection establishment is for the *Client* to send out all its pending data messages - whatever had happened while he was out of sync with his agent. This action is suited for an online-offline scenario where a *Client* goes offline at any moment and still allows the application to partially function. This is the moment where all the data messages should be sent towards the agent, allowing the rule engine to reason upon their receipt.

When the Agent has accepted all the data messages from the client, the client goes into the next phase of the synchronization process. Here, it asks the Agent for any changes that occurred after the last time they actually communicated. If that is true, the agent sends out all the pending data messages for the client. Should there be no changes, the synchronization process completes.

We define a data message as a transition on the state graph of a record. A *state* of a record is the value of the record at a given time. We hold on both the agent side and on the client side a list of all versions for each of the records.

In spite of the existence of such merging and conflict detection/resolution and advanced algorithms for handling these kinds of problems, the general recommendation is the avoidance of such situations.

The recommendations for avoiding replication conflicts include [8–10] unique row identification by a global unique identifier, deactivation rather than actual deletion of rows from the physical store, update avoidance techniques through portioning the dataset in such a manner that only one entity can modify its contents.

From a more general point of view, the chosen database system provides two basic mechanisms: dataset changed signaling - observing changes in the dataset - and dataset patching - notifying about changes. In the proposed system, we are relying upon rule engines to perform clear routing of messages between system nodes.

Upon receipt of a message from its assigned client, an agent attempts to perform the actual routing of the specified message. In the case of a data message, the agent performs its data synchronization steps and algorithm as described previously in this chapter. Upon solving the possible conflicts, the agent might assert a new fact into the fact-base enforcing that a propagation of the mitigated and merged conflict occurs. The agent is prone to communicate with another system node in order to inform it of the change that has currently occurred.

We describe the following rule template that could easily be applied in any context - in pseudocode - :

```
ON: MESSAGE_TYPE AND MPredicate(?input)

IF

USING( ?message_context = GetMessageContext(?input,
?message_context);

?data_context = GetRelatedDataContext(?input,
current_data_context);)

GPredicate(?input, ?message_context, ?data_context)

THEN

Assert (MMap(?input, ?message_context, ?data_context))

Perform(MAction( ?input, ?message_context, ?data_contex
t))

ELSE

Assert (MMap2(?input, ?message_context, ?data_context))

Perform(MAction2( ?input, ?message_context, ?data_conte
xt))
```

In Listing 1. Sample rule in pseudocode, MPredicate stands for a predicate that takes as sole parameter the input message, GetMessageContext is a function that gets the current message context form the global message repository, GetRelatedDataContext is a function that gets the entities related to the current message, GPredicate is a predicate on all the aforementioned variables, MMap and MMap2 is a map of the current contextual values to a new message to be added to the repository, while MAction and MAction2 are actions (parameterized functions) to be executed in case of success or failure.

6   Implementation

The implementation provided is a proof of concept for the specified requirements and encompasses, alongside the middle-tier system described, an exemplary Desktop Client and a Desktop application which plays the role of a backend server.

For implementing the described system, we have chosen to employ the Java programming language while the implementation for handling rule-based processing is *JBOSS Drools*. At the moment, the system has been tested to perform online-offline replication and conflict mitigation based on centrally available rules. Since it is only a proof-of-concept for the described architecture, it is still lacking functionality and has not been thoroughly tested in complex environments.

The messaging services described throughout this paper were implemented on top of HTTP technologies, while the storage and signaling is handled through the JPA (Java

Persistence API) [15] which facilitates an object oriented approach towards abstracting datasets.

The agent side processing model is based on rules and resides in a global stateless session - the request processor and a per-user stateful session - the synchronization engine.

Every event is issued by a running process. A user managed process changes the current user's state. An event that occurs for a user might be of interest for another user in the system inside the same application. It is the responsibility of the Agent to route the significant event to all interested users' agents.

7   Conclusion and Further Development

Documenting and designing the system presented in this paper was a chance to explore multiple paradigms in programming as well as multiple architectural patterns regarding loosely-coupled computer architecture. The problems raised by the distributed nature of the networked computer systems reside in the tradeoffs one has to make in order to ensure integrity between the components and in the same time to keep high performance standards.

The solution described in this paper has many advantages. However, in practice, the outlined desiderates are much harder to achieve than they are on paper. The primary obstacle in getting the most of a computer system lies in the limited nature of its resources.

We list some of the advantages of the proposed approach when designing a data consistency management unit.

Message-based communication is a very flexible approach to designing a distributed system, since the propagation of a message throughout the system is made not only on a local level, but also on a global level. Persisting data at client or agent level is accomplished using common abstractions, independent of platform or database implementations.

It is simple to implement a protocol using a rule-based engine, because the language offers a high level of flexibility and an important degree of readability. It is possible to extend the current functionalities with further enhancements. Currently, the exemplary solution presented has been deployed on a modest home computer with good results.

In the following paragraph, the disadvantages of using a rule-based approach for accomplishing data synchronization are enumerated. Resource-intensive computing is required since all rule engines reason upon facts stored in the working memory. Current implementation has no built-in security mechanism. The current implementation needs further testing and assessment.

The provided proof-of-concept implementation is just a starting point for a more powerful and reliable solution. Future development should provide thorough testing of all functionalities and comparative benchmarking against existing solutions.

Another important aspect that must be taken into account is that of providing multi-user simulations for validating system integrity. Currently, the hardware limitations make it impossible to simulate a highly dynamic environment.

References

1. The OpenGroup: SOA Reference Architecture Technical Standard: Basic Concepts. http://www.opengroup.org/soa/source-book/soa_refarch/concepts.htm
2. Microsoft TechNet: Understanding Data Synchronization with External Systems. https://technet.microsoft.com/en-us/library/jj133850(v=ws.10).aspx
3. Oracle: Oracle Database Mobile Server Documentation Release 12.1. http://docs.oracle.com/cd/E60418_01/index.htm
4. Hammarberg, E., Gustafsson, T.: A Partial Database Synchronization Scheme between a Centralized Server and Mobile Units. Thesis: University of Gottenborg, Gottenborg (2011)
5. Ramya, S.B., Koduri, S.B., Seetha, M.: A stateful database synchronization approach for mobile devices. Int. J. Soft Comput. Eng. **2**(3), 316–320 (2012)
6. Liu, T. J., Greene, E., Ahamed, V.: Scalable Rule-based Data Synchronization Systems and Methods. USA Patent US20120023074, 26 January 2012
7. Winstein, K., Balakrishnan, H.: Mosh: An interactive remote shell for mobile clients. In: Proceedings of the 2012 USENIX Conference on Annual Technical Conference, pp. 177–182, Boston (2012)
8. Oracle: Conflict Resolution Concepts and Architecture. Oracle Database Advanced Replication. http://docs.oracle.com/cd/B12037_01/server.101/b10732/repconfl.htm
9. Couch DB: Conflict Management. CouchDb - The Definitive Guide (2015). http://guide.couchdb.org/draft/conflicts.html
10. Microsoft Azure: Conflict Resolution When Synchronizing. https://msdn.microsoft.com/en-us/library/azure/hh667306.aspx
11. Forgy, C.L.: Rete: a fast algorithm for the many pattern/many object pattern match problem. Artif. Intell. **19**(1), 17–37 (1982)
12. CLIPS, CLIPS Basic Programming Guide. http://clipsrules.sourceforge.net/documentation/v630/bpg.pdf
13. JBOSS Drools, Drools Documentation. http://docs.jboss.org/drools/
14. Toussaint, A.: JSR-000094 Java(TM) Rule Engine API 1.0a Final Release, API Specification: Java Community Process (2003)
15. Oracle, The Java EE 6 Tutorial. http://docs.oracle.com/javaee/6/tutorial/doc/javaeetutorial6.pdf

Data-driven Approach to New Service Concept Design

Min-Jun Kim[1], Chie-Hyeon Lim[1,2], Chang-Ho Lee[1], Kwang-Jae Kim[1(✉)], Seunghwan Choi[3], and Yongsung Park[3]

[1] Pohang University of Science and Technology, Pohang, Republic of Korea
{minjun,arachon,dlckdgh,kjk}@postech.ac.kr
[2] University of California, Merced, USA
clim28@ucmerced.edu
[3] Korea Transportation Safety Authority, Hwaseong, Republic of Korea
{shchoi,katrieng}@ts2020.kr

Abstract. Various types and massive amounts of data are collected in multiple industries. The proliferation of data provides numerous opportunities to improve existing services and develop new ones. Although data utilization contributes to advancing service, studies on the design of new service concepts using data are rare. The present study proposes a data-driven approach to designing new service concepts. The proposed approach is aimed at helping service designers to understand customer behaviors and contexts through data analysis and then generate new service concepts efficiently on the basis of such understanding. A case using bus driving data is introduced to illustrate the process of the proposed approach. The proposed approach provides a basis for the systematic design of new service concepts by enabling efficient data analysis. It also holds the potential to create a synergetic effect if incorporated into existing approaches to designing new service concepts.

Keywords: Big data · Data utilization · Service concept design · Customer understanding

1 Introduction

We live in an information economy in which data are increasingly exchanged globally [1]. With the advancement of information and communication technologies, various types and massive amounts of data are collected in multiple industries [2]. Such data proliferation provides new opportunities for companies to improve existing services and to develop new ones. Automobile manufacturers analyzed driving records collected from inboard devices to develop various services (e.g., safety, entertainment, and consumable replacement information) for enhancing the experience of the drivers [3]. Heavy equipment manufacturers analyzed equipment condition data to provide services that cope with unexpected product breakdowns and maximize product availability for stakeholders [4]. In building system, many kinds of data, such as energy resource consumption (e.g., electricity, gas, and water) and external situation (e.g., external temperature, amount of rainfall, and solar insolation) were collected and analyzed to

© Springer International Publishing Switzerland 2016
T. Borangiu et al. (Eds.): IESS 2016, LNBIP 247, pp. 485–496, 2016.
DOI: 10.1007/978-3-319-32689-4_37

extract energy consumption patterns of building; then the analysis results were used to reduce energy cost and improve energy utilization efficiency [5]. Insurance companies analyzed patient data to understand their health-related behaviors and to develop services for high-risk patients to improve their healthcare safety [6]. Companies producing wearable fitness tracking devices, such as Fitbit, collected and analyzed people's fitness activity data (e.g., step achievement, active minutes, and awaken or restless time) to support them achieve specific fitness-related outcomes, such as walking 10,000 steps [7]. Such cases are becoming increasingly relevant in the current data-rich economy [8, 9].

Existing studies have demonstrated that using data is key to improving the design activities including a customer understanding and designing service concepts [10]. The design of adequate and innovative service concepts is the core of successful new service development [11]. A service concept indicates what to offer to customers and how to offer it and mediates between customer needs and the strategic intent of a company [12]. Several studies have explored the approaches to designing new service concepts, including a computer-based tool to design the functions of a service concept [13], a morphological approach to designing new smart service concepts [14], and a knowledge-based method for designing product service system concepts [11]. However, studies on the design of service concepts starting from data are rare despite the expected contribution of this topic to data-rich economies. Therefore, developing a systematic and efficient aid for new service concept design starting from data is obviously necessary.

This study proposes a data-driven approach to designing new service concepts that integrates insights from the literature related to big data and service concept design. The proposed approach aims to enhance the effectiveness and efficiency of new service concept design starting from the data. The proposed approach consists of five steps: (1) collecting available data and integrating the collected data for analysis, (2) developing an analysis model that aids in efficient data analysis, (3) analyzing data to understand customer behaviors and contexts, (4) identifying service ideas on the basis of insights gained from the data analysis, and (5) designing new service concepts. The proposed approach is illustrated using bus driving data to show its working process.

The proposed approach contributes to the systematic design of new service concepts by enabling efficient data analysis and further creating a synergetic effect when incorporated into existing approaches to service concept design.

2   Research Background

2.1   Data Utilization to Advance Service

Massive amounts of data in various formats are collected consistently and non-intrusively with the advancement of technologies of data collection and storage, such as the Internet of Things. In particular, data that indicate customer behaviors and contexts are recorded and tracked [15]. For example, automobile manufacturers collect drivers' driving records to monitor their driving behaviors [3]. Companies that produce wearable fitness tracking devices collect people's fitness activity data to help them attain specific fitness-related outcomes [7].

Customer data provide service companies with new opportunities to design new service concepts. In particular, such data help companies in understanding their customers and generating various service contents for customers. Ostrom et al. [9] indicated that companies today can easily get to know their customers in terms of what they did, when they did it, and where they did it through a constant flow of data from multiple sources. Lim et al. [10] indicated that data can be used to understand customer behaviors and produce the information contents required by customers. Opresnik and Taisch [16] similarly noted that the utilization of data from customers can facilitate the development of services in manufacturing industries. Huang and Rust [15] indicated that service companies can leverage and transform customer data into useful information about customers for strategic marketing planning.

The aforementioned studies demonstrate that data utilization contributes to the design of service concepts for customers. Although data utilization is a key for designing new service concepts, studies on service concept design starting from data are rare, and the understanding of the mechanism behind such design is limited. The current research addresses this limitation.

2.2   Existing Approaches to New Service Concept Design

In developing new services, designing service concepts is the first and foremost issue [11]. A service concept is defined as a bridge between the "what" and the "how" of a new service [17], which mediates between customer needs and the strategic intent of a company [12]. The importance of designing new service concepts has gradually increased because of various customer demands, competitive environment, and globalization of services.

Service concepts are commonly designed through intuitive, investigative, and analytic approaches [14]. In the intuitive approach, service concepts are designed on the basis of the intuitions of service designers, which are gleaned from activities such as brainstorming. The investigative approach designs new service concepts by asking for customers' ideas directly, for example, through customer surveys or interviews. The analytic approach uses engineering methodologies and tools for designing new service concepts. For example, Sakao and Shimomura [13] proposed a computer-based tool to design the functions of a service concept for satisfying customer needs. Kim et al. [11] established a methodology for product service system (PSS) concept generation that includes a list of general customer needs, a list of PSS models, a PSS concept generation support matrix, and a PSS case book. Geum et al. [14] proposed an approach to designing new smart service concepts using morphological analysis.

The aforementioned studies can support the design of new service concepts using data. However, the applicability of the results is limited because these studies do not focus on the use of data to design service concepts. By contrast, the present study focuses on service concept design starting from the data, which is a significant issue in data-rich economies. The approach suggested in this work is aimed at providing a systematic procedure that links data analysis to service concept design. Therefore, the approach will assist service designers in efficiently generating new service concepts.

3 Data-Driven Approach to New Service Concept Design

This study proposes a data-driven approach to designing new service concepts. The approach involves (1) collecting available data and integrating the data for efficient analysis, (2) defining variables related to customers and services and estimating the physical or statistical relationship among the variables, (3) analyzing data to understand customer behaviors and contexts, (4) identifying target customers and producing various service contents based on the results of the data analysis, and (5) designing new service concepts by considering the delivery process of service contents (Fig. 1). The following subsections describe each step in detail.

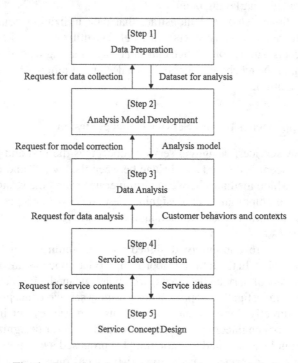

Fig. 1. Procedure for data-driven service concept design

3.1 Step 1. Data Preparation

Step 1 aims to collect proper data from multiple sources, such as the Internet, sensors, and social network activities. Although various types of data exist, this study uses data generated by customers, which include information on customer behaviors and contexts. Driver's driving data, fitness activity data, and patient behavior data are the examples of data used in this study. Moreover, the collected data also feature different formats and structures because of various data sources. Thus, the first step also aims to transform various types of data into a format that can be used to analyze data efficiently.

3.2 Step 2. Analysis Model Development

A prerequisite for customer understanding using data is defining the variables related to the customers and services in question, which indicate customer behaviors and contexts. Therefore, Step 2 aims to define three types of variables that can be measured using the collected data. If the collected data are not sufficient to define the variables, then Step 1 should be repeated to collect the data required to define such variables. To facilitate the understanding of such variables, we briefly describe three types of variables used in each type by using a driving safety enhancement service as an example.

The first type is a service objective variable that includes the goals of both service designers and customers. For example, minimizing accident rates is a goal of service designers for enhancing driving safety. In this case, accident rate is defined as the objective variable. The second type is the customer behavior variable, which indicates people's behaviors or the operation of objects, such as driving while drowsy or engine speed, respectively. Considering this type of variable, service designers can analyze customer behaviors and then identify "the behaviors that should be managed through the service." The third type is the customer context variable, which indicates customers' characteristics (i.e., demographic information) and situations (i.e., time and location), such as gender and driving time, respectively. By analyzing the variables, service designers can identify "when and where to offer the service and to whom it should be offered."

This step also aims to develop an analysis model for customer understanding, which is defined as a model that represents the relationship among the three types of variables. It aids in the analysis of data for identifying customer behaviors and contexts. The relationship among the variables may exist statistically or physically, and this relationship is estimated in this step. For example, a physical or statistical relationship between customer behavior variables and customer context variables may exist. The customer behavior variables are highly relevant to the customer context variables because customer behavior changes depending on customer types (e.g., gender and age) and situations (e.g., weather and time). Thus, analyzing the two types of variables enable service designers to understand customer behaviors and contexts comprehensively. Moreover, changes in customer behaviors under various contexts and differences in customer behaviors across diverse customer types can be analyzed.

3.3 Step 3. Data Analysis

Step 3 aims to analyze data to identify customer behaviors and contexts on the basis of the analysis model. For the data analysis, some variables in the analysis model are selected because of their potential to influence the results of the data analysis. Variable selection is conducted with several domain experts and through a literature review. If undefined variables are needed for the data analysis, then Step 2 should be repeated to define the variables. The statistical or physical relationship among the variables estimated in Step 2 is identified by analyzing the data with respect to the selected variables. The distribution of each selected variable or the relationship among the variables can be analyzed. Figure 2 shows the example of variable selection for analyzing risky driving behaviors that can be used to gain insights for designing driving safety enhancement services. Figure 3 shows analysis results considering selected customer behavior variables and customer context variable in Fig. 2.

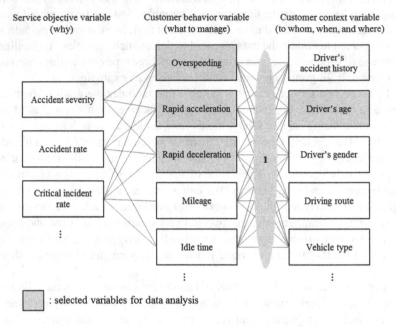

Fig. 2. Example of variable selection for analyzing risky driving behaviors

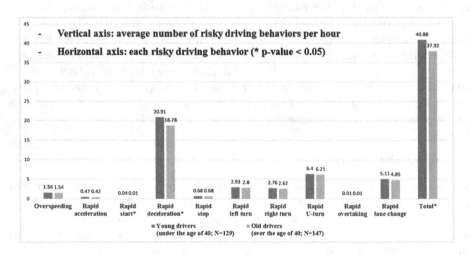

Fig. 3. Comparison of risky driving behaviors of young drivers and old drivers

3.4   Step 4. Service Idea Generation

Various studies explained that defining target customers should be the first stage of designing a service concept because different target customers require different service concepts [18]. Moreover, existing studies emphasized the understanding of target customers' behaviors and requirements in designing customized service concepts for them [19, 20]. Therefore, Step 4 aims to define the target customers of a service (to whom) and the motivations for such a service (why) on the basis of the insights gained from the data analysis in Step 3. For example, identifying the relationship between customer behaviors and customer context variables, which shows the change in customer behaviors considering various contexts, helps to define when and where to offer a service and to whom it should be offered.

This step also aims to produce various service contents because identifying appropriate information in terms of its contents and form is a key factor in improving service value creation [15, 21]. A service content is defined as a function or information that can be provided to target customers. Such function or information is derived from the results of the data analysis in Step 3. For example, the relationship between customer behaviors and context variables can be used to provide information on the comparison or classification of customers because it indicates changes in behaviors in different contexts. If data analysis results are needed to produce a service content, then Step 3 should be repeated to analyze the data.

3.5   Step 5. Service Concept Design

Building on existing studies on the definition of service concepts (see Sect. 2.2), the present study defines a service concept by indicating which contents (what) to offer to target customers (to whom) so as to enhance their experience (why) based on which data (how) and by which delivery process to employ (when, where, and how). The service concept is designed sequentially from Step 4 to Step 5. Step 4 indicates why to offer a service concept to whom (i.e., motivation and target customers) as well as what to offer through the service concept (i.e., service contents). Step 5 aims to define the primary components of the service content delivery, namely, when, where, and how to offer the service contents. In case a service content not produced in Step 4 is needed to design the delivery process, Step 4 should be repeated to produce the service content.

"When" represents the timing of the provision of a service content (i.e., before, during, and after customer process). Using the define, prepare, execute, monitor, and conclude steps of the universal job map [22], the customer process can be identified. This process helps identify the timing of the provision of a service content. "Where" indicates the delivery channels of the service content (i.e., machine and human). Smart devices and managers are examples of delivery channels. Finally, "how" indicates the delivery types of the service content (i.e., push and pull). The push type describes a communication in which the request for a given service content is initiated by service providers. By contrast, the pull type means that the initial request for a content originates from customers.

4 Illustrative Example: The Use of Bus Driving Data

Using the proposed approach, the authors designed service concepts for enhancing the driving safety of bus drivers with the Korea Transportation Safety Authority (TS) of the South Korean government. TS collects operational data of buses through digital tachograph (DTG) to manage the driving behaviors of bus drivers. All bus companies must install DTG on their buses and regularly upload the recorded operational data to TS. As a result, TS now maintains a database called DTG DB. TS uses this database to provide new services that will enhance the driving safety of bus drivers.

The three types of data prepared in Step 1 include DTG (e.g., speed and mileage), accident (e.g., accident type, time, and place), and driver (e.g., driver's age, driving date, and car plate number) data. DTG data are collected every second and then archived in TS. Accident data are collected and managed by the National Police Agency. Driver data are collected and managed by transportation companies. With assistance from TS, this study collected DTG data, accident data, and driver data related to 276 bus drivers of one transportation company covering the periods of April to May 2013, 2004 to 2013, and 2013, respectively. The collected data were then integrated. Through the data integration, we were able to analyze the differences in the driving behaviors of the 276 drivers. Moreover, we were able to analyze the changes in their driving behaviors by considering various driving contexts, such as driving route.

The three types of variables used to understand the driving behaviors of the bus drivers were defined in Step 2. First, we defined the service objective variables, which indicate driving performance such as the accident rate of a driver. Second, we defined the customer behavior variables, which explain driving behavior such as overspeeding and rapid acceleration. Third, we defined the customer context variables, which indicate drivers' characteristics and driving environment. After the variables were defined, an analysis model was developed. Figure 2 indicates an example of the analysis model.

On the basis of the opinions of transportation experts, 10 types of risky driving behaviors defined by the Korean government were selected as customer behavior variables. Driver's age, accident history, and driving routes were selected as customer context variables. The data analysis results in Step 3 include the correlations among risky driving behaviors, the frequency of risky driving behaviors in specific routes, and the comparison of different driver groups according to their risky driving behaviors. Figure 3 shows an example of data analysis results. Specifically, the figure indicates the results of the analysis of the differences between the driving behaviors of young drivers (i.e., under the age of 40) and old drivers (i.e., over the age of 40).

The data analysis results exemplified in Fig. 3 provided insights for defining the target customers of a service and the motivation for such service in Step 4. As shown in Fig. 3, the total number of risky driving behaviors per hour in the young driver group is higher than that in the old driver group (p-value < 0.05). Moreover, the average numbers of rapid start and deceleration per hour in the young driver group are higher than those in the old driver group (p-value < 0.05). These results indicate that driving safety enhancement services should be provided to the young driver group instead of the old driver group. In particular, the services for reducing rapid start and deceleration should be presented intensively relative to other risky driving behaviors.

The service contents for young drivers were also produced in Step 4. Examples of service contents include a service content that indicates the distribution of the risky driving behaviors of a young driver (Fig. 4) and a service content that indicates the ability of a young driver to drive safely (Fig. 5).

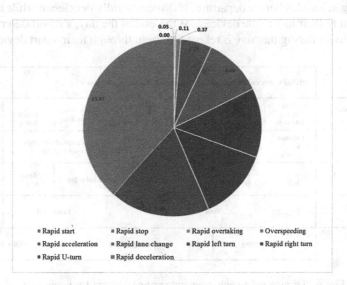

Fig. 4. Distribution of the risky driving behaviors of Driver A (young driver) on a given day

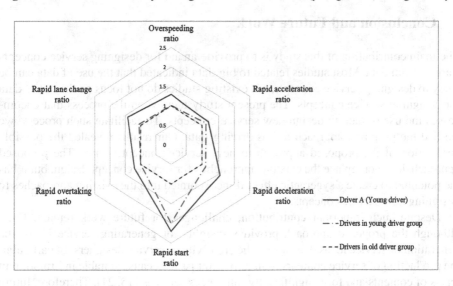

Fig. 5. Distribution of the driving performance of Driver A (young driver) in terms of driving safety

The concept of a driving safety enhancement service that delivers such service contents to young drivers was designed in Step 5 (Fig. 6). Through the service, drivers can receive an educational content about the necessity of safe driving and a feedback content describing their previous driving behaviors through a manager when they check their driving schedules before departure. If drivers rapidly decelerate while driving, an alarm is sent to their in-vehicle devices. At the end of the day, a report describing their driving behavior during that day is relayed to them through their smart devices.

Driving safety enhancement service concept for young drivers							
Driver actions (when)	Check driving schedules	Review previous driving	Drive to the destination	Adjust driving based on the guide, alarm	Arrive at the destination	Review today's driving	Take a rest
Service contents (what)	Education for safe driving	Feedback on previous driving	Interventions for driving safety (especially rapid start and deceleration)			Reports about today's driving behavior	Training for safe driving
Service channel (where)	Smart devices	Manager (strictly)	In-vehicle devices (e.g., navigation and radio)			Smart devices	Manager (strictly)
Delivery types (how)	Push					Push or pull	Push
	Before driving		During driving			After driving	

Fig. 6. Driving safety enhancement service concept for young drivers

5   Conclusion and Future Work

The main contribution of this study is to provide an aid for designing service concepts starting from data. Most studies related to big data indicated that the use of data can be a key to designing service concepts, but existing studies do not focus on the use of data for designing service concepts. The present study focuses on the process that encompasses the use of data to design new service concepts. To facilitate such process, we applied the proposed approach to bus driving data. Our results revealed the possible application of the proposed approach to new service concept design. The proposed approach does not replace the existing approaches for service concept design, but it has the potential to create a synergetic effect if incorporated into the existing approaches to designing new service concepts.

Despite such important contribution, challenges for future work remain. First, although the proposed approach provides insights for generating service ideas, the generation of service ideas depends on the creativity of service designers. In particular, the production of service contents is an important issue because suitable information in terms of contents and form significantly influences services [15, 21]. Therefore, future research should develop a tool for supporting service content production. Second, the proposed approach can be applied to various data in multiple industries. Thus, additional case studies on new service concept design using various data should be conducted.

Finally, our approach could be advanced further by incorporating it into the existing approaches to designing service concepts.

Acknowledgments. This research was supported by the Urban Architecture Research Program through a grant funded by the Ministry of Land, Infrastructure, and Transport (15PTSI-C064868-03) and by the Basic Science Research Program through the National Research Foundation of Korea (NRF) through a grant funded by the Ministry of Science, ICT and Future Planning (NRF-2014R1A2A2A03003387).

References

1. Karmarkar, U.S., Apte, U.M.: Operations management in the information economy: information products, processes, and chains. J. Oper. Manag. **25**(2), 438–453 (2007)
2. Atzori, L., Iera, A., Morabito, G.: The Internet of Things: a survey. Comput. Netw. **54**(15), 2787–2805 (2010)
3. Lim, C.H., Kim, K.J.: IT-enabled information-intensive services. IT Prof. **17**(2), 26–32 (2015). IEEE
4. Lee, J., Kao, H.A., Yang, S.: Service innovation and smart analytics for industry 4.0 and big data environment. Procedia CIRP **16**, 3–8 (2014)
5. Dounis, A.I., Caraiscos, C.: Advanced control systems engineering for energy and comfort management in a building environment—a review. Renew. Sust. Energ. Rev. **13**(6), 1246–1261 (2009)
6. OECD: ICTs and the Health Sector: Towards Smarter Health and Wellness Models. OECD Publishing (2013)
7. Takacs, J., Pollock, C.L., Guenther, J.R., Bahar, M., Napier, C., Hunt, M.A.: Validation of the fitbit one activity monitor device during treadmill walking. J. Sci. Med. Sport. **17**(5), 496–500 (2014)
8. Saarijärvi, H., Grönroos, C., Kuusela, H.: Reverse use of customer data: implications for service-based business models. J. Serv. Mark. **28**(7), 529–537 (2014)
9. Ostrom, A.L., Parasuraman, A., Bowen, D.E., Patrício, L., Voss, C.A., Lemon, K.: Service research priorities in a rapidly changing context. J. Serv. Res. **18**(2), 127–159 (2015)
10. Lim, C.H., Kim, M.J., Heo, J.Y., Kim, K.J.: Design of informatics-based services in manufacturing industries: case studies using large vehicle-related databases. J. Intell. Manuf. 1–12 (2015) (Online First)
11. Kim, K.J., Lim, C.H., Lee, D.H., Lee, J., Hong, Y.S., Park, K.: A concept generation support system for product-service system development. Serv. Sci. **4**(4), 349–364 (2012)
12. Goldstein, S.M., Johnston, R., Duffy, J., Rao, J.: The service concept: the missing link in service design research? J. Oper. Manag. **20**(2), 121–134 (2002)
13. Sakao, T., Shimomura, Y.: Service engineering: a novel engineering discipline for producers to increase value combining service and product. J. Clean. Prod. **15**(6), 590–604 (2007)
14. Geum, Y., Jeon, H., Lee, H.: Developing new smart services using integrated morphological analysis: integration of the market-pull and technology-push approach. Serv. Bus. 1–25 (2015) (Online First)
15. Huang, M.H., Rust, R.T.: IT-related service a multidisciplinary perspective. J. Serv. Res. **16**(3), 251–258 (2013)
16. Opresnik, D., Taisch, M.: The value of big data in servitization. Int. J. Prod. Econ. **165**, 174–184 (2015)

17. Clark, G., Johnston, R., Shulver, M.: Exploiting the Service Concept for Service Design and Development. New Service Design, pp. 71–91. Sage, Thousand Oaks (2000)
18. Schmenner, R.W.: How can service businesses survive and prosper? MIT Sloan Manag. Rev. **27**, 21–32 (1986)
19. Roth, A.V., Menor, L.J.: Insights into service operations management: a research agenda. Prod. Oper. Manag. **12**(2), 145–163 (2003)
20. Edvardsson, B., Olsson, J.: Key concepts for new service development. Serv. Indus. J. **16**(2), 140–164 (1996)
21. Lim, C.H., Kim, K.J.: Information service blueprint: a service blueprinting framework for information-intensive services. Serv. Sci. **6**(4), 296–312 (2014)
22. Bettencourt, L.A., Ulwick, A.W.: The customer-centered innovation map. Harvard Bus. Rev. **86**(5), 109–114 (2008)

Queuing-Based Processing Platform for Service Delivery in Big Data Environments

Florin Stancu, Dan Popa, Loredana-Marsilia Groza, and Florin Pop[(✉)]

Computer Science Department, Faculty of Automatic Control and Computets,
University Politehnica of Bucharest, Splaiul Independentei 313,
Sector 6, 060042 Bucharest, Romania
{florin.stancu,dan.popa,loredana.groza}@hpc.pub.ro, florin.pop@cs.pub.ro

Abstract. Service Delivery is one of the most important aspects in every nowadays platforms. Big Data and all analytics processes and services are responsible for new models of service delivery. In this paper we propose an architecture based on message queues for communication between various data sources (e.g. sensors) and a central application, providing stability of delivered services in case of faults: if the central application does not work, messages from the sensors will remain unused in queue and be consumed when the application will be back on-line. Implementation was achieved with RabbitMQ. Also, we have proposed a web application that will generate statistics based on a large volume of data. When we add a new filter (that will generate new statistics), considered as a new task, it must be taken up by a scheduler. The interface is able to configure how many such tasks can run in parallel. Finally, we implemented the proposed architecture to support faults and to be scalable.

Keywords: Queuing systems · Batch processing · Real-time processing · Big data processing · Smart cities

1 Introduction

Nowadays batch processing system can handle huge volume of data but this is not enough because many situations impose real-time or near real-time decisions on Big Data and in these cases we realize that Hadoop is not suitable anymore. Smart cities analytics on top of data from city services, water, electricity and gas management, garbage collection, traffic control, weather, pollution, natural disasters prediction, security threats, etc., all need to be processed in real time as data streams in order predict if citizens lives are in danger or if something happens in the city that needs immediate actions from various stakeholders. If the data would not be processed in real time for these systems then we would be in the case that nothing can be done because is too late.

We need analytics for real-time systems, in order to predict events that appear in a matter of minutes and act immediately base on them, practically the time makes the difference. So in this case another paradigm is coming into

© Springer International Publishing Switzerland 2016
T. Borangiu et al. (Eds.): IESS 2016, LNBIP 247, pp. 497–508, 2016.
DOI: 10.1007/978-3-319-32689-4_38

discussion the queuing systems, which are very important regarding the services that need to be done and the costs associated while waiting to be fulfilled.

There are many traditional enterprise messaging systems like the ones described in papers (ActiveMQ [1], Kafka [2], Websphere MQ [3], Oracle Enterprise Messaging Service [4], TIBCO Enterprise Message Service [5] or Web services message broker architecture [6]) and they have an crucial role in processing asynchronous data flows because they represent the way the events are transported from systems to applications. When communicating in a distributed system the messages are queued asynchronously, multiple providers can post them to a queue [7], in our case data comes from multiple sensors and we can have multiple consumers attached to a single queue, so different stakeholders can take actions based on the output of a single queue. The queuing infrastructure comes with benefits like the messages are delivered once, they can be posted in a queue even the consumers are offline, it is scalable and reliable.

Service Delivery is one of the most important aspects in every nowadays platforms. Big Data and all analytics processes and services are responsible for new models of service delivery. Starting with a simple and generic service delivery model we can create complex models based on advanced Big Data processing (collection, aggregation, cleaning, reducing and retrieval) in order to become more agile in the market [8].

This paper presents the design of an architecture based on queuing-based processing model that can receive and store a large amount of data from multiple sensors located in different geographical locations, but also that can perform various scientific workflows. The novelty of the proposed solution is represented by using RabbitMQ message broker [9,10], which was able to receive and deliver more than one million messages per second on Google Compute Engine [11]. We consider several case-studies oriented on smart cities, smart home automation, smart farming, and advanced application for visualization and analysis of national hydro-graphic network.

The main contributions of this paper are as follows:

- we proposed an architecture based on message queues for communication between various data sources (e.g. sensors) and a central application, providing stability in case of faults: if the central application does not work, messages from the sensors will remain unused in queue and be consumed when the application will be back online. Implementation was achieved with RabbitMQ.
- we have proposed a web application that will generate statistics based on a large volume of data; when we add a new filter (that will generate new statistics), considered as a new task, it must be taken up by a scheduler [12]. The interface is able to configure how many such tasks can run in parallel.
- we implemented the proposed architecture to support faults and to be scalable.

The paper is structured as follows. Section 2 presents the related work and the main open issues in the field. Then, in Sect. 3 the system architecture is introduced and the main components are described. Several case studies that can uses the proposed architecture for batch processing with soft real-time constraints. These studies are related to smart cities application, smart home automation, smart farming and advanced application for visualization and analysis of national hydro-graphic network. The experimental results and performance analysis are presented in Sect. 5. The paper ends with conclusions and future works, which are presented in Sect. 6.

2   Related Work

Distributed sensor networks, web and mobile applications require a new kind of data collection and analytics infrastructure that can take care of massive amounts of data. The researchers and also big companies reached to the same conclusion that the best way to get big data processed in real-time is by using a middleware that takes care of message queuing and delivery [13]. In this case the applications and sensors that publish messages in the queues can send data in a simple manner and they dont care anymore where it should go or how it should get there. Everyone works to get more insights from their big data and in order to do that they try to integrate various sources, as many as possible, with different data [14]. Big companies like Yahoo! and Twitter realize that it is not enough to apply analytics on batch systems for the needs they have, so they developed distributed real time data processing platforms: S4 [15], respectively Storm [16], which are scalable, can process continuous streams, are inspired by MapReduce programming paradigm and they use keyed streams.

In [17] was proposed D-Streams which was prototyped in an extension to Spark Streaming, which allows in the same time streaming, batch and interactive queries. The main idea given by D-Streams (discretized streams) is to consider a streaming computation as a series of deterministic batch computations on small time intervals.

As we mentioned in the introduction, sensor-based architecture are the main subject of this paper. Although there is a low level of consensus on what the term *Smart House* should represent, we see its implementation being similar to a living organism. We have sensors that represent the sensory receptors of the body, actuators that represent the muscles, controllers that represent the brain. Recent studies confirm that an important part of Domotics is the research for a low-energy, low-cost and an efficient network design [18] that will act as the backbone for all the sensors and actuators used in a home automation and ambient assisted living [19,20].

Gomez *et al.* in [21] does an exhaustive survey of current architectures and technologies that can be used in home automation systems. When we think of the concept of *Internet of Things (IoT)* we believe that any architecture or technology used in home automation must be in some way interoperable with the Internet. This survey showed us that out of the existing and relevant technologies on the market only 6LoWPAN [22] can be directly connected to a rooter and to the Internet. We believe that one of the most important factor in a successful home automation solution is knowing the residents that will interact with the automated house. For this to be achieved a wireless body area network (WBAN) [23] can be used. A network composed of sensors placed on the body that will provide ubiquitous information to the automation system.

A broad range of applications exists in the field of home automation. In his paper [24], Hargreaves analysed data gathered from 4 homes that were involved in a home automation field trial. The analysis concluded that the residents of those 4 houses used the home automation technology to improve their house energy efficiency or to enhance the house security. Applications like Vera^{TM} Z-Wave [25] systems were used for improving the electricity usage or RWE Smarthome^{TM} systems for monitoring and home security. Gill *et al.* showed us in his paper [26] a home automation architecture based on ZigBee [27] hardware where they managed to create interoperability between ZigBee and WiFi (and the Internet respectively) using a PC as a bridge between a ZigBee controller and a WiFi router.

A recent study by Ghaffarian Hoseini *et al.* [28] shows that although the term *Smart House* was something that represented the future, it is in fact more connected to the present as we start to see more and more smart houses being part of our lives. Although right now smart houses adapts and embeds ICT applications they will have to ultimately be build as systems adaptable to their residents needs and will have to be part of intelligent buildings or smart cities.

3   System Architecture

We built a system that can receive and store a large amount of data from multiple sensors located in different geographical locations, but also that can perform various scientific workflows. If we try to simplify this problem, we can view it like the problem of producers and consumers, with the number of producers (sensors) much greater than the consumers [29]. Another important thing is that the producer is more fast than the consumer and we can not afford to lose data.

Adding a new sensor in the system should be done relatively easily and it does not need to know more than the endpoint where it must send the data and a unique key so we can identify the sensor. Starting from this premise we thought that between producers and consumers must exist another layer of abstraction, a message broker server. Using this server we can achieve asynchronous messaging between the sensors and the central application. We chose RabbitMQ (http://www.rabbitmq.com) for this job because it can be clustered, is open source, runs on all major operating systems and supports many programming languages. The sensor should know only the name of the queue where it should send the data and a the key that is generated by the web portal when the sensor is register. Base on this key the system associates data with the sensor (Fig. 1).

The message broker between producers and consumers also make the system to be fault-tolerant. If the central application that should store and process the data is not working properly, the data will remain unused in queue until the problem is solved. The messages on this queue will be sent in the order in which they came. If a node stops working when processing data, the message broker will

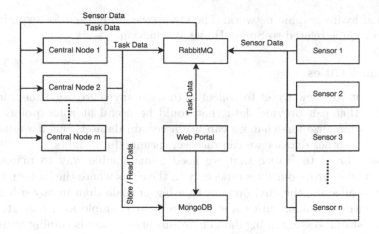

Fig. 1. System architecture.

try to send the data to another node. All those things are made automatically by RabbitMQ.

The data is stored on a NoSQL database because we have a large volume of data without a fixed structure. We chose MongoDB (https://www.mongodb.org), a key-value database system that scales well horizontally. The scaling is achieve by the "sharding" technique, the process of writing the data on multiple servers to distribute the work and storage.

Until now we have a RabbitMQ server that can be clustered, a database that distribute the data on multiple servers for scaling - the only thing left to do is to run the central application on different machines and create a protocol to be able to process data. This central application is more like a micro-service that can only do certain tasks: store the data from a particular sensor, perform some scientific work on a set of data, split a task to multiple tasks or it can merge the result of multiple tasks.

When a sensor data come in our system, the RabbitMQ server can send a message with this data to a free node or it can keep the data until we have one free. There will be cases when a new data will generate the recalculation of some reports. To cover this scenario, the nodes should be able to send tasks to another nodes. We can achieve this using a special queue for tasks in RabbitMQ. Every time we have a task, we send it on RabbitMQ queue and from here will be redirected to a free node.

We can also create tasks using the web portal. This portal is deployed on a single machine because it does not use any computational intensive code.

4   Case Studies

We consider several case-studies oriented on smart cities, smart home automation, smart farming, and advanced application for visualization and analysis of national hydro-graphic network. The main case study used for experimental demonstration is related to Smart Home automation.

4.1 Smart Cities

Nowadays, it is a new trend to collect data from anywhere, anytime and from everything that can provide data that could be useful at some point. Sometime we dont realize for what we can use a certain dataset, but if we use it in correlation to other dataset we can discover meaningful insights.

People started to realize that we need a sustainable way to manage our resources and improve our lives especially in the cities where the footprint of the activities is affecting the environment to a bigger scale than in any other parts of the countries. Making cities smarter is a great example as a case study for real time data processing in big data environments because is coming with many challenges like security, the right data, in the right time, analysis of huge volumes of machine-generated data in real time [30,31]. Lately, stream computing became the fastest and most efficient solution to obtain insights from big data.

Technology has the power to transform the transportation services by using real time data and batch data. We can reduce traffic congestions, influence citizens decisions related to which paths should take but the most important we should return the city to pedestrians, to people that use bicycles every day and to the one that use public transportation because they care about the environment, we should think to build green infrastructure which uses renewable energy in order to reduce pollution.

When we think to sustainability we should think to urban planning and management in such a way that problems given by population growth and resource constraints should be solved using a new urban model, where the public spaces, green areas and city services are merged together. In order to build a smart city many stakeholders should involve and collaborate to provide a platform that could for real bring efficiency and better lives. Interoperability is a key factor and we need it to be able to integrate data produced by many sources, in order to optimize the urban services and bring value to citizens. Technology, but especially real time data processing can help up to create smarter cities. One important application is analyzing events and anomalies in indoor air quality [32].

Take as an example the IBM City Heartbeat which provides insights of the city using a set of indicators, but in the same time is showing the location of events in real time. IBM helps a mayor to know what is happening in the city in real time, how to make the right choice. Practically he needs to know all about the city regarding security, safety, citizen sentiments related to different actions, transportation, water management, buildings management, and all this should be presented in a simple manner to avoid losing time in critical situations or when fast access is needed to get the appropriate data and to inform the structure that should handle a particular situation. Most of the time the data is there but it is dispersed on many systems which is highly un-efficient when you trying to get an overview of the city.

The data, on which we apply analytics, predictions, and cognitive computing make from this application a great tool for decision makers and help them to take the right actions in real time, and provides the opportunity to take advantage from data at the right moment.

4.2   Smart Home Automation

Smart House recently became a part of our present through the improvement of current technology [28]. A *Smart House* is usually made "smart" through the installation of home automation systems. This type of systems are designed to control the house environment and interact with its residents for the sole purpose of improving the quality of life for its residents. Home automation systems are usually composed out of five device categories

- Sensors - small devices that reads data from the environment and transmits it to the system;
- Actuators - execution devices that take action and interacts and modify the environment;
- Controllers - contains the algorithms that reads data from the sensors and based on that data they control the actuators.
- Human interfaces - devices that facilitate the human to machine communication;
- Networks   the protocol used for data communication between sensors, actuators, controllers and human interfaces.

Although all parts of an automation system are important, the part that will make the difference on how efficient an automation system is on energy consumption and quality of life improvement is the **Controller**. We focus on controllers governed by machine learning (ML) algorithms as this kind of controllers have the ability to adapt based on the environment they control. Before we could successfully use a ML algorithm to control the environment, we will have to put the algorithm through a learning process using some predefined models.

To simulate data coming from a sensor we will have to start from the mathematical model of the process where the sensor reads its data from. In consequence if we want to simulate a sensor that reads the temperature from a room we will have to deduct the mathematical model of the temperature for that room. The same procedure we will have to apply also when simulating sensor data for humidity and CO_2 concentration.

Temperature sensor simulation. For the temperature simulation we will use in our paper the process-driven approach to obtain the model of the room when controlling the temperature [33].

We start from the heat balance equation: $\Delta E = Q - U$, where the energy supplied to the system Q can be split into two different components:

1. Energy exchange between the room (our system) and the heater/cooler (our actuator) trough convection

$$\frac{dQ}{dt} = hA\Delta T \tag{1}$$

2. Heat exchange between the room and exterior environment trough conduction

$$\frac{dQ}{dt} = kA\frac{\Delta T}{\Delta x} = kA\frac{T_h - T_l}{l} \tag{2}$$

Using the first law of thermodynamics and replacing the heat exchange rate from Eqs. (2) and (1) we obtain the state equation for our system:

$$\dot{x} = \left(\frac{hA}{C} - \frac{kA}{Cl}\right) + \begin{bmatrix} \frac{hA}{C} & \frac{kA}{Cl} \end{bmatrix} \begin{bmatrix} u_1 \\ u_2 \end{bmatrix} \tag{3}$$
$$y = x$$

The discrete state equation of (3) can be used to generate the exact system response, and use it for generation of large data quantities that is usually needed in the learning phase of empiric control algorithms.

Humidity sensor simulation. The same principle can be applied for humidity when using a process-driven approach for obtaining the system equations.
We start by applying the mass balance principle:

$$V\frac{dx}{dt} = f_{HUM}(x_{HUM} - x) + \frac{n}{\rho_a}p \tag{4}$$

From Eq. (4) we can obtain the transfer function for our system by approximating it with a first order plus dead-time system [34]:

$$P(s) = \frac{1}{\frac{V}{f_{HUM}}s + 1}e^{-\frac{L_0}{f_{HUM}}s} \tag{5}$$

The discrete transfer function obtained from Eq. (5) can be used to generate the system response for humidity and used in the learning phase of empiric control algorithms.

CO_2 sensor simulation. When simulating the CO_2 concentration in a room a simple equation can be used as determined by Lachapelle *et al.* in [35]:

$$u(k) = \frac{G \cdot 10^6 \cdot P_z + \frac{V}{\Delta T}u(k-1) + V_{sa}C_{sa}}{\frac{V}{\Delta T} + V_{sa}} \tag{6}$$

where: G is CO_2 generation rate per person (L/s), P_z is number of occupants, V is volume of the room (L), ΔT is time step (s), V_{sa} is air flow rate (L/s), C_{sa} is supply air duct (*ppm* - parts per million), $u(k)$ is current CO_2 level (*ppm*), $u(k-1)$ is previous CO_2 level (*ppm*). The Eq. (6) can be used to simulate a system model for CO_2 concentration.

4.3   Smart Farming

The management of large farms are done by intelligent, integrated, cloud services-based systems, using advanced computer technology, automation and communications to increase product quality and business development in the area of farming. The integrated system for controlling the process in greenhouse crop production, using the services available on mobile devices requires queuing based system for messages processing services. The services also offer simple and cheap integration of the existing infrastructure in various types of companies involved in agriculture. In this case the processing platform is an intelligent system designed to increase the quality of the greenhouse grown products and to support the development of businesses in domains related to agriculture, based on cutting-edge IT&C technologies. Its components are: information infrastructure; the data acquisition subsystem; and sub-system for intervention in process (turning on/off water sources, adjusting temperature, etc.).

4.4   Advanced Application for Visualization and Analysis of National Hydro-Graphic Network

Water is an essential, limited and sensitive life resource, and it is in focus of various persons or groups, from simple citizens to decision persons at country/world level, and, of course, also of scientists from different research fields. Our current research activities in the water management field are focused on the water-energy nexus by addressing both energy and water consumption reduction. Reduction of energy consumed in relation to water processing is addressed by current researches, benefiting from IT support, dealing with several challenges like: energy recovery, demand forecasting and management, leakage detection and localization, reuse and cascaded use of water. Reduction of water consumption is a broad issue that includes improving the management of the water distribution network in order to reduce non-revenue water and reducing water consumed by customers (demand management), by taking into account several parameters: availability of water resources, changing demands, current state of the distribution network, energy consumption required. To achieve this, end-user awareness has to be increased and their behaviour has to be influenced by ensuring near real-time metering of WDN (Water Distribution Network) and real-time metering of households as well as collection of contextual information. In this context, visualization and analysis applications require a processing platform based on queues to support WDNs.

5   Experimental Results and Performance Analysis

RabbitMQ is a powerfull message broker. On an experiment [36] made by Google and Pivotal we can see the ability of this engine to receive and deliver more than one million messages per second. Unfortunately we didn't had the power of Google Compute Engine while testing the system but with our resources we delivered almost 1000 messages per seconds using 4 machines with 1 GB ram and 2 core processor. In Fig. 2 we can observe that if we increase the number of the central nodes, the number of delivered messages grow up. Each node has been set to receive up to 10 messages simultaneously. We observe that the system scale very well horizontally. Due to the status of the project, we tested only how many messages the system can handle, without a hard processing of them.

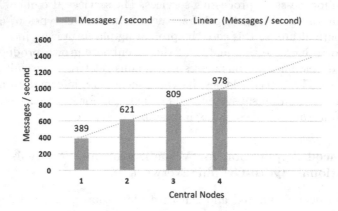

Fig. 2. Delivered messages.

6   Conclusions

We presented in this paper a system that can receive and store a large amount of data from multiple sensors located in different geographical locations. We described several scenarios focusing on smart house sensors simulation. Messages processing in a queuing-based platforms represents the direct way for service delivery for any Big Data platform. The proposed solution provides stability in case of faults and scalability regarding the number of processed messages per second. As future work, we will extend the proposed model with a formal modeling and validation and we will extend the systems to may other scenarios.

Acknowledgment. The research presented in this paper is supported by projects: *DataWay*: Real-time Data Processing Platform for Smart Cities: Making sense of Big Data - PN-II-RU-TE-2014-4-2731; *CyberWater* grant of the Romanian National Authority for Scientific Research, UEFISCDI, project 47/2012; *clueFarm*: Information system based on cloud services accessible through mobile devices, to increase product quality and business development farms - PN-II-PT-PCCA-2013-4-0870.

We would like to thank the reviewers for their time and expertise, constructive comments and valuable insight.

References

1. Snyder, B., Bosnanac, D., Davies, R.: ActiveMQ in Action. Manning (2011)
2. Kreps, J., Narkhede, N., Rao, J., et al.: Kafka: a distributed messaging system for log processing. In: Proceedings of the NetDB, pp. 1–7 (2011)
3. Lampkin, V., Leong, W.T., Olivera, L., Rawat, S., Subrahmanyam, N., Xiang, R., Kallas, G., Krishna, N., Fassmann, S., Keen, M., et al.: Building Smarter Planet Solutions with mqtt and IBM Websphere MQ Telemetry. IBM Redbooks (2012)
4. Krafzig, D., Banke, K., Slama, D.: Enterprise SOA: Service-Oriented Architecture Best Practices. Prentice Hall Professional, Upper Saddle River (2005)
5. Hohpe, G., Woolf, B.: Enterprise Integration Patterns: Designing, Building, and Deploying Messaging Solutions. Addison-Wesley Professional, Upper Saddle River (2004)
6. Brydon, S.P., Singh, I.: Web services message broker architecture. US Patent 7, pp. 702–724, 20 April 2010
7. Fiosina, J., Fiosins, M.: Resampling based modelling of individual routing preferences in a distributed traffic network. Int. J. Artif. Intell. **12**(1), 79–103 (2014)
8. Demirkan, H., Delen, D.: Leveraging the capabilities of service-oriented decision support systems: putting analytics and big data in cloud. Decis. Support Syst. **55**(1), 412–421 (2013)
9. Videla, A., Williams, J.: Rabbitmq in action: distributed messaging for everyone. Rabbit MQ in action (2012)
10. Dossot, D.: RabbitMQ Essentials. Packt Publishing Ltd (2014)
11. Krishnan, S., Gonzalez, J.L.U.: Google compute engine. In: Building Your Next Big Thing with Google Cloud Platform, pp. 53–81. Springer (2015)
12. Vasile, M.A., Pop, F., Tutueanu, R.I., Cristea, V., Kolodziej, J.: Resource-aware hybrid scheduling algorithm in heterogeneous distributed computing. Future Gener. Comput. Syst. **51**(C), 61–71 (2015)
13. Makpaisit, P., Marurngsith, W.: Griffon-gpu programming apis for scientific and general purpose computing (extended version). Int. J. Artif. Intell. **8**(S12), 223–238 (2012)
14. Costa, Â., Novais, P.: Mobile sensor systems on outpatients. Int. J. Artif. Intell. **8**(S12), 252–268 (2012)
15. Neumeyer, L., Robbins, B., Nair, A., Kesari, A.: S4: distributed stream computing platform. In: Proceedings of the 2010 IEEE International Conference on Data Mining Workshops. ICDMW 2010, pp. 170–177. IEEE, Washington, DC (2010)
16. Toshniwal, A., Taneja, S., Shukla, A., Ramasamy, K., Patel, J.M., Kulkarni, S., Jackson, J., Gade, K., Fu, M., Donham, J., Bhagat, N., Mittal, S., Ryaboy, D.: Storm@twitter. In: Proceedings of the 2014 ACM SIGMOD International Conference on Management of Data. SIGMOD 2014, USA, pp. 147–156. ACM (2014)
17. Zaharia, M., Das, T., Li, H., Shenker, S., Stoica, I.: Discretized streams: an efficient and fault-tolerant model for stream processing on large clusters. In: Proceedings of the 4th USENIX conference on Hot Topics in Cloud Ccomputing, p. 10. USENIX Association (2012)
18. Sun, Q., Yu, W., Kochurov, N., Hao, Q., Hu, F.: A multi-agent-based intelligent sensor and actuator network design for smart house and home automation. J. Sens. Actuator Netw. **2**(3), 557–588 (2013)
19. Oliveira, T.J.M., Costa, Â., Neves, J., Novais, P.: A comprehensive clinical guideline model and a reasoning mechanism for aal systems. Int. J. Artif. Intell. **11**(A13), 57–73 (2013)

20. Benazzouz, Y., Chikhaoui, B., Abdulrazak, B.: An argumentation based approach for dynamic service composition in ambient intelligence environments. Int. J. Artif. Intell. 4(S10), 137–152 (2010)

21. Gomez, C., Paradells, J.: Wireless home automation networks: a survey of architectures and technologies. IEEE Comm. Mag. 48(6), 92–101 (2010)

22. Shelby, Z., Bormann, C.: 6LoWPAN: The Wireless Embedded Internet. John Wiley & Sons, New York (2011)

23. Cao, H., Leung, V., Chow, C., Chan, H.: Enabling technologies for wireless body area networks: a survey and outlook. IEEE Comm. Mag. 47(12), 84–93 (2009)

24. Hargreaves, T., Hauxwell-Baldwin, R., Coleman, M., Wilson, C., Stankovic, L., Stankovic, V., Murray, D., Liao, J., Kane, T., Firth, S., et al.: Smart homes, control and energy management: how do smart home technologies influence control over energy use and domestic life? European Council for an Energy Efficient Economy (ECEEE) 2015 Summer Study Proceedings, pp. 1022–1032 (2015)

25. Johansen, N.T.: Z-wave protocol overview (zensys), document no. sds 10243 (2006)

26. Gill, K., Yang, S.H., Yao, F., Lu, X.: A zigbee-based home automation system. IEEE Trans. Consum. Electron. 55(2), 422–430 (2009)

27. Alliance, Z.: ZigBee Home Automation Public Application Profile (2007)

28. Ghaffarian Hoseini, A.H., Dahlan, N.D., Berardi, U., Ghaffarian Hoseini, A., Makaremi, N.: The essence of future smart houses: From embedding ict to adapting to sustainability principles. Renewable and Sustainable Energy Reviews 24, 593–607 (2013)

29. Bessis, N., Sotiriadis, S., Pop, F., Cristea, V.: Optimizing the energy efficiency of message exchanging for service distribution in interoperable infrastructures. In: 2012 4th International Conference on Intelligent Networking and Collaborative Systems (INCoS), pp. 105–112. IEEE (2012)

30. Dragoicea, M., Patrascu, M., Serea, G.A.: Real time agent based simulation for smart city emergency protocols. In: 2014 18th International Conference on System Theory, Control and Computing (ICSTCC), pp. 187–192. IEEE (2014)

31. Patrascu, M., Dragoicea, M., Ion, A.: Emergent intelligence in agents: a scalable architecture for smart cities. In: 2014 18th International Conference on System Theory, Control and Computing (ICSTCC), pp. 181–186. IEEE (2014)

32. Skön, J.P., Johansson, M., Raatikainen, M., Haverinen-Shaughnessy, U., Pasanen, P., Leiviskä, K., Kolehmainen, M.: Analysing events and anomalies in indoor air quality using self-organizing maps. Int. J. of Artif. Intell. 9(A12), 79–89 (2012)

33. Ellis, C., Hazas, M., Scott, J.: Matchstick: A room-to-room thermal model for predicting indoor temperature from wireless sensor data. In: Proceedings of the 12th International Conference on Information processing in Sensor Networks, pp. 31–42. ACM (2013)

34. Yamazaki, T., Kamimura, K., Kurosu, S., Yamakawa, Y.: Air-conditioning PID control system with adjustable reset to offset thermal loads upsets. In: Yurkevich, V.D., (Ed.) Advances in PID Control, InTech.INTECH (2011)

35. Lachapelle, A.C., Love, J.A.: Simulink® model of single co2 sensor location impact on CO2 levels in recirculating multiple-zone systems. In: Proceedings of eSim 2012: The Canadian Conference on Building Simulation, ESIM.CA, pp. 189–201 (2012)

36. Kuch, J.: Rabbitmq hits one million messages per second on google compute engine, point of view (2014). https://blog.pivotal.io/pivotal/products/rabbitmq-hits-one-million-messages-per-second-on-google-compute-engine

A Service-Oriented Framework for Big Data-Driven Knowledge Management Systems

Thang Le Dinh[1(✉)], Thuong-Cang Phan[1], Trung Bui[2],
and Manh Chien Vu[1]

[1] Research and Intervention Laboratory on Business Development in
Developing Countries, Université du Québec à Trois-Rivières, C.P 500,
Trois-Rivières, QC G9A 5H7, Canada
{Thang.Ledinh,Thuong-Cang.Phan,Manh.Chien.Vu}@uqtr.ca
[2] Adobe Research, Adobe Systems Incorporated,
San Jose, CA 95110-2704, USA
Bui@adobe.com

Abstract. Enterprises nowadays are intensifying their efforts to create value through big data initiatives as well as knowledge management systems to outperform their competitors. Big data is considered as a revolution that transforms traditional enterprises into Data-Driven Organizations (DDOs) in which knowledge discovered from big data will be integrated into traditional organizational knowledge to improve decision-making and to facilitate organizational learning. This paper proposes a service-oriented framework for designing a new generation of big data-driven knowledge management systems to help enterprises to promote knowledge development and to obtain more business value from big data. The key artefacts of the framework are presented based on design science research, including constructs, model, and method. The objective of the framework is to promote both knowledge exploration and knowledge exploitation that need to take place simultaneously in DDOs.

Keywords: Big data analytics · Knowledge management system · Service-oriented · Design science research

1 Introduction

In the knowledge-based economy, the use of Information and Communication Technologies (ICT) for creation, management, dissemination and exploitation of organizational knowledge is extremely critical because knowledge is a vital factor for managers in modern and networked organizations [1].

Big data is a popular term used to describe the exponential growth and availability of data, both structured and unstructured from traditional and new digital sources inside and outside enterprises [8]. In order to transform big data into organizational knowledge, a new generation of knowledge management systems (KMSs) is required to enable insight discovery and to promote organizational learning [9]. Big data is considered as a revolution that drifts toward data-driven discovery and decision-making [10]. This revolution transforms traditional enterprises into a new generation of

© Springer International Publishing Switzerland 2016
T. Borangiu et al. (Eds.): IESS 2016, LNBIP 247, pp. 509–521, 2016.
DOI: 10.1007/978-3-319-32689-4_39

knowledge-intensive enterprises: *Data-Driven Organizations* (DDOs) in which managers can translate knowledge discovered from big data into organizational knowledge to improve decision-making and enterprise performance [11].

This paper proposes a service-oriented framework for designing a new generation of big data-driven KMSs to help enterprises to promote knowledge development and to obtain more business value from big data. The paper is organized as follows. Section 2 describes the theoretical background and the related work. Section 3 introduces the research design. Section 4 proposes the fundamental of the framework based on design science research, including the constructs, model, and method. Section 5 presents an illustrative example of the framework. Section 6 ends the paper with the conclusions and future work.

2 Background

Knowledge is defined as 'information possessed in the mind of individuals related to facts, procedures, concepts, interpretations, ideas, observations, and judgments' [2]. Based on the knowledge-component classification, there are different types of *knowledge components* such as know-what (declarative), know-how (procedural), know-why (causal), and know-who (possessive) [3, 4].

Knowledge Management is considered as "...the art of performing knowledge actions such as organizing, blocking, filtering, storing, gathering, sharing, disseminating, and using knowledge objects..." [5]. *Organizational Knowledge* is the capability of members of an organization that have developed to draw distinctions in the process of carrying out their work, in particular, and concrete contexts, by enacting sets of generalizations whose application depends on historically evolved collective understandings [6]. Enterprises require having an effective knowledge management system that renders them more competitive [2]. Knowledge-intensive enterprises offer to the market the use of sophisticated knowledge or knowledge-based products and services [7]. DDOs are a specific type of knowledge-intensive enterprises in which knowledge captured from big data needs to be integrated with traditional knowledge to promote both knowledge exploration as well as knowledge exploitation.

Through *Knowledge Management Systems* (KMSs), enterprises are not only collecting and storing large amounts of knowledge, but also they are using it to develop intellectual capital, to improve customers' experiences, and to make better business decisions [2]. KMSs nowadays are being confronted with a variety and unprecedented amount of data, resulting from different business and ICT-based services, called "*big data*". Big data, which is high volume, velocity, or variety information assets or all, provides a new source of knowledge about the business environment. Therefore, big data is considered a challenge but also an opportunity for enterprises. In order to integrate knowledge extracted from big data into organizational knowledge, there are several studies that separately concentrated on specific aspects such as knowledge management, business intelligence and business analytics [11], data mining and knowledge discovery [12, 13]. However, most enterprises spend more time, money and effort to build and manage their big data infrastructure than to create applications that solve their own business problems [9]. In other words, current applications of big data concentrate on knowledge exploration, but have not been fully supported knowledge exploitation yet.

In addition, the emerge of service science has directed KMSs research towards service-based knowledge management systems [14–17]. In our observation, there is still a little effort to study both the trends in service orientation and in big data in order to promote the whole process of organizational knowledge management, including knowledge exploration and knowledge exploitation [18].

Consequently, we propose a novel service-oriented framework for designing big data-driven KMSs. The new generation of KMSs forms the knowledge infrastructure [5] of a DDO that supports different activities in the knowledge development process in order to provide a unified way of working, learning and innovating in the big data era. This framework is fundamental for DDOs, in which both knowledge exploration and exploitation need to take place simultaneously [18]. The framework helps DDOs to create more business value by discovering more knowledge, obtaining more customer/user experience, and making more accurate business decisions.

3   Research Design

The main research question of this study is *"How to design a service-oriented knowledge management system for a data-driven organization?"*.

In order to respond to this question, we propose a framework that has two main objectives. Firstly, the framework presents a new viewpoint on knowledge management research by introducing the service orientation as an architectural approach for managing organizational knowledge. Secondly, the framework allows DDOs to capture knowledge discovered from big data and to integrate it with traditional organizational knowledge. Therefore, the proposed framework addresses two major challenges: *Service orientation for organizational knowledge management* [18] and *Unification of organizational knowledge discovered from diverse data sources, including big data.*

The service-oriented framework for designing big data-driven KMSs, hereafter called the SO-KMS (service-oriented knowledge management system) framework, aims at providing a knowledge infrastructure to support the knowledge development process in a data-driven organization. The specification of the framework (Table 1) is based on the principles of design science research, including artefacts such as constructs, model, method, and instantiations [19].

Table 1. Artefacts of the SO-KMS framework.

Artefact	Description
Constructs	Different types of concepts related to knowledge objects in a data-driven organization and its business environment.
Model	A set of statements expressing the relationships between knowledge objects at different levels in the knowledge base.
Method	A set of activities that supports the process of knowledge development.
Instantiations	Best practices related to the operationalization of the framework.

4 Service-Oriented Framework for Designing Big Data-Driven KMSs

This section presents the key artefacts of the framework, including the constructs, model and method. The instantiations will be developed in our future work based the validation and experimentation of the framework with real-world applications [25].

4.1 Framework Constructs

The *constructs* of the framework are based on the existing typologies of knowledge for knowledge creation [20] and knowledge components for knowledge organization [3, 4]. The knowledge infrastructure for a DDO is composed of different knowledge components that are used to represent knowledge objects and to form the semantic context of knowledge creation.

In our approach, knowledge is constituted from objects, called *knowledge objects*. These knowledge objects are classified based on their level of development such as data, information, knowledge or wisdom [48]. In addition, the knowledge development process covers organizational activities in an organization that promotes the learning process and develops the intellectual capital. The main activities of this process are knowledge capture, knowledge organization, knowledge transfer and knowledge application [4].

Concerning the development view, a knowledge object is a highly structured, interrelated set of data, information, knowledge, and wisdom (Fig. 1). In our approach, we prefer the term "understanding" instead of "wisdom" [18] because our research just focuses on the first level of understanding. At this level, enterprises understand how to create or increase values by using their knowledge and knowing [26]. A knowledge object may concern some organizational, management or leadership situation and provides a viable approach for dealing with that situation [48]. Concerning the structure view, a knowledge object is constructed based on a set of knowledge components such as know-what, know-how, know-who and know-why. Organizational knowledge could be explicit knowledge or tacit knowledge, individual or collective [18]. Systems and people can use and share organizational knowledge of knowledge objects by using different knowledge conversion processes such as socialization, externalization, combination and internalization [20].

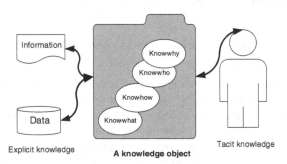

Fig. 1. A knowledge object.

Knowledge development process supports both knowledge exploration and knowledge exploitation. The *knowledge exploration* creates and stores knowledge through individual's cognitive processes (tacit knowledge) or collaboration processes (explicit knowledge) [2, 20]. The *knowledge exploitation* enhances the intellectual capital of an enterprise with existing knowledge in the knowledge base [23]. The process of knowledge exploration, including *knowledge capture* and *knowledge organization*, concerns the capture and organization of different knowledge (tacit and explicit) in the organization memory. The process of knowledge exploitation, including *knowledge sharing* and *knowledge application*, concerns the transfer and application of classified and organized explicit knowledge in the knowledge base.

4.2   Framework Model

The *model* of the framework is based on four aspects of knowledge that forms the knowledge structure of a DDO: structure, transition, possession, and governance [4]. The structure of knowledge is represented by know-what that describes knowledge artefacts known and related to a phenomenon of interest [3]. The transition of knowledge is represented by know-how that describes the understanding of the generative processes constituting phenomena [3]. The possession of knowledge is represented by know-who that refers to individuals, groups, or organizations that work on knowledge objects [4]. The governance of knowledge is represented by know-why that describes the understanding of principles of the underlying phenomena [3].

Recently, we have witnessed a rapid progress in a paradigm shift from the object-oriented computing paradigm to the service-oriented paradigm, which aims at structuring enterprises around services [27–29]. Consequently, the model of the framework (Fig. 2), which determines the knowledge infrastructure for a DDO, includes four levels: service-oriented computing (know-what), service-oriented architecture (know-how), service-oriented enterprise (know-who), and service-oriented paradigm (know-why).

Service-Oriented Computing (SOC) is a computing paradigm that utilizes services to process data as the basic constructs to support the rapid and low-cost development of distributed applications in heterogeneous environments [28]. *Service-Oriented Architecture* (SOA) is a design framework for the construction of information systems by "combination of services" to transform data into useful information. *Service-Oriented Enterprise* (SOE) aims at transforming information into organizational knowledge by combining business processes in a horizontal fashion [30, 31]. *Service-Oriented Paradigm* (SOP) aims at improving business services by applying organizational knowledge that is based on the principles of service science, including Service management, Service science, and Service engineering [26, 32].

In addition, the framework model should also match the requirements of the new-generation of KMSs as mentioned before, such as the support of the service-oriented activities, and the unification of knowledge derived from diverse (big) data sources in a DDO. Designing the framework based on service orientation leads to more shareable, reusable, efficient and flexible KMSs. Besides, one of the most

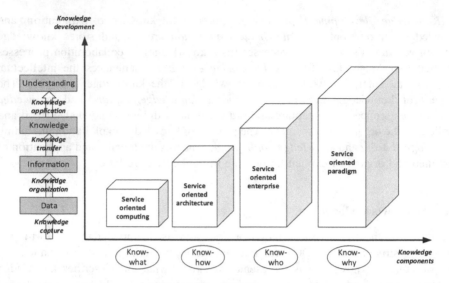

Fig. 2. Framework model.

important characteristics of those KMSs is *big data-driven* that leverages all available data to gain a competitive advantage in the big data era.

An overall architecture of the SO-KMS based KMSs includes four layers: Data Services, Information Services, Knowledge Services, and Business Process layers (Fig. 3).

Business layer, corresponding to the SOP, includes the process representation and provides the structure for aggregating knowledge-intensive services to form a knowledge-intensive process that is aligned with a subset of business goals [7, 26]. A business is now constructed by a flow of knowledge-intensive processes realized by corresponding services. The flow contains the logic for the sequence in which the services need to be invoked and executed. To access a capability provided by a service, a process needs to be aware of the existence of the service. This requirement is generally achieved by executing queries on the service registry or by using other means of service discovery. The business layer finally allows users to develop their service-oriented way of working through supplying a workflow of processes and associating each process with corresponding services in different layers.

Knowledge layer, corresponding to the SOE, provides knowledge services to support processes that are also called *Knowledge-as-a-Service* (KaaS). This layer is a conceptual bridge between *Business layer* and *Information layer*. Its primary work is to transfer the information from *Information layer* into the knowledge based on their semantic contexts. The organizational knowledge of this layer is delivered on request by using different services such as knowledge-based, collaboration, discovery and decision-making services. *Knowledge base service* is a high-level composite service realized by the data migration and analytics services. *Collaboration service* allows the creation, sharing and application of the knowledge from the knowledge base service. *Discovery service* provides functions such as search, retrieval, mining, mapping,

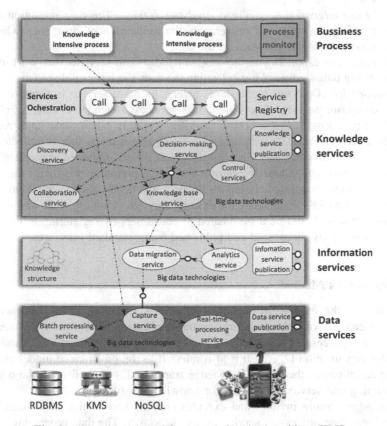

Fig. 3. A service-oriented framework for big data-driven KMSs.

navigation, and presentation of the knowledge from the knowledge base service. *Decision-making service* devises an increased understanding about a business situation, and provides a guideline to make the most effective and strategic business decision. *Control services* ensure the high-quality performance for business processes and their corresponding services. These services are published thanks to a *knowledge service publication*. In addition to the services listed above, a service orchestration enables the layer support different processes by orchestrating existing services. Some of those services are the services of the organization and others of which may be provided by external organizations. A service registry function stores information and specification about all the available services (e.g. service artifacts, description, configuration and policies) to advertise for service clients.

Information layer, corresponding to the SOA, contains information services that carry out isolated business functions, which are also known as *Information-as-a-Service* (IaaS). These services provide a bridge between the higher-level layers and the data layer. They structure and analyze the disorder, disparate and obscure data from data layer into linked, integrated, and organized information. Thus, this information is delivered on demand as a service throughout the organization. The information services consist of *Data migration service* and *Analytics service*. The data migration service manages the data structure and implements the unification of data; meanwhile, the analytics service performs analytics on the data.

Data layer, corresponding to the SOC, includes data services that work directly with diverse big data sources. After collecting the data, the layer publishes the available *Data-as-a-Service* (DaaS) to higher-level layers. Its main service is *Capture service* that is a composite service of two individual services: *Batch processing service* and *Real-time processing service*. Those services capture batch data and real-time streaming data. The batch data is data of existing applications that is collected, processed, and stored in databases. The real-time data is data delivered immediately after the collection from continuous inputs in a short time period or near real time.

Thanks to loose coupling between the services, the layers can be adapted to specific requirements of a DDO by updating the existing services or adding some new ones. All these new services should be disseminated to consumers by registering to the service registry and be easily discovered and published using standard interfaces.

4.3   Framework Method

In this section, the framework method is presented according to its main activities: knowledge capture, organization, transfer and application. The *framework method* is based on the process of knowledge development and organizational learning for knowledge organization [2, 21]. It is also referred to the governance model enhanced from the coordination theory for knowledge transfer [22] as well as to the organizational learning and service innovation for knowledge application [23, 24].

Knowledge capture invokes and executes *capture service* that is realized by the batch and real-time processing services in the data layer. The data processing services then call user-defined functions to collect data from the diverse data sources such as big data, existing KMSs, and traditional information systems. It notes that both the data sources and volume of data collected have exploded for the time being, especially the case of social network data. These sources lead to the formation of new useful information that can be mined to glean insights into organizations, products, services and customers. In contrast, there would be great challenges in capturing, analysing and processing them.

Knowledge organization calls *data migration service* and *analytics service* to receive, unify and analyze the data from *capture service* and then transforms it into semantic information stored in a large-scale distributed knowledge base. In detail, the *data migration service* maps the batch and real-time data from the *capture service* into semantic information stored in the knowledge base, which is organized based on the knowledge structure. Meanwhile, the *analytics service* creates more knowledge for decision-making thanks to analytic tools and techniques used by data scientists, predictive modelers and other analytics professionals. In addition, cluster analysis is used to segment the information into groups based on similar attributes. Once these groups are discovered, organizations can fulfill targeted actions. These capabilities as mentioned above have been untapped by conventional KMSs.

Knowledge transfer invokes and executes the *discovery and collaboration services* to retrieve, transform and infer the semantic information into knowledge that is stored in the knowledge base. The actual knowledge structure is designed once (under the supervision and revision of the designer) and must be updated when the data schema is changed. In contrast, knowledge views in the knowledge base are built on demand. The *discovery service* can incorporate rules and the knowledge views in the design of updatable knowledge views that represent inferred knowledge. The collaboration service provides functions such as discussion, feedback, personal note, comment, and rating to facilitate the collaboration in a DDO.

Knowledge application uses *decision-making services* to create a new application of the knowledge. Moreover, the activity may also communicate the services of external application systems through standard service interfaces. The services of this activity can query the knowledge views, and represent the result in several ways, such as virtual personalized file system views in the form of folder hierarchy, graph views, and array views. Finally, users can use tools to visualize and analyze their query result. Besides, the result can be published on the desktop of the end-user through a knowledge explorer or a web browser.

5 Illustrative Example

The SO-KMS framework is built based on the service orientation that supports loosely coupled services to enable business flexibility in an interoperable and technology-agnostic manner. From the technical perspective, the framework is an application architecture wherein services are defined using a description language with callable interfaces. Those services are implemented in different programming languages to support various knowledge-intensive processes in a DDO.

In order to demonstrate the applicability of the framework, we present an illustrative example based on our on-going project that builds a Customer Knowledge Management System (CKMS) for SMEs (small-and-medium-sized enterprises). The purpose of this application is to construct and leverage a knowledge structure as an ontology to organize information assets efficiently so that they can be used and shared to facilitate the decision-making and organizational learning. We are developing an open-source software prototype based on the current open-source tools and systems for developing big data applications. This prototype can assist DDOs, especially SMEs, to take the benefits of exploring and exploiting business value from their data as well as big data.

At first, Web service technology has been chosen for implementing CKMS because it is the most popular and well-known technology for implementing SOA, both in the industry and academia [33]. The main triad of Web services standards is [34]: WSDL (Web Service Definition Language) for defining the interfaces of the services, SOAP (Simple Object Access Protocol) for invoking the services, and UDDI (Universal Description, Discovery, and Integration) for publishing and querying the registry of services. To specify a knowledge structure, OWL (Web Ontology Language), which is the most powerful of the ontology languages [35], adds a semantic layer to the descriptions of Web services.

The semi-structured and unstructured data sources are not often processed in traditional KMSs and enterprise systems, which are generally based on relational databases. Furthermore, these existing KMSs are not able to handle on sets of big data that are updated frequently or even continuously. In Table 2, we, therefore, investigate emerging open-source big data technologies used for this application to overcome these challenges.

Table 2. List of emerging open-source big data software tools.

Name	Description	Implementation
Apache Hadoop [36]	A large-scale parallel data processing framework across clusters traditionally, used to run MapReduce jobs. It has become dominant in the area of big data processing with large infrastructures being deployed and used in manifold application fields [37, 38].	Capture service, Batch processing service, Data migration service, and analytics service.
Apache Spark [39]	A cluster-computing framework for big data processing. Spark has emerged as the next-generation big data processing engine. It is faster, easier to program, and better to support a variety of computing-intensive tasks [40, 41].	Capture service, Real-time processing service, Data migration service, Analytics service, Knowledge base service, Discovery service, Decision-making service, Control service, and Collaboration service.
Apache Jena Elephas [42]	A set of libraries that provide various basic building blocks to write Hadoop based applications, which work with RDF or OWL data. Jena is a leading Semantic Web programmers' toolkit [43, 44].	All the services of the information and knowledge layers
Apache Hive [45]	A data warehouse software facilitates querying and managing large datasets residing in distributed storage assembled on top of Hadoop. It is widely used for data warehouse systems with Hadoop, and big data analytics applications [46].	Capture service, Data migration service, Analytics service, and Knowledge base service.
Apache Axis2/Java [47]	A Web Services/SOAP/WSDL engine, the successor to the widely used Apache Axis SOAP stack.	All the services of the framework

6   Conclusion

We presented a novel service-oriented framework, called the SO-KMS framework, for designing big data-driven knowledge management systems (KMSs) that aims at providing a knowledge infrastructure to support the knowledge development process in a data-driven organization. The purpose of this approach is to add more business value from big data and to facilitate the whole knowledge development process. According to our knowledge, our approach is one of the first that focuses on unifying big data with knowledge management systems based on the perspective of knowledge structure [18]. Besides, applying the principles of service orientation and big data to knowledge management, we can achieve more agile and flexible KMSs and make knowledge more available, consistent and trustworthy. The approach also enables access to complex, heterogeneous data within organizations and deployment of that information as reusable services. As a result, the framework focuses not only on providing a loosely coupled infrastructure for service enablement, but also effectively designing and managing loosely coupled business processes, which are aggregations of knowledge-intensive services.

With regard to practical and theoretical implications, our approach helps enterprises to unify big data and KMSs to gain a competitive advantage in the big data era. By proving the different categories of knowledge components, the artefacts of our framework can be adapted to some real-world scenarios of innovation and decision-making in which each category of knowledge components could be more or less important. Unifying big data within KMSs following our framework helps practitioners to make better use of their data in traditional information systems and new information assets, and to accumulate organizational knowledge. When an enterprise intends to build its own knowledge infrastructure that covers big data applications and KMSs, the framework provides a starting point for capturing, classifying, integrating and organizing knowledge, and for sharing them within and among organizations through services.

Concerning the future work, the suggested framework could be applied and refined by researchers to improve its generalizability and to broaden its scope. We have stressed on validating the framework in practice, especially to manage knowledge related to customers and the business environment. The open-source customer KMS is currently being built to support customer knowledge management in digital marketing. Furthermore, we continue to complete the instantiations of the framework. Besides, process optimization problems of the framework should also be thoroughly considered.

References

1. Le Dinh, T., Ho Van, T., Moreau, É.: A knowledge management framework for knowledge-intensive SMEs: the NIFO approach. In: Proceedings of the 16th International Conference on Enterprise Information Systems, pp. 435–440. Scitepress, Lisbon, Portugal (2014)
2. Alavi, M., Leidner, D.E.: Review: knowledge management and knowledge management systems: conceptual foundations and research issues. MIS Q. **25**, 107–136 (2001)
3. Garud, R.: On the distinction between know-how, know-why, and know-what. In: Advances in strategic management, pp. 81–101. JAI Press Inc (1997)

4. Le Dinh, T., Rinfret, L., Raymond, L., Dong Thi, B.T.: Towards the reconciliation of knowledge management and e-collaboration systems. Interact. Technol. Smart Educ. **10**, 95–115 (2013)
5. Sivan, Y.Y.: Nine keys to a knowledge infrastructure: a proposed analytic framework for organizational knowledge management. In: WebNet, pp. 495–500 (2000)
6. Tsoukas, H., Vladimirou, E.: What is organizational knowledge? J. Manag. Stud. **38**, 973–993 (2001)
7. Doloreux, D., Shearmur, R.: Collaboration, information and the geography of innovation in knowledge intensive business services. J. Econ. Geogr. **12**, 79–105 (2012)
8. McAfee, A., Brynjolfsson, E.: Big data: the management revolution. Harv. Bus. Rev. **90**(10), 60–68 (2012)
9. Beyer, M.: Gartner says solving "big data" challenge involves more than just managing volumes of data (2011). http://www.gartner.com/newsroom/id/1731916
10. Lohr, S.: The age of big data (2012). http://www.nytimes.com/2012/02/12/sunday-review/big-datas-impact-in-the-world.html
11. Chen, H., Chiang, R.H.L., Storey, V.C.: Business intelligence and analytics: from big data to big impact. MIS Q. **36**, 1165–1188 (2012)
12. Wu, X., Zhu, X., Wu, G.-Q., Ding, W.: Data mining with big data. IEEE Trans. Knowl. Data Eng. **26**, 97–107 (2014)
13. Begoli, E., Horey, J.: Design principles for effective knowledge discovery from big data. In: Joint Working IEEE/IFIP Conference on Software Architecture (WICSA) and European Conference on Software Architecture (ECSA), pp. 215–218 (2012)
14. Woitsch, R., Karagiannis, D.: Process oriented knowledge management: a service based approach. J. UCS **11**, 565–588 (2005)
15. Šaša, A., Krisper, M.: Knowledge management in service-oriented systems. In: Proceedings of the 2010 Conference on Information Modelling and Knowledge Bases XXI. pp. 89–104. IOS Press, Amsterdam (2010)
16. Tsui, E., Cheong, R.K.F., Sabetzadeh, F.: Cloud-based personal knowledge management as a service (PKMaaS). In: 2011 International Conference on Computer Science and Service System (CSSS), pp. 2152–2155 (2011)
17. Abdullah, R., Eri, Z.D., Talib, A.M.: A model of knowledge management system for facilitating knowledge as a service (KaaS) in cloud computing environment. In: 2011 International Conference on Research and Innovation in Information Systems (ICRIIS), pp. 1–4 (2011)
18. Le Dinh, T., Rickenberg, T.A., Fill, H.-G., Breitner, M.H.: Enterprise content management systems as a knowledge infrastructure: the knowledge-based content management framework. Int. J. e-Collab. **11**, 49–70 (2015)
19. Hevner, A.R., March, S.T., Park, J., Ram, S.: Design science in information systems research. MIS Q. **28**, 75–105 (2004)
20. Nonaka, I., Takeuchi, H.: The Knowledge-Creating Company: How Japanese Companies Create the Dynamics of Innovation. Oxford University Press, New York (1995)
21. Spender, J.-C.: Organizational knowledge, collective practice and penrose rents. Int. Bus. Rev. **3**, 353–367 (1994)
22. Malone, T.W., Crowston, K.: The interdisciplinary study of coordination. ACM Comput. Surv. **26**, 87–119 (1994)
23. Choo, C.W., Bontis, N. (eds.): The Strategic Management of Intellectual Capital and Organizational Knowledge. Oxford University Press, New York (2002)
24. Bitner, M.J., Ostrom, A.L., Morgan, F.N.: Service blueprinting: a practical technique for service innovation. Calif. Manage. Rev. **50**, 66–94 (2008)
25. Fan, W., Bifet, A.: Mining big data: current status, and forecast to the future. SIGKDD Explor. Newsl. **14**, 1–5 (2013)

26. Le Dinh, T., Thi, T.T.: Information-driven framework for collaborative business service modelling. Int. J. Serv. Sci. Manage. Eng. Technol. (IJSSMET) 3(1), 1–18 (2012)
27. Erl, T.: Service-Oriented Architecture: Concepts, Technology, and Design. Prentice Hall PTR, Upper Saddle River (2005)
28. Papazoglou, M.P., Traverso, P., Dustdar, S., Leymann, F.: Service-oriented computing: state of the art and research challenges. Computer 40, 38–45 (2007)
29. Yang, X.: Principles, Methodologies, and Service-Oriented Approaches for Cloud Computing. IGI Global, Hershey (2013)
30. Bose, S., Walker, L., Lynch, A.: Impact of service-oriented architecture on enterprise systems, organizational structures, and individuals. IBM Syst. J. 44, 691–708 (2005)
31. Schroth, C.: The service-oriented enterprise. J. Enterp. Archit. 4, 73–80 (2007)
32. Spohrer, J., Maglio, P.P., Bailey, J., Gruhl, D.: Steps toward a science of service systems. Computer 40, 71–77 (2007)
33. Chollet, S., Lalanda, P.: A Model-Driven Approach to Service Composition with Security Properties. Service Life Cycle Tools and Technologies: Methods, Trends and Advances, pp. 154–174. IGI Global (2011)
34. Booth, D., Haas, H., McCabe, F., Newcomer, E.: W3C Working Group Note 11: Web Services Architecture. http://www.w3.org/TR/ws-arch/#stakeholder
35. Sireteanu, N.-A., Sîrbu, C.-F.: Semantic integration of knowledge management systems. In: 10th IBIMA Conference on Innovation and Knowledge Management in Business Globalization, Kuala Lumpur, Malaysia (2008)
36. Apache Hadoop. http://hadoop.apache.org
37. Fotaki, G., Spruit, M., Brinkkemper, S., Meijer, D.: Exploring big data opportunities for online customer segmentation. Int. J. Bus. Intell. Res. 5, 58–75 (2014)
38. Yao, Q., Tian, Y., Li, P.-F., Tian, L.-L., Qian, Y.-M., Li, J.-S.: Design and development of a medical big data processing system based on hadoop. J. Med. Syst. 39, 1–11 (2015)
39. Apache Spark - Lightning-Fast Cluster Computing. https://spark.apache.org
40. Zaharia, M., Das, T., Li, H., Hunter, T., Shenker, S., Stoica, I.: Discretized streams: fault-tolerant streaming computation at scale. In: Proceedings of the Twenty-Fourth ACM Symposium on Operating Systems Principles, pp. 423–438. ACM, New York (2013)
41. Shanahan, J.G., Dai, L.: Large scale distributed data science using apache spark. In: Proceedings of the 21th ACM SIGKDD International Conference on Knowledge Discovery and Data Mining, pp. 2323–2324. ACM, New York (2015)
42. Apache Jena - Apache Jena Elephas. https://jena.apache.org/documentation/hadoop
43. Grobe, M.: RDF, Jena, SparQL and the "semantic web." In: Proceedings of the 37th Annual ACM SIGUCCS Fall Conference: Communication and Collaboration, pp. 131–138. ACM, New York (2009)
44. Wang, H., Zhang, R., Wang, Z.: JenaPro: A distributed file storage engine for jena. In: Proceedings of the Fifth International Joint Conference on Computational Sciences and Optimization, pp. 610–613. IEEE Computer Society, Washington, USA (2012)
45. Apache Hive. https://hive.apache.org
46. Huai, Y., Chauhan, A., Gates, A., Hagleitner, G., Hanson, E.N., O'Malley, O., Pandey, J., Yuan, Y., Lee, R., Zhang, X.: Major technical advancements in apache hive. In: Proceedings of the 2014 ACM SIGMOD International Conference on Management of Data, pp. 1235–1246. ACM, New York (2014)
47. Apache Axis2. http://axis.apache.org/axis2/java/core
48. Bellenger, G.: Creating Knowledge Objects (2004). http://www.systems-thinking.org/cko/guide.htm

Towards a Platform for Prototyping IoT Health Monitoring Services

Mădălina Zamfir[1]([✉]), Vladimir Florian[1], Alexandru Stanciu[1],
Gabriel Neagu[1], Ştefan Preda[1], and Gheorghe Militaru[2]

[1] National Institute for Research and Development in Informatics,
B-dul Averescu 8-10, 011455 Bucharest, Romania
{madalina,vladimir,alex,gneagu,stefanalex}@ici.ro
[2] University Politehnica of Bucharest,
Splaiul Independentei 313, 060042 Bucharest, Romania
gheorghe.militaru@upb.ro

Abstract. The Internet of Things (IoT) is a priority topic for research and innovation in ICT as well as a major trend for its development in the next period. Due to the large variety of IoT based solutions and their economic and social impact, the healthcare is among most relevant application domains to illustrate this trend. The paper presents the main adopted design and development decisions to build a platform for prototyping IoT based assistive applications with health monitoring capabilities. The prototyping approach is expected to improve the quality and speed up the deployment of these interdisciplinary solutions. A special emphasis was put on the platform architecture which is based on an IoT reference model and a reference architecture to take advantage of, and be compliant with relevant solutions in this field. The functional and information views of the platform architecture are detailed and the main development solutions are outlined.

Keywords: IoT · Health monitoring · Prototyping platform · Architecture reference model · Architecture views · IoT services

1 Introduction

In recent years, the Internet of Things (IoT) has been a priority topic for both R&D and Innovation communities. A major advantage of the IoT is the large variety of deployment models, depending on the configuration, location and interaction between their major components [1].

In this context, the efforts focused on providing IoT architectural solutions, either general or domain specific ones, play an important role. Well-conceived reference architectures (RAs) generate significant cost reductions and efficiency in delivering particular architectures, enhanced flexibility and extendibility for systems designed and built in compliance with these solutions [2]. Relevant results were delivered by the EU funded IoT-A project: the IoT Architectural Reference Model (ARM), the derived IoT reference architecture and its implementing guideline [3].

© Springer International Publishing Switzerland 2016
T. Borangiu et al. (Eds.): IESS 2016, LNBIP 247, pp. 522–533, 2016.
DOI: 10.1007/978-3-319-32689-4_40

In healthcare the IoT is anticipated to enable a variety of services, including health monitoring ones like ambient assisted living (an IoT platform powered by artificial intelligence that support people with special needs in their daily routine), Internet of m-health things (IoT based on mobile computing and wearable medical sensors) or embedded gateway configuration (network nodes communicating in the Internet and with other medical equipment) [4].

Implementing an IoT system is an interdisciplinary project. To facilitate and speed up the development of a target system it is reasonable to start from a generic solution that could facilitate its rapid prototyping, with several obvious benefits: improved quality of design solutions, better communication and understanding at the development team level, effective exploitation of former experience and results.

The research objective is a platform for prototyping IoT health monitoring services where the required generic level is implemented through its architectural solution. To derive this solution an architectural model is proposed with the aim to integrate service oriented and event driven paradigms which are relevant for the IoT specificity.

The paper is presents the preliminary results in implementing this approach. The remaining part of the paper is organized as follows: Sect. 2 briefly argues the idea of diversity as specific feature of the IoT area. Section 3 overviews the specificity of the intelligent health monitoring area with the aim to define the functional profile of the IoT platform. Section 4 is devoted to the IoT architectural framework. Reference solutions for the Service Oriented Architecture (SOA) and Event Driven Architecture (EDA) are presented first and their relevant features are emphasized. Then, the proposed IoT ARM capable to integrate these features is described. Section 5 starts with the presentation of the adopted RA which is compatible with ARM and is used to instantiate the IoT platform architecture. Then, the main features of the functional and information views of this architecture are emphasized. Section 6 outlines the major development solutions of the IoT platform. Finally, Sect. 7 formulates some concluding remarks about the reported results and highlights the further research work aiming to use the IoT platform into two concrete projects for health monitoring.

2 Addressing the IoT Diversity

In the IoT European Research Cluster (IERC) view, the IoT is "a concept and a paradigm that considers pervasive presence in the environment of a variety of things/objects that through wireless and wired connections and unique addressing schemes are able to interact with each other and cooperate with other things/objects to create new applications/services and reach common goals" [5]. What makes IoT a strong and extremely disruptive solution is "the combination of a technological push and a human pull for more and ever-increasing connectivity with anything happening in the immediate and wider environment" [3]. This trend is being confirmed at the market level: according to the survey results presented in [6, 7], IT professionals from 17 domains included IoT among their priority initiatives for 2015.

In the case of Healthcare the most impacted field is patient monitoring, where the taxonomy of IoT based services includes: vital parameters monitoring (blood pressure, blood glucose, heart rate, temperature, EKG, weight, and walking pace), body monitoring (intelligent sensors attached to the body), activity monitoring (steps taken, speed, calories burned, rest time), ambient monitoring. In its Hype Cycle for the IoT in 2015, Gartner places wearables on the peak of the hype [8]. According to [9] it is estimated that the use of IoT technologies in human health applications could have an economic impact up to $1.6 trillion globally in 2025.

At the deployment level, the variety of the adopted solutions is generated by IoT devices for remote sensing, actuating and monitoring capabilities; software components installed on IoT devices for accessing, processing and storing sensor information; controller services of these devices to communicate with Web services which links the device level with remaining IoT system components; administration solutions for data generated by the IoT devices; analysis components providing easy to understand results based on sensing data; applications embedding user interface for monitoring and control functions [1]. Data administration facilities may be focused on structured data or may be adapted to Big Data requirements. Similarly, data analysis capabilities may be compliant with data warehouse standards or may include advanced analytics approaches.

Considering this large diversity of approaches in configuring IoT solutions it is not surprising that various initiatives have been launched to coordinate activities in the domain. At the European level, the IERC aims at addressing the large potential for IoT-based capabilities in Europe (http://www.internet-of-things-research.eu/). The Alliance for Internet of Things Innovation has the aim of creating a dynamic European IoT ecosystem which is built on the IERC work, with participation of various IoT players, to support innovation across industries (http://www.aioti.eu/).

3   Intelligent Health Monitoring

Ambient Assisted Living (AAL) provides assistive solutions for people with a wide range of physical, age-related, and cognitive impairments. One major concern of AAL systems is monitoring of health conditions (like chronic illness) in order to provide predictive measures, alarming and reminder services. In order to provide these functionalities AAL systems are relying on sensing technologies embedded in objects, or in the environment or worn by the person. The data gathered by sensors is analyzed to detect activity and infer knowledge about the physical, cognitive, or affective state of the person, recognizing and classifying patterns, detecting trends and unusual or anomalous behavior.

An AAL system is characterized by being connected, context-aware, pervasive, personalized, adaptive and anticipative. Context awareness is the capability of systems and applications to be aware of the occurrence of user activities and of the environment characteristics. A system is context-aware if it can extract, interpret and use context information to adapt its functionality to the current context. In assistive environments, contextual information might refer to user context (e.g., special user requirements, user status and location, etc.), the environment context (e.g., floor plan and existing indoor furniture, outdoor configuration), and the hardware context (e.g., type of body sensors or monitoring devices used, network status, etc.).

Ambient Intelligence (AmI) is a desirable AAL characteristic enabling the system to provide a digital environment that proactively, but sensibly, supports people in their daily lives [10]. Based on AmI and context awareness capabilities, the assistive applications can implement intelligent health monitoring functionalities like: Activity Recognition, Behavioral Pattern Discovery, Anomaly Detection, Planning and Scheduling and also Decision Support. The challenge of such applications lies in dealing with the complexity of capturing, representing and processing contextual data.

The objective of this research is to develop a platform for easy development and delivery of ambient intelligent and context-aware services, as a mean to provide support for the implementation of various assistive applications with health monitoring capabilities.

4 IoT Architectural Framework

IoT devices are unique in that they are focused on physical interfaces, contrasting to desktops and handheld devices, which are primarily focused on human interfaces. Implementing this concept leads to interconnecting a plurality of sensors and the emergence of data transfers between them, in addition to transfers to the upper levels of the system.

Sensor generated data has specific characteristics. By chaining and interconnecting data sources, the capacity to generate data is multiplied, both in volume and in speed. Because the interconnected sensors are very diverse in type and in measured property types, data from sensor networks are also highly heterogeneous. These characteristics entitle the data to be considered as "Big Data".

Real-time streaming sensor data flows constantly and continuously from sources to network. A large amount of these sensor events could be irrelevant or not useful, therefore there might be necessary to be filtered out. For achieving intelligent capabilities, an IoT application system must be able to: analyze and filter sensor data, reason on sensing events, trigger responding actions. Trends, patterns and exceptions must be identified and acted upon immediately, even where the data are arriving from many different sensor types and locations, collection channels and data formats. Consequently, the architecture of an IoT system needs to address many data management capabilities like scalability (adaptability to the exponential increase of traffic and storage requirements), interoperability, reliability and quality of services.

SOA is focusing on implementing synchronous request-response interaction patterns to connect components in distributed systems. EDA is based on an asynchronous message-driven communication model to propagate information throughout the system layers. It is more fitted for describing event processing applications where a higher degree of local autonomy is needed, and does not bind functionally disparate components into the same centralized management model.

In contrast with SOA, where services must be aware of each other before interacting, the components of EDA do not interact directly, so they are not required to be aware of each other. Instead, they constitute event producers and consumers interacting through an intermediary: a publish/subscribe event broker or event manager, an enterprise service bus (ESB), a message/event bus, or business process orchestration engine. Event producers publish notifications of events to the broker. Event consumers subscribe with the broker and receive them as they are published.

A real time service provision platform should combine SOA and EDA function-alities, ensuring that EDA can trigger events as events happen and loosely coupled services can be quickly accessed and queried by the event consumers.

The conceptual model of an event processing system introduced in [11] provides valuable concepts for development of reference architecture. Among them, there are the Event Processing Network (EPN) and the Event Channel (EC). An EPN describes how events received from producers are directed to the consumers through agents/managers that process these events by performing transformation, validation or enrichment. An EC is a mechanism for delivering events or event streams from event producers and event managers to event consumers and other event managers.

In order to provide a separation of concerns needed to facilitate implementing a SOA, the SOA Reference Architecture [12] provides a logical view that groups the various architectural building blocks into several logical layers. The first three layers address the implementation and interface definition of a service. The other layers support the consumption of services. In contrast, the EDA Reference Architecture [13] is flow oriented, depicting the functional elements that compose the event stream processing flow. These are: Event Generators, Event Channels, Event Processing Building Blocks and other Downstream Event driven Activities.

One of the challenges of this research project was to integrate these two archi-tectural views into an actionable IoT architecture.

According to the European Commission group of experts on IoT [14], this domain encompasses an extremely wide range of technologies. It is unlikely that single ref-erence architecture can be developed and used as a blueprint for all possible concrete implementations. In this context, an ARM is conceived as the initial conceptual model of the future system structure that facilitates the evaluation of existing architectural variants and the adoption of the final architectural solution.

A middleware based IoT model comprising five functional layers is presented in [15]. They are: Perception layer (or Device layer), Network layer, Middleware layer (responsible for the management of devices and resources), Application layer (service management layer) and the Business layer, responsible for the management of overall IoT system including the applications and services.

The research in [16] emphasizes the distinction between the "Middleware based" approach and the "Service oriented" approach in structuring a model description.

A comprehensive IoT ARM was proposed by the Architecture Committee of the IoT World Forum (IoTWF), which includes prominent industry leaders [17]. The model is decomposing IoT systems into parts and levels. IoTWF is structured on seven functional levels. Level 1 – Physical devices and their controllers: includes intelligent edge nodes that can be queried and/or controlled. Level 2 – Connectivity: provides communications and connectivity capabilities, including the management of IP-less legacy devices and translation between protocols. Level 3 – Edge (Fog) Computing: it is based on the fog computing principle (information processing is done as early and as close to the edge of the network as possible). Data flows are converted into information suitable for storage and higher level processing. Level 4 – Data Accumulation: converts data in motion to static data ("at rest"). It bridges the differences between the real-time, event-driven components and the query based data consumption and processing. It also determines if data must be combined with other sources, what data should be persisted and what type of storage is needed. Level 5 – Data Abstraction: supports data representation and rendering at enterprise or even global scale. It requires different storage systems, possible clustered and/or distributed, adapted for IoT device data alongside with enterprise and legacy data. Level 6 – Application level: components on this level interact only with data at rest on Levels 4 and 5. Domain specific application services like monitoring, control, analytics and reporting are provided on this level. Level 7 – Collaboration and processes: integrates the business logic and user interaction with the applications.

The architecture reference model elaborated within this research project is presented in Fig. 1. It draws from the previously cited ones and is aiming to integrate the service oriented approach with the event-driven architecture in order to better respond to the requirements of Big Data real time stream processing and analysis (mining and deep learning).

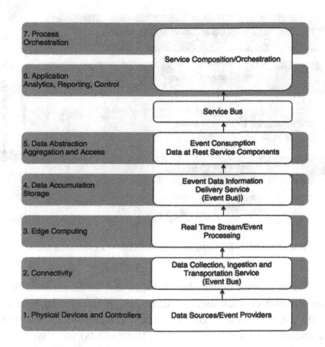

Fig. 1. The IoT architecture reference model

5 IoT Platform Architecture

5.1 Adopted Reference Architecture

There is a broad consensus regarding the advantages generated by using RA as starting point to instantiate a complex system particular architecture: it encapsulates best practices filtered from many previously developed solutions, provides a common framework for designing new consistent solutions, helps in improving quality and reducing risks in the solution development cycle [2]. Therefore the first step in designing the IoT platform architecture was to adopt a reference solution compatible with the adopted architecture reference model. The WSO2 RA was selected in this regard as it covers most of the requirements of the IoT systems and platforms [18].

The next two sections present the functional and information views of the particular architecture for the IoT platform which were instantiated from this reference solution.

5.2   Functional View

The architecture is structured on a physical (device) and a services layers (Fig. 2).

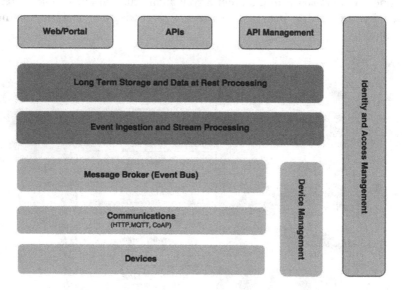

Fig. 2. The IoT Platform Architecture – Functional view

The physical layer contains wearable devices and other medical devices used to monitor the user's health or track user's activity, but it can also include environmental sensors which are found in smart homes or intelligent buildings. Network controlled devices (web cameras, security devices, smart thermostats) are also part of this layer.

On top of the physical layer a service layer of software components is conceived, which control and support the user interaction with those physical devices. The building blocks are dedicated software stacks that provide specialized functionalities, for example: a data storage facility, a predictive modeling and automation service, client components and agents running on the physical devices, and a network based service interface to glue together all these parts with the user interface implemented in various forms like the web, desktop or mobile applications.

The main decision made with regard to the functional view was to split the event processing and analytics level into two separate components, according to the Data accumulation concept introduced by the IoTWS reference model. The Event Ingestion and Stream Processing level contains the components that ingest a large volume of real-time events generated by the lower levels. It accomplishes the data processing that realizes the transformation from data in motion to data at rest. The Long Term Storage and Data at Rest Processing level provides support for advanced functionalities like data mining and Big Data analytics.

5.3 Information View

The information view is built from several modules which are implemented independently and exposed as services (Fig. 3).

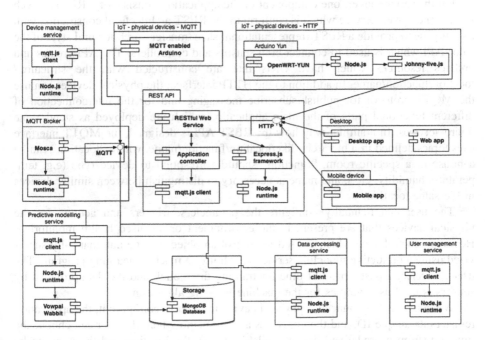

Fig. 3. The IoT platform architecture – Information view

These modules correspond to the functional view levels. The Device management service performs the tasks associated with the Device Management layer. The User management service implements the Identity and Account Management requirements. The processing of a large volume of data on the Event Ingestion and Stream Processing level is done by a Data processing service. Data analytics provide support for the intelligent operation of IoT devices, and is implemented by a predictive modeling service.

These services are interconnected by an Enterprise Service Bus (ESB) which is deployed as a MQTT broker. The application controller orchestrates these services as necessary in order to provide the required functionality.

6 Development Solutions

On the physical layer, the sensors, controllers and smart physical devices are modeled using Arduino boards which can be connected with different monitoring components or actuators in order to command other objects. Arduino is an open-source hardware and software project that provides a microcontroller based kit which can be used to design various IoT enabled sensors and controllers. Arduino based products are covering a wide range of devices from miniature wearables [19, 20] to combined microcontroller and microprocessor boards [21].

On the service layer, one component of the application consists of a RESTful web service (i.e. a web service which is conform to the REST architectural constraints) with the purpose to provide a REST (representational state transfer - architectural style of the web) API which is used to connect both sensors and controllers. The API creates and updates resources which have URIs that are constructed with the structure:/ location/function/name. In addition to the HTTP interface, the physical devices can use the MQTT protocol for publish/subscribe messaging and for the interconnection of different functional parts of the main application which are deployed as stand-alone micro-services. In a similar way how the REST API is designed, the MQTT interface uses topics defined in a hierarchy like/location/function/name, where "location" can be a house or a specific room, "function" should correspond to device type (e.g. temperature, humidity, etc.), and name is necessary to distinguish between similar devices in the same location.

The user can manually configure the parameters, triggers and actions for the physical devices that are present in the environment or are used health monitoring. However, each device which is used to control an object can be automatically supervised using a predictive modeling service which uses a machine learning program. The user can select a past period of time for training the model, and the data provided by sensors is used as examples for the machine learning algorithm.

When a user first connects a physical device in order to configure it, the application registers its unique ID, and then provides a setup menu where the user can choose the function (from a predefined list of available types), the location and the name to be assigned to the device. Subsequently, a new resource which corresponds to the device is created using the REST API. Next time when the device connects to the application, it is recognized and configured based on its location, function (type) and its name which were previously defined by the user (Fig. 4).

The IoT platform implementation in based on Javascript technologies and each component is briefly described as follows. The REST API which provides services to Arduino clients and user applications uses a stack based on MongoDB database [22], Node.js runtime [23] and the Express.js framework [24]. The predictive modeling application uses mqtt.js Javascript library to connect to the MQTT broker and it employs the Vowpal Wabbit [25] machine learning library running in daemon mode.

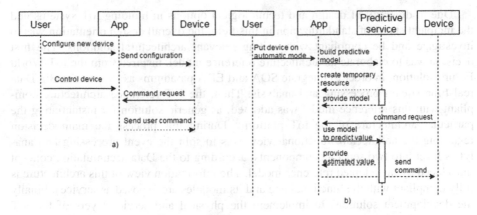

Fig. 4. Device configuration: (a) user manually controls the device; (b) automatic control of the device using a predictive model which learns from previous experience

The MQTT broker is implemented with Mosca [26] which is a Node.js module. Arduino clients are either implemented with MQTT or HTTP native support, or by using Firmata protocol [27] with Johnny-Five.js library [28] in the case of Arduino Yun board that runs OpenWrt-Yun [29] Linux distribution.

The user interface is available as a web application, but the user can access the service with a desktop or a mobile application as well. These applications are designed for different form factors and platforms, or use a single code base in case of a specialized framework like Apache Cordova [30]. Therefore, the user interface is common to all platforms and is implemented using React.js Javascript UI toolkit [31].

As a final remark, it is envisaged to have complete Javascript implementation in addition to off-the-shelf components in order to facilitate the development of the first prototype iteration. Several alternative technologies were investigated, such as the development of the RESTful web services in Java or Go languages, which are currently widely used in similar applications. However, due to perceived advantage in using a common language for the implementation of all system's components, it was decided to build the first prototype with only-Javascript frameworks and toolkits. The application's REST API adopts the MEAN software stack model (MongoDB as a NoSQL database, Express.js as a web application framework which runs on Node.js, Angular.js MVC framework and Node.js execution environment), but uses a different UI framework, as Angular.js is replaced with React.js toolkit.

7 Conclusions and Future Research

The paper presents the main adopted design and development decisions to build a platform for prototyping IoT based assistive applications with health monitoring capabilities. Considering the interdisciplinary character of health monitoring projects, the main reason to build this IoT platform was to take advantage of the prototyping approach in improving the quality and shortening the deployment period of instantiated particular solutions.

Due to diversity of design and technological options in building IoT systems and the incipient status of standardization in this field, the overall design orientation was to investigate and be compliant with exiting relevant architectural solutions. The first decision was to elaborate an architecture reference model, inspired from the IoT World Forum solution, in order to integrate SOA and EDA paradigms as support for Big Data real time stream processing and analysis. Then, the IoT reference architecture compliant with this reference model was adopted, as generic solution for instantiating the particular architecture of the IoT platform. During this process the main decision regarding the architecture functional view was to split the event processing and analytics level into two separate components, according to the Data accumulation concept introduced by the adopted reference model. The information view of this architecture is fully compliant with the functional one and its modules are exposed as services. Finally the development solutions to implement the physical and service layers of the IoT platform architecture were assessed and adopted.

To exploit the obtained results two concrete projects are envisaged: home monitoring services for elderly people with dementia and a health monitoring platform for patients with asthma.

Acknowledgments. This work was supported by the institutional research programme PN 0923 "TEHSIN - Advanced technologies and services for the Information Society development", 2015.

References

1. Bahga, A., Madisetti, V.: Internet of Things: A Hands-On Approach (2014)
2. Godinez, M., Hechl, E., Koenig, K., Lockwood, S., Oberhofer, M., Schroeck, M.: The Art of Enterprise Information Architecture - A Systems-Based Approach for Unlocking Business Insight. IBM Press, Pearson Education Inc., Boston (2010)
3. Bassi, A., Bauer, M., Fiedler, M., Kramp, T., Kranenburg, R.V., Lange, S., Meissner, S. (eds.): Enabling Things to Talk - Designing IoT solutions with the IoT Architectural Reference Model. Springer, Heidelberg (2013)
4. IslamS, M.R., Kwak, D., Kabir, H., Hossain, M., Kwak, K.S.: The internet of things for health care: a comprehensive survey. IEEE Access **3**, 678–708 (2015)
5. Vermesan, O., Friess, P. (eds.): Internet of Things – From Research and Innovation to Market Deployment. River Publishers, Denmark (2014)
6. Burton, B., Willis, D.A.: Gartner's Hype Cycles for 2015 - Five Megatrends Shift the Computing Landscape. Garner, 12 August 2015. https://www.gartner.com/doc/3111522?ref=unauthreader&srcId=1-3478922254
7. Schlack, M.: 2015 IT Priorities Editorial Global. TechTarget (2015). http://docs.media.bitpipe.com/io_10x/io_102267/item_465972/2015%20IT%20Priorities%20Global.pdf
8. Velosa, A., Schulte, W.R., Lheureux, B.J.: Hype cycle for the Internet of Thinks, 2015. Gartner, 21 August 2015. https://www.gartner.com/doc/3098434?ref=ddisp
9. Manyika, J., Chui, M., Bisson, P., Woetzel, J., Dobbs, R., Bughin, J., Aharon, D.: The Internet of Things - Mapping the Value Beyond the Hype. McKinsey Global Institute, Zürich (2015)

10. Acampora, G., Cook, D.J., Rashidi, P., Vasilakos, A.V.: A survey on ambient intelligence in healthcare. Proc. IEEE **101**(12), 2470–2494 (2013)
11. Moxey, C., Edwards, M., Etzion, O., Ibrahim, M., Iyer, S., Lalanne, H., Stewart, K.: A conceptual model for event processing systems. IBM Red guide publication, REDP-4642-00 (2010)
12. The Open Group: SOA Reference Architecture. Technical standard (2011)
13. Michelson, B.M.: Event-Driven Architecture Overview. Patricia Seybold Group, Boston (2006)
14. Internet of Things Expert Group (E02514): Internet of Things Factsheet Architecture (2013). http://ec.europa.eu/information_society/newsroom/cf/dae/document.cfm?doc_id=1750
15. Khan, R., Khan, S.U., Zaheer, R., Khan, S.: Future internet: the internet of things architecture, possible applications and key challenges. In: 10th International Conference on Frontiers of Information Technology, pp. 257–260. IEEE (2012). http://www.computer.org/csdl/proceedings/fit/2012/4946/00/4927a257.pdf
16. Al-Fuqaha, A., Guizani, M., Mohammadi, M., Aledhari, M., Ayyash, M.: Internet of things: a survey on enabling technologies, protocols, and applications. IEEE Commun. Surv. Tutorials **17**(4), 2347–2376 (2015). http://suanpalm3.kmutnb.ac.th/teacher/FileDL/DrSunantha2011255810194.pdf
17. Green, J.: The Internet of Things Reference Model. Internet of Things World Forum (IoTWF) White Paper (2014). http://cdn.iotwf.com/resources/71/IoT_Reference_Model_White_Paper_June_4_2014.pdf
18. Fremantle, P.: A Reference Architecture for the Internet of Things. WSO2 White Paper (2014)
19. Arduino Gemma. https://www.adafruit.com/gemma
20. Arduino LilyPad. http://lilypadarduino.org
21. Arduino Yun. https://www.arduino.cc/en/Main/ArduinoBoardYun
22. MongoDB for GIANT Ideas — MongoDB. https://www.mongodb.org/
23. Node.js. https://nodejs.org/en/
24. Express - Node.js web application framework. http://expressjs.com/en/index.html
25. Vowpal Wabbit (Fast Learning). http://hunch.net/vw/
26. Mosca - MQTT broker as a module. http://www.mosca.io
27. Firmata protocol. http://www.firmata.org/
28. Johnny-Five. https://github.com/rwaldron/johnny-five
29. OpenWrt-Yun. https://github.com/arduino/openwrt-yun
30. Apache Cordova. https://cordova.apache.org/
31. React.js. https://facebook.github.io/react/index.html

Web Service Design
and Service-Oriented Agents

A Freight Brokering System Architecture Based on Web Services and Agents

Florin Leon[1(✉)] and Costin Bădică[2]

[1] Technical University "Gheorghe Asachi" of Iaşi, Iaşi, Romania
fleon@cs.tuiasi.ro
[2] University of Craiova, Craiova, Romania
cbadica@software.ucv.ro

Abstract. The aim of this paper is to introduce the architecture of a system that combines the strengths of agents and web services to address the practical application of freight brokering. This is an important real-life business problem which aims to provide matchmaking services that facilitate the connection of the owners of goods with the freight transportation providers. The paper presents the general architecture of the system including agents and web services, as well as the use cases and the details of its main operations. Our system can be beneficial to logistics companies by increasing the quality of provided services and by reducing costs.

Keywords: Web services · Agents · Architecture · Freight brokering

1 Introduction

The integration of web services and agents tries to combine the strengths of both techniques. On the one hand, web services have the advantages of interoperability, flexibility in heterogeneous systems and the ability to automate service discovery and invocation with appropriate service description. On the other hand, agents are capable of autonomous and intelligent behaviour in order to represent the interests of their human users in an appropriate way [1]. In this paper, we aim to present the architecture of a system that combines these two computing paradigms. As a practical application, we address freight brokering, which is an important real-life business problem. The cargo owners and the providers of freight transportation services are continuously seeking new transport opportunities. This has led to the emergence of a new business model of freight transportation exchanges, which includes matchmaking services that facilitate the connection of the owners of goods with the freight transportation providers, in addition to online announcement and appropriate contracting. There are many virtual logistics platforms that operate in the domain of freight transport, exploiting the prospects provided by the requirements of goods that need to be transported, as well as of the availability of free vehicles, e.g. www.eurofreightexchange.com, www.bursadetransporturi.ro, www.europeancargo.ro, www.easycargo.ro, ro.trans.eu, www.timocom.com. The users are invited to register and post their offers in public directories. Then, potential customers can easily browse, search and manually inspect these directories in order to determine

T. Borangiu et al. (Eds.): IESS 2016, LNBIP 247, pp. 537–546, 2016.
DOI: 10.1007/978-3-319-32689-4_41

appropriate offers that suit their business needs. The available information contains real-time transport and goods postings in many, diverse fields of activity [2].

The main contribution of the present paper is the architecture of a brokering system for the delivery of smart logistics services, which integrates the concepts of web services and agents.

We organize it as follows. Section 2 presents some previous research in the field of intelligent brokering solutions. Section 3 describes the proposed architecture of the system. Section 4 contains the conclusions of our work and some ideas for future investigations.

2   Related Work

A freight broker coordinates transportation arrangements between transport customers, usually shippers and consignees, and transport resource providers or carriers. Their revenue model is based on transaction fees or commissions. For a successful, sustainable operation, freight brokers create and manage a vast network of customers. The goal is a convenient, efficient matchmaking of freight and transport availability according to various customer specifications, which allows customers to find the best terms and conditions for fulfilling their specific needs, including e.g. price, loading and unloading points, duration and safety [3].

This logistic problem has been addressed by means of web services, e.g. a freight transportation systems based on SOAP web services [4], a service-oriented architecture for long distance logistics and supply chain management [5] or a semantic web service discovery and selection system for the logistic operators domain [6].

There is also a quite rich research literature on the use of multiagent systems for modelling and development of domain-independent or domain-specific brokering services, as well as for the design of e-business applications in the logistics sector.

A sound taxonomy of domain-independent middle-agents based on formal modelling using process algebras and temporal logic is proposed in [7]. In particular, the formal details of a domain-independent broker agent are presented and its differences from matchmaker and front-agent types of middle-agents are highlighted.

An agent-based domain-independent brokering service is presented in [8], where the focus of the research is set on the semantic capabilities of the broker using rules and ontologies, rather than on its formal behavioural features. Domain-specific semantics in the logistics sector are described in [9].

A new agent and cloud-based model for the logistics chain is proposed in [10], where the SMART cooperation model is introduced, which allows companies to collaborate during the logistics process, thus improving the overall system intelligence.

Another study that suggests the use of agent-based negotiation for logistics management systems is [11], where the focus is on the whole supply chain, rather than on brokering of logistics services. The use of multiagent systems is motivated by the interactivity, responsiveness and social characteristics of this domain.

The integration of agents and web services has been investigated e.g. by [12], with the aim of reusing agent-based reasoning capabilities by making them available for invocation as web services. The EMERALD framework [13] for agent-based reasoning interoperability in the semantic web was extended with a web service interface. In the context of semantic web, ontologies for the freight transportation brokering domain have also been proposed [14] and evaluated with prototypical use case scenarios [15].

3   The Proposed Architecture

A key feature of a freight broker is the ability to negotiate with both transport providers and customers to efficiently choose among the many delivery segments that define a certain transport task such that each segment is covered and the vehicles do not travel without cargo on the delivery segments. A delivery segment is defined as the distance travelled by the vehicles of a transport provider between two locations in order to deliver the goods from one place to another.

Typically, a freight broker acquires an address on the Internet and sets up a web application, i.e. an e-marketplace, to communicate more effectively with transportation providers and customers. This e-marketplace allows the registration of actors that represent legal persons or individuals. Each actor may subsequently register the availability of certain vehicles or certain transport applications, respectively. The goal of the broker is the efficient automation of allocating freight requests to transport resources. Transport providers can register for the e-marketplace with several transport vehicles. A transport request is allocated to a transport vehicle owned by a specific transport provider. While the e-marketplace is mainly perceived as a user-friendly interface by the clients, the actual functionality behind this interface is provided by our proposed system.

An intelligent service is able to create an optimal transport route such that a vehicle does not move without cargo or, at least, that the movement without cargo is kept at a minimum on the road segments between two loading points. The actual implementation of the designed system can benefit from existing mathematical optimization methods developed for the freight brokerage industry [16].

In a previous study [2], an agent-based freight brokering system was proposed. In the present paper, we extend this model by describing an architecture which integrates both agents, as representatives of customers and of transport providers, and RESTful web services for a more efficient, scalable solution that can handle a large number of requests.

The general architecture of the system is presented in Fig. 1. The agents represent both individual clients and individual transport providers. They connect to specific web services in order to interact with the matchmaking system.

It is important to distinguish between the agents and the service they use in the first step of interaction. That is why we named the agents *Clients* and the web service *Customer* for the beneficiary part, and we named the agents *Transporters* and the web service *Provider* for the supplier part, respectively.

The *Customer* and the *Provider* web services further send the requests and offers of the *Clients* and *Transporters* to the *Broker* web service, which acts as a mediator. It is here that the requests and offers are matched and a tentative schedule is computed. The results must be communicated to the *Clients* and *Transporters*. This is made by email notification, with the help of an *Email* web service and an *EmailNotifier* agent which

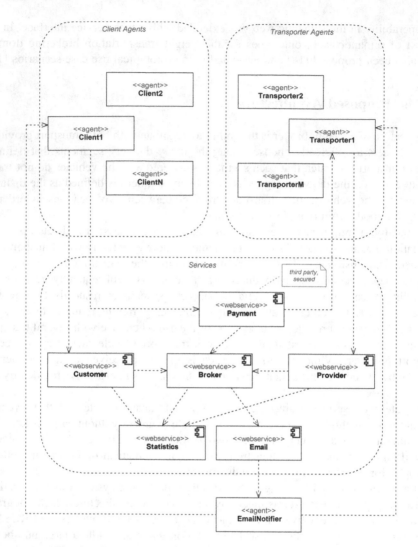

Fig. 1. The general architecture of the freight brokering system

sends direct messages to the *Clients* and *Transporters* agents. Both *Clients* and *Transporters* can accept or reject a solution proposed by the *Broker*. Also, after a task has been completed, a *Client* may optionally assess the quality of the transportation. All this information is communicated to the *Statistics* web service, which aggregates it in an appropriate way.

The *Broker* eventually receives the transport requests from the *Customer* (including vehicle description and points of loading and unloading) and the list of available vehicles that are capable to perform the transport requests from the *Provider* (including vehicle description as well as location and date of availability) and has to establish convenient terms and conditions for the tasks, e.g. a lower price and/or a convenient date and time. The *Broker* determines the list of potential freight providers matching a given transport request or a list of potential travel requests matching a given freight transport resource provision and proposes convenient matches for both parties.

The *Statistics* web service collects the data about past transactions and satisfaction reports and performs a post-action analysis that can be used to improve the decision making process.

Finally, when a *Client* must pay for the transportation service, it accomplishes this by using a third-party, secure *Payment* web service. The *Transporter* receives the payment and the brokering system receives a fee for matching offers and scheduling tasks.

3.1   Integrating Web Services and Agents

The integration of web services and agents is an active area of research. One of the most popular middleware frameworks for the development of multiagent systems is JADE [17]. It has the capability of defining services provided by agents, listed in a "yellow pages"-like directory called *Directory Facilitator* (DF). There are several ways in which these agent-based services can be exposed as actual web services. Also, it is important to enable the agents to access external web services.

One method is to use Web Services Integration Gateway (WSIG), proposed by the creators of JADE [18]. Its objective is to expose services provided by agents and published in the JADE DF as web services with no or minimal additional effort from the part of developers. The process involves: the generation of a suitable Web Service Definition Language (WSDL) file that represents the interface of each service registered with the DF, and possibly the publication of the exposed services in a Universal Description, Discovery, and Integration (UDDI) registry.

Another method is WS2JADE [19], a two-layer architecture composed of a dynamic interconnection layer containing web service agents (WSA), capable of communicating with web services and offering web services as their own, and a static management layer responsible for active service discovery and registration.

Both these methods are based on a service-oriented architecture and technically use SOAP web services.

However, JADE agents can be also integrated with RESTful web services, which are simpler in terms of implementation and resource addressing.

One example of a specific integration of agents with RESTful web services is presented in [20]. In this case, the architecture of the REST publisher is more complex than the WSDL publisher. The authors suggest the use of an automatic generator for simple services and the use of a dedicated, manually created mapping for more complicated services. In order to use external web services from within the agent middleware, a wrapper component can be used, which mimics the original service interface and also complies with the asynchronous requirements of the middleware. The implementation of the provided service is represented by a specific forward mechanism that dispatches the call to the external web service.

Due to the overall simplicity and scalability of RESTful web services, this is the approach we adopted for our system.

3.2   The Broker

Unlike the previous approach [2] that relies on direct agent negotiation to obtain a solution, in this paper we assume a centralized matchmaking process encapsulated in the *Broker* web service. The centralized approach has the main disadvantage of complexity, but the clear advantage of more accurate solutions. The negotiation with the agents is still present in the form of accepting or rejecting solutions, as presented in Sect. 3.3.

Regarding the internal functionality of the *Broker*, a combination of heuristics and optimization by linear programming can be used, adapted from the methodology described in [16].

The first heuristic step is to eliminate the invalid pairings between clients and transporters: (1) pairings with conflicting shipping dates and times; (2) pairings with conflicting requirements, i.e. the trucks which do not match the necessary equipment for a particular load; (3) pairings in which the load origin and the empty location of a truck are too far away, i.e. when a truck needs to come empty from a long distance, e.g. 500 km, in order to pick up a load; (4) pairings in which the empty time and location of a truck preclude its ability to arrive at the client by the specified time, considering e.g. an average speed of 60 km/h and a minimum of 2 h to load the freight.

The second step is to add a "phantom" pairing for each load with a non-existing, very expensive truck. The purpose of these pairings is to guarantee a feasible solution to the optimization problem.

The third step is to express the matchmaking as a zero-one linear programming optimization problem and solve it using for example one of many tools freely available, e.g. *lpsolve* [21]. The optimization problem can be expressed as follows:

$$\underset{j \in P}{\text{Min}} \ c_j x_j \tag{1}$$

such that:

$$\sum_{j \in P} x_j \delta_i^j = 1, \ \forall i \in L \tag{2}$$

$$\sum_{j \in P} x_j \gamma_k^j \leq 1, \ \forall k \in T \tag{3}$$

$$x_j, \ \delta_i^j, \ \gamma_k^j \in \{0, \ 1\}, \ \forall j \in P, \ \forall i \in L, \ \forall k \in T \tag{4}$$

where L is the set of all loads, T is the set of all trucks, P is the set of all possible pairings and c_j is the cost of pairing j. x_j is 1 if pairing j is selected and 0 otherwise. δ_i^j is 1 if load i is part of pairing j and 0 otherwise. γ_k^j is 1 if truck k is part of pairing j and 0 otherwise.

Equation 2 guarantees that each load is part of one and only one pairing and Eq. 3 guarantees that each truck is used at most once in the set of pairings.

3.3 Use Cases for Agents as User Representatives

We assume that the *Customer* provides the following services to a *Client*: (1) register or deregister; (2) send or update requests; (3) accept or reject a schedule solution; (4) send satisfaction report.

Also, the *Client* can make payments using the *Payment* web service. Figure 2 presents an UML use case diagram for these operations.

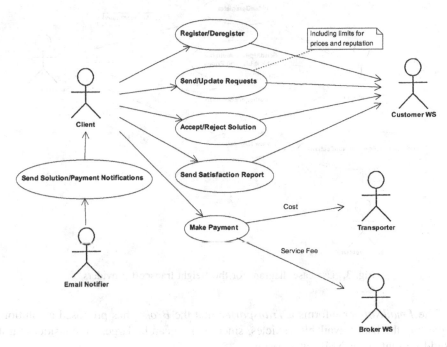

Fig. 2. Use case diagram for the customers

When a *Client* sends or updates a request, the call to the web service also includes possible limits for the acceptable price range or a minimum required level of reputation for the transporter.

The *EmailNotifier*, which informs a *Client* that the *Broker* has proposed a solution, is also an actor.

A *Client* agent needs information from the user that describes his/her request of a transport service, including: date of request, point of dispatch, point of destination, proposed date of loading, proposed date of unloading, weight, volume, special transport constraints, lifetime. The interaction with the *Broker* is performed exclusively through the *Customer* web service. In the end, possibly after several rounds of proposals from the *Broker*, sent by means of notifications by the *EmailNotifier* agent, the *Client* agent may succeed or fail in finding an appropriate transport deal for its user. If successful, it will present its user with a suitable transport deal including negotiated dates of loading and unloading, as well as other specific details, depending on the request.

A similar diagram is presented in Fig. 3 for a *Transporter*, which can interact with the *Provider* web service in the following ways: (1) register or deregister; (2) send or update the list of available vehicles; (3) accept or reject a schedule solution; (4) only view information about its reputation, based on the satisfaction reports sent by the *Clients*.

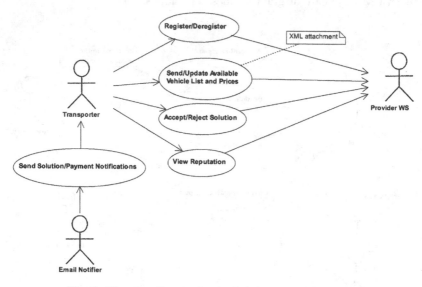

Fig. 3. Use case diagram for the freight transport providers

The *EmailNotifier* informs a *Transporter* that the *Broker* has proposed a solution. Regarding the list of available vehicles, since its size can be large, we consider that it should be sent as an XML attachment.

A *Transport* agent needs information from its user about the vehicle description, including: type of vehicle (e.g. regular truck, tanker truck, van), vehicle dedicated for a special type of freight (e.g. regular cargo, logs, cars, animals, etc.), type of fuel (e.g. petrol, diesel), carrying capacity, length, width, height, as well as special characteristics such as: canvas vehicle, hydraulic tailgate vehicle (hydraulic lift). It also needs information about the transport resource availability, including location, date and time. Like in the *Client* case, the interaction with the *Broker* is performed exclusively through the *Provider* web service, and it is notified by the *EmailNotifier* agent about the proposals of the *Broker*. Finally, it will present the possible solution to its user.

3.4   Details of the Main Operations

In this section, we describe the main operations in more detail. Regarding the process where the system receives requests/offers and searches for matches between them, the *Clients* and *Transporters* can access their corresponding contact points, *Customer* and *Provider*, respectively, at any time. The two web services work in parallel and notify the *Broker* that updates have been performed. The *Broker* accesses the actual data through some file links, because the volume of information may be too high to be sent directly. After the *Broker* has solved the optimization problem given the current constraints, it informs the *Email* web service, which sends email messages to the involved parties. This process is facilitated by the *EmailNotifier* agent.

Another important process is the way in which the agents, as user representatives, decide whether a proposed solution is acceptable. This is also performed in an asynchronous way. Both a *Client* and a *Transporter* must accept a solution in order for a contract to be established. Since the system is based on email notifications, and many users can be present in the system while some users/agents may simply give up a previous request or offer without explicitly informing the brokering system, a timeout is introduced, such as if the two parties do not confirm their commitment in a predefined period of time, the solution is considered to be automatically rejected. After a contract has been established, the client must pay. The payment method is not enforced by our architecture, because it may depend on the parties: some may require advanced payment while others may accept payment after the service has been successfully completed, or even payment into an escrow account may be used.

4 Conclusions

In this paper we described the architecture of a freight brokering system that integrates the use of web services and agents. Such a system can be beneficial to logistics companies by increasing the quality of provided services and by reducing costs. As future directions of investigation, we aim at specifying additional details about the information required by each component of the system which will help the implementation of the system and its use for real-world transportation case studies.

References

1. Betz, T., Cabac, L., Wester-Ebbinghaus, M.: Gateway architecture for web-based agent services. In: Klügl, F., Ossowski, S. (eds.) MATES 2011. LNCS, vol. 6973, pp. 165–172. Springer, Heidelberg (2011)
2. Luncean, L., Bădică, C., Bădică, A.: Agent-based system for brokering of logistics services – initial report. In: Nguyen, N.T., Attachoo, B., Trawiński, B., Somboonviwat, K. (eds.) ACIIDS 2014, Part II. LNCS, vol. 8398, pp. 485–494. Springer, Heidelberg (2014)
3. Bowersox, D.J., Closs, D.J.: Logistical Management: The Integrated Supply Chain Process. McGraw-Hill, New York (1996)
4. Ji, C., Li, M., Li, L.: Freight transportation system based on web service. In: Proceedings of the 2004 IEEE International Conference on Services Computing, pp. 567–570 (2004)
5. Cho, H., Woo, J., Ivezik, N., Jones, A., Denno, P., Peng, Y.: An integration technology for long distance logistics and supply chain management. In: Proceedings of the 18th International Conference on Management of Technology (2009). http://ebiquity.umbc.edu/_file_directory_/papers/559.pdf

6. Carenini, A., Cerizza, D., Comerio, M., Della Valle, E., De Paoli, F., Maurino, A., Palmonari, M., Sassi, M., Turati, A.: semantic web service discovery and selection: a test bed scenario. In: Proceedings of the 6th International Workshop on Evaluation of Ontology-based Tools and the Semantic Web Service Challenge, CEUR Workshop Proceedings, vol. 359, paper no. 3 (2008). http://ceur-ws.org/Vol-359/Paper-3.pdf

7. Bădică, A., Bădică, C.: FSP and FLTL framework for specification and verification of middle-agents. Appl. Math. Comput. Sci. 21(1), 9–25 (2011)

8. Antoniou, G., Skylogiannis, T., Bikakis, A., Doerr, M., Bassiliades, N.: Dr-brokering: a semantic brokering system. Knowl.-Based Syst. 20(1), 61–72 (2007)

9. Scheuermann, A., Hoxha, J.: Ontologies for intelligent provision of logistics services. In: Proceedings of the Seventh International Conference on Internet and Web Applications and Services, ICIW 2012, pp. 106–111 (2012)

10. Kawa, A.: SMART Logistics Chain. In: Pan, J.-S., Nguyen, N.T., Chen, S.-M. (eds.) ACIIDS 2012, Part I. LNCS, vol. 7196, pp. 432–438. Springer, Heidelberg (2012)

11. Guanghai, Z., Runhong, Y.: Multi-agent supply logistics intelligent management system based on negotiation. Comput. Sci. Appl. Educ. 3(1), 476–481 (2013)

12. Bădică, C., Bassiliades, N., Ilie, S., Kravari, K.: Agent reasoning on the web using web services. Comput. Sci. Inf. Syst. 11(2), 697–721 (2014)

13. Kravari, K., Kontopoulos, E., Bassiliades, N.: EMERALD: a multi-agent system for knowledge-based reasoning interoperability in the semantic web. In: Konstantopoulos, S., Perantonis, S., Karkaletsis, V., Spyropoulos, C.D., Vouros, G. (eds.) SETN 2010. LNCS, vol. 6040, pp. 173–182. Springer, Heidelberg (2010)

14. Luncean, L., Bădică, C.: Semantic modeling of information for freight transportation broker. In: Proceedings of the 2014 16th International Symposium on Symbolic and Numeric Algorithms for Scientific Computing, SYNASC, pp. 527–534 (2014)

15. Luncean, L., Becheru, A., Bădică, C.: Initial evaluation of an ontology for transport brokering. In: Proceedings of the 2015 IEEE 19th International Conference on Computer Supported Cooperative Work in Design, CSCWD, pp. 121–126 (2015)

16. Silver, J.L.: Optimization tools for the freight brokerage industry. Master's thesis, Massachusetts Institute of Technology, Engineering Systems (2003). http://hdl.handle.net/1721.1/28574

17. Bellifemine, F.L., Caire, G., Greenwood, D.: Developing Multi-Agent Systems with JADE. Wiley Series in Agent Technology. Wiley, Chichester (2007)

18. JADE Board: JADE Web Services Integration Gateway (WSIG) Guide. Telecom Italia (2008). http://jade.tilab.com/doc/tutorials/WSIG_Guide.pdf

19. Nguyen, X.T., Kowalczyk, R.: WS2JADE: integrating web service with Jade agents. In: Huang, J., Kowalczyk, R., Maamar, Z., Martin, D., Müller, I., Stoutenburg, S., Sycara, K. (eds.) SOCASE 2007. LNCS, vol. 4504, pp. 147–159. Springer, Heidelberg (2007)

20. Braubach, L., Pokahr, A.: Conceptual integration of agents with WSDL and RESTful web services. In: Dastani, M., Hübner, J.F., Logan, B. (eds.) ProMAS 2012. LNCS, vol. 7837, pp. 17–34. Springer, Heidelberg (2013)

21. Berkelaar, M., Eikland, K., Notebaert, P.: lpsolve, Open source (Mixed-Integer) Linear Programming system. http://sourceforge.net/projects/lpsolve/

Automated Identification and Prioritization of Business Risks in e-service Networks

Dan Ionita[1(✉)], Roel J. Wieringa[1], and Jaap Gordijn[2]

[1] Cybersecurity and Safety Group, University of Twente - Services, Drienerlolaan 5,
7522 NB Enschede, The Netherlands
{d.ionita,r.j.wieringa}@utwente.nl
[2] Vrije Universiteit Amsterdam, De Boelelaan 1105,
1081 HV Amsterdam, The Netherlands
j.gordijn@cs.vu.nl
http://scs.ewi.utwente.nl/
http://e3value.few.vu.nl/

Abstract. Modern e-service providers rely on service innovation to stay
relevant. Once a new service package is designed, implementation-specific
aspects such as value (co-)creation and cost/benefit analysis are investigated. However, due to time-to-market or competitive advantage constraints, innovative services are rarely assessed for potential risks of fraud
before they are put out on the market. But these risks may result in loss
of economic value for actors involved in the e-service's provision.

Our $e^3 fraud$ approach automatically generates and prioritizes
undesired-able scenarios from a business value model of the e-service,
thereby drastically reducing the time needed to conduct an assessment.
We provide examples from telecom service provision to motivate and
illustrate the utility of the tool.

Keywords: e-services · Value models · Risk assessment · Fraud

1 Introduction

Many services are *commercial* services. That is, they are of economic value to
someone, and are paid for. As a result, end users and enterprises may be tempted
to commit fraud or abuse, which we refer to as non-ideal behaviour. Such non-
ideal behavior of actors involved in the acquisition or consumption of the service
can lead to undesirable losses for the provider or undeserved gains for other
actors. Examples include but are not limited to misusing the service, bypassing
payments and exploiting unintended interactions between services. For example,
in the field of telecom service provision, "simboxing" involves acquiring telephone
services from multiple providers and setting up a composite service that disguises
international calls as local traffic, thereby undercutting termination fees [1].

The problem is exacerbated because many services are in fact electronic
services, which are provisioned via the Internet or other digital means [2].
These electronic services are characterized by short time-to-market (typically

© Springer International Publishing Switzerland 2016
T. Borangiu et al. (Eds.): IESS 2016, LNBIP 247, pp. 547–560, 2016.
DOI: 10.1007/978-3-319-32689-4_42

a few months). But these e-services are provisioned over complex networks, that increases the opportunity for malicious actors to commit fraud or otherwise misuse e-services [3]. Risk assessment thus becomes more complex, and this creates a tension with the desire of marketeers to put out innovative e-services fast. Thus, there is a need to speed up and enhance the capability of e-service risk assessment.

Service innovation commonly consists of three phases: Service exploration, where potential new or improved services are identified; Service Engineering, where one or more of the options are explored in detail; and Service Management, which deals with implementation and continuity [4]. The Service Engineering phase carries particular importance, as errors introduced in the early phases of service design can have significant (financial) consequences later on [5,6]. E-service risk assessment should therefore be done in the service engineering stage. This requires quantifying the cost of misuse and designing prevention or detection mechanisms, which in turn requires projections, usage estimates and financial computations [7]. Doing this in a way that does not unduly slow down service innovation requires efficient tool support.

Business risks for a provider include fraudulent violations of contracts by clients, violations of agreements or terms of service, as well as the creation, by clients, of false expectations with the provider with regard to usage. We define **fraud** as the intentional misrepresentation by a client of his or her intentions, in order to acquire something of value from a provider. Fraud may be legal or illegal. We call the actor performing a fraud a **fraudster.** In our assessment of fraud risk we sidestep the issue of legality but focus on the potential loss for the provider and potential gain for the fraudster. In other words, we focus on what is observable for the provider (his loss) and on what can be estimated about the fraudster, given a business model (his potential gain). The potential loss is the negative impact that the risk can have on the provider, and the potential gain for the fraudster indicates the likelihood that the fraud will be committed.

Previously, we introduced e^3fraud as a model-based approach to assessing business risks in e-service networks [8]. In that paper, we introduced three basic fraud operations, namely not paying for a delivered service, performing a hidden value transfer, and colluding with another actor; and we introduced different ways to estimate loss for a service provider and profit for a fraudster. Non-payment breaks transactional reciprocity (and causes loss) [9], hidden transfers can encourage misuse (by providing hidden gains) [10] and collusion allows exploiting unintended interactions between atomic services [11]. Our goal in this paper is to scale up these techniques to non-trivial scenarios by *automatically* generating fraud scenarios from a business value model. We will see that for realistic business models, the sheer number of possible variations is staggering, so the ability to filter, rank and group risks so as to zoom in on the most risky scenarios, becomes critical. With this paper, we aim to provide scalable tool support for generating, quantifying and ranking business risks directly from a business model of the given service.

Our approach to fraud risk assessment is constructive in the sense that we analyze the architecture of a business model, in particular a business model represented in e^3value , to construct possible mechanisms to commit fraud. This distinguishes it from statistical approaches to assess fraud risk [12], which use patterns of past client behavior to assess fraud risks in new business models. Since the new business model has by definition not contributed to the statistical data on which this assessment is based, statistics-based fraud assessment leaves one with unknown and un-estimated risks. Therefor, our approach is able to discover fraud scenarios a priori, while statistical models identify fraud a priori.

e^3fraud is based on the e^3value method for representing business models, and allows the generation of possible fraud mechanisms in new business models. The e^3fraud tool (available at: https://github.com/danionita/e3fraud) can automatically generate misuse scenarios based on configurable heuristics, such as collusion, non-payment and hidden payments. Furthermore, it can group and rank such scenarios on various criteria, such as loss to a service provider or profit to a fraudster. Finally, it can help visualize the financial results across a range of projected usage levels. We illustrate the tool using examples from telecom service provision.

The paper is structured as follows: Sect. 2 introduces the underlying e^3value language, the e^3fraud extension, and the new e^3fraud tool. Section 3 describes the application of the approach to a telecom service and showcases the results provided by the tool. Finally, Sect. 4 draws some conclusions with regard to the approach, its applicability and future development.

2   The e^3fraud Methodology and Tool

2.1   Starting Point: e^3value

Value co-creation modeling is aimed at showing that a given business model is profitable for all (or most) of the parties involved in its provision and consumption. One established method for building value models and doing profitability computations is e^3value [13]. An e^3value model describing a flat-rate telephony service is shown in Fig. 1. A flat rate, also referred to as a flat fee or a linear rate, is a pricing structure that charges a single fixed fee for a service, regardless of usage. [14]

An e^3value model represents how actors exchange commercial services in an ideal world during a period of time called the **contract period.** For example, Fig. 1 may represent the way actors exchange services during a period of one month. An e^3value model assumes that all actors trust each other and all transactions occur as specified. It consists of several basic elements:

Actors are profit-loss responsible entities, such as organizations, customers and intermediaries. In Fig. 1, the "Provider A", "Provider B", "User A" and "User B" are actors.

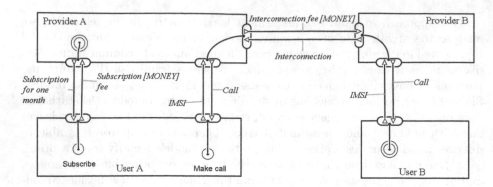

Fig. 1. e^3value model of flat-rate telephony service

Value objects are things of economic value, such as money, services, products, knowledge or experiences. In Fig. 1 "Subscription for one month", "Subscription fee", "IMSI" (International Mobile Subscriber Identity, used to identify the user of a cellular network and is a unique identification associated with all cellular networks. [15]), "Call", "Interconnection fee", "Interconnection" are all value objects.

Value transfers are transfers of value objects, such as a payment or the delivery of a service. In Fig. 1, all the lines between two actors are value transfers.

Economic transactions are transactional groups of two or more (reciprocal) value transfers. In Fig. 1, there are several such groups. E.g. "Subscription fee" in exchange for "Subscription for one month" and "IMSI" in exchange for "Call". Transactionality here means atomicity: if one transfer in a transaction occurs, all of them occur. Once we include the possibility of non-ideal worlds, as in e^3fraud , transactionality may be broken, because one actor may not deliver the value that is expected of it. In e^3value , however, transactionality is maintained

Dependency paths are chains of economic transactions. In Fig. 1, there are two dependency paths: one for the subscription and one for the calling. Dependency paths do *not* represent processes [16]. They merely indicate that in the contract period, a consumer need triggers a certain combination of economic transactions, without saying when or how these transactions are performed. This is sufficient for doing profitability computations.

Consumer needs trigger a chain of economic transactions. In Fig. 1, "Subscribe" and "Make call" are such needs.

Each value object has an associated monetary value (for each actor). Each consumer need has an associated occurrence rate (per contractual period). Both the monetary value and the expected occurrence rate need to be estimated by the user before any computations can be carried out. Together, these numbers can be used by the tool to estimate the financial result of each actor per contractual period.

e^3value is used to estimate whether a business model can be profitable under ideal circumstances of trusted actors. After the business model is fully understood, the next step is assess the risk(s) that not all actors behave as expected.

2.2   The e^3fraud Methodology

In previous work [8] we've shown how an e^3value model can be extended to describe fraud. The resulting e^3fraud models differ from the original e^3value model in several ways, as described below (see Fig. 1).

- An e^3fraud model takes the point of view of one actor in the network, dubbed the **Target of Assessment** or ToA and marked with a thick border. This is needed to define the concept of hidden transactions, introduced below, and to assist with ranking the possible fraud models according to the potential loss for the ToA (further described in Sect. 2.3). In Fig. 2, "Provider A" is the ToA.
- Value transfers may not take place and are marked using dashed lines. In Fig. 2, the "Subscription Fee" transfer does not take place.
- Hidden transfers may occur between secondary actors, not involving the ToA and are marked using dotted lines. In Fig. 2, a "Revenue Share" is being paid out by Provider B to User A for each call received. The ToA cannot directly observe these hidden transactions.
- Actors might collude, which means that they pool their budgets. In Fig. 2, User A and User B are colluding. Collusion is usually kept hidden for the ToA.

Figure 2 shows that User A has a flat-fee subscription with provider A, and colludes with User B, who has a revenue-sharing subscription with provider B. An example of a revenue-sharing subscription is a subscription for an 0900 number, where the client is paid by the provider for being called. Provider B receives a large fee for providing access to an 0900 number, and shares some of this revenue with User B. The dotted line in Fig. 2 shows that this revenue-sharing payment is invisible to the ToA. By making the maximum number of calls to himself, User A+B can generate more income from the revenue-sharing subscription than the cost of the flat-fee contract. However, to increase profit, User A+B does not even pay the flat fee, as shown by the dashed line in figure 1.

This is just one possible sub-ideal model derived from the value model of a flat-rate show in Fig. 1. The e^3fraud approach involves building several of these sub-ideal models, and comparing their financial outcomes to that of the ideal model in order to estimate the potential impact of each instance of fraud or misuse [8].

Manually creating these models and re-running the analysis is time-consuming, especially since the search space is potentially infinite. Furthermore, deciding which scenarios should be mitigated implies comparing a large number of models, and this cannot be done manually. In the following section, we describe our approach to delegate the time- and resource-intensive tasks of generation and ranking to a computer.

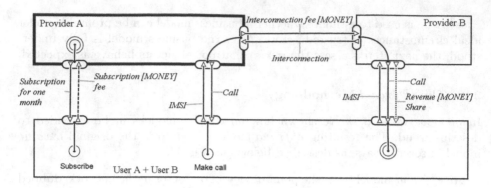

Fig. 2. e^3fraud model of flat-rate fraud

2.3   The e^3fraud Tool

In this paper, we present a (tool-based) extension to the e^3fraud approach which allows the user to quickly and effectively generate, rank and compare possible sub-ideal variations of a given value model, based on several heuristics. The tool is open-source and publicly available at https://github.com/danionita/e3fraud. It performs three tasks:

1. Generating e^3fraud models, representing various fraud scenarios;
2. Ranking the generated e^3fraud models, so that the business model designer can zoom in on the most risky ones;
3. Computing and plotting the profit/loss of each actor across a given usage projection.

Generation. Given a valid e^3value model, the tool generates all combinations of possible deviations: *hidden transactions, non-occurring transactions and collusions*. These patterns were previously found to be the building blocks of several telecom fraud scenarios [17]. Each valid combination is then instantiated as new sub-ideal model. A sub-ideal model may contain any number of hidden transactions and non-occurring transactions but only one collusion. The number of actors colluding is configurable.

Hidden transactions are generated in three steps.

- First identify pairs of transactioning secondary (non-ToA) actors.
- Then, for each such pair, the profit/loss resulting from the dependency path of which this transaction is part, is computed for each actor.
- Finally, for the actor(s) with a positive result, a new outgoing transaction is added: this transaction takes a value of one third and two thirds of the positive result, respectively. The reasoning behind this is that if an Actor makes some profit on a dependency path, he might be be willing to pass on 1/3 or even 2/3 of that value to another actor, B, if that would motivate B to generate more traffic. This models an established practice in the services industry called Revenue Sharing [18].

The generation of hidden transactions is thus bound by the number of actors and transactions in the ideal model.

Non-occurring transactions are created by invalidating individual monetary transfers (that is, transfers marked as type *MONEY*). The restriction to monetary transfers is to limit state space explosion, but this assumption could be dropped in the future. The user may indicate that certain *MONEY* transfers will always occur by marking them as as type *MONEY-SECURE*. This can be either because they are initiated by the provider itself, because safeguards are in place or simply to reduce the search space of sub-ideal models. This will prevent these transfers from being invalidated by the generation engine. The generation of hidden transactions is thus bound by the number of monetary transfers in the ideal model.

Collusion takes place when two actors are acting as one: they pool their budgets and collectively bear all expenses and profit. By colluding, actors might deceive controls and invalidate expectations by appearing independent but in fact working together against the best interests of the provider. Therefore, only secondary actors (not the ToA) can collude. To generate collusions, pairs of secondary actors are merged into a single actor. The number of actors allowed to part of a colluding group is configurable. The generation of collusions is thus bound by the number of actors in the ideal model.

Ranking. Depending on the complexity of the initial ideal model, hundreds of even thousands of models might be generated. Many of these might not be possible due to existing controls or might be unlikely because they are not profitable for any of the actors.

To aid with selection and prioritization of risks, the tool provides several ways of ranking and grouping the set of generated models, described below. The prioritization is always carried out from the perspective of a single actor (the Target of Assessment), as described below.

In terms of value creation, non-ideal behavior causes a disruption in the financial result of the actors involved. This means that a non-ideal scenario can (1) cause a loss for the service provider and (2) trigger an unexpected gain for one of its customers or users. As such, the software tool allows ranking based on Loss for the ToA, Gain for the secondary actors and Loss+Gain. Gain for a secondary actors is defined as the difference between the financial result of a that actor in the ideal case versus the sub-ideal case.

Ranking on Loss+Gain ranks risks on negative impact for the ToA (Loss) and profitability for the potential fraudster (Gain). This is similar to the classical definition of risk as Impact times Likelihood of an event, except that we do not use Likelihood of the fraud but Gain to the fraudster. We use Gain to estimate the attractiveness of a fraud to a potential fraudster. A fraud with a higher gain for the fraudster is more attractive to the fraudster, and therefore more likely, than a fraud with a lower gain.

Furthermore, to allow for "what-if" analyses and easier navigation through the long list of sub-ideal models, results can be grouped based on who is colluding with who. Since each group is ranked independently, this allows investigating the most risky way each pair or group of actors can collude.

Visualization. The ranked list of generated sub-ideal models is presented by the $e^3 fraud$ tool as a list of textual descriptions. If grouping was selected, the list is nested and collapsible. This facilitates the exploration of the state space. Additionally, the financial results of the ideal models and any of the sub-ideal modes can also be visualized as a 2D plot showing the profit/loss across a range of usage levels for the fraudster and for the ToA. The user may select which usage indicator (i.e. consumer need) to be represented on the X-axis, as well as its range. We provide a detailed illustration later in Fig. 5. These representations can be understood by marketeers and product managers without having to learn $e^3 value$ or $e^3 fraud$.

The results contain several useful pieces of information. Firstly, they show the loss for the ToA across the given occurrence range, as both a plot and an average. Loss is a direct indicator of the potential impact that each of the particular fraud risks can bring about. Secondly, the gain experienced by all other actors in the model is also shown as both a plot and an average. This gain can be used as a proxy for likelihood: the higher potential gain for some actor, the more likely it is that he will attempt that specific fraud scenario. Finally, the slope of all the plots are estimated, which gives an indication of how the loss and gain of the fraud scales with usage, outside the given range, and therefore how the impact and likelihood vary. Visualizing the result as a plot also allows for easy, visual identification of break-even points and thresholds.

3   Preliminary Evaluation Results

The approach has been applied to several telecom service packages known to be exploitable. In this section, we present one of these cases: call forwarding to other networks via post-paid subscription.

The (ideal) value model of this service is shown in Fig. 3. Provider A is our target-of-assessment, i.e. the entity who is offering the service and conducting the assessment. User A is a customer of Provider A. In this case, he is using a pre-paid SIM card to make calls to some other customer of Provider A: User B. User B, in turn, has a post-paid subscription with Provider A. This subscription involved a fixed monthly payment, plus an incremental payment based on his usage. In this simple example, he does not initiate any calls and has set his device to forward all received calls to User C. User C is a customer of Provider B, and therefore User B will have to pay for the connection from his own Provider, A, to User C. Since Provider B is a separate commercial entity, we do not know his contractual structure nor his usage pattern, so we only model the fact that User C can receive calls.

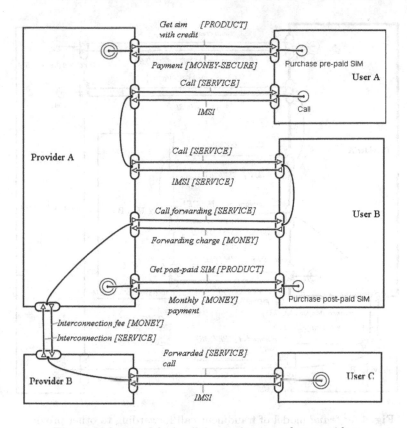

Fig. 3. Value model of call forwarding to other provider

A known fraud scenario (shown in Fig. 4) for this case is as follows: User A initiates a very large number of calls to User B. The calls are usually charged at a preferential rate, as the two users are on the same network. User B, as the forwarding party will have to pay for the call outside the network. He will receive a very large bill at the end of the month, which he does not pay. In reality, User A commonly pays User B a small amount of money to start a post-paid subscription using fake credentials, so that User B cannot be traced by Provider A. Finally, User C, the end-recipient of the call would have a Revenue Sharing agreement with Provider B, by which he receives a pay-out for every call that comes through. This is common with 0900 numbers but also available with some "budget" subscriptions.

By running the model in Fig. 3 through the e^3fraud tool using default settings, we obtain the fraud scenario described above and visualized in Fig. 4 as the 7th highest ranked scenario. Figure 5 shows a screen-shot of the actual output. The left part of the screen describes the 7th highest ranked risk as:

Average of **-11.23** (instead of **25.82**) for Provider A due to:
Colluding actors "User A" and "User C"

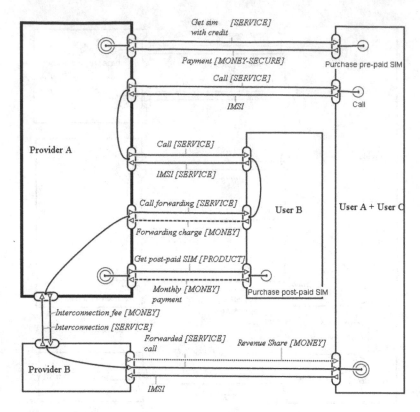

Fig. 4. e^3fraud model of fraudulent call forwarding to other provider

Non-occurring exchange Forwarding charge
Non-occurring exchange Monthly Payment
Hidden transfer of value 0.02 (out of 0.03) from "Provider B" to "User A + User C"

The value in brackets of 25.82 is the average profit for the ToA in the ideal case (i.e. the model provided as input to the tool). The assumption is that this value is what the ToA would have expected to obtain given its own estimates. However, in this scenario, the ToA will only obtain an average of -11.23 across the same occurrence rate. The reasons for this are also given by the tool: two actors (Actor A and Actors C) are colluding, User B will not pay his bill this month (consisting of a Monthly Payment and a Forwarding charge, and Provider B is passing two thirds of his revenue per call to the now colluding Users A and C. The tool uses the total incoming value per occurrence rate as a basis for this last estimation of 0.02 out of 0.03.

The right part of the screen shows the evolution of the risk with the number of (forwarded) calls per contractual period. The x-axis represents the number of calls by User A and the y-axis represents the corresponding profit and loss for the actors. The steepest upward line is "User A + User C" (the fraudsters).

The next steepest upward line is "Provider B". The horizontal line is User B, and the downward line is Provider A (the ToA). The graph therefore shows that this particular scenario allows the two colluding actors to obtain a sizable profit, that scales very well. It also shows that this would cause an unexpected loss for the provider, which gets significantly worse with the number of minutes called. Provider B maintains a positive financial result, and User B does not incur any loss or profit from participating in this scenario.

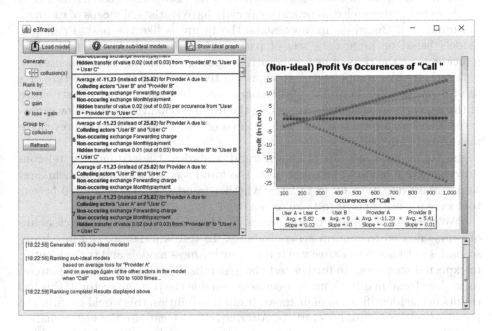

Fig. 5. Screen-shot of the e^3fraud tool's output for the value model in Fig. 3.

The higher ranked risks (numbers 1 to 6 in the list) trigger the same loss for the provider, but yield a higher profit for other groups of colluding actors at the detriment of other secondary actors, making them unrealistic. For instance, it makes no (financial) sense for Actor A to initiate the calls in the first place if he is in on the fraud. Furthermore, other highly ranked risks imply a User colluding with Provider B, thus also obtaining Provider B's legitimate interconnection income. While collusion between user and providers is not impossible, in this case it is extremely unlikely. Grouping the results per collusion would help in this case to eliminate unrealistic collusions from the analysis.

These results can help design fraud detection thresholds, identify transaction that require (further) procedural or technical controls or even trigger a re-design of the service in order to eliminate or mitigate business value risks [7].

4   Discussion and Future Work

This $e^3 fraud$ approach described in this paper provides a novel, constructive, semi-automated method for conducting quantitative risk assessments of value models. The approach relies on a small set of misuse patterns commonly seen in telecom fraud, that so far has been sufficient to generate known fraud scenarios. Our results highlight the potential of automating the identification, quantification and ranking of business risks associated with one or more service offerings.

As noted earlier, telecom providers already have statistical means of estimating fraud [12]. But these means assume the future is like the past. Predictive models based on large data sets of past service deliveries do not necessarily indicate what the risks of new, innovative e-service provision arrangements are. $e^3 fraud$ provides a supplementary approach that analyzes the architecture of a service provisioning network and identifies risks that follow from the structure of the network, by actually constructing the fraud mechanisms. This allows marketeers and managers to identify the source of these risks and take preventive measures, before the risks materialize.

So far we have only found known fraud scenarios. Understandably, telecom providers are reluctant to disclose all of the fraud scenarios known to them, and so it will be very hard for us to know whether fraud scenarios generated by our tool were already known to them or not.

We've shown feasibility in other cases [8]. However, more real-world cases are of course needed to confirm generalizability. To test whether we can find fraud scenarios not known to *us,* we will collect new business models and try to identify unexpected scenarios. To further test the generalizability of our ideas, we intend to analyze fraud in other kinds of e-services, outside the telecom sector. If this too results in the identification of unknown fraud possibilities, this would confirm the power of our basic fraud operations. Alternatively, we can use the new scenarios to distill a more complete set of fraud patterns and heuristics. Implementing them into the tool's generation and ranking modules in a customizable way would further the flexibility and applicability of the approach. For instance, it might be the case that in certain scenarios, higher gain does not necessarily imply higher likelihood. Therefor, it is worth exploring alternative heuristics in future research.

Finally, a larger search space also raises issues of resource exhaustion; care must be given to trimming the search space and streamlining code. One way of limiting the search space seems to be to differentiating between clients and providers. Then, only clients can be assumed to collude or attempt to bypass payments. Another way of managing the potentially very large lists of results is filtering. Therefore, one of the main topic for improvement in the future is integrating a filter functionality in the tool. Examples filters are: removing sub-ideal models that do not cause a loss, removing sub-ideal models that are not profitable for any of the actors and only showing the most profitable or costly sub-ideal model per collusion type. Furthermore, integrating a model editor into the tool might further increase its usability: firstly, users would need not go through the export/import process for every instance of a model and secondly, users would be able to visualize the fraud directly on the value model.

References

1. Reaves, B., Shernan, E., Bates, A., Carter, H., Traynor, P.: Boxed out: Blocking cellular interconnect bypass fraud at the network edge. In: 24th USENIX Security Symposium (USENIX Security 15), pp. 833–848. Washington, D.C., USENIX Association, August 2015
2. Mohan, K., Ramesh, B.: Ontology-based support for variability management in product and families. In: Proceedings of the 36th Annual Hawaii International Conference on System Sciences, pp. 9–18, January 2003
3. Carbo, J., Garcia, J., Molina, J.: Trust and reputation in e-services: concepts, models and applications. In: Lu, J., Zhang, G., Ruan, D. (eds.) E-Service Intelligence. Studies in Computational Intelligence, vol. 37, pp. 327–345. Springer, Berlin Heidelberg (2007)
4. Tan, Y.H., Hofman, W., Gordijn, J., Hulstijn, J.: A framework for the design of service systems. In: Demirkan, H., Spohrer, J.C., Krishna, V. (eds.) Service Systems Implementation. Service Science: Research and Innovations in the Service Economy, pp. 51–74. Springer, New York (2011)
5. Soomro, I., Ahmed, N.: Towards security risk-oriented misuse cases. In: La Rosa, M., Soffer, P. (eds.) BPM Workshops 2012. LNBIP, vol. 132, pp. 689–700. Springer, Heidelberg (2013)
6. Yu, E.S.K.: Models for supporting the redesign of organizational work. In: Proceedings of Conference on Organizational Computing Systems, COCS 1995, pp. 226–236. ACM, New York (1995)
7. Cahill, M., Lambert, D., Pinheiro, J., Sun, D.: Detecting fraud in the real world. In: Abello, J., Pardalos, P.M., Resende, M.G.C. (eds.) Handbook of Massive Data Sets. Massive Computing, vol. 4, pp. 911–929. Springer, New York (2002)
8. Ionita, D., Wieringa, R.J., Wolos, L., Gordijn, J., Pieters, W.: Using value models for business risk analysis in e-service networks. In: Ralyté, J., et al. (eds.) PoEM 2015. LNBIP, vol. 235, pp. 239–253. Springer, Heidelberg (2015). doi:10.1007/978-3-319-25897-3_16
9. Ruch, M., Sackmann, S.: Customer-specific transaction risk management in e-commerce. In: Nelson, M.L., Shaw, M.J., Strader, T.J. (eds.) AMCIS 2009. LNBIP, vol. 36, pp. 68–79. Springer, Heidelberg (2009)
10. Dritsoula, L., Musacchio, J.: A game of clicks: Economic incentives to fight click fraud in ad networks. Perform. Eval. Rev. **41**, 12–15 (2014)
11. Pieters, W., Banescu, S., Posea, S.: System abuse by service composition: Analysis and prevention. In: CESUN 2012: 3rd International Engineering Systems Symposium Delft University of Technology, The Netherlands, pp. 18–20, June 2012
12. Bolton, R.J.: Statistical fraud detection: A review. Stat. Sci. **17**(3), 235–249 (2002)
13. Gordijn, J., Akkermans, H.: Designing and evaluating e-business models. IEEE Intell. Syst. **16**(4), 11–17 (2001)
14. Gerpott, T.J.: Biased choice of a mobile telephony tariff type: Exploring usage boundary perceptions as a cognitive cause in choosing between a use-based or a flat rate plan. Telematics Inform. **26**(2), 167–179 (2009)
15. Scourias, J.: Overview of the global system for mobile communications. Technical report (1995)

16. Gordijn, J., Akkermans, H., van Vliet, H.: Business modelling is not process modelling. In: Mayr, H.C., Liddle, S.W., Thalheim, B. (eds.) ER Workshops 2000. LNCS, vol. 1921, pp. 40–51. Springer, Heidelberg (2000)
17. Ionita, D., Koenen, S.K., Wieringa, R.J.: Modelling telecom fraud with e3value. Technical report TR-CTIT-14-11, Centre for Telematics and Information Technology, University of Twente, Enschede, October 2014
18. Ross, S.: How does revenue sharing work in practice? Investopedia (2015). http://www.investopedia.com/ask/answers/010915/how-does-revenue-sharing-work-practice.asp. Accessed 12 December 2015

The Sharing Economy Revolution and Peer-to-peer Online Platforms. The Case of Airbnb

Linda Meleo[✉], Alberto Romolini, and Marco De Marco

International Telematic University Uninettuno,
corso Vittorio Emanuele II, 39, 00187 Rome, Italy
{l.meleo,a.romolini,
m.demarco}@uninettunouniversity.net

Abstract. The "sharing revolution" would not be possible without digital technologies and the diffusion of ICT worldwide. ICT has created a new level playing field also thanks to peer-to-peer (P2P) platforms, and a new concept, the "sharing and collaborative consumption online", is expanding. This concept is based on what can be called CASH - "collaboration", "access", "sharing" rather than "ownership" meant also as a chance to collect money in addition to monthly salary. This paper aims to describe a successful P2P platform that well reflect the CASH concept, Airbnb, currently the leader of the online accommodation marketplace, using the case study approach and the SWOT analysis methodology. This analysis is useful in order to understand the main features and functioning of such a platform and what to expect for the years to come. Results show that Airbnb is growing at high speed in terms of users and profits but some challenges have to be faced in the next future linked to regulatory issues and to traditional accommodation market and citizens reactions.

Keywords: Sharing economy · Collective consumption · ICT · Peer-to-peer · Airbnb

1 Introduction

In recent years, the sharing economy has opened new opportunities for individuals and companies. There is not a unique notion of sharing economy and there is some confusion about the activities that can be linked to this concept i.e. on-demand, social economy, cooperative economy, etc. (see i.e. [1, 2, 3, 4]). In general, the term sharing economy indicates different forms of exchange that can involve for-profit and non-profit activities and the main goal is to maximize the usage of under-utilized resources. Despite the debate on how the sharing economy should be defined, the "sharing revolution" would not be possible without digital technologies and the diffusion of ICT worldwide. In fact, ICT usage has dramatically increased the spread of information and reduced transaction costs, especially searching and bargaining costs. This had been possible especially thanks to Internet platforms that keep a myriad of individuals and businesses all over the world in contact, via a peer-to-peer relationship

© Springer International Publishing Switzerland 2016
T. Borangiu et al. (Eds.): IESS 2016, LNBIP 247, pp. 561–570, 2016.
DOI: 10.1007/978-3-319-32689-4_43

where actors interact providing, requesting or sharing resources for [co-]creating value [5]. In this scenario, the active contribution of Information Management in developing value-added services may transform IT from a perceived cost center to a perceived profit [6].

Peer-to-peer (P2P) platforms are nothing new on the Internet; in the past many other attempts were made such as the late nineties' Napster for music sharing (even if some authors argued that it was not a true example of "sharing economy" as ownership of the music changed from one user to another [7]). Given the rapid access of people to the Internet thanks to the reduction of the so called digital divide, and to the diffusion of pc and mobile devices with internet access, these platforms are well known worldwide and in different sectors [8]. In this scenario, where also the Public Administrations develop innovation-friendly business environment with appropriate ICT investments [9, 10], there is an higher propensity of consumers to use the Internet and all the services offered by the Internet through the access to several digital platforms [11], having an ubiquitous relationship with different applications and business services [12].

In short, P2P platforms have created a new level playing field where a new concept, based on what can be called CASH - "collaboration", "access", "sharing" rather than - "ownership", forms the basis for what is called "sharing and collaborative consumption online", as well as for new work opportunities. As a consequence, the acronym CASH has a twofold nature and accurately reflects these two points, namely a new way of consumption and the chance for individuals to collect money in addition to their monthly salary. The P2P platforms that reflect the CASH concept, mainly the not for profit ones, are several and represent the source of "disruptive" innovation among markets and business models.

Collaborative consumption, in particular, is based on the P2P online marketplace. The core idea of this kind of platform is renting or swapping different types of goods or services such as housing, cars, study materials and even food. Collaborative consumption has affected many sectors (see i.e. [13, 14]), and, as one of the most successful business developments has been experienced by the accommodation industry, an analysis of the main characteristics, strategies and business models adopted in this sector is an aid to understanding the forces at work.

Given this importance of understanding the main features of the "CASH platforms", this paper aims to analyze the strengths, weaknesses, opportunities, and threats (SWOT analysis) of the successful P2P platform Airbnb, currently the leader of the online accommodation marketplace. The high levels of diffusion and use of the Airbnb platform worldwide together with the economic effects created for both consumers and producers reflect the CASH paradigm described above and make it an appropriate case study. In fact, Airbnb get in touch hosts and users reducing transaction costs and let hosts rent assets (rooms or houses) that would be otherwise underused, collecting additional money, and guest to find cheaper alternatives to "traditional" accommodations such as hotels.

Section 2 provides a short theoretical background to collaborative consumption, and Sect. 3 illustrates the Airbnb case. Section 4 shows the Airbnb SWOT analysis, and, finally, Sect. 5 closes the paper with conclusions and a number of indications for further research.

2   Methodology

The sections below examine one of the most successful examples of collective consumption, Airbnb, using a case study approach and the SWOT methodology. In details, this paper uses an illustrative approach based on the analysis of 3 main aspects: 1. Airbnb investment strategy; 2. Airbnb business model; 3. Airbnb main legal and debated issues. Data are collected from different sources. For point 1 this paper refers to Marketline database [15], CBInsights database [16], Airbnb website and economic newspapers, and for point 2 Airbnb website, economic literature and economic newspapers. Finally, for point 3 data are gathered from economic literature, internet sources and economic newspapers. The information collected is finally used to develop the SWOT matrix.

3   Results and Discussion

3.1   Airbnb, History and General Information

Airbnb (formerly named AirBed & Breakfast) is a P2P platform launched in October 2007, with headquarters in San Francisco, California. Since then, it has experienced a rapid expansion and growing number of listed accommodation all over the world. Data provided by the company indicates that more than 6 million nights have been booked in more than 190 countries and more than 34 thousand cities [17] since its start. Data from a 2015 survey indicates that almost 12 % of leisure and business travellers have chosen Airbnb at least once to find accommodation, and that, among the 41 % of the sample aware of Airbnb, 25 % has used its services [18]. For 2016, demand is expected to grow further reaching 18 % of both leisure and business travellers [18]. The company is currently worth 25 billion dollars, more than the Marriott group [18].

The idea was the fruit of the personal experience of the 3 founders who wanted to make enough money to attend a conference and decided to rent out their airbed as accommodation. The company has since expanded to offer apartments, houses, rooms, and other types of accommodation with or without onsite hosts.

The Airbnb platform represents the typical case of "two-sided" market with positive network externalities on both sides; the more the one side grows the higher the benefits for the other side [19]. Given the importance to improve the number of guests and hosts due to these network externalities, the platform is user-friendly. Once becoming a validated member by providing a scan of an identity card or passport, the user can be a host and a guest at the same time and receive and provide feedback on his experience. Guests can look for accommodation by selecting the date and destination and thus obtaining a list of solutions and the price charged. The user then chooses a solution and sends a request to the owner of the property. When he accepts, the transaction is closed. The arrival and the departure times are at the host's agreement. Money is transferred by Airbnb to the host on the day of the guest's arrival.

Airbnb currently owns roughly 4 % of the market share of the Vacation Rental and P2P rental sector [7]. The economic performance experienced by the company saw important revenues increase from its launch. Estimates indicate that revenues were approximately 423 million dollars in 2014 and 675 million in 2015 (+55 %) [7]. This growth is due to a demand increase but also to specific and on-going investment strategies that rely on significant financial funding (see Sect. 3.2.).

3.2   Investment and Financial Strategies

Looking at the company financial strategy, it is expected that Airbnb will expand its activity in efforts to catch other market segments. The aim is probably to enrich the platform options by offering new and integrated travelling and accommodation services. This differentiation strategy is probably needed in order to improve Airbnb's reputation and brand fidelity and to counter growing competition from other platforms offering similar services such as Homeaway (its main competitor), Couchsurfing, or Roomrama.

In 2010 the company secured $7.2 million in Series A funding from 3 main investors, Sequoia Capital, Greylock Partners, and a third, undisclosed source [15]. Then, in 2011, it started a fund-raising campaign that enabled Airbnb to enlarge its international network and acquire the majority of shares on 1 June, in Accoleo, a German company providing the same hosting services locally as Airbnb. In July of the same year, Airbnb secured an additional $112 million in Series B round of venture funding led by Andreessen Horowitz. On 20th November 2015, total funding was equal to 2493.8 million dollars vis-a-vis 711.5 million dollars of Homeaway [16].

The expansion policy of Airbnb continued with the acquisition of [15]: 1. Crash-padder, a British online marketplace for individuals to list accommodation to be rented out only for short periods of time (21st March 2012); 2. Dailybooth a website where people can find photo and blogging services (24th July 2012); 3. Localmind, a question and answer platform where users can ask what is happening in any country in the world and provide replies to these questions (13th December 2012); 4. Pencil Labs, a firm that develops calendar and messaging applications (1st December 2014); 5. and Lapka, a Russian start-up producing manufacturing sensors (29th September 2015).

There is also a plan to acquire Vamo Labs, a platform for planning and booking travel, in future months.

3.3   Airbnb Business Model

As mentioned in Sect. 3.1., the Airbnb business model is quite simple. Thanks to its platform, Airbnb matches the supply and demand for accommodation. In this way, transaction costs are dramatically reduced, and will continue to fall as more individuals sign up to the platform (network externalities) [20]. Membership is free of charge and requires only identity card verification. When a person books a room or an apartment and the host accepts the reservation, he will be charged a sum. This sum includes the price per night that is decided by the hosts (that can include also a cleaning fee), and revenues for Airbnb. These revenues are calculated as below:

– Revenues from guest that is charged by a 6–12 % fee, according to the type of accommodation, and to the length of the stay.
– Revenues from the host that is also charged by a 3 % credit card transaction fee.

Hosts can be individuals and bed and breakfast (B&B) owners can also register. However, listing a block of identical rooms is forbidden [21]. This means that the platform enables small and less well-known accommodation to access demand [22].

Trust and reputation are two fundamental principles for enhancing and protecting any online business and allowing the company to grow. The basic strategy adopted by Airbnb to foster the trust is not a novelty as they introduced online reviews in a similar manner to hotel. However, for Airbnb there is a double review mechanism as for other platforms (such as eBay), one for the host and one for the guest. The platform offers a number of additional special features, such as the opportunity to send messages and questions directly to the host [20], see pictures, and other personal information linked to Facebook or LinkedIn hosts and guests' profiles.

Data indicates that business travellers currently prefer to book traditional hotels due to safety and services offered in this type of accommodation [20]. Airbnb is trying to conquer part of this market segment by investing in client satisfaction launching a 24/7 telephone concierge service. Guests can call for advices, book tickets, for example, and generally receive the same type of information as they would in a hotel. The entrance strategy of Airbnb in business and luxury travellers segments, traditionally managed by hotels, has started in July 2014 after the partnership with Concur, an American travel management enterprise that offers travel and expenses management services to companies [23].

3.4 Legal Issue on Safety and Tax

Airbnb is a pioneer in P2P accommodation platforms and this is the main reason why the company is encountering problems on both legal and regulatory grounds. In fact, it is facing several legal actions as the result of damage and vandalism by guest travelers, especially in the US. This has led the company to establish rules to protect hosts, and design strategies in order to discourage dishonest and hazardous behaviour [17]. This represents a fundamental step in order to preserve the trustworthiness of the platform and overall reputation. Airbnb is already defining a number of measures to improve safety and identification mechanisms, such as a 24-hour hotline. The company has insurance coverage for damage caused during the stay.

Other problems are linked to the tax issues as many local government complained against Airbnb because the platform represents a way to elude local taxes, mainly city hotel taxes. This issue is still controversial, even if Airbnb has reached several agreements in order to gather and remit these taxes to local authorities (i.e. San Francisco, Chicago and Amsterdam) [20].

3.5 Regulatory Issues and the Impact on the Accommodation Market

Legal issues are not the only obstacles encountered by Airbnb; there are also those of a regulatory nature. As a P2P accommodation marketplace, the company lowers transaction costs, and allows individuals to offer a tangible service (the room) by means of an intangible asset (the platform), enhancing the growth of the so-called "Internet of things". As a consequence, barriers to entry to the accommodation market are dramatically lower. Referring to the contestable market theory [24], this means that more competitors are offered an incentive to enter the market, thus lowering the price for the stay.

This situation generates a twofold effect. On the one side, Airbnb is becoming an attractive, cheaper alternative to hotels, and consumers on a tight budget have a greater opportunity to travel. Morgan Stanley 2015 survey [18] indicates price is the main reasons for which travellers chose Airbnb (55 % of respondents), even if for more than 1 night stays. Guttentag [25] showed that in selected cities of the North America, the average Airbnb price for a private room is roughly equal to the average room price of 1–2 star hotel accommodation. However, the average of the 10 lowest Airbnb prices for a home-apartment are comparable to the price of 1–2 star hotel room, whereas for a single private room, Airbnb prices are as low as those offered by hostels. Rental costs are lower than hotels because the host generally lives in the house and already pays the fixed costs (i.e. utilities).

That being said, there is also a significant impact on competition. The market entry of private accommodations is creating drawbacks for the hotel and online travel agencies (OTAs) sectors, which can be considered as part of the same relevant market. Morgan Stanley 2015 survey [18] indicates that 42 % and 20 % of travellers have decided to rent an Airbnb listed accommodation to the expense of hotels and OTAs respectively. Despite the fact that the services offered are not totally comparable with hotels, Airbnb is perceived as an alternative with a number of additional features, such as the chance to experience the cultural and every-day life of the destination, a value that appears to be more and more important for travellers [26], and is expanding to catch also business travellers as already mentioned. It is therefore generating "disruptive innovation" in the accommodation market that could lead to the same degree of change as that experienced when OTAs such as Expedia began to challenge High Street travel agencies, many of which went out of business because they could not exploit the same cost advantages as the online agencies ([25, 27]).

There is also a problem of a level playing field in regulatory terms. At the time of the writing, there is a regulatory gap to fill as a shared set of rules or strategies worldwide has yet to be devised, with the result that the business model of Airbnb, and other P2P platforms, has opened up new challenges in terms of regulation.

As well documented in the literature (i.e. [28]), regulation could incentivize proper behaviour if adequately defined. To avoid the situation of over- or under-regulation, one fundamental step is the definition of *ex-ante* regulatory goal(s). At the moment, it seems that policy makers all over the world do not yet have a clear picture of the "acceptability" of the sunrise of such a phenomenon as the collective consumption platforms, especially when considering the tax payment issue as mentioned in the previous section. This uncertainty is quite clear when observing what is going on in different countries. In San Francisco and New York, for example, there have been significant knock-on effects.

In details, a number of San Francisco citizens, aided by hotel associations, are arguing that rents in the city have risen because of Airbnb (data indicates a 40 % price rise since 2010, [29]). This has been explained by the fact that households find it more profitable to rent on a short stay basis, causing a shortage of long term rental properties and an increase in rent prices which forces long-term tenants, especially those of middle to low income, to leave. Some proposals have been under review by San Francisco authorities over recent months. One of them, "proposition F", proposes a reduction in short term rentals to 75 days per year from 90 if the host does not live in the same place, but no limitation if the owner lives in the house listed on the Airbnb platform.

The issue was temporary resolved by referendum on 4th November 2015 in favour of Airbnb (55 % of citizens voted against proposition F) [30], but there is an uncertain scenario for the months to come as Airbnb could be a factor influencing long term rent prices in other cities. The shortage of houses could be a problem especially in cities where rents are already high. For example, in February 2016, the average Airbnb price for an accommodation for a one month stay in Rome is equal to 2,766.00 euros (Airbnb list, last access 19th December 2015). This price is considerably higher than the average long term monthly rental of 864.00 euros [31]. At the time of the writing, additional legal disputes have been registered in New York City [32]. Long term rental prices have increased substantially. Local authorities and a part of the population alleged that this is due to the fact that Airbnb lists also short-term accommodation that infringes local regulation. In fact, New York law settles that less than 30 days stays are forbidden in case the host does not live in the rented accommodation. This is the reasons for which, in January 2016, several house previously listed were cancelled from Airbnb site [33].

Finally, regulation should also determine how competition should flow in the accommodation market as a whole and how to handle competition with hotels. In fact, it is important to recall that, given the Airbnb expansionary strategy (see Sects. 3.2 and 3.3), hotels associations joint the local population causes against Airbnb above described. As a consequence, it is expected that some regulatory actions will be introduced in order to set rules to settle an appropriate competitive framework.

4   Airbnb SWOT Analysis

The sections above provide an examination of the strategy and problems encountered by Airbnb since its foundation and form the basis of the SWOT analysis illustrated in Table 1.

As the SWOT analysis shows, Airbnb still has a number of important opportunities for growth linked for the most part to the possibility of enforcing price competition and increasing market shares to the detriment of "traditional" accommodation, but adding an everyday life experience that you would not have in a hotel. Airbnb would benefit from a strong brand reputation, facilitated by a dual rating system, and from growing network externalities thanks to its user-friendly platform where hosts and guests can interact. The brand is currently well known and new services have been introduced to overcome some quality issues.

However, Airbnb still has to face a number of weaknesses, such as opposition from the hotel industry, whose future is jeopardized by this new type of business. Other weaknesses are related to the growing legal disputes linked for the most to vandalism or other guests' moral hazard behaviour. This issue represents a threat if episodes of

Table 1. The SWOT matrix (Source: own elaboration)

Strengths	Weaknesses
- Low prices	- Lobby action from hotel industry
- Low transaction costs	- Legal disputes
- Network externalities	- Low entry and exit barriers to enter online rental
- Daily-life experience	markets
- Direct exchange of information between host and guest	
- Easy to use the platform	
- Clear fees and charges	
- Dual rating system	
- High brand reputation and new services	
Opportunities	Threats
- Tourism flow can increase due to lower prices	- Regulation across different countries
- Demand could grow especially where hotels are expensive	- Tax issue
- Venture capital	- Rise in prices of long-term rents as owners find short-term stays more profitable
- Expansion initiatives in related markets to diversify offer	- Increasing episodes of vandalism, and other moral hazard behaviour
- Growing number of travellers in addition to tourists	- Increasing number of competitors

this kind are not limited and if individuals are discouraged from listing property on Airbnb, affecting the system and the effects of the network externalities. Another weakness is related to the fact that entry and exit barriers for the online marketplace are quite low and consequently new entrants could easily copy the Airbnb model, thereby reducing profitability.

On the other hand, Airbnb can exploit several opportunities in the future. The more competitive prices of the company compared with hotels, especially in more expensive cities, would attract new demand; the Airbnb expansion strategy, as evidenced by the financial operations carried out over recent years, will permit the company to enter related markets and enable Airbnb to diversify its core business and offer higher quality and integrated services. Finally, the number of people who can be defined as travellers rather than tourists is increasing and means that individuals are increasingly interested in experiencing the local culture and way of life, the fundamental idea behind Airbnb's proposal of staying in private accommodation.

Nevertheless, the analysis has highlighted a number of threats linked mainly to the local regulatory uncertainty regarding the Airbnb business, including the tax issue. Other threats are related to the issues coming from citizens in places where long-term rent prices have increased due to the higher profits guaranteed by short-term stays, increasing vandalism and other moral hazard behaviour of guests and hosts. Finally, the number of competitors is growing and forcing Airbnb to invest in quality and other services in order to preserve its accommodation market share.

5 Conclusions

The analysis developed in this paper on Airbnb case study of "collaborative consumption", has highlighted several points for discussion.

At first, even if the definition and the borders of what can be called "sharing economy" are still an open debate, there is strong evidence that this kind of model is going to improve and spread over time. The case study on Airbnb is a good description of the innovative solutions and the growing success of online marketplace platforms and perfectly realizes the CASH concept described in the introduction. In fact, Airbnb experiences all the features of CASH: 1. Collaboration as it keeps in contact persons that desire to use underutilized resources (an entire house, a room, etc.) and persons that need accommodation; 2. Access as Airbnb provides the chance to find accommodation opportunities also at lower prices than B&B and hotels, thanks to its platform; 3. Sharing as property owners choose to share their accommodation with unknown hosts knowing that they would exploit the same benefits in case of leisure or business travels; 4. Hosts gain extra-cash from renting their properties.

The main findings of the analysis suggest that Airbnb platform appears to work properly and they are supposed to grow further as data shows. However, there are still many challenges to manage linked to reputation, to the reactions of the main competitors (hotels for the most) to Airbnb expansion, to the future regulatory decisions, and to the competitive forces that will characterize the accommodation market in the next future. For these reasons, this paper represents a useful starting point for understanding and monitoring the evolution of online P2P platform markets and for further studies on Airbnb and similar platforms.

References

1. Belk, R.: Sharing. J. Cons. Res. **36**, 715–734 (2010)
2. Gansky, L.: The Mesh: Why the Future of Business is Sharing. Portfolio Penguin, New York (2012)
3. Ritzer, G., Jurgenson, N.: Production, consumption, prosumption: the nature of capitalism in the age of the digital "Prosumer". J. of Consum. Cult. **10**, 13–36 (2010)
4. Morozov, E.: The "sharing economy" undermines workers' rights. The Financial Times, 14 October 2013
5. Za, S., Marzo, F., De Marco, M., Cavallari, M.: Agent based simulation of trust dynamics in dependence networks. In: Sampaio da Nóvoa, H., Dragoicea, M. (eds.) Exploring Services Science, pp. 243–252. Springer, Heidelberg (2015)
6. Ricciardi, F., De Marco, M.: The challenge of service oriented performances for chief information officers. In: Snene, M. (ed.) Exploring Services Science. Lecture Notes in Business Information Processing, vol. 103, pp. 258–270. Springer, Heidelberg (2012)
7. Piper Jaffray: Sharing Economy. An In-Depth Look At Its Evolution & Trajectory Across Industries. Piper Jaffray Investment Research (2015)
8. Carillo, K., Scornavacca, E., Za, S.: An investigation of the role of dependency in predicting continuance intention to use ubiquitous media systems: combining a media sytem perspective with expectation-confirmation theories. In: Proceedings Twenty Second European Conference on Information Systems (ECIS 2014) (2014). http://aisel.aisnet.org/ecis2014/proceedings/track16/11/

9. Sorrentino, M., De Marco, M.: Implementing e-government in hard times: when the past is wildly at variance with the future. Inform. Polity **18**, 331–342 (2013)

10. Dameri, R.P., Benevolo, C., Rossignoli, C., Ricciardi, F., De Marco, M.: Centralization vs. decentralization of purchasing in the public sector: the role of e-procurement in the italian case. Contemporary Research on E-business Technology and Strategy. Communications in Computer and Information Science, vol. 332, pp. 457–470. Springer, Heidelberg (2012)

11. Resca, A., Za, S., Spagnoletti, P.: Digital platforms as sources for organizational and strategic transformation: a case study of the Midblue project. J. Theor. Appl. Electron. Commer. Res. **8**, 71–84 (2013)

12. Za, S., D'Atri, E., Resca, A.: Single sign-on in cloud computing scenarios: a research proposal. In: D'Atri, A., Ferrara, M., George, J.F., Spagnoletti, P. (eds.) Information Technology and Innovation Trends in Organizations, pp. 45–52. Springer-Verlag, Berlin Heidelberg (2011)

13. Botsman, R., Rogers, R.: What's Mine Is Yours: The Rise of Collaborative Consumption. Harper Business, New York (2010)

14. Geron, T.: Airbnb and the unstoppable rise of the share economy. Forbes, 23 January 2013

15. Marketline database. http://www.marketline.com

16. Cbinsights database. https://www.cbinsights.com

17. Airbnb web site. https://www.airbnb.it/

18. Morgan Stanley: Internet, Lodging, Leisure and Hotels. Global Insight: Who Will Airbnb Hurt More - Hotels or OTAs?. Morgan Stanley, 15 November 2015

19. Lin, M., Wu, R., Zhou, W.: Platform Pricing with Endogenous Network Effects (2015). SSRN, http://ssrn.com/abstract=2426033

20. Henter, A.H., Windekilde, I.M.: Transaction costs and the sharing economy. Info **18**, 1–15 (2016)

21. The Economist: Airbnb in New York City: After the fine, 28 May 2012

22. Vermeulen, I.E., Seegers, D.: Tried and tested: the impact of online hotel reviews on consumer consideration. Tourism Manage. **30**, 123–127 (2009)

23. Concur Business Travel & Expense Management, https://www.concur.com/blog/en-us/concur-airbnb-sharing-economy

24. Baumol, W.J., Panzar, J.C., Willig, R.D.: Contestable markets and the theory of industry structure. Am. Econ. Rev. **72**, 1–15 (1982)

25. Guttentag, D.: Airbnb: disruptive innovation and the rise of an informal tourism accommodation sector. Curr. Issues Tour. **18**, 1192–1217 (2013)

26. PricewaterhouseCoopers: The Sharing Economy. Consumer Intelligence Series (2015). http://download.pwc.com/ie/pubs/2015-pwc-cis-sharing-economy.pdf

27. Law, R.: Disintermediation of hotel reservations: the perception of different groups of online buyers in Hong Kong. Int. J. Contemp. Hospit. Manag. **21**, 766–772 (2009)

28. Stigler, G.J.: The Theory of Economic Regulation. Bell J. Econ. **2**, 3–21 (1971)

29. Hall, B.S.: Airbnb Fights Back Against An Increasingly Hostile San Francisco. Forbes, 24 September 2015

30. Money CNN. http://money.cnn.com/2015/11/04/technology/san-francisco-prop-f-airbnb-results/

31. Case.trovi.it. http://case.trovit.it/136/prezzo-affitto-casa-provincia-roma

32. Airbnb action. https://www.airbnbaction.com/data-on-the-airbnb-community-in-nyc/

33. The Guardian. http://www.theguardian.com/technology/2016/feb/10/airbnb-new-york-city-listings-purge-multiple-apartment-listings

IoT and Mobile Apps. for Public Transport Service Management

Dynamic Service Capacity and Demand Matching in a Holonic Public Transport System

Theodor Borangiu[✉], Silviu Răileanu, Iulia Voinescu,
and Octavian Morariu

Department of Automation and Industrial Informatics, Research Centre in CIM
and Robotics - CIMR, University Politehnica of Bucharest,
313, Spl. Independentei, Sector 6, Bucharest, Romania
{theodor.borangiu,silviu.raileanu,
iulia.voinescu}@cimr.pub.ro

Abstract. The paper describes the development of a fleet management system for public transport services, operating in semi heterarchical mode: (1) hierarchical on long term, with optimal activity planning and resource scheduling; (2) heterarchical– agile and robust at disturbances, with real-time rescheduling of unavailable drivers, not operational busses and blocked routes. The holonic paradigm is used; the holonic transport control architecture, the types of holons and the basic cooperation rules between them are presented. The paper describes the Service Scheduler, as centralized, hierarchical information system used for optimized, long-term capacity managing. The decentralized, heterarchical Delegate MAS (Multi-agent System) performs real-time change management for capacity and demand matching, based on intelligent devices embedded on resources. An implementing MAS framework based on JADE is proposed.

Keywords: Service management · Matching capacity and demand · Dynamic environment · Holonic Public Transport System · Multi-agent framework

1 Introduction

A systemic approach of complex services relies on two basic principles: (1) Designing initial, long-term service capacity in an open perspective that considers the first two stages of the **service's lifecycle** (Managing Service Set-up and Configuring – for *efficiency* and *profitability*; Customer Order Management – for *value co-creation*) and (2) Modelling service operations, resources and interdependencies as **dynamic,** closed loop **system** reacting to changes in service demand and capacity (in the last two stages of the service's lifecycle: Service Monitoring and Evaluation – for *observability* and *reactivity*; Service Operations Management – for *controllability, robustness, agility*).

This open systemic approach is necessary especially when services are delivered in a dynamic environment such as public transport, and can be materialized through an information system acting as Service Scheduler (operations planner, human resources scheduler and physical resources allocator) with variable operating mode, which is capable to switch from centralized, hierarchical operating mode (assuring optimality on

© Springer International Publishing Switzerland 2016
T. Borangiu et al. (Eds.): IESS 2016, LNBIP 247, pp. 573–589, 2016.
DOI: 10.1007/978-3-319-32689-4_44

long term) to decentralized, heterarchical one (providing robustness to disturbances and agility to temporary changes in service demand) [1, 2].

Such an approach preserves the optimality with which initial capacity investment has been made, while allowing real-time adaptability to disturbances and variations in service demand, due to special, sometimes unforeseen situations. For public transport systems, disturbances may have internal causes, i.e. human resources not available, transport means not operational or external causes, i.e. traffic accidents, closed routes etc. To cope with such situations, there is need to assure a high level of instrumenting resources through network embedded systems, i.e. access to elements of the physical world any time from any level using an unified communication environment (such as fast, broadband Internet) in an Internet of Things (IoT) and Internet of Services (IoS) vision [3–5].

In the service lifecycle analysis, the Service Management stage corresponds to the Design and Development core service activity, being covered by the Service Configuring and Set-Up (SCSU) component of aggregate service activities; in information based service systems SSyst, the core activities in the SCSU Management stage are: *service planning* and *scheduling*, which consist in scheduling the operations of a composite service, respectively in allocating capacity and resources (human, technology).

Service planning consists in assigning the necessary time interval and capacity corresponding to the service specifications requested by the customer and settled in the Service Level Agreement (SLA); these specifications may refer, in the most general case, to the number of users for which a simple (1-activity) or composite (n-activity, $n \geq 1$) service is requested and its delivery must be started at a certain time moment or must be finished at a certain time moment. We shall refer to such task as "service set" with $\dim(service\_set) = n$, and

$$delivery(service\_set) = \begin{cases} t_{start\_delivery}, & start\ imposed \\ t_{finish\_delivery} & termination\ imposed \end{cases}$$

The service planning and scheduling function of the SCSU is related to matching capacity and demand; several strategies and methods have been proposed and can be included in the Shared Information repository (methods, algorithms and tools) of the Service Scheduler [6, 7]. *Chase demand* and *level capacity* are two generic strategies available for service planning. For the chase demand strategy, a number of operations-oriented strategies such as workshift scheduling to vary capacity to match the changing levels of customer demand are proposed [8]. *Level capacity* strategy uses marketing-oriented strategies, such as price incentives to smooth customer demand to utilize better fixed capacity, but is not adequate for public transport service. *Yield management* is a hybrid strategy using real-time information to maximize revenue [9]. Finally, to test the acceptance of rush transport orders received from the customer (e.g., the municipality), the Early Deadline First (EDF) strategy may be considered [10].

Level capacity is a second generic strategy for capacity management, providing generally low customer waiting for long-run public transport forecasting; it is characterized by moderate utilization of employees having a high labour-skill level and for whom high training and low supervision is necessary; there is also low labour turnover

[11]. Service capacity is defined in terms of an achievable level of output per unit time (e.g., bus arrival rate each day, repetitive during a week). For a public transport service provider the measure of capacity is based on busy bus drivers; however, service capacity can be also defined in terms of the supporting facility (e.g., number of busses); capacity can be limited by several factors such as: available labour by skill classification, equipment or environment.

For the public transport service, demand cannot be smoothed very effectively; therefore, control must come from adjusting service capacity to match demand.

Future public transport systems need to cope with frequent changes and disturbances. As such, their control requires constant adaptation and high flexibility. Holonic transport, derived from holonic manufacturing is a highly distributed control paradigm that promises to handle these problems successfully. It is based on the concept of autonomous co-operating agents, called "holons" [12]. Inspired by ideas of the HMS (Holonic Manufacturing Systems) consortium [13] which translated the concepts that Koestler developed for social organisations and living organisms into a set of appropriate concepts for manufacturing industries, the present work aims at attaining in the domain of public transport services the benefits that holonic organisation provides to living organisms and societies: robustness at disturbances, adaptability and flexibility at change in demand, and efficient use of available human and technology resources. The Holonic Public Transport (HPTS) concept developed for this purpose combines the best features of hierarchical and heterarchical organisation [14]. It preserves the stability of a hierarchy while providing the dynamic flexibility of a heterarchy.

The rest of the paper is organized as follows: Section 2 presents the structure of the holonic transport control architecture, the types of holons and the basic rules for the cooperation between holons. Section 3 describes the Service Scheduler as centralized, hierarchical information system used for optimized, long-term capacity managing. In Sect. 4 we detail the organization of the decentralized, heterarchical Delegate MAS (Multi-agent System) performing the real-time change management for capacity and demand matching. An implementing framework, solutions and conclusions are included in Sect. 5.

2 The Holonic Public Transport Control Architecture

Applying the Holonic paradigm to Transport Systems (HTS) and Service-Oriented Architectures (SOA) are at present two of the most studied and referenced solutions for the next generation of Holonic Public Transport Systems (HPTS); both of these solutions offer the necessary features to create open, flexible and agile control environments for the smart, digital and networked transport (activities planning, resource scheduling and allocation, operations monitoring).

The Holonic paradigm has been recognized in industry, academia and research, as providing the above mentioned attributes by means of a decentralized control architecture composed by a social organization of intelligent entities, called holons, with specific behaviours and goals defined by reference architectures such as PROSA [15], HABPA [16], CoBASA [17], ADACOR [18]. On the other hand, the Service-oriented paradigm defines principles for conceiving decentralized informational architectures for the control of public transport that decompose computational processes into sub-processes called services, to later distribute them among the different available resources available. Its focus is to leverage the creation of reusable and interoperable function blocks in order to reduce the amount of reprogramming efforts.

The interpretation of the holon as a whole particle refers to an entity which is entirely stand-alone or supreme (a whole), but belongs to a higher order system as one basic individual part (a particle). If a limited number of parts (holons) fail, the higher order system should still be able to proceed with its main task by diverting the lost functionality to other holons [19]. The following holonic attributes have been considered in the present research: *autonomy* (the capability of an entity to create and control the execution of its own strategies) and *cooperation* (a set of entities develops and executes mutually acceptable plans).

In the context of public transport services, a holon is defined as an autonomous and co-operative building block of a public transport system for transforming, transporting, storing and/or validating information and physical items (e.g., passengers, busses). It consists of an information- and physical-processing part; a holon can be part of another holon.

The combination of holonic and SOA paradigms appears to be a very attractive solution for the new generation of smart public transport systems, thanks to the flexibility provided by:

- HPTS at a structural level in the control architecture, and by
- SOA at a process level,

with decomposition and encapsulation of manufacturing processes allowing their distribution among resources. The holonic approach is the main engine for the digital transformation of public transport in what concerns "Distribution" and "Intelligence". The HTS paradigm is based on defining a main set of assets: *resources* (technology - busses, humans - bus drivers, reflecting the service provider's profile, capabilities, skills), *routes* (reflecting the client's needs, value propositions) and *orders* (reflecting the business solutions) – represented by holons communicating and collaborating in *holarchies* according to a set of rules to reach a common goal – expressed by orders.

Due to the fact that:

$$[\text{Holon}] \leftarrow [\text{Physical Asset}] + [\text{Agent} = \text{Information counterpart}]$$

it becomes possible to solve at informational level all specific activities of the **Service Configuring and Set-Up** and **Service Delivery and Monitoring** components of aggregate service activities in a public transport service system [20]: activities planning, resource scheduling and allocation, process and environment (e.g., route) monitoring, preventive resource maintenance, service evaluation and QoS control:

- Triggered by real-time events gathered from the transport processes, resources and environment or customer's requests;
- Controlled in real-time, with orchestration and choreography assured by SOA in standard, secure mode.

Thus, the holarchy created by the holons defined for the HPTS acts as a "Physical Multi-agent System – PMAS", transposing in the physical realm the inherent distribution induced by agent implementation framework, according to a predefined transport ontology.

The proposed HPTS covers aspects of both hierarchical as well as heterarchical control; also, the structure of the transport system is decoupled from the control algorithm, and logistical aspects can be decoupled from technical ones. The control architecture of the HPTS is illustrated in Fig. 1.

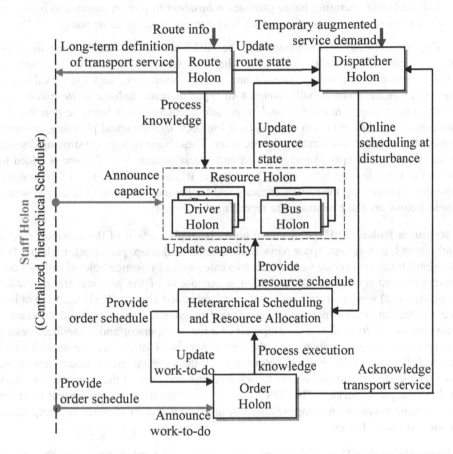

Fig. 1. Control architecture of the HPTS, basic building blocks and their relationships

The control system is in charge with:

1. Offline, long term set up and configuring of transport service (SCSU): defining the global service capacity from customer specification and environment characteristics, establishing feasible duties and pieces of work, sequencing activities (bus driving/care/preventive maintenance, drivers' health control), daily and weekly workshift scheduling. This initial planning of the long term public transport is

performed using algorithms that *optimize the cost of fixed capacity investment*, while interacting with the customer (the municipality) in a value co-creation process.

2. Online resource scheduling in case of deviations from normal conditions off line planned (driver not available, bus not operational, route blocked) and temporary changes in demand (rush orders); real-time monitoring resource and service status. In order to rapidly detect these deviations, resources are instrumented with mobile or embedded devices which can send information and event alerts over fast and secure communication networks to a decision system with distributed intelligence. This real-time operating mode provides *robustness to perturbations* and *agility to demand variations*, dynamically matching service capacity to demand.

Physical entities/human operators in the HPTS are represented by their informational counterparts, which take part in the processes of global activity planning, reactive resource scheduling, control and online monitoring, and QoS evaluation. The HPTS architecture is built around four types of **basic holons**: *route holons*, *resource holons*, *dispatcher holons* and *order holons*, each of them being responsible for one aspect of public transport control, be it logistics, technological planning, resource capabilities or route specifications respectively. These basic holons are structured using object-oriented concepts like aggregation and specialisation. A *staff holon* is added to assist the basic holons with expert knowledge; it allows for the use of centralised algorithms optimizing the service capacity and for the incorporation of legacy systems. These holons are their relations are represented in Fig. 1:

- **Resource Holon (ReH).** A resource holon is an abstraction of the transport means such as: bus, bus garage, spare parts, maintenance workshop, personnel, fuel, etc. For the global transport service we consider two categories of resource holons: vehicles and drivers (human operators). A *bus holon* is composed of the physical transportation mean (the bus) equipped with an Intelligent Embedded Device (IED) used for online event detection, status monitoring, automated diagnosis, traceability and preventive maintenance. A *driver holon* is composed of a human operator and a handheld device for real-time communication with the dispatcher. ReH offers service capacity and functionality to the other types of holons; it holds the mechanisms to allocate resources, and the knowledge and procedures to organise, use and control the transport resources to drive the public service. The HPTS does not separate the transport system from the service control system; it comprises both. A physical transport resource is incorporated inside a resource holon.

- **Route Holon (RoH).** It holds the process and service knowledge to assure the correct making of the transport service with sufficient quality. A *route holon* contains consistent and up-to-date information on the road and stops configuration, traffic particularities, user requirements, service configuring, process plans, bill of materials, quality assurance, procedures, etc. As such, it contains the "service model" of the public transport, not the "transport service state model" of one service instance being delivered. RoH acts as an information server to the other holons in the HPTS. The route holon comprises functionalities which are traditionally covered by service operations management, process planning and quality assurance.

- Order Holon (OH). It is composed of a particular bus and named human operator, a detailed route, a timing and time interval in which the route must be serviced. An *order holon* represents a task in the public transport service system; it is responsible for performing the assigned service correctly and on time. It manages the service being delivered, the produced, the transport service state model, and all logistical information processing related to the job. An order holon may represent customer orders, rush orders for temporary capacity update, orders to check the drivers' health, orders to clean maintain and repair busses, etc. The OH performs tasks traditionally assigned to a dispatcher and a short term scheduler based on negotiation and collective decision. It is a result of an aggregation process managed by the dispatcher holon and performed through negotiation in the heterarchical scheduler (see Fig. 1) which integrates in transport service task a temporary demand for route(s) with particular timing, vehicle (s), driver(s), and servicing aspects. Both the drivers and busses are monitored during service delivery (OH execution) and eventually replaced if their state or quality of services requires it.

- Dispatcher Holon (DH). It coordinates the process of rescheduling the transport service in case of temporary blocked routes, not available drivers and not operational vehicles, or dynamically matching the transport capacity with a temporary increased demand by assigning additional transport resource on short, peak time periods. The *dispatcher holon* is responsible with online monitoring of the transport activities, state of OH execution, validating schedules asked for in rush orders and real-time resource scheduling in case of deviations from normal conditions as described above.

The HPTS includes also a **Staff holon** (SH) to assist the basic holons in performing their work. The SH provides the basic holons with sufficient information such that these can take the correct decision to solve the online scheduling problem. The staff holon allows for the presence of centralised elements and functionality in the HPTS architecture to solve the long-term global transport service planning problem. The SH represents the centralized Service Scheduler which provides optimal long-term schedules; these schedules are taken as advice. The basic holons will follow this advice as well as possible; when, due to disturbances and changes in the service demand, the hierarchical SH performs badly, the advice may be ignored by the basic holons, which again take autonomous actions to do their collaborative scheduling work. On the other hand, when disturbances are absent, the HPTS is configured such that the basic holons do follow (in a hierarchical way) the advice of the staff holon. This semi-heterarchical operating mode is determined by a meta-controller, which defines the basic rules for cooperation of the holons present in the holarchy.

This design principle does not introduce a hierarchical rigidity into the HPTS, since the final decision on capacity scheduling is still to be taken by the basic holons. This concept of basic holons, enhanced with staff holon giving advice, decouples robustness and agility from service optimization.

3 Optimizing Global Capacity with Centralized Service Scheduler

This section presents a centralized approach for off line optimal computing the fixed public service transport capacity that meets the customer's requirements and scheduling the transport resources (drivers, busses) on long-term horizon. Numerical results are provided for the Service Scheduler's computational stages; they represent advice to be followed by the basic holons in normal service delivery mode, i.e. in the absence of an internal perturbation (resource unavailability, poor QoS) or external one caused by a temporary increased service demand (unforeseen, rush order).

During this off-line stage, the staff holon solves the following global problems:

- Planning the daily transport service on an hourly basis, 7 day from 7.
- Sequencing the activities which compose the public transport service: bus driving on established route with specified timing; bus cleaning, bus maintenance, etc.
- Human, material and financial resource scheduling and allocation (drivers, busses, fuel, spare parts) to meet the quality requirements imposed to the service with cost optimization (salaries, infrastructure, tooling, consumables, authorizations, etc.).

3.1 Planning the Transport Service on Long Term

The following requirements are formulated for public transport service in a city district: total route length: 12 km; number of bus stations on the route: 15; average bus stop duration in a bus station: 1.2 min.; number of crossroads with semaphore on the route: 22; average bus stop duration at a crossroad with semaphore: 30 s; upper limit speed of busses on route: 50 km/h; daily peak transport demands: (a) Monday–Friday: 6:00 h–10:00 h and 14:00 h–18:00 h; (b) Saturday: 18:00 h–22:00 h; (c) Sunday: 18:00 h–22:00 h.

From this data, the total stop duration in bus stations is $t_{ss} = 15 \cdot 1.2$ min $= 18$ min, the total stop duration in crossroads is $t_{si} = 22 \cdot 0.5$ min $= 11$ min, the total foreseen bus stop duration on the route is $t_s = t_{ss} + t_{si} = 29$ min ≈ 30 min, and for an average bus speed of 25 km/h the 12 km are covered in 30 min., and the route with stops is covered in 60 min. Imposing a high rate of bus arrivals in stations every 4 min., a minimum transport capacity of 15 busses is necessary (Table 1), which is increased to 20 busses for preventive maintenance and backup reasons.

Planning the basic activities of the public transport service refers to scheduling the tasks implying the material resource - the bus fleet (BF), and the tasks performed by the human resource working with busses - the personnel employed as bus drivers (BD). This activity scheduling consists in:

1. Defining the types of tasks or *duties* which must be performed by/for the BF units, respectively which are assigned to the BD people by joining sets of *pieces of work* (PoW) in individual *daily duties*. PoW results by dividing the daily bus exploiting time interval in task units; they begin and finish in *change points*, i.e. in places where bus drivers replace one another [21].
2. Configuring these PoWs and duties: number (BF units respectively BD people), BF utilisation regime, work program for BD members, duration.

Table 1. No. of busses necessary for imposed arrival rates in stations

Day of the week	Hourly time interval	Time interval between arrivals	No. of busses necessary
Monday - Friday	22:00 h - 6:00 h	12 min.	5
	10:00 h - 14:00 h and 18:00 h - 22:00 h	6 min.	10
	6:00 h - 10:00 h and 14:00 h - 18:00 h	4 min.	15
Saturday	22:00 h - 6:00 h	12 min.	5
	6:00 h - 18:00 h	6 min.	10
	18:00 h - 22:00 h	4 min.	15
Sunday	22:00 h - 18:00 h	12 min.	5
	18:00 h - 22:00 h	6 min.	10

3. Defining the set of *feasible duties* that cover all *daily tours* (*shifts*) for the route, by concatenating the tasks defined at point and configured at point 2 above.
4. Defining the *weekly program* exploiting the BF respectively the *weekly workshift* of the BD members with days-off constraints.
5. Defining the monthly *program* exploiting the BF respectively the *monthly workshift* of the BD members with the objective of balancing the utilization of the BF units and respecting equity requirements concerning the timing of days off and the assignment of overtime work which involves extra payment.

To schedule the basic activities of the public transport service according to points 1–5 above, it is necessary to assign both the available capacity (in BF) and the personnel (in BD) such as to satisfy the demand in the following three working regimes: (a) normal traffic at day; (b) traffic at night; (c) peak transport demand. In this context, two **roles** are defined for bus drivers:

- *Category A*: a driver operates a bus at day time;
- *Category B*: a driver operates a bus at night time,

and two types of **tasks**: (1) bus driving; (2) bus verification and maintenance in the garage, as two categories of PoW.

A "bus driving" PoW can have two possible durations:

- 8-hour PoW, feasible in the normal traffic at day and traffic at night regimes;
- 4-hour PoW, feasible only in peak demand regime; this type of bus driving is always followed by a 4-hour PoW for bus verification and maintenance.

The "bus verification and maintenance" PoW has always a duration of 4 h.

A daily workshift of a BD employee has a duration of 8 h; it can be composed either by an 8-hour "bus driving" PoW or by two successive 4-hour PoW: one 4-hour "bus driving" PoW followed by a 4-hour "bus verification and maintenance" PoW. There are defined 3 8-hour *tours* (shifts) representing various start and end times of work, so that they aggregate to the top line profile (diagram indicating the number of drivers that add up each hour to the number required by the service demand curve): A1: day tour 1, category A, hourly interval 6:00 h–14:00 h; A2: day tour 2, category A, hourly interval 14:00 h–22:00 h; B: night tour, category B, hourly interval 22:00 h–6:00 h. Related to tour scheduling, the constraint is imposed that after doing a tour B, a driver should not immediately begin an A1 tour in the morning of the next day.

In what concerns scheduling the activities that exploit BF units, a uniform vehicle utilisation during each month is imposed, which implies using each week in "bus driving" other 15 busses from the 20 ones composing the BF (each week other 5 busses remain in the garage, or can be eventually used only in 4-hour PoWs of increased peak demands of service – to satisfy rush orders).

Also, for each bus circulating in the current week, the PoW "bus verification and maintenance" will be realized 3 times in the interval Monday–Friday.

4   Scheduling the Human Resource for the Transport Service

The problem of human resource scheduling for transport services is NP-hard, being solved through combinatorial optimization. To avoid the big computational effort of such an approach, heuristic procedures are considered which offer a good compromise between processing time and quality of results. The following stages are considered:

1. Daily Workshift Scheduling: determine the necessary staffing levels at the start of each feasible duty to cover the service demand for the associated hourly interval.
2. Weekly Workshift Scheduling: planning the weekly tours with 2 consecutive days-off for all bus drivers.
3. Determine the total number of bus drivers to be employed in the BD set.
4. Compute the cost of personnel per week and month considering the roles A and B assigned to the members of the BD set in the "bus driving" PoW.
5. Hourly, daily, weekly and monthly scheduling of BF units to satisfy the transport requirements.
6. Assign drivers in daily and weekly tours to the busses scheduled in stage 5.
7. Hourly, daily, weekly and monthly scheduling of BF units to verification and maintenance tasks in the garage.

5   Heterarchical Control for Variable Demand Matching

In the situations when deviations from the off-line computed resource schedule are detected, the optimal advice calculated by the staff holon is updated through a collaborative decision handled by the dispatcher holon which uses a heterarchical short-term resource scheduling and allocation algorithm (see Fig. 1). The DH receives permanent information from the route holons about the state of the routes and traffic (normal, temporarily blocked, etc.), from the bus holons via their intelligent embedded devices about the vehicle's operational state, from the driver holons via the mobile devices about the driver's availability, and monitors the execution state of the order holons.

As shown in Fig. 1, the basic holons exchange knowledge about the transport service system. Route holons and resource holons communicate process knowledge, route holons and order holons exchange service knowledge, and resource holons and order holons share process execution knowledge.

- *Process knowledge* contains the data, information and methods on how to perform a certain process on a certain resource. It is knowledge about the capabilities of the resource, which processes it can perform, the relevant process parameters, the process quality, possible outcomes of a process, etc.
- *Service knowledge* represents the information and methods on how to deliver a particular transport service using certain human and physical resources. It is knowledge about the possible sequences of processes or operations to be executed on the resources, data structures to represent the outcome of the processes, methods to access information of process plans, etc.
- *Process execution knowledge* contains the information and methods regarding the progress of executing service operations on resources (e.g., "bus driving", "bus verification and maintenance", etc.). It is knowledge about how to request the starting of processes on the resources, making reservations on resources, how to monitor the progress of service execution, how to interrupt a process, the consequences of interrupting a process or service, suspending and resuming processes.

The composing entities of the holonic transportation control system, as described in Fig. 1, interact based on the time diagram shown in Fig. 2.

The HPTS has in heterarchical operating mode a flat structure, being composed of independent entities called agents. As discussed, these agents typically represent the transport resources (human, material), service specifications and tasks, and have local intelligence to adapt to unforeseen situations. Instead of a master-slave relationship as in the hierarchical mode supervised by the global Service Scheduler, information and commands are exchanged by the use of a negotiation protocol, initiated by the dispatcher holon, in which resources can accept or refuse certain jobs.

The Contract Net Protocol (CNP) is used as negotiation mechanism [22]. It consists of five steps: service (task) announcement by a dispatcher holon, potential contractors evaluate task announcements from several dispatcher holons, potential contractors (resource holons) bid upon the selected task, the dispatcher holon acting as task manager awards the contract to one of the bidding contractors, finally manager and contractor communicate to execute the contracted service. This protocol is applied to the public transport context as follows: managers (dispatchers) represent services offering work and contractors are resources bidding to get this work assigned.

This yields a simple and fault-tolerant system, since none of the agents need a priori information about the other agents. As a consequence, several disturbances and changes can easily be handled. When a resource is malfunctioning, it just doesn't take part in the bidding process (market); when a resource is able to perform new operations, the associated agent starts responding to bids for such tasks; new resources only require the creation of an additional agent in the market.

The global transport service control is implemented through three operating regimes as described in Fig. 2: (i) *normal, long-term operating regime* when the bus fleet is formed and transport services are optimally scheduled according to permanent requirements (here both busses and drivers are tested for availability before OH creation), (ii) permanent, *monitoring regime* when the RoH, ReH and OH are tested in real-time to detect perturbations or changes in the service demand, and (iii) *temporary updated regime* that is entered when one of the following conditions occurs: <u>internal event</u> - driver not available, bus not operational, or <u>external</u> event: route cannot be used or rush order detected (an increased service demand, such as additional service request not foreseen at global planning or unexpected transport peak).

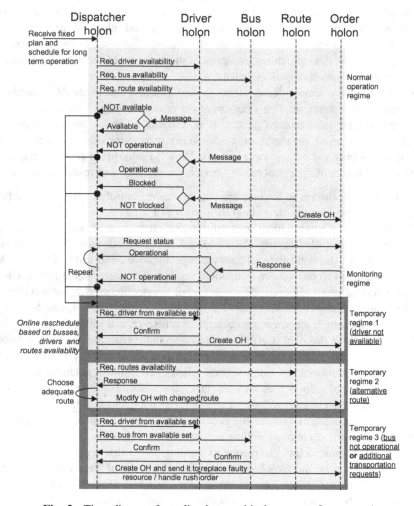

Fig. 2. Time diagram for online heterarchical transport fleet control

6   Implementing Solution and Conclusions

The implementation of the informational part of the holons will be done using a multi-agent platform JADE (Java Agent Developing Environment), [23] for *holon interaction* and *real-time decision making* and the ILOG commercial optimization application [24] based on constraint programming for *online scheduling of vehicles and crew*. These applications will be disposed on a layered structure as depicted in Fig. 3, each layer responsible with control on a certain time interval such as: (i) *strategic layer* - long term operation, (ii) *tactical layer* - day to day operation, OH creation and monitoring, and (iii) *operational layer* - real-time fleet update; short-term ILOG-based optimization is used in this operating mode.

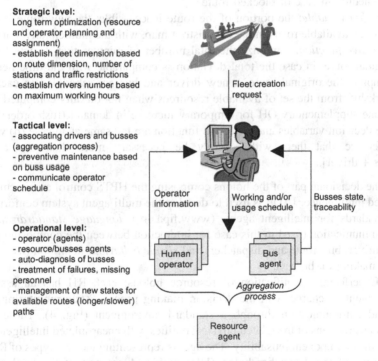

Strategic level:
Long term optimization (resource and operator planning and assignment)
- establish fleet dimension based on route dimension, number of stations and traffic restrictions
- establish drivers number based on maximum working hours

Fleet creation request

Tactical level:
- associating drivers and busses (aggregation process)
- preventive maintenance based on buss usage
- communicate operator schedule

Operator information

Working and/or usage schedule

Busses state, traceability

Operational level:
- operator (agents)
- resource/busses agents
- auto-diagnosis of busses
- treatment of failures, missing personnel
- management of new states for available routes (longer/slower) paths

Human operator

Bus agent

Aggregation process

Resource agent

Fig. 3. Layered implementation of the holonic transport control system

The real-time optimization problem based on bus, driver and route availability in case of perturbations has the following implementation:

Given: The global driver allocation for busses circulating on specified routes and the available set of spare drivers and busses for the current day.

Requested:

(a) Reschedule drivers on busses in case a scheduled driver becomes unavailable
    Decision variables: the driver to do the current job. He is chosen from the limited set of drivers waiting on duty.

Objective function: minimize the total number of hours that deviate from the offline long-term schedule; the drivers involved will switch work shifts and the objective function will refers to the two deviations: |waiting hours when not on duty - waiting hours when not on duty computed offline.

(b) Reschedule in case of faulty bus

Decision variables: the driver to conduct the bus to the location where the faulty one stopped; this driver is chosen from the set of drivers waiting on duty based on the criteria that he should return in time for his shift.

Objective function (independent): (1) maximize the time difference between the chosen driver's return and the beginning of his shift, and (2) for the chosen bus maximize the time difference between completing the additional task and re-entering to normal schedule.

(c) Reschedule in case of blocked route

Decision variable: the portion of the route inaccessible; the new route is chosen from the available roads in the city district map, with the municipality's approval.

Objective function: minimize the total number of minutes that deviate from the original route; in case the total deviation is comparable with the time needed to complete the original route, a new driver and bus are scheduled to each daily workshift from the set of available resources when not on duty computed offline.

(d) Create supplementary OH for temporary increase in demand (rush order)

The decision variables and objective function are the same as in case (b) with the difference that there will possibly be necessary more than one assigned [bus + driver].

For the decisional part of the holons composing the HPTS control architecture with distributed intelligence, JADE is used to develop the multi-agent system conforming to FIPA standards for intelligent agents (www.fipa.org): *language standardization* for agent communication (used in this case for interaction between the composing control entities: driver, bus, route and dispatcher) and *simple behaviour definition* (used for the decision making on busses).

JADE performs agentification of resource holons: each RH has an associated software agent in charge with the decision making process, state monitoring, alarm rising and communication through a standard environment (Fig. 4). These agents represent abstractions of the related physical entities with encapsulated intelligence [25] allowing thus component reusability. The agents representing the two types of RH (bus and driver) and the dispatcher holon (DH) in Fig. 4 are part of the implementing solution.

The RH representing the driver is formed of a human operator equipped with hand-held device for real-time communication with the dispatcher about its availability. The data communicated concerns the long and short term schedule of the driver computed by the dispatcher and last minute notifications of the driver. The agent running on the handheld device is a simple GUI capable of sending/receiving this information. The handheld device can be any type of smartphone or tablet with an operating system capable of running the original Java Virtual Machine from Oracle (e.g., all devices running an Android version newer than 2.3.3 [26].

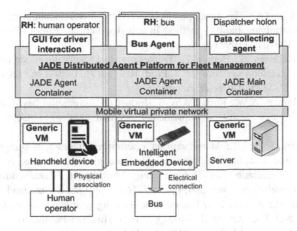

Fig. 4. Details of RH and DH hardware and software for heterarchical control

The RH representing the bus is composed of the physical vehicle together with an IED running a deliberative agent in charge with traceability, diagnostics, maintenance and participation in bids for online job assignment based on its current state. The IED has sensors connected to the vehicle's main parts (engine, doors, air conditioning, a.o.) so that the bus agent processes the acquired information for both state evaluation and reporting to the dispatcher, and schedule negotiation. Just like in the case of the handheld device, the IED can be any type of real-time processing device capable of running original Java Virtual Machine from Oracle in order to run JADE (e.g., Overo AirSTORM) [27]; it must also be able to handle digital and analogue I/O signals.

In order for the agents to communicate they must be on the same network. For security reasons a mobile VPN is proposed to interconnect the agents, which allows remote access to entities composing the HPTS (the fleet management system).

The paper has reported the research aiming at developing a fleet management system based on the holonic paradigm and implemented in a multi-agent framework. The semi-heterarchical control system sets up the transport capacity and optimizes on long term workshift scheduling using a centralized Service Scheduler; the dynamic demand variations due to internal (human and material faulty states) and external (route and demand changes) causes are treated in real-time by distributed intelligence composed by the agents representing physical entities (resources, routes) and managed by a dispatcher. Currently, tests are performed with the mobile and IED on resources interacting with the dispatcher holon in the MAS. In the future there will be developed a simulation platform to run the online scheduling with distributed intelligence.

References

1. Novas, J.M., Bahtiar, R., Van Belle, J., Valckenaers, P.: An approach for the integration of a scheduling system and a multiagent manufacturing execution system. Towards a collaborative framework. In: Proceedings of the 14th IFAC Symposium INCOM 2012, Bucharest, pp. 728–733. IFAC PapersOnLine (2012)

2. Ou-Yang, C., Lin, J.S.: The development of a hybrid hierarchical/heterarchical shop floor control system applying bidding method in job dispatching. Robot. Computer-Integrated Manuf. **14**(3), 199–217 (1998)
3. Borangiu, T., Răileanu, S., Berger, T., Trentesaux, D.: Switching mode control strategy in manufacturing execution systems. Int. J. Prod. Res. **53**(7), 1950–1963 (2014). doi:10.1080/00207543.2014.935825. Taylor & Francis
4. Leitão, P., Colombo, A.W., Karnouskos, S.: Industrial automation based on cyber-physical systems technologies: prototype implementations and challenges. Comput. Ind. (2015). Elsevier
5. Babiceanu, R.F., Seker, R.: Manufacturing operations, internet of things, and big data: towards predictive manufacturing systems. In: Borangiu, T., Thomas, A., Trentesaux, D. (eds.) Service Orientation in Holonic and Multi-agent Manufacturing. Studies in Computational Intelligence, vol. 594, pp. 157–164. Springer, Switzerland (2015)
6. Chen, M., Niu, H.: A model for bus crew scheduling problem with multiple duty types. Discrete Dyn. Nat. Soc. Article ID 649213 (2012). Hindawi Publishing Corporation
7. Borangiu, T., Dragoicea, M., Oltean, V.E., Iacob, I.: A generic service system activity model with event-driven operation reconfiguring capability. In: Borangiu, T., Trentesaux, D., Thomas, A. (eds.) Service Orientation in Holonic and Multi-agent Manufacturing. Studies in Computational Intelligence, vol. 544, pp. 159–175. Springer, Switzerland (2014)
8. Fitzsimmons, J.A., Fitzsimmons, M.J.: Service Management: Operations, Strategy, and Information Technology, 7edn. Irwin Professional Publications (2010)
9. Daskin, M.S.: Service Science. Wiley, New York (2010). ISBN 978-0-470-52588-3
10. Borangiu, T., Gilbert, P., Ivanescu, N.-A., Rosu, A.: An implementing framework for holonic manufacturing control with multiple robot-vision stations. Eng. Appl. Artif. Intell. **22**, 505–521 (2009)
11. Johnston, R., Clark, G.: Service Operations Management. Improving Service Delivery, Third Edition edn. Prentice Hall, Harlow (2008)
12. Bongaerts, L., Wyns, J., Detand, J., Van Brussel, H., Valckenaers, P.: Identification of manufacturing holons, In: Albayrak, S., Bussmann, S. (eds.) Proceedings of the European Workshop for Agent-Oriented Systems in Manufacturing, vol. 9/26–27, pp. 57–73. Berlin (1996)
13. Valckenaers, P., Van Brussel, H., Bongaerts, L., Wyns, J.: Results of the holonic control system benchmark at the KU Leuven, In: Proceedings. of the CIMAT Conference (Computer Integrated Manufacturing and Automation Technology), pp. 128–133. Rensselaer Polytechnic Institute, Troy, 10–12 Oct 1994
14. Kaminsky, P., Kaya, O.: Centralized versus decentralized scheduling and due date quotation in a make-to-order supply chain. In: Proceedings of the MSOM 2005 Conference. North-Western University Evanston, Illinois (2005)
15. Van Brussel, H., Wyns, J., Valckenaers, P., Bongaerts, L., Peeters, L.: Reference architecture for holonic manufacturing systems: PROSA. Comput. Ind. **37**(3), 255–274 (1998)
16. Panescu, D., Pascal, C.: HAPBA – a holonic adaptive plan-based architecture. In: Borangiu, T., Thomas, A., Trentesaux, D. (eds.) Service Orientation in Holonic and Multi-agent Manufacturing Control. Studies in Computational Intelligence, vol. 402, pp. 61–74. Springer, Heidelberg (2012)
17. Barata, J.: The Cobasa architecture as an answer to shop floor agility. In: Kordic, V., Lazinica, A., Merdan, M. (eds.) Manufacturing the Future, Concepts, Technologies and Vision, pp. 31–76. InTech, Rijeka (2006). ISBN 3-86611-198-3

18. Leitão, P., Colombo, A.W., Restivo, F.: An approach to the formal specification of holonic control systems. In: Mařík, V., McFarlane, D.C., Valckenaers, P. (eds.) HoloMAS 2003. LNCS (LNAI), vol. 2744, pp. 59–70. Springer, Heidelberg (2003)

19. Deen, S.: A cooperation framework for holonic interactions in manufacturing. In: Proceedings of the 2nd International Working on Cooperating Knowledge Based Systems (CKBS 1994) (1994)

20. Koestler, A.: The Ghost in the Machine. Arkana Books, London (1989)

21. Van Brussel, H: Holonic manufacturing systems, the vision matching the problem. In: Proceedings of the 1st European Conference on Holonic Manufacturing Systems, IFW-Hannover (1994)

22. Dias, G., de Sousa, T.J.P., e Cunha, J.F.: Genetic algorithms for the bus driver scheduling problem: a case study. J. Oper. Res. Soc. 53(3), 324–335 (2002)

23. FIPA (1996). www.fipa.org/index.html. Accessed Dec 2015

24. Bellifemine, F., Caire, G., Greenwood, D.: Developing Multi-agent Systems with JADE. Wiley, Wiltshire (2007). ISBN 978-0-470-05747-6

25. IBM ILOG. http://www-01.ibm.com/software/websphere/ilog/. Accessed Aug 2013

26. Obitko, M., Mařík, V.: Ontologies for Multi-agent Systems in Manufacturing Domain. In: DEXA Workshop, pp. 597–602 (2002)

27. Caire, G., Iavarone, G., Izzo, M., Heffner, M.: JADE programming for Android (2014). http://jade.tilab.com/doc/tutorials/JadeAndroid-Programming-Tutorial.pdf

28. Overo AirSTORM. https://store.gumstix.com/coms/overo-coms/overo-airstorm-com.html. Accessed Jan 2016

Specifying Modernization into Service-Oriented SaaS System in a Case of Public Transport Document Generator

Muhammad Ghufron Mahfudhi[✉] and Teresa Galvão Dias

Faculty of Engineering, University of Porto, Rua Dr. Roberto Frias s/n, 4200-465 Porto, Portugal
{mesg1301167,tgalvao}@fe.up.pt

Abstract. The alignment of the information technology implementation with the ever-changing business strategies in an enterprise drives modernization of the legacy system. However, the existing modernization contexts have not adequately addressed the focus of customer experience and service-orientation within the SaaS system development. This paper investigates the modernization process of legacy system into SaaS system using services concept through multidisciplinary approach. Several best practices are discussed to propose the Service-Oriented Modernization Framework (SOMF) which involves the maturity model for evolution roadmap identification, the service-oriented SaaS reference architecture, and the User-Centered Service-Oriented Software Reengineering (UCSOSR) methodology. An industrial case study is demonstrated by applying the framework to develop the public transport document generator as a service. The modernization process described in the framework provides a comprehensive and systematic guideline in developing a scalable system. In conclusion, this research, by integrating service analysis and design with SOA towards the SaaS modernization, enables the creation of an agile business model to achieve competitive advantages.

Keywords: Business modernization · Service-Oriented Modernization Framework · SaaS · SOA · Public transport document generator

1 Introduction

Cloud computing promotes the use of cloud services to gain cost reduction and agility and provide accessibility and flexibility to customer [1]. Software Equity Group predicts that Software as a Service (SaaS), as one model of cloud computing, will represent the 25 % revenues of the overall software market until 2019, thus giving a promising results for achievements [2]. The form of accessing software features and functionalities through the internet will give more added value for business companies to compete. Therefore, modernization into SaaS system enables the service innovation which promotes better experience to customers, business goals achievement, and competitive advantages.

Moreover, services concepts contribute in SaaS development to create a scalable and customer-oriented system. Industrial and software engineering disciplines involve services under two different perspectives: business and technological [3]. In business perspective services represent the economic values delivered by the companies to

© Springer International Publishing Switzerland 2016
T. Borangiu et al. (Eds.): IESS 2016, LNBIP 247, pp. 590–603, 2016.
DOI: 10.1007/978-3-319-32689-4_45

customers through strategies and channels [4], while in technological perspective services represent the software components as encapsulation of business processes under Service-Oriented Architecture (SOA) [5]. Both definitions support the development of services system which enables the value propositions delivery to customer through configuration of people, technology, and information. Therefore, the development of services system in SaaS model allows the establishment of a service-oriented SaaS system, emphasizing the customer experience, using SOA as architectural strategy and SaaS as on-demand business model.

In spite that modernization into service-oriented SaaS system involves multiple disciplinary, current research is still scarce in providing examples of a holistic approach putting business, technology, and customer in development process. To the best of our knowledge, the presentations of framework and methodology for legacy system modernization into service-oriented SaaS system are still separated apart on different aspects. Most studies limit the context of modernization either only into SaaS or SOA, only showing the technical part, or lack of comprehensiveness, even though the combination of SaaS and SOA is quite common for service system development from scratch. Moreover, despite that SaaS emphasizes the services delivery, the studies rarely discuss about the customer experience, and instead focus on the architecture development using SOA. This raises the concern of integrating several characteristics within modernization, SaaS, and the whole services concept to gain a comprehensive modernization framework.

In the same way, a Portuguese consulting firm in transportation was also interested in evolving its Information for Public (Infopub) solution into Public Transport Document Generator as a Service. The on-premise delivery model limits the Infopub's flexibility and interoperability, causing high maintenance cost for the firm and inefficiency for clients. Meneses [6] proposed a solution to develop the system in a web-based environment. However, the proposal only focuses on the web-based software development, whereas the transformation also can affect the business model and service delivery. The application of SaaS in Infopub can enrich the proposal by providing an on-demand model based on a flexible service-level agreement (SLA) and centralized management platform. This transformation serves to demonstrate how the foregoing modernization model can be applied in the industrial case.

Based on the foregoing motivation, this research aims to investigate the modernization process of a legacy system into service-oriented SaaS system using multidisciplinary approach. The contribution comes in the development of a conceptual framework designed from the key aspects derived by correlating the services concept under business and technological perspectives into SaaS modernization. The Infopub case then serves as demonstration of the framework, aiming to develop the modernization requirement and design specification for the Public Transport Document Generator as a Service. Finally, the modernization process can lead to the impact analysis of the services concept application in business and technological aspects and changes in an enterprise.

The remainder of the paper is organized as follows. Several literatures are reviewed within the modernization contexts and followed by the methodology, including the conceptual modernization framework. The case study is then demonstrated to show the modernization process and the findings and followed by the discussion and conclusion.

2   Background and Related Work

Legacy modernization is necessary to improve the efficiency and support easy maintenance from an expensive and outdated infrastructure and technology. Modernization
involves reengineering process with several transformations in code, functional, and
architectural aspects [7]. The reengineering process aims to find the best solution, either
through redevelopment, wrapping, migration, or replacement, based on the legacy
system's abstraction and the target system analysis.

Since there are different contexts of modernization, the literatures related to the
modernization process need to be carefully selected to cover the research motivation
concerning a solution based in SaaS and services. Despite the difference between SaaS
and service-orientation, both are actually intertwined and hold the key success factor to
achieve competitive advantage. As a delivery model, SaaS is connected to the company's
business model to determine the customer experience, including how customers access,
interact with, and assess the offered services through web browser [8, 9]. The customer
experience innovation can be reach through the alignment between business and technology. Accordingly, SOA serves as the bridge to represent the loosely-coupled abstraction between business and application services, creating separation of concern to
promote enterprise agility and interoperability [5].

Furthermore, the studies on both SaaS and services developments emphasize the
important of maturity model, reference architecture, and development life cycle. The
SaaS maturity model [10] and the Open Group Service Integration Maturity Model
(OSIMM) [11] shows the connection of their characteristics on the highest level to create
an improvement roadmap. These characteristics contributes to the general component
identification to design the architecture of the SaaS and SOA system through their
development life cycles. For instance, Kommalapati and Zack [12] proposed an SaaS
development life cycle to guide the SaaS development process in a systematic way.
Likewise, Mohammadi and Mukhtar [13] compared several SOA modeling approaches
and pointed out a comprehensive approach combining Service-Oriented Modeling and
Architecture (SOMA) [14] methodology and Service-Oriented Architecture Modeling
Language (SoaML) [15] to design the SOA solution. Moreover, the concern on customer
experience as key of service innovation can be reached by applying service design and
user-centered design [16, 17].

Most studies of modernization into service-orientation and SaaS often illustrate the
application of cloud computing as foundation inside SOA, which is in contrary to this
research's motivation. Apparently, Chauhan and Babar [18] shows the suitable mean of
this research context by extending the SOA-based software into SaaS model. However,
the described process is too practical without a systematic procedure. The context can
be extended by putting a systematic methodology combining several approaches
described in the SOA and SaaS development life cycles to create a comprehensive
methodology.

One of the best practices to evolve the legacy system into service-oriented system
is transforming the legacy system into SOA and then into cloud-based SaaS environment
[19]. This transformation uses an integrated Service-Oriented Software Reengineering
(SOSR) method to evolve the legacy system into SOA [20, 21]. Then, the deployed

services can be orchestrated as SaaS system components and the platform can be developed using PaaS and/or IaaS cloud providers, either with public, private, or hybrid cloud, with concern to SaaS principles, especially, multi-tenancy, scalability, and security.

In summary, SaaS and services characteristics are the essential components of the modernization process in question, utilizing service design and modeling as service development method, SOA as service design model, and SaaS as service delivery model.

3   Methodology

This research is based on the Design Science Research Methodology (DSRM) [22]. This methodology is chosen because it allows the creation of an artifact as solution to a problem. Since this research requires a comprehensive discussion of the modernization context, DSRM serves to design a conceptual framework to address the research problem and it is also applicable for the context of information and service system. Following the pattern, this research is a client/context initiated project with the proposed demonstration from the conceptual framework.

After designing the framework as solution artifact, the industrial setting of Infopub system acts as demonstration in an instrumental case study. The demonstration illustrates how to execute the framework using the described methods related to the modernization process. The data for the development process were acquired through interviews with the director and technical director of the company, legacy system exploration, documents review, and additional research through internet. The required data were analyzed and put into the development of artifacts described in the framework to design the target system. To summarize, this research composes two main contributions: the modernization conceptual framework as an academic contribution and the design structure and specification of the Public Transport Document Generator as a Service as an industrial contribution.

Based on the research objectives, Service-Oriented Modernization Framework (SOMF) is proposed to guide the modernization process [23]. SOMF was designed from the investigation and integration of multidisciplinary approaches and best practices for business and technical modernization into service-oriented SaaS system. SOMF provides an integrated blueprint for consultants, businesses, and IT practitioners for making architectural, design, and implementation decisions in the development of modernization solution. The intertwined characteristics between SaaS and SOA underlay the conception of this framework, resulting in three main artifacts: maturity model, reference architecture, and development life cycle.

SaaS and SOA Maturity Model. SOMF facilitates the transformation from legacy into basic SaaS and SOA, and even further to the highest maturity level, based on the business targets. The gap between the current and the target models identifies the evolution roadmap which determines the necessary capabilities for modernization. Wherever the position within SaaS maturity model, the goal is to achieve the virtualization level to leverage the use of service-orientation to its extent by implementing multi-tenant database scheme and cloud computing. As a consequence, the SOA principle needs to be applied to achieve the services level in OSIMM and can be further extended into the dynamically re-configurable services level by applying the proper services technologies.

Service-Oriented SaaS Reference Architecture. The reference architecture represents the template solution for designing the solution architecture based on the predefined components. The architecture describes three sides of SaaS architecture, including the layered-SOA within the SaaS platform side, the service customer side, and the service provider side, and also the interaction with the main stakeholder in each side.

User-Centered Service-Oriented Software Reengineering (UCSOSR). This methodology was designed as a reliable and systematic guideline for the modernization process from legacy into service-oriented SaaS system. UCSOSR describes a comprehensive six main phases reengineering process through model-based development from modernization provisioning, service development, and SaaS development, as shown in Fig. 1. The UCSOSR design is based on SOMA methodology configured with SOSR, and integrated with the SaaS development life cycle. Underlining the best practices in each methodology, UCSOSR also provides several suggested methods to carry out and develop the corresponding artifacts.

The modernization provisioning acts as the project initiation. The business modeling and transformation phase holds the foundation to identify the modernization strategy from business opportunities based on business architecture and strategy. This phase involves business architecture and model development using Business Motivation Model [24], Business Model Canvas [9], and SaaS and SOA maturity model analysis. Then, the organization determines the modernization strategy in corporate, business, and operational level [25]. Furthermore, the project plan is organized based on the identified strategies and followed by specifying the requirements from the stakeholder needs, legacy system, documents, standards and regulation, and domain information, to be compiled into a formal specification document.

The core of the modernization process lies in the reengineering process. The reengineering begins with the reverse engineering to analyze the legacy system through visual model based on the application, source code, and documents investigation. Then, the forward engineering process identifies the required services to be developed using particular services technology as components for the SaaS system. Firstly, the candidate services are identified from the goal-service model, the domain decomposition focused on customer experience and service blueprint, the legacy system analysis, and the SaaS component analysis. Secondly, the candidate services are specified to elaborate the higher level view of the service design model. Thirdly, the services are realized into a detailed SOA solution design which defines the services components composition. Fourthly, the services are implemented into a particular platform using services technology. Finally, the developed services are deployed into cloud servers to be used in the SaaS system development. Additionally, the services development can be supported by the market-available CASE tool which allows inter-model transformation based on SoaML. Above all, the SaaS system then can be developed and deployed into the identified cloud server.

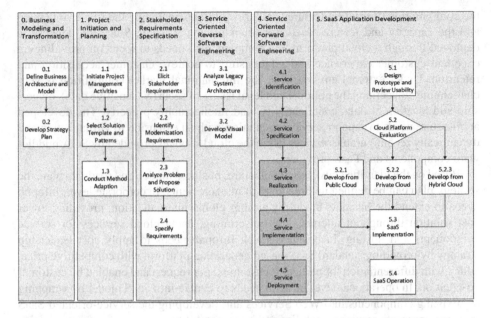

Fig. 1. Workflow of User-Centered Service-Oriented Software Reengineering Methodology

4   Case Study

Infopub is a public transport document generator system developed in a desktop-based client-server architecture which automates the production of public transport information. Public transport document generator system is part of public information system which serves to provide transport information to public travelers [26]. The context of Infopub concerns on a holistic information system, involving the organization, technology, people, and knowledge. It acts as the main physical evidence of a product-service system to deliver the graphical documents production service with advanced design which adapts to the data contents. The automatic production of public information creates a standardization of format and media, reducing cost, increasing the efficiency of the mass documents production for transport companies, and providing better visibility and accessibility for public passengers.

This case study aims to demonstrate the execution of SOMF in an industrial environment by modernizing the Infopub system into Public Transport Document Generator as a Service (PTDGAAS). The case study is presented based on the structure in the UCSOSR methodology. The constraint of the case study is that the modernization only focuses to produce the system design specification, without concerning the detailed implementation and deployment phases.

Business Modeling and Transformation. The company aims to evolve the development platforms and deliver the solution via the web to attract new market opportunities with a flexible service offer. The evolution involves business model expansion with more variants of value propositions and customer segments. The on-demand model enables the configuration of solution features and price options, including the free trial version and the capacity and feature-based freemium pricing strategy. Since the delivery is deployed through a cloud platform, the company also needs to focus on providing an excellent customer experience and relationship to achieve customer acquisition and retention. Under external environment, the international market competition is very challenging, concerning the political and legal issues of security (sensitive data), ownership and location of data, confidentiality, and intellectuality property. The developed architecture needs to support service orientation with an extension to virtualization and dynamically reconfigurable services using the cloud services provided by SOA middleware components and PaaS providers.

Based on the identified business architecture, business model, and roadmap plan, the strategy plan can be defined in three level of managements. In corporate level, Infopub needs to extend the business model by aiming global internalization, providing lower cost solution throughout internet, and outsourcing, using cloud services for service components and hosting. In business level, Infopub needs to apply cost leadership strategy by providing standard SaaS-based generation platform with competitive price, added with differentiation for particular customers per request and enabled by customer co-creation. In operational level Infopub needs to evolve into SaaS model by wrapping the existing components into Web Services and developing the service-oriented SaaS system to promote service reusability and interoperability.

Project Planning and Requirements Specification. With the situation of the industry competition, the company envisioned the need to modernize the Infopub system into SaaS model using the latest supporting technology to achieve high accessibility, cost reduction, and business agility. The modernization requirements were elicited from different sources: the company stakeholder, Infopub documentations, the Infopub system, domain literature study. Then, the PTDGAAS services development was executed through a series of processes into the provisioned service technology using the IBM's Rational Software Architect (RSA).

Reverse Engineering. The legacy Infopub consists of three main elements: data manager, generation engine, and document. The main component lies on the data manager information system with an integrated database to store and manage network data, schedule, and graphics (routes, paths, stops, landmarks, zoning, colors, and pictograms). The information system is connected to the graphic generation engine, as second component, for rapid development of configurable document templates generation. The engine will automatically generate the documents, which is the third component, to be put as displays in the stops or clients' websites.

As a desktop-based application, Infopub is deployed in the customer side with the network connection to OPT's servers. The support services of Infopub is still being managed manually by contacting the company, thus creating a non-efficient dedicated-personalized service agreement. The company needs to focus on maintenance and innovation of the document generator system, providing the best services to customer with every needed insight.

Forward Engineering. In service identification phase, the service candidates of PTDGAAS are determined based on the service-goal model, domain decomposition, legacy system analysis, and SaaS components analysis. Firstly, the goal of PTDGAAS emphasizes four main points: easy and effective public transport document generation, low cost solution system, highly accessible system through cloud and SaaS, and business agility supported system. Secondly, the PTDGAAS domain is decomposed based on the following customer journey: access the site, purchase the services, manage network data, customize template, generate document, review and maintenance, and post document in bus stops or websites. The customer journey leads to the detailed services blueprint development which exhibits the interaction of processes between customers, the frontend of generator platform, and the backend, involving the generator platform, CRM, and platform management. Thirdly, the legacy system analysis in reverse engineering leads to the capabilities from the Infopub's modules. Fourthly, the identified SaaS capabilities in accordance to the customer journey consist of: service management, user management, and payment. Finally, eight candidate services can be identified from the four approaches, which consist of instruction processing, data management, template customization, document generation, CRM, service management, user management, and payment.

In service specification phase, the candidate services are composed into service architecture model. Figure 2 illustrates the connection of service consumption and provision between participants through service contracts. The identified participants consist of customer, instruction handler using ESB as hub, the legacy Infopub (wrapped into data manager and document generator modules), CRM for creating customer relation and loyalty, PaaS provider for deploying the application, and bank as payment service provider. Furthermore, the message data structure and the sequence diagram of

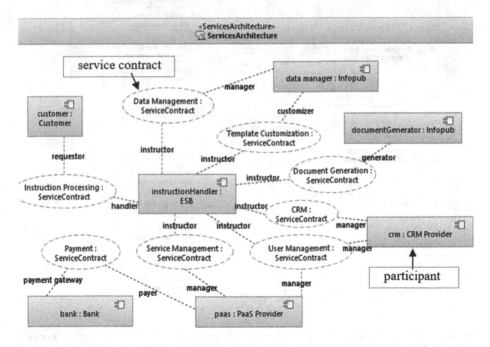

Fig. 2. Service architecture of public transport document generator as a service

the service contract, which are not presented in this paper, also need to be designed to represent the information and process specification.

In service realization phase, the specified services are realized into detailed design specification to identify the required services components which are represented by the identified participants, as illustrated in Fig. 3. Each participant has service and request ports which represent the service interfaces to interact between the services through service channel. The participants are structured by connecting the corresponding service and request ports. Furthermore, the layered SOA, which is not covered in this paper, also needs to be designed to illustrate the components in each building block based on the service-oriented SaaS reference architecture.

In service implementation and deployment phases, the services components can be implemented into web services and further deployed into web servers. RSA supports the UML-to-SOA model transformation tool to generate the web services structure from

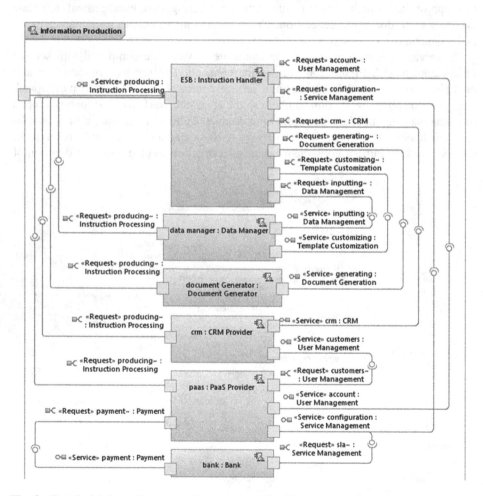

Fig. 3. Detailed information production structure of public transport document generator as a service in participant diagram

SoaML diagrams, involving the business objects (XSD), interfaces (WSDL), module assemblies (SCA), and processes (BPEL4WS) generations. Figure 4 illustrates the generated web services structure from the services components in Fig. 3. The generation produces the WSDL files from the identified service interfaces and the components definition (SCA) files from the specified participants. Then, the web services can be further implemented by developing the implementation codes, which associate the service and component interface with the access to the Infopub's API and the other necessary outsourced components. In short, this process illustrates the generation feature of Model-Driven Development (MDD) for SOA which is supported by the available tools.

SaaS Development. The SaaS system is developed using the deployed web services as functional components. The first step is to design and develop the prototype. Figure 5 illustrates the user interface mock-up of PTDGAAS as low fidelity prototype. Furthermore, the mock up can be developed into a high fidelity prototype to better perform usability testing for customer experience improvement. After designing the prototype, developer needs to evaluate the cloud platform providers to decide the development and deployment strategy. For SaaS and services development, the software application and web services need to be deployed in a network infrastructure to be accessed widely. There are three choices of deployment: public cloud, private cloud, and hybrid cloud [27].

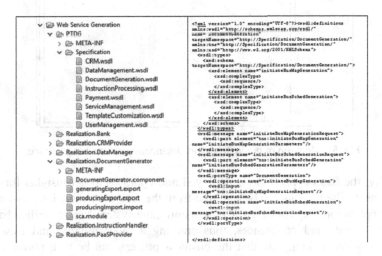

Fig. 4. Generated web services and WSDL example of document generator interface

The PTDGAAS web services and SaaS application should be deployed in a hybrid cloud. Since the company already has an in-house server, the sensitive web services related to the core value propositions can be deployed in the company's existing in-house servers to keep efficient maintenance and configuration, promoting the security of the code implementation. Moreover, the company can use the outsourced resources from the public cloud server to increase the software processing. Additionally, the SaaS application can be deployed in outsourced PaaS providers which already provide the required services for database management system and service management. The combination of both deployment style will provide the benefit of security with additional on-the-go resources supported by computing and storage rental.

Then, the implementation of the SaaS application is executed based on the designed prototype and defined cloud platform environment using the web services as main components. The developer develops the graphical user interface of the application in web-based technology on a multiplatform environment, such as web, desktop, and mobile. Furthermore, the implementation can be extended to create a community for co-creation. The services development needed to be well-documented to provide the infor-mation about the API for clients to integrate within their server. Therefore, the service ecosystem can be developed, including the application and co-creation system between customers. After developing the application, the system is migrated into the targeted server with concern on change management, including the database and application.

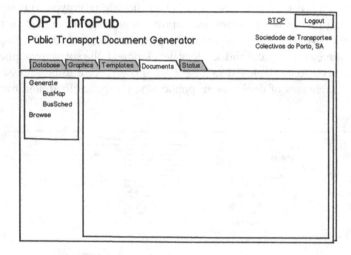

Fig. 5. Mock-up of public transport document generator as a service

Finally, the SaaS application is deployed and operated to get insights for further improvement. The insights can be acquired from the services evaluation, subscription, and the application usage behavior. Consequently, the system can be verified based on customers' needs and preferences, thus creating a more reliable and trustworthy ecosystem. After making sure that the business process can be well performed, the application can be launched and operated with continuous monitoring, performance evaluation, and tuning to keep serving the best experience to customers.

5   Discussion

This research proposes a comprehensive framework for a modernization process from legacy system into service-oriented SaaS system by integrating multidisciplinary approaches. The framework can be applied in a wide-range of industrial cases as it serves as general guideline of modernization and development process in general, with consideration to the identified business strategy. In this research, the framework was demonstrated in an industrial case study of modernization process of Infopub system. The demonstration was supported by the CASE tool to improve the development process by creating automatic generation and a traceability between each artifact. The demonstration produced a modernization and design specification of the Public Transport Document Generator as a Service. The specification points out several artifacts, which were developed through several best practice methods. The artifacts emphasize the modernization course through service innovation, involving the business transformation, architectural transformation, and functional evolution.

This research covers the benefits of integrating several best practices. The framework improves the context of modernization within [18] in a more comprehensive and systematic way. This research is focused on the business process and on the service architecture development, whereas [18–21] concern on the technical detail and quality attributes of SaaS system. Similarly, this research follows the best practice in [19–21], combining the advantages described in those researches.

Furthermore, the application of modernization also raises several issues. The decision of choosing the public, private, and hybrid cloud solution also needs to be concerned in regards with data privacy and security. Deployment in public cloud will decrease the concern on infrastructure and platform system, but increase the issues on security and control system. Whereas deployment in private cloud will keep the security and maintain the efficient maintenance, it will increase the inflexibility issues. The combination of both deployment style into hybrid cloud would give benefit of security with additional resources on-the-go by renting computing and storage requirements. However, managing both clouds would be difficult since the security on the private cloud needs to be extended to be accessed by public cloud and there might be different protocol and policy. Moreover, the change management within modernization context also involves with the bureaucracy, administration, and management issues from the organization. Therefore, every decision in the modernization process needs to be considered carefully to gain the most benefits of SaaS and service-orientation.

6 Conclusion

Modernization is the key of success to survive in business competition since business requirements and technology always evolve in an unpredictable way. This paper provides a configurable modernization guideline into service-oriented SaaS system applicable in a wide-range industry, emphasizing the alignment of business and IT strategy. This solution contributes in both academic and industry areas, providing a modernization framework to enrich the service and software engineering body of knowledge, and a guideline to develop the architecture model and prototype as requirement and design specification for modernization process especially in system of information for public.

Further research involving both service engineer and software engineer is needed to improve the validation and verification of the modernization framework. The framework context can be further extended to the detailed technical view within realization, implementation, and deployment phases to allow a thorough functional and code transformation as expansion on the current transformation scopes. Further methods, techniques, and tools development also supports this expansion, with concern on model-driven development to promote reuse and efficiency within modernization process.

Acknowledgment. The authors would like to thank our colleagues from Optimização e Planeamento de Transportes, S.A. for granting permission to use Infopub system as a case study on which our research was based on and also the insight and expertise that greatly assisted the research.

References

1. Khanjani, A., Rahman, W.N.W.A., Ghani, A.A.A.: Feature-based analysis into the trend of software technologies from traditional to service oriented architecture and SaaS cloud. J. Comput. Sci. **10**, 2408–2414 (2014)
2. The Business Journals: Advision of ACBJ. http://www.bizjournals.com/bizjournals/how-to/funding/2014/12/how-the-saas-business-model-affects-valuations.html?page=all
3. Chen, H.M.: Towards service engineering: service orientation and business-IT alignment. In: Proceedings of the 41st Annual Hawaii International Conference on System Sciences, p. 114 (2008)
4. Lovelock, C., Wirtz, J.: Services Marketing: People, Technology, Strategy. Prentice Hall, Englewood Cliffs (2011)
5. Erl, T.: Service-Oriented Architecture: Concepts, Technology, and Design. Prentice Hall, Upper Saddle River (2005)
6. Meneses, A.D.C.: InfoPub na web. Departamento de Engenharia Informática. Faculdade de Engenharia da Universidade do Porto, Porto (2009)
7. Seacord, R.C., Plakosh, D., Lewis, G.A.: Modernizing Legacy Systems: Software Technologies, Engineering Process and Business Practices. Addison-Wesley, Boston (2003)
8. Hagins, J.: Making the SaaS decision: the threats, opportunities, and challenges of moving to SaaS. SoftSummit 2008. Mural Consulting Corporation (2008)
9. Osterwalder, A., Pigneur, Y.: Business Model Generation: A Handbook for Visionaries, Game Changers, and Challengers. Self Published (2010)
10. Kang, S., Myung, J., Yeon, J., Ha, S., Cho, T., Chung, J., Lee, S.: A general maturity model and reference architecture for SaaS service. In: Kitagawa, H., Ishikawa, Y., Li, Q., Watanabe, C. (eds.) DASFAA 2010. LNCS, vol. 5982, pp. 337–346. Springer, Heidelberg (2010)
11. The Open Group: The Open Group Service Integration Maturity Model (OSIMM), Version 2. The Open Group, Reading (2011)
12. InfoQ. http://www.infoq.com/articles/SaaS-Lifecycle
13. Mohammadi, M., Mukhtar, M.: A review of SOA modeling approaches for enterprise information systems. Procedia Technol. **11**, 794–800 (2013)
14. Arsanjani, A., Ghosh, S., Allam, A., Abdollah, T., Ganapathy, S., Holley, K.: SOMA: a method for developing service-oriented solutions. IBM Syst. J. **47**, 377–396 (2008)
15. OMG: Service Oriented Architecture Modeling Language (SoaML) Specification Version 1.0.1, pp. 1–132. Object Management Group, Inc. (OMG), Needham (2012)
16. Patricio, L., Fisk, R.P., Falcao e Cunha, J., Constantine, L.: Multilevel service design: from customer value constellation to service experience blueprinting. J. Serv. Res. **14**, 180–200 (2011)

17. Saini, A., Nanchen, B., Evequoz, F.: Putting the customer back in the center of SOA with service design and user-centered design. In: Lau, K.-K., Lamersdorf, W., Pimentel, E. (eds.) ESOCC 2013. LNCS, vol. 8135, pp. 94–103. Springer, Heidelberg (2013). doi:10.1007/978-3-642-40651-5_8

18. Chauhan, M.A., Babar, M.A.: Migrating service-oriented system to cloud computing: an experience report, pp. 404–411 (2011)

19. Ionita, A.D.: Introduction to the migration from legacy applications to service provisioning. In: Ionita, A.D., Litoiu, M., Lewis, G. (eds.) Migrating Legacy Applications: Challenges in Service Oriented Architecture and Cloud Computing Environments, pp. 1–11. IGI Global (2013)

20. Khadka, R., Saeidi, A., Idu, A., Hage, J., Jansen, S.: Legacy to SOA evolution: a systematic literature review. In: Ionita, A.D., Litoiu, M., Lewis, G. (eds.) Migrating Legacy Applications: Challenges in Service Oriented Architecture and Cloud Computing Environments, pp. 40–71. IGI Global (2012)

21. Chung, S., Chul An, J., Davalos, S.: Service-Oriented Software Reengineering: SoSR, p. 172c (2007)

22. Peffers, K., Tuunanen, T., Rothenberger, M.A., Chatterjee, S.: A design science research methodology for information systems research. J. Manag. Inf. Syst. **24**, 45–78 (2008)

23. Mahfudhi, M.G.: From Legacy System into SaaS-Based System: A Public Transport Document Generator. Departamento de Engenharia e Gestão Industrial. Faculdade de Engenharia da Universidade do Porto, Porto (2015)

24. OMG: Business Motivation Model Version 1.3, pp. 1–104. Object Management Group, Inc. (OMG), Needham (2015)

25. Johnson, G., Scholes, K., Whittington, R.: Exploring Corporate Strategy. Prentice Hall, Essex (2008)

26. IMTT: COLECÇÃO DE BROCHURAS TÉCNICAS/TEMÁTICAS: Sistemas de Informação ao Público. In: Pacote de Mobilidade: Conferência em Território, Acessibilidade e Gestão de Mobilidade, pp. 1–17 (2011)

27. Cloudyn. http://learn.cloudyn.com/who-moved-my-cloud/

Improving the Service Level of Bus Transportation Systems: Evaluation and Optimization of Bus Schedules' Robustness

Joana Hora[✉], Teresa Galvão Dias, and Ana Camanho

Faculdade de Engenharia da Universidade do Porto and CEGI – INESC TEC,
Porto, Portugal
{joana.hora, tgalvao, acamanho}@fe.up.pt

Abstract. This study proposes an optimization model to improve the robustness of an existing bus schedule. Robustness represents the ability of schedules to absorb deviations from the timetable and to prevent their propagation through the daily operations. The model developed proposes an optimal assignment of arrival times and distribution of slacks among Time Control Points of a bus line, in order to minimize delays and anticipations from schedule. This required the use of data collected through GPS devices installed in buses, informing the location of buses during their daily operation. The robustness of bus schedules was evaluated through the quantification of delays and anticipations of real observations of bus shifts by comparison with the timetable. The performance measures used to evaluate robustness are the average delay (or anticipation) of buses by comparison with the timetable, and the probability that a passenger that arrives on time according to the timetable will miss the bus or have to wait more than a specified threshold at a Time Control Point. We also compared the improvement of the schedule proposed by the optimization model with the original schedule. The results obtained in a real-world case study, corresponding to a bus line operating in Porto, showed that the model could return an improved schedule for all performance measures considered when compared with the original schedule.

Keywords: Robust scheduling · Transportation systems · Optimization

1 Introduction

Transportation systems play a central role in modern societies, accounting for 5 % of GDP and employing around 10 million people in EU [1]. A significant share of governments' budget is spent in public transports. Local transportation authorities face challenges such as the reduction of pollutant emissions [2–4], the satisfaction of an increased demand for quality and reliable public transport [5], and the design of networks with improved accessibility and mobility of citizens in urban areas [6].

Bus services have a significant impact on the life of citizens, mostly in areas with high population density [5, 7]. The demand for urban transports, particularly by bus,

© Springer International Publishing Switzerland 2016
T. Borangiu et al. (Eds.): IESS 2016, LNBIP 247, pp. 604–618, 2016.
DOI: 10.1007/978-3-319-32689-4_46

has increased considerably during the last decades, together with the growth of cities. This created the need for higher capacity and improved access to bus transports [6, 8]. Citizens expect bus transportation systems to satisfy their needs with quality, efficiency, low-cost, minimum travel time, punctuality and availability [9, 10].

The planning of bus transportation systems is a complex problem, normally addressed using optimization tools. This problem may consider the minimization of operating costs, waiting time of passengers, the total route length or inconvenience of delays and anticipations from schedule [11]. It can incorporate the dynamics of several features, such as the coordination of buses, the interaction of buses with passengers, constraints of traffic or unforeseen events causing instability [12]. Moreover, the planning of bus systems must consider the specificities of the geographic area to respond adequately to the specific needs, constraints, demand and topology of each case study [5, 13, 14]. A transportation system carefully planned leads to lower costs and increased clients' satisfaction.

Bus schedules are normally built with optimization methods aiming to minimize cost, originating rigid schedules with few slack time [15]. However, the daily operations of bus systems are highly exposed to uncertainty, arriving from non-foreseen events such as traffic, accidents, weather conditions, road block, road work, strikes, accidents, bus breakdown and unexpected peak of demand [6, 14–16]. Delays and disruptions impact negatively the quality of the transportation service, and often trigger expensive recovery actions [15, 16]. Non-foreseen events lead to the occurrence and propagation of delays, and sometimes to the disruption of the service. Delays can be classified into two categories: primary and secondary delays. A primary delay cannot be prevented and induces the later arrival of a service trip that has departed on time [16]. A secondary delay occurs when an already delayed bus trip leads to the delayed start of the next bus trip. This inheritance of delays is called delay propagation. Delay propagation results from dependencies of consecutive trips whose slack time is not sufficient to absorb preceding delays [15, 16]. Only secondary delays can be minimized by adjusting the bus schedule [17, 18].

The management of uncertainty in bus systems can be strengthened with techniques of robust planning (planning phase) and of dynamic re-planning (operational phase) [17]. This paper addresses the robust planning of bus schedules. The most common approach to address this issue is the incorporation of slack time in schedules to absorb delays. Although the allocation of slack time is an approach that can successfully improve the robustness of timetables, its implementation entails the increase of operational costs [16].

This work aims to prevent the occurrence of disruptions due to uncertainty by improving the robustness of bus schedules. A set of real observations is used to define the range in which uncertainty fluctuates, which is a standard approach in robust optimization [19]. The optimization model minimizes deviations of real data from the current schedule. The decision variables correspond to the set of slack time to be added to the mean travel time between two adjacent time control points. The restrictions impose that the total slack of the original schedule and the optimized schedule is the same, implying that the two schedules have identical operational costs.

The robustness of bus schedules is assessed with the quantification of the Average Delay (AD) and the Probability of Delay (PD) per Time Control Point (TCP). Analogously, the Average Anticipation (AA) and the Probability of Anticipation (PA) are also computed. These measures are compared between the optimized schedule and the current schedule, to evaluate the relative performance of the schedule proposed by the optimization model developed in this paper.

The model was applied to a real case study concerning a bus line operating in Porto, Portugal. The bus line under study operates with five coordinated shifts and with non-even headways. The dataset for this case study was obtained through GPS devices installed in all buses. The model was implemented using the CPLEX solver.

A comprehensive literature review on this topic is provided in Sect. 2. The optimization model is described in Sect. 3. The robustness indicators used to assess the schedules obtained with the model are detailed in Sect. 4. The case study is described in Sect. 5. The results obtained and their implications are presented in Sect. 6, and the main conclusions are drawn in Sect. 7.

2   Optimization of Robustness in Bus Transportation Systems

One of the main challenges faced by bus transportation systems is to manage uncertainty occurring at the operational stage, and to minimize its negative impacts (e.g., failure in complying with scheduled times, bunching of buses or the disruption of the service) [20]. An adequate approach to address this problem is the improvement of robustness in bus schedules at the planning phase. The objective is to develop schedules that will minimize negative impacts after the occurrence of uncertainty events at the operational phase. In this context, more robust schedules have an enhanced ability to absorb or minimize the propagation of deviations (delays and anticipations) from the timetable. The implementation of robust schedules improves the quality of the transportation service delivered to passengers, leading to a more reliable service.

However, the definition of robustness of transportation schedules is not consensual in literature [15, 21, 22]. There is a panoply of approaches designed to address the needs of specific case studies, leading to a diversity of robustness definitions and measurements. Whilst studies with applications to bus systems are still scarce [15–17, 23], the literature devoted to railway systems is more advanced.

The robustness of a bus schedule can be defined as its ability to absorb secondary delays, considering penalties every time a Primary Delay causes the later start of the next bus trip (i.e., when the slack time is not able to compensate a delay). Naumann, Suhl and Kramkowski [16] applied this concept with the simulation of disruption scenarios designed with stochastic programming, and pursuing the minimization of total costs (i.e., planned costs plus the costs caused by disruptions). The study concluded that robust scheduling significantly reduces the total expected costs (plan and disruption costs) when compared with the sole minimization of planned costs or with the simple addition of fixed slack time between trips. This approach can be unfeasible in large scale problems.

Kramkowski, Kliewer and Meier [17] considers that bus schedules are robust when they are able to reduce the propagation of the effects of unforeseen events. [17] pursued this concept with a measure for delay-tolerance in bus schedules (including planned costs and costs of delays), to obtain schedules with optimized distribution of buffer times, improving the absorption of disruptions and preventing delay propagation. Similarly, [15] applied this concept for the integrated Vehicle Schedule Problem and

Crew Schedule Problem, building a bus schedule with increased delay-tolerance by redistributing its buffer time and minimizing its costs.

A related concept considers that schedules are more robust when they return minimum time deviations from planned. This approach was explored by Yan et al. [23] with an optimization model returning the distribution of slack time that minimizes time deviations, including delays, anticipations and overall variability from schedule. This approach was illustrated using data obtained from a Monte Carlo simulation. Hora, Dias and Camanho [24] proposed an optimization model adapted from [23], which optimizes the slack time distribution in order to minimize both delays and anticipations from schedule, using data from historic records.

An associated concept is the "recoverable robustness", when bus schedules are recoverable by limited means in all likely scenarios, proposed by Liebchen et al. [19].

Finally, it is important to clarify the differences between alternative robust optimization techniques, all of which can be used to address problems whose information is uncertain to some extent. This is the case of bus daily operations that are often unable to comply with the schedule planned. Strictly Robust Optimization returns the best feasible solution for any realization of uncertainty within a convex set [25, 26]. The formulation of strictly robust concepts for public transportation timetables is provided in [27]. A Strictly Robust Optimization model is deterministic, set-based and solved through traditional optimization concepts and algorithms [28]. Moreover, uncertainty is not considered to follow a specific probabilistic distribution, from where Strictly Robust Optimization diverges from Stochastic Optimization [28]. However, strictly robust solutions are often considered too conservative, as they imply a great loss of optimality in order to guarantee robustness [27]. As an alternative to Strictly Robust Optimization, Fischetti and Monaci [29] proposed the approach of Light Robustness Optimization, whose solutions comply with an established quality level whilst maximizing robustness [27]. Models of Light Robustness are solved with heuristic methods, which require the initial specification of parameters such as "robustness goal" and "maximum objective function deterioration" to be accepted in the model [29].

3 Optimization Model to Improve Robustness of Bus Schedules

This section presents a model aiming to improve the robustness of an existing bus schedule. This model is an adapted formulation of the model proposed in [23]. The model can be applied to a bus line integrating several bus stops, some of which are monitored by the bus operating company, called Time Control Points (TCPs). The optimization model considers the entire set of sequential TCPs to be covered during a daily bus shift. A bus schedule is optimized by minimizing the deviation of a set of real observations ($k = 1, ..., K$) from the timetable planned. The decision variables of the optimization model shown in (1) are the values of slack time (stored in vector τ) to be allocated between two adjacent TCPs (TCP_m and TCP_{m+1}) in the schedule under construction. This model can be converted by standard techniques into an equivalent Mixed Integer Linear Programming (MILP) model [30].

The objective function quantifies, for all TCPs, the time deviations of a set of real observations from a given schedule under assessment. The objective function penalizes earlier arrivals at each TCP with weight γ_1 and later arrivals with weight γ_2.

This model has several features that differentiate it from the approach proposed by Yan, et al. [31]. It involves the optimization of non-cyclic bus schedules adopting a daily perspective. The component of the objective function associated with the minimization of the absolute value of deviations, included in [31], was removed from our formulation as the quantification of deviation variability was considered to have a high degree of redundancy with the other two components of the objective function. This term would also increase considerably the computation complexity of the optimization model (changing from quadratic complexity to cubic complexity). The total time of the daily trips (Ψ) is not allowed to change, in order to ensure that the original schedule and the new one returned by the optimization model have the same operational cost. Furthermore, it was imposed a minimum travel time between adjacent TCPs ($N_{m,m+1}$), to ensure the feasibility of the schedule proposed.

Minimize:

$$\mathrm{F}(\tau, \gamma_1, \gamma_2) = \frac{1}{K} \sum_{m=1}^{M} \sum_{k=1}^{K} \gamma_1 \cdot max(0, SD_{m,k}) + \gamma_2 \cdot max(-SD_{m,k}, 0) \qquad (1)$$

Subject to:

$$SD_{1,k} = 0 \qquad (1.1)$$

$$SD_{m+1,k} = E(T_{m,m+1}) + \tau_{m,m+1} - T_{(m,m+1),k} + (1 - \beta_{m,m+1}) * SD_{m,k} \qquad (1.2)$$

$$E(T_{m,m+1}) + \tau_{m,m+1} \geq N_{m,m+1} \qquad (1.3)$$

$$\sum_{m=1}^{M-1} (E(T_{m,m+1}) + \tau_{m,m+1}) = \Psi \qquad (1.4)$$

Where:

- $M \in \mathbb{Z}$: number of TCPs;
- $K \in \mathbb{Z}$: number of real observations of the system (i.e., days);
- $\gamma_1 \in \mathbb{R}$: weight for earlier arrivals, $\gamma_1 \in [0,1]$;
- $\gamma_2 \in \mathbb{R}$: weight for later arrivals, $\gamma_2 \in [0,1]$;
- $\Psi \in \mathbb{R}$: total time for the daily trip (in time units);
- $\tau = [\tau_{m,m+1}] \in \mathbb{R}^{M-1}$: vector of slack time to be allocated in each segment between two consecutive TCPs [$m,m+1$] (decision variables - in time units);
- $\beta = [\beta_{m,m+1}] \in \mathbb{R}^{M-1}$: vector of dimension ($M-1$) storing the Adjustment Factor of Driver between each pair of adjacent TCPs (input data, percentage);
- $E(T) = [E(T_{m-1,m})] \in \mathbb{R}^{M-1}$: vector of dimension ($M-1$) storing the expected value of Travel Time in each segment (in time units);
- $N = [N_{m,m+1}] \in \mathbb{R}^{M-1}$: vector of dimension ($M-1$) storing the minimum travel time needed by a vehicle to travel between two adjacent TCPs (input data, in time units);

- $T = [T_{(m,m+1),k}] \in \mathbb{R}^{(M-1) \times K}$: array of dimension $(M-1) \times K$ storing the Travel Time in each segment $[m,m+1]$ at each day k (input data, in time units);
- $SD = [SD_{m,k}] \in \mathbb{R}^{M \times K}$: array of dimension $M \times K$ containing in each position the Schedule Deviation at TCP m in day k (in time units); $SD_{m,k} < 0$ indicates a delay, $SD_{m,k} > 0$ indicates an anticipation and $SD_{m,k} = 0$ indicates full compliance with the schedule.

Constraint (1.1) considers that the system starts on time at the first TCP, for all observations ($SD_{1,k} = 0$). Constraint (1.2) defines each value of Schedule Deviation ($SD_{m,k}$) as the accumulated deviation from schedule in observation k at TCP_m (considering all preceding TCPs). This constraint quantifies delays and anticipations in each TCP for each observation with respect to the planned schedule and accounts for deviation recovery through the behavior of drivers. When deviations from schedule occur, the model considers that drivers will adapt the average velocity (always complying with regulation) as an attempt to recover. This is included in the model through vector β, which stores a recovery percentage for each segment composing the daily path. A value of $\beta_{m,m+1}=0$ means the driver cannot recover from deviations during the course between TCP_m and TCP_{m+1}, and a value of $\beta_{m,m+1}=1$ means the driver would recover completely from the deviation during that segment. $SD_{m,k}$ is defined as the difference between the expected time ($E(T)_{m,m+1} + \tau_{m,m+1}$) and the real time ($T_{(m,m+1),k}$), plus the accumulated SD from the previous moment ($SD_{m,k}$) multiplied by the percentage of recovery from drivers ($1 - \beta_{m,m+1}$). Values of $SD_{m,k} < 0$ indicate a delay from schedule, $SD_{m,k} > 0$ indicate that the bus is ahead from schedule, and $SD_{m,k} = 0$ indicate that the bus is on time.

Values composing the vector $E(T)$ correspond to the current schedule. The values composing array T concern the real observations, which include the arrival time retrieved at each TCP in each day. The vector τ stores the slack time assigned to each TCP which optimizes the problem (decision variables).

Constraint (1.3) ensures that the arrival time for each TCP is always greater or equal to the arrival time of its antecedent TCP plus the minimum travel time necessary to travel that segment ($N_{m,m+1}$). Note that the value of $N_{m,m+1}$ is strictly positive. The slack time assigned to a specified TCP can assume a positive or negative value, provided that its joint duration with the correspondent expected time ($E(T)_{m,m+1} + \tau_{m,m+1}$) comply with the minimum time necessary to travel between two adjacent TCPs ($N_{m,m+1}$).

Constraint (1.4) allows the user to define the total schedule time through the definition of parameter Ψ. In our empirical study this parameter was set to be equal to the total travel time of the daily trips in the original schedule.

4   Measuring Robustness of Bus Schedules

This section details the performance measures proposed in this study to assess the robustness of bus schedules. The indicators AD (Average Delay) and AA (Average Anticipation) represent the absolute values of delays and anticipations per TCP, respectively. The indicators PD and PA represent the proportion of delays and the proportion of anticipations per TCP, respectively. These indicators are also compared between the optimized schedule and the original schedule, to obtain relative performance measures, indicating the improvement attained through the optimization procedure. These other measures were called AD_r, AA_r, PD_r and PA_r, where the subscript r intends to highlight their relative nature, involving a comparison between the new schedule with the base schedule. The computations involved in the estimation of these measures are detailed in Table 1.

Table 1. Measures used to assess robustness of schedules.

Measuring Delays	$AD = \frac{1}{M \cdot K} \sum_{m=1}^{M} \sum_{k=1}^{K} |SD_{m,k}|$, $if\ SD_{m,k} < 0$	(2)
	$AD_r = 100 \cdot \frac{AD_R}{AD_N}$	(3)
	$PD = 100 \cdot \frac{\sum_{m=1}^{M} \sum_{k=1}^{K} D_{m,k}}{K \cdot M}$, $\begin{cases} D_{m,k} = 1 & if\ SD_{m,k} < -\varepsilon\ ,\ \varepsilon \geq 0 \\ D_{m,k} = 0 & if\ SD_{m,k} \geq -\varepsilon\ ,\ \varepsilon \geq 0 \end{cases}$	(4)
	$PD_r = 100 \cdot \frac{PD_R}{PD_N}$	(5)
Measuring Anticipations	$AA = \frac{1}{M \cdot K} \sum_{m=1}^{M} \sum_{k=1}^{K} |SD_{m,k}|$, $if\ SD_{m,k} > 0$	(6)
	$AA_r = 100 \cdot \frac{AA_R}{AA_N}$	(7)
	$PA = 100 \cdot \frac{\sum_{m=1}^{M} \sum_{k=1}^{K} A_{m,k}}{K \cdot M}$, $\begin{cases} A_{m,k} = 1 & if\ SD_{m,k} > \varepsilon\ ,\ \varepsilon \geq 0 \\ A_{m,k} = 0 & if\ SD_{m,k} \leq \varepsilon\ ,\ \varepsilon \geq 0 \end{cases}$	(8)
	$PA_r = 100 \cdot \frac{PA_R}{PA_N}$	(9)

Where:

- M: number of TCPs;
- K: number of days in the sample (i.e., observations);
- SD: Schedule Deviation at TCP_m under day k (in time units); $SD_{m,k} < 0$ indicates a delay, $SD_{m,k} > 0$ indicates an anticipation (see Eqs. (1.1) and (1.2));
- ε: tolerance threshold defining the amount of time from which a delay or anticipation should be accounted (e.g., $\varepsilon = 1$ min), $\varepsilon \geq 0$;
- D: number of delays observed given a set of real observations, considering the threshold ε;
- A: number of anticipations observed given a set of real observations, considering the threshold ε;
- R: indicates a Robust schedule obtained with the model;
- N: indicates the Nominal schedule currently in use by the transportation operator.

The measure AD, detailed in expression (2), returns the average time that the transportation service was delayed at each TCP. Analogously, measure AA, which is detailed in expression (6), returns the average duration of the anticipations per TCP.

The measure PD returns the proportion of delays observed in TCPs of the bus line during the period studied, which is computed according to expression (4). The transportation service is considered delayed when a bus arrives at a TCP after what was planned in the schedule and the amount of time delayed exceeds a tolerance threshold (ε) specified by the analyst or decision maker. This measure represents the probability that a client arriving on time at a TCP of the bus line will have to wait for a bus more than the time threshold specified. Similarly, the measure *PA* represents the proportion of anticipated arrivals in TCPs of the bus line. According to expression (8), a bus service is considered anticipated when its arrival at the TCP occurs before what was planned in the timetable, with a deviation from schedule larger than the tolerance threshold (ε).

Relative measures AD_r, PD_r, AA_r, and PD_r are adequate to assess the robustness of a schedule when compared with another schedule used as reference. In this study, the indicators associated with the schedule obtained using the optimization model (identified with an *R*, representing a Robust schedule) are compared with the schedule currently in use by the bus operator (identified with an *N*, representing the Nominal schedule). When these measures return values lower than one, it means that the new schedule performs better than the reference schedule.

5 Case Study

The case study used in the empirical part of this paper relates to a bus route operating in the city of Porto (Portugal). This section briefly presents this route, describing its geographic path and the shifts operating during a day. This section also describes the dataset used.

Figure 1 shows the map with the path travelled by this route, including the six TCPs selected by the bus company. The six TCPs of this route are: TCP_1 "*Campanhã*", TCP_2 "*Campo 24 de Agosto*", TCP_3 "*Marquês*", TCP_4 "*Carvalhido*", TCP_5 "*Viso*" and TCP_6 "*Br. Sto. Eugénio*". The total distance between TCP_1 and TCP_6 (one way path) is 11.1 km, and it includes a total of 37 bus stops.

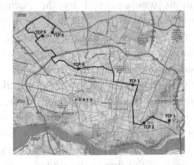

Fig. 1. Map of route 206 with identification of the six TCP.

On working days, the schedule of this bus route is organized into 5 shifts. The 5 shifts are coordinated to satisfy the demand of passengers as shown in Fig. 2. Table 2 provides information characterizing each shift, concerning the start, end and length of daily trips, alongside with the corresponding daily slack time, total number of bus stops

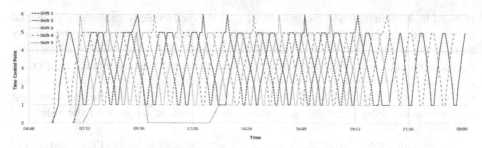

Fig. 2. Current schedule of route 206 including the five shifts for working days.

Table 2. Information of schedules currently operating in all shifts.

Shift	Daily start	Daily end	Total daily length (Ψ)	Daily slack time	M	M·K
1	TCP₁ (06 h 56)	TCP₅ (20 h 47)	13 h 51 = 831 min.	166 min.	99	1287
2	TCP₁ (06 h 02)	TCP₅ (00 h 08)	18 h 06 = 1086 min.	211 min.	141	1833
3	TCP₆ (07 h 00)	TCP₁ (20 h 46)	13 h 46 = 826 min.	161 min.	100	1300
4	TCP₅ (06 h 00)	TCP₅ (23 h 38)	17 h 38 = 1058 min.	207 min.	137	1781
5	TCP₁ (07 h 32)	TCP₅ (19 h 24)	11 h 52 = 712 min.	232 min.	67	871

composing the daily path of each shift (M) and the number positions under assessment for the case study ($M{\cdot}K$).

A set of real observations was gathered by the Portuguese company *"OPT - Optimização e Planeamento de Transportes SA"*, collected from GPS devices installed in all buses operating in Porto. The process of data collection was operationalized with a script gathering information automatically from each bus, with a periodicity of 5 min, during 3 weeks. Each record includes the identification code of the bus, the time of the observation and the estimated time that the bus would spend to achieve each TCP.

The resulting dataset was used to feed the model, including K daily observations with the arrival time at each TCP for each shift. The dataset encompasses the surveillance of 13 working days (i.e., excluding holidays, Saturdays and Sundays).

Figure 3 shows the daily observations (grey lines) alongside the current schedule (continuous black line) for each of the five shifts under study. It is possible to see that buses of all shifts typically arrive early and leave delayed from the inversion spot TCP₅. They are often delayed when arriving to TCP₆. In general, the shifts are able to comply reasonably with the plan during the first half of the day. The trips observed between 14 h 00 and 21 h 00 are systematically delayed. The last trip of shift 1 is an exception, as it always ends earlier than the schedule. Shift 3 has the most irregular pattern, including severe deviations from schedule throughout the day.

6 Results and Discussion

This section presents the results obtained with the optimization model implemented using IBM ILOG CPLEX Optimization Studio, version 12.6, for the case study analysed.

The optimization model is endowed with freedom to reallocate slack time, preserving the total daily time of the current schedule, defined by Ψ (i.e., the total time between the beginning and the end of the daily trips). This constraint allows a fair comparison between the current schedule and the schedules obtained with the optimization model, as both have the same total duration of the daily trips, implying identical operational costs. All runs used a value of β equal to zero, meaning that efforts of drivers to minimize deviations from schedule are not accounted for. Thus, it is assumed that drivers adopt a similar behaviour in all trips between two given TCPs.

The model optimizes the robustness of individual shifts. Different viewpoints regarding the relative importance of delays and anticipations can be adopted. A neutral perspective is labelled as R[1, 1] ($\gamma_1 = 1$; $\gamma_2 = 1$), the exclusively minimization of anticipations as R[1;0] ($\gamma_1 = 1$; $\gamma_2 = 0$), and the fully minimization of delays as R[0;1] ($\gamma_1 = 0$; $\gamma_2 = 1$).

The measures defined in Table 1 were used to assess the robustness of the different schedules obtained with the optimization model. The results are summarized in Table 3, including different values for the tolerance threshold ε, allowing a broad depiction of the sensibility of the performance measures to changes in the threshold used for the evaluation of deviations from schedule.

Considering the length of deviations from schedule, when all shifts are taken into account we can observe that the average delay and anticipation from schedule is around 1.5 min. However, the delays and anticipations occur with different patterns in different shifts. For example, in shift 5 the average length of delays is considerably longer than the length of anticipations (2.6471 vs. 1.2874), whilst the reverse occurs for the other shifts. In the optimized schedules, the length of deviations from schedule could be reduced to values around one minute, which represents a notable overall improvement in relation to the current schedule, with an overall reduction between 67 % and 73 % of the length of delays of the original schedule and an overall reduction between 79 % and 82 % of the length of anticipations of the original schedule, depending on the scenario considered. The greatest improvements in terms of delays occurred for shift 5, whereas for shift 3 the improvements are less significant. Regarding anticipations, the improvement pattern is more homogeneous among the shifts, although shifts 1, 2 and 3 have slightly better results for the indicator AA_r than shifts 4 and 5.

The analysis of the three scenarios with different priorities for the reductions of delays or anticipations (R[1;1], R[1;0], R[0;1]) revealed that the performance of the schedules obtained is not very sensitive to the specification of parameters γ_1 and γ_2.

Regarding the indicator evaluating the proportion of delayed or anticipated arrivals of the buses to the TCPs, we can see that the optimized schedule is particularly good in terms of avoiding extreme values of delays and anticipations. Thus, as the threshold of delays and anticipations increases, the performance of the optimized schedule in terms of the proportion of delays and anticipations improves significantly. For example, considering a

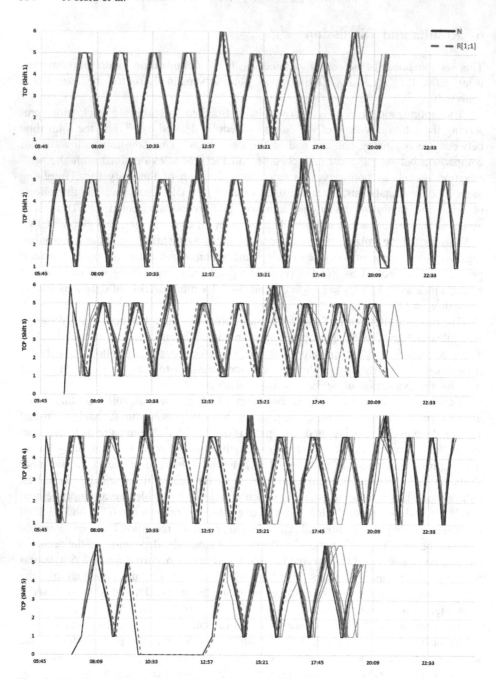

Fig. 3. Nominal schedule (black line), robust schedule R[1;1] (dashed blue line) and real observations (grey lines) for the five shifts of the case study (Color figure online).

Table 3. Robustness measures obtained for the five shifts.

	AD (min)	AA (min)	AD,	AA,	ε=0 minutes PD (%)	PA (%)	PD,	PA,	ε=1 minute PD (%)	PA (%)	PD,	PA,	ε=3 minutes PD (%)	PA (%)	PD,	PA,	ε=6 minutes PD (%)	PA (%)	PD,	PA,
					Shift 1															
N	1.3249	1.6711	--	--	38.31	60.30	--	--	29.60	48.64	--	--	17.79	24.01	--	--	5.67	3.81	--	--
R[1;1]	0.9023	1.2501	0.68	0.75	39.32	57.19	1.03	0.95	26.81	40.79	0.91	0.84	8.70	15.00	0.49	0.62	2.49	1.32	0.44	0.35
R[1;0]	0.9005	1.2497	0.68	0.75	39.01	58.20	1.02	0.97	26.88	40.79	0.91	0.84	8.70	14.76	0.49	0.61	2.49	1.32	0.44	0.35
R[0;1]	0.9049	1.2527	0.68	0.75	39.78	57.26	1.04	0.95	27.12	40.95	0.92	0.84	8.55	14.84	0.48	0.62	2.33	1.24	0.41	0.33
					Shift 2															
N	1.0807	1.2621	--	--	28.75	39.83	--	--	23.13	33.88	--	--	12.98	18.44	--	--	5.46	3.93	--	--
R[1;1]	0.7438	0.9605	0.69	0.76	27.50	39.99	0.96	1.00	19.69	30.61	0.85	0.90	7.69	11.89	0.59	0.64	2.62	1.47	0.48	0.37
R[1;0]	0.7516	0.9551	0.70	0.76	27.99	39.55	0.97	0.99	19.75	30.50	0.85	0.90	7.75	11.84	0.60	0.64	2.62	1.47	0.48	0.37
R[0;1]	0.7364	0.9656	0.68	0.77	27.28	40.21	0.95	1.01	19.59	30.61	0.85	0.90	7.69	11.95	0.59	0.65	2.56	1.53	0.47	0.39
					Shift 3															
N	1.5263	1.6770	--	--	40.62	56.38	--	--	31.92	46.31	--	--	17.00	23.77	--	--	6.85	4.69	--	--
R[1;1]	1.5154	1.1376	0.99	0.68	46.85	48.46	1.15	0.86	35.31	35.62	1.11	0.77	16.08	13.00	0.95	0.55	6.46	2.77	0.94	0.59
R[1;0]	1.5749	1.1041	1.03	0.66	48.62	46.85	1.20	0.83	37.00	34.62	1.16	0.75	16.46	12.31	0.97	0.52	6.85	2.69	1.00	0.57
R[0;1]	1.2096	1.3588	0.79	0.81	40.15	55.62	0.99	0.99	27.54	40.46	0.86	0.87	12.08	16.46	0.71	0.69	5.46	3.23	0.80	0.69
					Shift 4															
N	1.0695	1.1730	--	--	31.33	39.92	--	--	24.20	31.95	--	--	13.53	16.40	--	--	5.00	2.70	--	--
R[1;1]	0.8354	0.9962	0.78	0.85	27.85	42.11	0.89	1.05	18.98	29.98	0.78	0.94	8.70	12.75	0.64	0.78	3.71	1.85	0.74	0.69
R[1;0]	0.8656	0.9627	0.81	0.82	28.75	41.27	0.92	1.03	19.93	28.80	0.82	0.90	8.93	12.30	0.66	0.75	3.71	1.74	0.74	0.64
R[0;1]	0.8182	1.0131	0.77	0.86	27.51	42.67	0.88	1.07	18.70	30.38	0.77	0.95	8.53	13.03	0.63	0.79	3.59	1.85	0.72	0.69
					Shift 5															
N	2.6471	1.2874	--	--	47.99	48.79	--	--	39.72	39.61	--	--	22.16	18.14	--	--	10.79	1.72	--	--
R[1;1]	1.0993	1.1443	0.42	0.89	41.91	53.85	0.87	1.10	30.31	39.38	0.76	0.99	11.60	11.94	0.52	0.66	3.21	1.26	0.30	0.73
R[1;0]	1.1384	1.1301	0.43	0.88	43.17	52.81	0.90	1.08	31.46	39.27	0.79	0.99	12.40	11.25	0.56	0.62	3.21	1.26	0.30	0.73
R[0;1]	1.0985	1.1434	0.41	0.89	42.14	53.73	0.88	1.10	30.08	39.61	0.76	1.00	11.37	11.94	0.51	0.66	3.21	1.26	0.30	0.73
					Average of all shifts															
N	1.5297	1.4141	--	--	37.40	49.04	--	--	29.71	40.08	--	--	16.69	20.15	--	--	6.75	3.37	--	--
R[1;1]	1.0192	1.0977	0.71	0.79	36.69	48.32	0.98	0.99	26.22	35.28	0.88	0.89	10.55	12.92	0.64	0.65	3.70	1.73	0.58	0.55
R[1;0]	1.0462	1.0803	0.73	0.77	37.51	47.74	1.00	0.98	27.00	34.80	0.91	0.88	10.85	12.49	0.65	0.63	3.78	1.70	0.59	0.53
R[0;1]	0.9535	1.1467	0.67	0.82	35.37	49.90	0.95	1.02	24.61	36.40	0.83	0.91	9.64	13.64	0.59	0.68	3.43	1.82	0.54	0.56

tolerance value of ε equal to 3 min in the scenario R[1;1] giving equal importance to delays and anticipations, the new schedule reduces the probability of delays and anticipations to around 65 % of the values associated to the nominal schedule. Regarding the individual shifts, the greatest improvements to these indicators are possible for shifts 1, 2 and 5.

The visualization of the schedules obtained with the optimization model considering a neutral perspective on the relative importance of delays and anticipations ($\gamma_1 = 1$ and $\gamma_2 = 1$) is provided in Fig. 3. This plot represents the schedules returned by the model with a blue dashed line and the corresponding nominal schedule with a continuous black line, for each of the five shifts. Whilst the current schedule allocates slack time exclusively at path inversion TCPs (i.e., TCP 1, 5 or 6), the schedules obtained from the optimization model redistribute the slack time through all TCPs.

7 Conclusions

The main objective of this work was to endow bus schedules the ability to absorb uncertainty through their adjustment to historical data of real bus trips collected by ICT technologies. This involves the use of optimization techniques for the robust planning of bus schedules. This study proposed an approach to enhance existing schedules based on a mathematical programming model applicable to bus routes performing non-cyclic daily trips with non-even headways. The model uses real observations to learn the best distribution of slack time to be incorporated in each TCP integrating the daily path.

A set of measures was proposed and applied to quantify the robustness of bus schedules. The assessment of delays was quantified with the Average Delay (*AD*) and the Proportion of Delays (*PD*) at each TCP. These measures were complemented with relative measures (*AD_r* and *PD_r*) allowing comparisons with a reference schedule. The assessment of anticipations was conducted using analogous measures: Average Anticipation (*AA*), Proportion of Anticipations (*PA*), and the relative measures *AA_r* and *PA_r*, involving direct comparisons with a reference schedule.

The validity of the optimization model was demonstrated with its application to a real-world case study, concerning a bus route operating in Porto, with five daily shifts. The schedules obtained with the model were able to minimize delays and anticipations in all shifts when compared with the corresponding original schedule. For the cases analysed in this work, the schedules obtained with different values of the parameters γ_1 and γ_2, reflecting the priorities assigned to improvements in delays or anticipations, were very similar. This demonstrates that this model does not need extensive experimentation for the calibration of the parameters.

The development of models and measures for the improvement of robustness of bus schedules is relevant to support managers in their effort to enhance urban transportation systems. The optimization model developed in this paper can contribute to improve existing schedules based on the data made available by ICT regarding the actual daily trips of buses. This type of quantitative modelling approaches, involving mathematical programming, can help translate the vast amounts of data currently collected by transportation companies into valuable information allowing the continuous improvement of mobility services provided to citizens.

Acknowledgments. This work was partially supported by the Project "NORTE-07-0124-FEDER-000057", funded by the North Portugal Regional Operational Programme (ON.2 – O Novo Norte), and by national funds, through the Portuguese funding agency, Fundação para a Ciência e a Tecnologia. This research was also supported by the Portuguese Foundation for Science and Technology (scholarship reference PD/BD/113761/2015).

References

1. COM: White Paper on Transport: Roadmap to a Single European Transport Area - Towards a Competitive and Resource-Efficient Transport System. Publications Office of the European Union, Luxembourg (2011)
2. Proost, S., Van Dender, K.: What sustainable road transport future? trends and policy options. OECD/ITF Joint Transport Research Centre Discussion (2010)
3. COM: Communication From The Commission - A sustainable future for transport: Towards an integrated, technology-led and user friendly system Commission of the European Communities (2009)
4. Tzeng, G.H., Lin, C.W., Opricovic, S.: Multi-criteria analysis of alternative-fuel buses for public transportation. Energy Policy **33**, 1373–1383 (2005)
5. Mulley, C., Ho, C.: Evaluating the impact of bus network planning changes in Sydney, Australia. Transp. Policy **30**, 13–25 (2013)

6. Farahani, R.Z., Miandoabchi, E., Szeto, W.Y., Rashidi, H.: A review of urban transportation network design problems. Eur. J. Oper. Res. **229**, 281–302 (2013)

7. Chua, T.A.: The planning of urban bus routes and frequencies: a survey. Transportation **12**, 147–172 (1984)

8. Schmid, V.: Hybrid large neighborhood search for the bus rapid transit route design problem. Eur. J. Oper. Res. **238**, 427–437 (2014)

9. Zhao, F., Zeng, X.G.: Optimization of transit route network, vehicle headways and timetables for large-scale transit networks. Eur. J. Oper. Res. **186**, 841–855 (2008)

10. Ceder, A., Wilson, N.H.M.: Bus network design. Transp. Res. Part B Methodol. **20**, 331–344 (1986)

11. Liu, G., Wirasinghe, S.C.: A simulation model of reliable schedule design for a fixed transit route. J. Adv. Transp. **35**, 145–174 (2001)

12. Hill, S.A.: Numerical analysis of a time-headway bus route model. Physica A **328**, 261–273 (2003)

13. Szeto, W.Y., Wu, Y.Z.: A simultaneous bus route design and frequency setting problem for Tin Shui Wai, Hong Kong. Eur. J. Oper. Res. **209**, 141–155 (2011)

14. van Oudheusden, D.L., Zhu, W.: Trip frequency scheduling for bus route management in Bangkok. Eur. J. Oper. Res. **83**, 439–451 (1995)

15. Amberg, B., Amberg, B., Kliewer, N.: Increasing delay-tolerance of vehicle and crew schedules in public transport by sequential, partial-integrated and integrated approaches. Procedia-Soc. Behav. Sci. **20**, 292–301 (2011)

16. Naumann, M., Suhl, L., Kramkowski, S.: A stochastic programming approach for robust vehicle scheduling in public bus transport. Procedia-Soc. Behav. Sci. **20**, 826–835 (2011)

17. Kramkowski, S., Kliewer, N., Meier, C.: Heuristic methods for increasing delay-tolerance of vehicle schedules in public bus transport. In: MIC 2009: The VIII Metaheuristics International Conference, Hamburg, Germany (2009)

18. Carey, M.: Ex ante heuristic measures of schedule reliability. Transp. Res. Part B Methodol. **33**, 473–494 (1999)

19. Liebchen, C., Lübbecke, M., Möhring, R., Stiller, S.: The concept of recoverable robustness, linear programming recovery, and railway applications. In: Ahuja, R.K., Möhring, R.H., Zaroliagis, C.D. (eds.) Robust and Online Large-Scale Optimization: Models and Techniques for Transportation Systems. LNCS, vol. 5868, pp. 1–27. Springer, Heidelberg (2009)

20. Xuan, Y., Argote, J., Daganzo, C.F.: Dynamic bus holding strategies for schedule reliability: optimal linear control and performance analysis. Transp. Res. Part B Methodol. **45**, 1831–1845 (2011)

21. Roy, B.: Robustness in operational research and decision aiding: a multi-faceted issue. Eur. J. Oper. Res. **200**, 629–638 (2010)

22. Salido, M.A., Barber, F., Ingolotti, L.: Robustness in railway transportation scheduling. In: IEEE (ed.) WCICA 2008 - 7th World Congress on Intelligent Control and Automation, pp. 2880–2885 (2008)

23. Yan, Y., Meng, Q., Wang, S., Guo, X.: Robust optimization model of schedule design for a fixed bus route. Transp. Res. Part C Emerg. Technol. **25**, 113–121 (2012)

24. Hora, J., Dias, T.G., Camanho, A.: Improving the robustness of bus schedules using an optimization model. In: Póvoa, A.P.F.D.B., Miranda, J.L. (eds.) Operations Research and Big Data - IO2015-XVII Congress of Portuguese Association of Operational Research (APDIO). Studies in Big Data, vol. 15, pp. 79–88. Springer, Heidelberg (2015)

25. Ben-Tal, A., Nemirovski, A.: Robust optimization–methodology and applications. Math. Program. **92**, 453–480 (2002)

26. Soyster, A.L.: Convex programming with set-inclusive constraints and applications to inexact linear programming. Oper. Res. **21**, 1154–1157 (1973)
27. Goerigk, M., Knoth, M., Müller-Hannemann, M., Schmidt, M., Schöbel, A.: The price of robustness in timetable information. In: OASIcs-OpenAccess Series in Informatics, vol. 20. Schloss Dagstuhl-Leibniz-Zentrum fuer Informatik (2011)
28. Bertsimas, D., Brown, D.B., Caramanis, C.: Theory and applications of robust optimization. SIAM Rev. **53**, 464–501 (2011)
29. Fischetti, M., Monaci, M.: Light robustness. In: Ahuja, R.K., Möhring, R.H., Zaroliagis, C.D. (eds.) Robust and Online Large-Scale Optimization: Models and Techniques for Transportation Systems. LNCS, vol. 5868, pp. 61–84. Springer, Heidelberg (2009)
30. Garfinkel, R.S., Nemhauser, G.L.: Integer Programming. Wiley, New York (1972)
31. Yan, Y.D., Meng, Q., Wang, S.A., Guo, X.C.: Robust optimization model of schedule design for a fixed bus route. Transp. Res. C-Emerg. **25**, 113–121 (2012)

Mobile Communication Solutions
for the Services in the Internet of Things

Sorin Zamfir, Titus Balan$^{(\boxtimes)}$, Florin Sandu, and Cosmin Costache

Faculty of Electrical Engineering and Computer Science,
"Transilvania" University, Politehnicii 1-3, Brasov 500024, Romania
{zamfir.sorin, titus.balan, sandu,
cosmin.costache}@unitbv.ro

Abstract. The Internet of Things paradigm has most of the times been associated with distributed devices directly connected to the Web, uniquely identifiable and with different sensing-processing-driving capabilities. The paper addresses this context, with focus on industry driven solutions for cloud communications, describing how these technologies impact the mobile telecommunications world as well as consumers, with a clear perspective on different service models for network operators. We present an implementation strategy and showcase two different scenarios to validate our service presentation solutions, with details on data representation for a semantic interfacing of heterogeneous connected devices.

Keywords: Internet of things · Mobile network operators · Cloud communications

1 Introduction

In order to fully understand the problematic of industry driven Internet of Things (IoT) technologies, we must first address the various definitions given to this term. While initially considered around the context of supply chain, the real meaning was often misunderstood and according to its' initial creator at the center of IoT relies information and of most importance are the providers of such data themselves. It was considered that IoT revolves around autonomous intelligence gathering by empowered computers [1]. While his definition is accurate, the actual "things" were later identified [2] as a collection of tags, sensors, actuators and mobile phones capable of interacting with each other to achieve common goals.

Simple data collection paradigm shifted to devices capable of taking decisions and becoming smarter. This became more and more visible by the amounts of gadgets the industry has thrown on the market and their relative diversity, from smart water bottles to intelligent thermostats and lightning systems.

To overcome the major challenges of addressing and ownership the information sources are identifiable through unique URIs (Uniform Resource Identifiers). The interesting aspects about collecting so much data, from connected devices, are hidden behind data analytics that could be used to predict different outcomes and take the optimum actions. In this sense the whole IoT ecosystem becomes a feedback loop for

© Springer International Publishing Switzerland 2016
T. Borangiu et al. (Eds.): IESS 2016, LNBIP 247, pp. 619–632, 2016.
DOI: 10.1007/978-3-319-32689-4_47

the autonomous world (self-driving cars, intelligent homes, adaptive networks etc.). Researches [3] pointed out that storing amounts of heterogeneous information requires a centralized storage, that should take into consideration factors such ownership and expiration date as well as capacity.

The paper explores the advantages that Telco operators bring (together with a big investment) in the IoT business, given the growing financial outcome (e.g. "Verizon announces its own IoT business has grown almost 50 % year over year, and enterprise IoT market is poised for strong growth, rising to 5.4 billion business-to-business connections across the globe by 2020") [4].

We were *motivated* by the great challenge of new commercial service models for mobile Telco that should include machine-to-machine (M2M) communications (given their increasing volume). The reciprocal benefit would be *mobility in the IoT*, extending a service-oriented approach, based on the mature Telco BSS (Business Support Systems).

Our *research goal* was to develop solutions for IoT *service presentation* in heterogeneous sub-nets of "smart objects", validated in complex scenarios and use cases. The Public Transportation System (PTS) demonstrator was chosen for the *intrinsic mobility* - not only of customers but even of the core sub-nets (e.g. GSMR - railways embarked GSM core-networks or modern airplanes, boats and other vehicles with own Pico- or Femto- radio base stations for cellular mobile Telco) cooperating with core sub-nets of road/metropolitan tunnels etc.

The *approach* is bilateral - Telco offers to IoT a modern range of commercially robust solutions for mobility and a service-organized IN (Intelligent Network) where customers (not only professionals of network producers or operators) can create, configure and run the services. Furthermore, an extended *charging model*, an *attach-detach model* of registration-deregistration of IoT smart objects (that can be unified as subscribers - humans & machines to an integrated *social network model*), *a roaming model* and, last but not least, a *call model* (with a generalized seizure-release of resources, based on subscriber profiles of features-capabilities) are all telco assets.

The mutual offer of IoT is a huge volume of communications that should be monetized, the opportunity of a *comprehensive business model* integrating M2M communications with H2H and H2M ones.

Our *objectives* were: a feasibility study on mutual enhancement Telco-IoT in the context of Cloud monetization; identification of best protocols for service presentation in *pervasive*(and mobile networked) computing (CoAP and MQTT detailed in the next section); proposal of an *interoperability* solution for smart objects with heterogeneous connectivity (a *semantic interfacing* via dedicated Ponte bridging); and accomplishment of a *demonstrator* for the aggregation of IoT services in the PTS to validate our solution.

The *research methodology* was driven by important international cooperation projects and calls of the standardization bodies.

Data-driven control was chosen for semantic integration of bridging and brokerage and state-of-the-art Telco models for subscriber identity and capabilities profiles were extended to IoT.

Organization of the paper was done in 5 sections. After the Introduction, the 2nd paragraph is dedicated to service-presentation solutions for the IoT (focusing on CoAP and MQTT). The 3rd section is dedicated to the Telco-IoT relationship aiming to consolidate the mutual advantages of mobility, reliability and security, in the challenging context of diversity while the 4th paragraph details the PTS proof-of-concept, with some implementation close-ups and code snippets. Last chapter presents the Conclusions and future developments.

2 Service Presentation in Industry-Driven IoT

We have seen so far that Internet of Things comes with a special set of requirements and while the endpoints of IoT (the Internet and the 'smart' objects) are explored in depth by the industry – given by the vast number of applications identified in the IoT related literature [5] – the communication in between has not sparked such a huge interest among enablers [6], giving birth to skepticism in what concerns the real value of this technology trend. As a result of these concerns, it is vital that existing Telco standardization bodies take a stand for uniformity across different "smart things" vendors and cloud-based implementations.

Governing bodies such as IETF (the Internet Engineering Task Force) and OASIS (Open Standards for the Information Society consortium) have already defined two approaches for *pervasive networked computing*.

While these two IoT-aimed protocols have been in-depth described in their standard specification, we consider it's important to detail their specific *service presentation* aspects and also summarize some key differences between them in the perspective of smart objects' capabilities exposure, searching/polling, discovery, seizure, aggregation etc.

2.1 The Constrained Application Protocol

In 2014 IETF published a RFC describing the Constrained Application Protocol (CoAP) specifically aimed for usage within resource/performance constrained nodes and low power networks [7]. One of the key focuses of CoAP was to easily integrate with existing web technologies such as HTTP and REST, while taking into account constraints such as low bandwidth and low power consumption due to less overhead.

An application level protocol that makes use of the existing UDP transport layer protocol, CoAP must enforce by its own reliability, more specifically using so called confirmable messages. Since in IoT we talk about M2M interactions, the client-server model is expanded with the help of CoAP to such an extent at which each node assumes at the same time both the client and server roles [8].

Nevertheless the addressing strategy relies on URIs (similar to HTTP) which uniquely identify a resource (with its *capability* or a set of capabilities – depending on the implementer needs). Two CoAP peers must speak the same resource-*dialect* in order to communicate.

2.2   The Message Queuing Telemetry Transport

While initially invented in 1999 and deployed in various industries, the MQTT protocol was only submitted for standardization in 2013 under the OASIS supervision. It was conceived as lightweight messaging protocol working under the *publish-subscribe* model (not under client-server model like CoAP) for low-bandwidth networks and constrained devices [9]. MQTT represents an application layer protocol for transferring *messages* between different peers and uses existing protocols that offer ordered, bi-directional connections [10]. Most implementations rely by default on TCP and a message *broker* responsible for *registering* each peer and managing the peer to peer communication as well as handling a *separate session state* per connected endpoint. MQTT defines QoS (Quality of Service), which inherently guarantees that a message will be delivered by the broker either no more than once(QoS 0), at least once(QoS 1) or exactly once(QoS 2), achieved through a series of acknowledgement control packets. Identification is based on peer UIDs (User Identifiers), subscription topics (corresponding to the "subscriber info" in mobile communications home-/visited- location registers, HLR/VLR) and *persistent* session tags which makes M2M interaction similar to the *chat* in social networks. This limited persistence has also an analogue as the *availability* in social networking – disposing of published offers if they aren't needed. Two peers must share the same dialect in order to communicate effectively.

3   Relationship Between IoT and Telco Industry

Constant drops in average revenue per user [11] force telecom operators to investigate new service models capable of underlining their unique capabilities and differentiating them from classical Internet service providers.

There are several aspects that make mobile networks as the "favorite" technology to be used for IoT, and the most important one is maturity. Mobile networks offered the first wireless services to consumers and industry over twenty years ago, and have been built reliable, available, secure, and cost effective. From availability point of view there is an accelerated technology shift to mobile broadband connections (i.e. 3G and 4G technologies) with already good wireless coverage area. These networks have solid identity mechanisms that could be successfully reused, like the SIM card that will become a dual-use component, capable of securing application communi-cations and the application itself.

SIM cards could be considered as computing trust anchors, capable of mitigating identity theft, passive interception, side-channel analysis, physical tampering.

Furthermore, 3G and 4G technologies use mutual authentication to verify the identity of the Endpoint and the network.

The evolved SIM cards, like the ones described by GSMA in the "Embedded SIM Remote Provisioning Architecture" are appropriate for deeper component level integration into IoT Endpoint devices optimizing production cost and management costs of connectivity via Over-The-Air (OTA) platforms.

Another argument for the dual-use of the SIM card is the introduction of mobile industry security specifications such as those provided by 3GPP, named Generic

Bootstrapping Architecture (GBA) for user authentication at HLR/HSS level (Home Location Register), but also adoption of other standards like OMA (Open Mobile Alliance) and oneM2M. The already developed and proved technologies from mobile networks ("no need for reinventing the wheel") and the extended mobile coverage area are the main reasons for the Telco operators to have confidence in investing in the IoT area.

3.1 Mobility

One of the most important benefits of having Internet provided by a telecom operator is the continuous service delivery while the end customer is moving. At a first glance, mobility seems transparent and somewhat implicit for all the applications independent of their implementer, (e.g. 3rd party) but for critical scenarios network driven insights provide a unique and valuable asset. Imagine for instance a scenario in which once an IoT control session is established, it is vital this is not interrupted (e.g. remote updating software on moving objects such as cars [13] or perhaps event health monitoring equipment). An insight such as network traffic load and mobility data of a certain subscriber could help determine when is the most appropriate time for such a control session to be established. Handling network disconnection and congestion can be achieved through caching methods on the IoT device, but this would imply high costs. As a result we cannot deny the benefit mobile networks offer through continuous service delivery mechanisms implemented by design, which makes the Telco ecosystem quite attractive for specific IoT use cases.

3.2 Reliability

Considered an important technological characteristic of the networks in general, the Telco industry crafted a standard (TL 9000) to specifically address the quality, reliability and performance of the telecom products and services around the world.

Telco was one of the first industries that achieved the Five-9 s availability (this is the equivalent of 99.999 % service availability), but this is a common expectation from computing equipment as well as other mission critical systems [14]. However, up until this point cloud providers have not been able to provide such a level of reliability on all of their services [15] mainly due to the complexity of the distributed computing systems that adds to the heterogeneous nature of the pipe between them and the end-users.

Even if cloud providers manage to enhance their datacenters availability (and considering the numbers it is quite feasible to assume this) they still do not have any control or insights on the network and still depend on ISPs for the distribution of their cloud hosted services.

This actually means that in a scenario like disaster monitoring, (e.g. earthquake and tsunami monitoring through high depth sensors or wildfire alarming through) even if the service is up and running within the cloud providers' datacenter, it is inaccessible because ISP failure. The Internet wasn't designed to be connection oriented and never offered the concept of QoS which seems is a major impediment for safety relevant use cases and for real time traffic.

3.3 Security

Last but not least security is one of the major concerns of the connected world in the last following years, especially considering the confidential information that can be stored. Some notable examples in relation to data are customer details required for issuing electric bills for instance, that represents the core of every customer relationship management system, and tie the customer to on-premises equipment such as a smart meter.

Security can be enforced by the service enabler through means of encryption and a private cloud, but traditional cloud providers solutions are targeted for multi-purpose applications which in fact is not enough for safety critical IoT scenarios as the one described above. Even so, the security aspect in standard cloud environments relies on the service creator which is the sole responsible for the authentication and encryption of that information being handled, thus often leading to more complex code residing on the endpoint devices.

Traditional mobile network environments were designed as a safe and reliable ecosystem for specific services that have critical needs when it comes to security, and as result, customer data is always protected by encryption and stored in contained environments. While security is not guaranteed by default, as per the GSMA IoT security guidelines recently released [16] network operators should enforce and control the *network level* security by:

- using the MILENAGE or TUAK mutual authentication scheme between endpoints and the RAN
- using different encryption algorithms for protecting data sent over the air (e.g. A5/3 with minimum 128 bit cipher, Kasumi, EEA1, EEA2 or EEA3)
- core network encryption for both user and data plane
- HLR/HSS/VLR denial of service protection including unintentional attacks such as signaling storms due to massive roaming in case of disaster scenarios
- secure management of UICCs (e.g. form factor embedded SIMs)
- deep packet inspection techniques that can detect anomalies within traffic flow and can trigger packet isolation
- differential service provisioning (e.g. limit access only to specific services even within the IP world)

This moves most of the security aspects towards the network layer, reducing the complexity of the software that needs to be deployed in the endpoint devices, and enabling also the separation of concerns: the IoT service provider is only interested in the data and not how this is handled over the network.

4 Implementing IoT Services in Public Transportation Systems

Network operators have unique capabilities when it comes to network insights but the grasp towards new service models within the Telco world is still limited. While some tend towards mobile payments and money transfers it is the closed type of ecosystem that makes the Telco unattractive to third party service providers and stops the creation of new revenue streams.

IoT has sparked quite an interest for the established cloud providers such as Amazon, Google and Microsoft that provide their own offering for integrating smart devices and creating such services. In contrast with telecom operators, public cloud offerings like these (widely accessible from the Internet), can be used quite facile by service providers to rapidly prototype and deploy their applications making them quite attractive because of reduced TCO (total cost of ownership), available third party services and automatic resource management.

Fundamentally the assets for offering an IoT platform are not different for a regular mobile operator: inventory and network management are already established and reliability along with enforced security come as an added bonus.

To explore in-depth the service models and their description process, we have chosen as domain of interest the public transportation systems, that represent a huge interest in the context of future intelligent cities. The choice of this use case is representative for our approach, as it leverages all three important capabilities of the commercial mobile networks (mobility, reliability and security).

As a first step we identify the sub-categories of Public Transportation Systems:

1. The vehicles (trains, buses, metro, trams)
2. The transportation network (roads, tunnels, railways, stations)
3. The center of operations (handling maintenance, distribution of tickets, billing etc.)
4. The passenger (the users of the PTS).

Humans (4) and machines (1) can be considered *service subscribers* in a larger perspective. *Deployment of smart devices* should enable these two kinds of subscribers with backend connectivity: the vehicles and, probably the most important, the passengers. Next we will explore different resulting service models. The specific of our solutions is the integration of *heterogeneous* IoT protocols that would require *brokerage*.

As a basis for our solution, a *bridge* was used for integrating the communication between two clients supporting different protocols (explored in depth in the following paragraphs). Our approach is based on the Eclipse IoT *Ponte* project [17] deployed on the *nodeJs* platform [18]. Additionally, for the two Java based clients, the *paho* and *californium* libraries [19, 20] were used, as they provide the basis of our communi-cation scenarios through MQTT and CoAP (Fig. 1).

The standard supported protocols are CoAP, MQTT as well as HTTP but their range can easily be extended with new protocol adapters. To accommodate various data formats and representations, the bridge component uses a non-relational database to store the messages.

Depending on the QoS level required by the clients, the messages can be persisted until all the subscribers have received the data. For high volume data and high availability, the bridge and database can be clustered and distributed databases can be used.

By leveraging the multi-protocol bridge, it is possible to develop flexible APIs accessible using the various communication protocols. For example, some smart

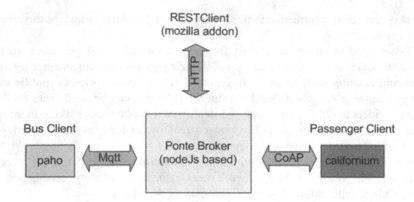

Fig. 1. The representative scenario and the implemented solutions

devices can publish data using the CoAP protocol, data that can be retrieved for example by subscribers using the MQTT protocol or even queried using HTTP REST.

After setting up the bridge we fire it up by entering the following shell command **ponte -v | bunyan** that will basically start listening on specific protocol ports for inbound connections.

Next we power up the two java clients by issuing the following commands:

```
java -jar pass-example-0.0.1-SNAPSHOT.jar
java -jar bus-example-0.0.1-SNAPSHOT.jar
```

As a result the Ponte bridge shell will display the following outputs.

```
INFO: ponte/2341 on linux.site: client connected (service = MQTT,
client = Bus17)
INFO: ponte/2341 on linux.site: subscribed to topic (service = MQTT,
client = Bus17, topic = Bus17Cmd, qos = 1)
INFO: ponte/2341 on linux.site: request received (service = CoAP,
url =/r/Bus17Info, code = 0.01)
```

The first two lines notify the connection of the bus client (MQTT - based) and the subscription to the commands queue (e.g. for registration purpose). Since MQTT is session-based it will always try to establish a connection to its broker before attempting any communication. The last line represents a GET request issued by the passenger's client (CoAP-based) to obtain update information; this is a preliminary method of checking whether this instance has connected to our bridge or not (this is due to the request-response nature of CoAP which doesn't keep alive a whole session throughout the conversation).

Next, the two clients exchange information (Fig. 2) through JSON objects which are encoded using the Jackson library, specifically for each scenario phase (e.g. Registration or UpdateInfo).

Current technologies encourage Internet driven service description through unique resource identifiers that are independent of the technology choice (in our case it's **technology://domain/resource/{bus}**) and pass the data encoding responsibility to the service designer.

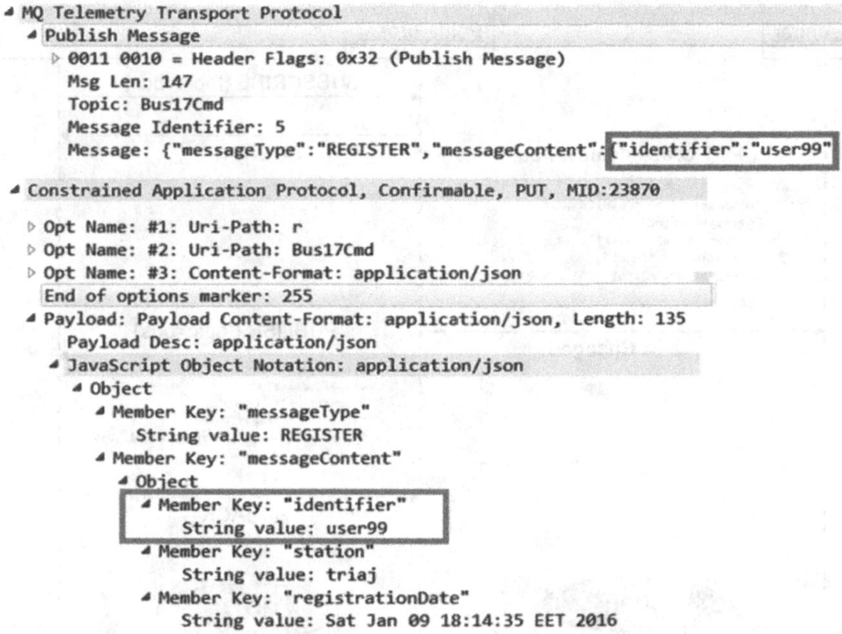

```
◢ MQ Telemetry Transport Protocol
  ◢ Publish Message
    ▷ 0011 0010 = Header Flags: 0x32 (Publish Message)
      Msg Len: 147
      Topic: Bus17Cmd
      Message Identifier: 5
      Message: {"messageType":"REGISTER","messageContent":["identifier":"user99"
◢ Constrained Application Protocol, Confirmable, PUT, MID:23870

  ▷ Opt Name: #1: Uri-Path: r
  ▷ Opt Name: #2: Uri-Path: Bus17Cmd
  ▷ Opt Name: #3: Content-Format: application/json
    End of options marker: 255
  ◢ Payload: Payload Content-Format: application/json, Length: 135
      Payload Desc: application/json
    ◢ JavaScript Object Notation: application/json
      ◢ Object
        ◢ Member Key: "messageType"
            String value: REGISTER
        ◢ Member Key: "messageContent"
          ◢ Object
            ◢ Member Key: "identifier"
                String value: user99
            ◢ Member Key: "station"
                String value: triaj
            ◢ Member Key: "registrationDate"
                String value: Sat Jan 09 18:14:35 EET 2016
```

Fig. 2. Registration request translated from CoAP to MQTT

4.1 The Passenger Registration Service

Fleet management services have always been of big interest for public transport organizations that need to track mobile entities with monitoring purposes in mind. However, since most services revolve around position relevant information - LBS (Location-Based Services) there was little attention for the interaction between the passengers and the actual transportation systems.

Let us consider the following simple bus example and then explore how an implementation strategy would look like:

- the bus notifies its presence and availability as a resource of transport in the Internet, publishing its capabilities
- the passengers waiting in different bus-stops register as users of this resource when they hop in the bus (e.g. by validating an electronic ticket)
- the bus sends load information for different stations to the operations center

This use-case would generate relevant real-time information about the load status of the transport network infrastructure and could help a public transport operator plan routes and schedules accordingly.

In terms of software this can be implemented using one of the standard IoT communication protocols such as CoAP or MQTT and any mix of these two considering an abstraction mechanism through resources identifiers provided by a framework such as Ponte (Fig. 3).

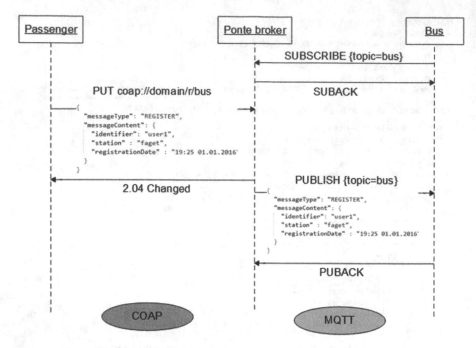

Fig. 3. CoAP to MQTT interfacing through Ponte - passenger registration

The code snippets in Table 1 show our approach of how the bus registration can be achieved using IoT enabled protocols.

The two clients are interfaced by a proxy-broker capable of transposing resources between URI format supported by CoAP and HTTP to publish/subscribe message queue supported by MQTT. The connection in between the two is the actual API endpoint specified by a unique identifier which in our case is **{bus}**.

It should also be noted that even though two or even three different application level protocols are used, the semantics between the IoT endpoints (passenger and bus) must be known in advance by each (e.g. the JSON schema of the document that is exchanged must be known by both clients).

This scenario is a proof-of-concept that can be complemented with an explicit de-registration ("detach") mechanism, adding also a security mechanism. The purpose was to demonstrate how special solutions for mobile connectivity of smart devices can empower modern services for the IoT. The passenger client code could reside on his/her smartphone and registration/deregistration could be triggered by means of local handover (e.g. if a mobile communications Femtocell is placed inside vehicles). Another solution for the emerging smart devices is a virtual "embedded SIM" proposed by GSMA (the GSM Alliance) [21] as a more direct implementation of subscribed identity in the mobile communications registers (HLR/VLR, HSS - Home Subscriber Systems etc.).

Table 1. Code snippets for passenger and bus residing software

Passenger client code snippet - publishing registration information (using Californium Java CoAP library)

```
. . . .
URI uri= new URI("coap://domain:5683/r/bus");
CoapCient client= new CoapClient(uri);
. . . .
IoTMessage<Passenger> msg= new IoTMessage<Passenger>();
msg.setMessageType("REGISTER");
msg.setMessageContent(Passenger);
response=client.put(message,50);
```

Bus client code snippet - subscribing to registration API (using Paho MQTT Java library)

```
. . . .
String uri= "tcp://domain:1883";
String id= "bus17"
MQTTClient client= new MQTTClient(uri,id,persistence);
MQTTConnectOptions connOpts= new MQTTConnectOptions();
connOpts.setCleanSession(true);
connOpts.setConnectionTimeout(30);
BusInfoPublisher pub= new BusInfoPublisher(client);
BusCmdSubscriber sub= newBusCmdSubscriber(pub);
client.setCallback(sub);
client.connect();
client.subscribe("bus");
```

4.2   The Bus Information Publisher Service

Obtaining real time bus information for the passengers could provide an important asset for some calculations enabling intelligent-transportation decisions.

It could be estimated the arrival time of a specific bus in a specific station, or checked if it is enough space for passengers and/or luggage versus vehicle capacity.

In this scenario we would have the following (Fig. 4):

- the bus periodically publishes relevant information about itself to the operations center
- the passengers poll for this data according to their need (H2M and/or M2M scenarios if smart devices facilitate this query).

Of course in this case the biggest concern relies with identifying the public transport system of interest and then monitoring its behavior over a period of interest. For this to happen using the same clients, our solutions include a separate coordinating entity that handles the published resources: this could be either a separate MQTT client that publishes aggregated messages in a separate queue or it could even be a manager deployed in the operations center (M2M/H2M alternatives).

Excluding (just for brevity) some secondary details of our implementation - we consider that the key for such services relies in identifying what kind of information is useful for the end user (a "user-centric" approach).

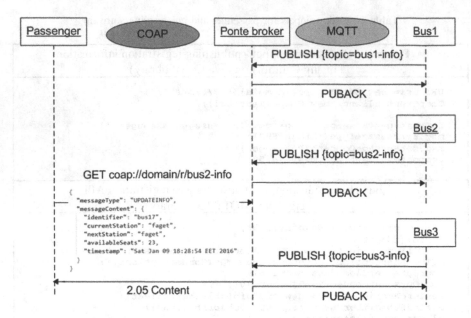

Fig. 4. Bus updates published through MQTT and polled via CoAP

In our case-study, passing tracking information from the public transport system to the passengers would provide a better user experience in terms of timing reliability (an example of driving services by QoE - Quality of Experience) (Table 2).

Table 2. Code snippet for bus update info publishing and receiving

Passenger client code snippet - receiving update information (using Californium Java CoAP library)
```\nclient.setURI("coap://192.168.0.100:5683/r/Bus17Info");\nCoapResponse response = client.get(50);\nhandleCoapResponse(response);\n```
Bus client code snippet - publishing update information (using Paho MQTT Java library)
```\nUpdateInfo info = new UpdateInfo();\ninfo.setCurrentStation(currentStation);\ninfo.setNextStation(currentStation)\ninfo.setIdentifier("bus17");\ninfo.setTimestamp(new Date().toString());\ninfo.setAvailableSeats(MAXIMUMPASSENGERS-pass.size());\n...\nmsg.setMessageType("UPDATEINFO");\nmsg.setMessageContent(info);\nMqttMessage message= new MqttMessage(msg.getBytes());\nmessage.setQos(1);\nmessage.setRetained(true);\nclient.publish("Bus17Info", message);\n```

5 Conclusions

Modern transportation has been granted an impressive attention - our PTS solutions can also contribute to better passenger-centric services that are putting at greater stakes concepts such privacy and security.

We have seen how easy services can be crafted using IoT technologies by implementing a demonstrator use-case, and also identified some key aspects that distinguish mobile networks from classical ISPs.

Furthermore we highlighted the heterogeneous nature of the smart devices in the whole Internet of things ecosystem and we proposed a strategy for decomposing existing service systems and also showcased the interoperability capabilities between different cloud communication protocols.

The solution proposed was a semantic interfacing ("northbound" in the protocol stack) between smart devices that are using different "southbound" protocols.

Last but not least we illustrated service identification inspired from the Internet world, leveraging the powerful nature of RESTful APIs and simple language independent data encoding.

In the end the registration-deregistration mechanism was associated with attach-detach scenario from cellular telecommunications domain and core abilities to manage such services enforcing mobile operators to be the leading technological poles in the M2M world.

Further development will address the automatic service discovery and management methods emphasizing the importance of the existing Telco ecosystem.

As the technical committee of UDDI decided to close its work in 2008 [22] since web service registries didn't spark the expected community interest, we now clearly see the need for similar solutions to handle the management of IoT services, considering the future of M2M communications in the scope of the semantic web.

We have also mentioned the important prospect for social networking - further development could unify aggregation of participants to a service run whatever they are (humans and/or machines).

Acknowledgement. Our research was supported by the Romanian Executive Agency for Higher Education, Research, Development and Innovation Funding, in the frame of the PN-II-PT-PCCA-2013-4-2023 project "NaviEyes" – nr 240/2014.

References

1. Ashton, K.: That 'Internet of Things' Thing. RFiD Journal (2009). http://www.rfidjournal.com/articles/view?4986
2. Giusto, D., Iera, A., Morabito, G., Atzori, L. (eds.): The Internet of Things. Springer, New York (2010)
3. Gubbi, J., Buyya, R., Marusic, S., Palaniswami, M.: Internet of Things (IoT) - A vision, architectural elements, and future directions. Future Gener. Comput. Syst. **29**(7), 1645–1660 (2013)

4. Billion Business IoT Connections by 2020. The Security Ledger, Verizon https://securityledger.com/2015/02/verizon-5-billion-business-iot-connections-by-2020/
5. Miorandi, D., Sicari, S., De Pellegrini, F., Chamlat, I.: Internet of things - Vision, applications and research challenges. Ad Hoc Netw. **10**(7), 1497–1516 (2012)
6. Atzori, L., Iera, A., Morabito, G.: The Internet of Things - A survey. Comput. Telecommun. Networking **54**(15), 2787–2805 (2010)
7. Valerio, P.: Is the IoT a Tech Bubble for Cities? IEEE Consum. Electron. Mag. **5**(1), 61–62 (2016)
8. Shelby, Z., Hartke, K., Bormann, C.: The Constrained Application Protocol (CoAP). IETF RFC7252 (2014). https://tools.ietf.org/html/rfc7252
9. Message Queuing Telemetry Transport - v3.1.1. OASIS MQTT TC (2014). http://docs.oasis-open.org/mqtt
10. Message Queuing Telemetry Transport Org (2013). http://mqtt.org
11. Digital agenda for Europe. EU Commission (2014). http://digital-agenda-data.eu
12. ICT Facts & Figures. ITU (2015). https://www.itu.int
13. De Boer, G., Engel, P., Praefcke, W.: Generic remote software update for vehicle ECUs using a telematics device as a gateway. In: Valldorf, J., Gessner, W. (eds.) Advanced Microsystems for Automotive Applications, pp. 371–380. Springer International Publishing, Heidelberg (2005)
14. Bauer, E.: Design for Reliability: Information and Computer-Based Systems. Bauer, Eric. Design for Reliability: Information and Computer-based Systems. John Wiley & Sons (2010)
15. Butler, B.: Which cloud providers had the best uptime last year? Network World (2015). http://www.networkworld.com/article/2866950/cloud-computing/which-cloud-providers-had-the-best-uptime-last-year.html
16. IoT Security guidelines for network operators v1.0. GSMA (2016). http://gsma.com/connectedliving/gsma-iot-security-guidelines-complete-document-set
17. The Ponte Project. Eclipse Foundation (2013). http://www.eclipse.org/ponte
18. The NodeJs Project. NodeJs Foundation (2015). https://nodejs.org/en
19. Kovatsch, M., Lanter, M, Shelby, Z.: Californium - scalable cloud services for the internet of things with CoAP. In: 2014 International Conference on the Internet of Things (IoT), Cambridge, MA, pp. 1–6. IEEE Press (2014)
20. Walker-Morgan, D.: Practical MQTT with Paho. InfoQ (2013). http://www.infoq.com/articles/practical-mqtt-with-paho
21. Embedded SIM Remote Provisioning Architecture v1.1. GSMA (2013). http://www.gsma.com/connectedliving/wp-content/uploads/2014/01/1.-GSMA-Embedded-SIM-Remote-Provisioning-Architecture-Version-1.1.pdf
22. McRae, M.: Closure of OASIS UDDI Specification TC. Oasis uddi-spec mailing list (2008). https://lists.oasis-open.org/archives/uddi-spec/200807/msg00000.html

E-Health Services and Medical Data
Interoperability

Improving the Introduction of Electronic Health Record: Lessons from European and North American Countries

Sabrina Bonomi[1][✉], Nabil Georges Badr[2], Alessandro Zardini[3], and Cecilia Rossignoli[3]

[1] eCampus University, Novedrate, CO, Italy
sabrina.bonomi@uniecampus.it
[2] Grenoble Graduate School of Business, Grenoble, France
nabil.badr@alumni.grenoble-em.com
[3] University of Verona, Verona, VR, Italy
{alessandro.zardini,cecilia.rossignoli}@univr.it

Abstract. The Electronic Health Record (EHR) has many advantages and its introduction is, at the moment, in different stages of progress in various European countries. Reasons such as historic paths, elements and procedures of her affect the progress stages, including issues of law, politics and economics strengths and weakness of national systems. A shared observation among countries underscores the value that can be co-created by the interaction between doctors, nurses, and patients. Certainly the technology has an important role in this value co-creation, facilitating the exchange of information, reducing errors, and enabling more effective and appropriate treatments. We present finally the concrete case of Kaiser Permanente, showing how the interaction between the healthcare providers, patients and demonstrating the ensuing value in improved health for people.

Keywords: EHR · EMR · Service science · Kaiser permanente

1 Introduction

An Electronic Health Record is a collection of data on a patient's digital health. According to [1], health information technology in general and EHRs in particular, are tools for improving the quality, safety and efficiency of health systems. Physicians, nurses and health workers add to EHR data, progressively, over the course of a patient's life. Data also includes information entered by the patients themselves.

The benefits of EHR are recognized worldwide, in developing and developed countries [2]. Developing countries has been slower to adopt due to high acquisition costs [2]. Post implementation maintenance could be prohibitive to the installation of the three key major ancillary department systems (laboratory, pharmacy, and radiology) [3]. The lack of skilled resources and the deficiency in the required infrastructure is seen as hindrance to implementation; the lack of computer user skills has been known to present a significant barrier [4]. Similarly, in the case of developed countries, such as Italy, United Kingdom (UK), and Northern Europe (NE - Norway, Finland, Denmark and

T. Borangiu et al. (Eds.): IESS 2016, LNBIP 247, pp. 635–648, 2016.
DOI: 10.1007/978-3-319-32689-4_48

Sweden), Canada and United States, we can observe that, despite many benefits, EHR has not uniformly proliferated. Jha et al. [1] explained that it is difficult for hospitals to obtain quality data, and that only a small fraction of hospitals (< 10 %), possessed the key components required by an EHR. Those components are known to include systems that track and document data on patient admission, pharmacy, medical record registration, archiving, laboratory, radiology, etc. On the other hand, the main scope of the new science of service is to classify and explain how different types of service systems interact and evolve in order to co-create value through a continuous chain of interactions between physicians and patients [4], i.e. service providers and consumers [5]. Human factors, management-economic factors, and engineering factors are involved in several interactions and in an interdisciplinary effort to co-create value [7].

To make advances in service innovation it is necessary that the service system has information about the capabilities and the needs of its clients, its competitors and itself. Indeed, not all interactions between service systems co-create value and service science seeks to understand the reasons that could be detected by observing and analysing different behaviours [6]. Thus, an approach of Service Science, Management and Engineering (SSME) could be applied to this topic. SSME is a concept that describes a whole domain of study that allows engineers, economists and managers to interact and cooperate in order to analyse, develop and exploit complex dynamic systems, i.e. the service systems [7, 8]. Indeed, e-health is in a continuous improvement process and it can reorganize processes and improve quality of service, in order to develop the performance management system [9]. For these reasons, in this paper we try to understand if and how service science can help the diffusion of EHR in different countries. Therefore, we present the case of Kaiser Permanente (KP), a nationwide Healthcare provider in the US, has succeeded in "breaking the ice" of EHR usage with an integrated patient health record portal, clinical transaction records, workflow, and account management [10].

2   Background

2.1   Electronic Health Record

The terms "electronic medical record" (EMR) and "electronic health record" (EHR) are often used interchangeably. This could be due to the fact that the word EMR was used historically to indicate the early stages of the concept [11].

The EHR is the first step and the reference point during the healthcare process for realizing the e-health project, since it provides a clear picture of a patient's state of health from birth onwards. It consists in a clinical document, digitally stored in repositories with cumulative indexing systems obtained from a full electronic medical record with access to authorized people [12]. The EMR is created through contributions from different health system authorities that have intervened during the care path and adopted the approach through processes to represent and share information [13]. This information can be shared across the continuum of healthcare services (Fig. 1) and the patient's progress can be followed in the various care settings [14]. A structured data approach that incorporates formatting for patient data (personal record), provenance

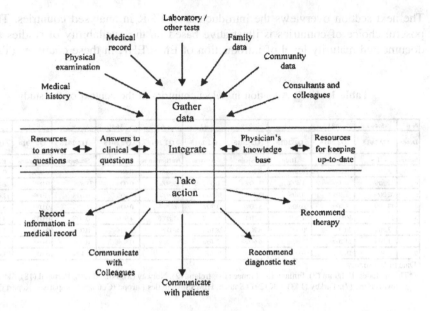

Fig. 1. The basis of value co-creation– A flow of information in primary care practice - Source: Bates D. et al. [14]

data for traceability (organization information), and a care record summary for the clinical data [15].

The main characteristics of the EHR [12] are: (1) the ability to enter and manage information about the health condition of patients in real time in order to develop their case history; adopting the EMR as the first point of reference to support the patients' care path; (2) A qualitative improvement in health services resulting from knowledge of data about past medical treatments; (3) Continuously redefining the use of resources and planning of health services; and (4) Possibility of investigating the population's health condition and promoting initiatives for public health protection.

Further studies show measurable benefits emerging from the adoption of EHR in the form of efficiency and effectiveness of care [1], patient safety [16], preventive care [17], and provider satisfaction specific to enhanced decision making capabilities [18], these benefits are often designated as measurement of value in the healthcare context [19]. The literature points out that the "human element" is critical to health IT implementation [20]. The interactions in clinic operations and physicians produce outcomes to patients and care providers leading to competitive advantages in the healthcare environment [21]. Further, the rate of adoption of EHR systems is an important indicator of the degree of national e-health. EHR adoption is faced with the perceived usefulness of EHR systems for executive decision makers [22] and the reluctance of medical practitioners based on the perceived interference with the prescriber–patient relationship [4, 23]. The literature on EHR introduction and adoption is copious in the context of NA, NE, and the UK. It also seems that practitioners have focused on the same global footprints for the mapping of the maturity of adoption of electronic medical.

The next section overviews the introduction of EHR in analysed countries. The purposeful choice of countries is illustrative based on the availability of studies and the documented maturity level of introduction of EMR/EHR in these countries (Table 1).

Table 1. EMR Adoption in Select countries in the context of the study

N =	5,464	641	211	229	42	63	164	9	24	1,321
Date*	Q2 2015	Q2 2015	Q2 2015	Q2 2015	Q2 2015	Q2 2015	Q2 2015	Q2 2015	Q2 2014	Q2 2014
Stage	US	Canada	Italy	Spain	Austria	Netherlands	Germany	Singapore	Denmark	Europe**
7	3.70%	0.20%	0.00%	0.40%	0.00%	0.00%	0.60%	0.00%	0.00%	0.20%
6	22.20%	0.90%	1.40%	3.90%	0.00%	9.50%	0.00%	77.80%	0.00%	2.60%
5	32.20%	1.10%	19.40%	42.40%	38.10%	11.60%	19.40%	0.00%	100%	17.00%
4	13.20%	3.40%	0.90%	5.20%	3.20%	6.70%	0.90%	11.10%	0.00%	5.60%
3	18.20%	30.90%	4.70%	1.70%	0.00%	1.60%	4.90%	0.00%	0.00%	3.70%
2	3.80%	30.70%	40.30%	26.20%	38.10%	46.00%	23.80%	0.00%	0.00%	33.40%
1	1.90%	14.20%	22.30%	6.60%	2.40%	1.60%	0.60%	0.00%	0.00%	13.80%
0	3.30%	18.60%	10.90%	13.50%	21.40%	0.00%	51.80%	11.10%	0.00%	23.80%

*Date of last survey
**This includes: Belgium (2), Finland (3), France (18), Ireland (2), Norway (3), Poland (20), Portugal (18), Slovenia (2), Switzerland (7), Turkey (143), UK (29) - Source: HIMSS Analytics Europe (Country Comparison Report Q2/2014)

2.2   The European Context

There are many differences concerning the introduction of the EHR and its implementation across the various countries such as timetable, mode of operations and procedures that require standardization and the aim of the European program is to establish common guidelines for implementing specific systems for administrative information [23]. Other research agree on a long list of barriers for adopting EHRs by physicians; namely time, cost, computer literacy, workflow disruption, interaction, data accuracy, reliability, patient acceptance, etc. [24].

Denmark is the new European leader in EHR/EMR adoption [25]. In mid-2014, a survey conducted in 24 hospitals found that 92 % of Denmark hospitals capture and evaluate system usage statistics to influence user behaviour and system enhancements, 96 % of hospital are entering 90 % of their orders electronically, and 100 % of hospitals indicate their imaging departments are fully automated. Still 75 % indicated they do not have clinical decision support present during physician documentation; 41.2 % stated that they are not providing clinical guidelines and pathways for nurses and physicians; and less than 40 % are checking for duplicate orders in medication administration; showing some advancements opportunity in closed loop medication administration, a key element of patient safety improvement.

In Denmark, Finland and Sweden, state governments matched investments made for information technologies in healthcare. Patient privacy is therefore one of the key factors; the information system must share information safely and ensure that it reaches the right people. A portal, "Sundhed" (Danish Ministry of Health) provides access to health information and uses a system of engineering controls, such as encryption, electronic identification and control registers.

The Finnish health care system is diversified; it uses inputs from several sources to support services and medical care [26]. Semantically interoperable infrastructures (such as HL7) enable users to send, access and use the data contained in the national archive, through EHR systems, pharmaceutical or online portals.

Sweden uses a decentralized health system; both central and local government authorities are responsible for most of the costs incurred at national level [27]. Regulatory changes promoted the construction of user-friendly systems, to support decision-making by supplying and sharing the required documents with other systems used by municipalities, regions or individuals Testo.

In 2010 the Italian Ministry of Health established the EHR guidelines aimed at implementing their use and aligning the Italian context with the international scenario. Italy is one of the countries, which invests less in healthcare. This situation contributes to the explosion of a lot of isolated investment, which is not integrated in a national system and is not sufficient to guide development [28].

In 1997, the British government began transforming the National Health Service (NHS) in England with the aim of creating a "person-based" health care system with the citizen as an actor in the treatment decision-making process [29]. In England, the implementation boasts a two level system: the Summary Care Record (SCR) covering the country and a Detailed Care Record (DCR). Among the obstacles reported are in the need for structural changes at organizational level and the lack of time and the human resources required for patient care [30] and practitioners acceptance of the new tool sometimes shown related to their age [31].

Greeks have implemented four regional health information networks (RHINs) in four regional health authorities (RHAs) [32]. EMR system implementations have not progressed as expected. Open Source based implementation is prevalent in this context, which could explain their slow adoption [33]. Documented issues are technical related to platforms and infrastructure, management issues regarding implementation and planning, and socio-organizational issues. Without formalization of the introduction process, which involves defining a policy and standards framework that can integrate public and private, local and central systems, the adoption of electronic medical records would not become part of the Greek national health system. The case in Spain is similar, different EHRs exist in each of the Spanish regions. The need for interoperability between different systems has become a major concern [34]. This might explain that, even though almost half (42.4 %) of Spanish hospitals have deployed a full complement of radiology PACS systems, only a small fraction (3.9 %) has incorporated complete physician documentation with structured templates and discrete data.

2.3   The Situation in USA and Canada

Healthcare is one of the largest segments of the US economy, approaching 20 % of GDP. Federal law requires all health insurance companies and health care providers to use EHRs by 2015. President Obama signed the Affordable Care Act, then on June 2012 the Supreme Court rendered a final decision to uphold the health care law. In addition to improving quality, safety and efficiency of healthcare, the legislation provided guidelines for complying with "Meaningful use" which is expected to lead to maintaining privacy and security of patient health information, better clinical outcomes, and more robust research data on health systems.

The privacy laws typically consist of technical controls, a written information security plan, and breach notification protocols. Particularly, EHR data is to be represented as discrete data elements (atomic data) with associated metadata, separating chart (data dissociated from the patient) and record data (patient data) for additional privacy, acknowledging the need to support clinical trials and clinical research while protecting patient privacy. US providers were found more likely to access EHR based information for higher-risk patients than for those who received less frequent care. Partial implementations of EHR functions such as closed loop medication administration (71.3 % of US hospitals) have proven the most significant progress. However, only 3.7 % of hospitals have reached full EMR implementations with cumulative capabilities supporting continuity of care data transactions across emergency, ambulatory, and paediatrics. KP hospitals are in the lead.

The 30.9 % of EMR implementations in Canada are at an early stage of maturity (Stage 3), with implementations covering main functions such as nursing, pharmacy, laboratory, and radiology with partial integration clinical data repository that provides physician access for reviewing all orders and results. In contrast, the US counterparts moved into stages 5 (32.2 %) and 6 (22.2 %) with a closed loop medication administration and complete physician documentation relying on clinical decision support a full imaging. In Canada, healthcare is organized at the provincial level and therefore each province has its own EMR adoption program and policies [35].

Obstacles to deployment of EMRs in hospitals setting are more complex as they include external and internal parameters such as structure, culture, resources, capabilities, stakeholders and politics of the hospital [36].

3   Our Contribution and Research Method

A patient in Europe is an actor in the healthcare system, while in North America is a private customer. Therefore, we are well aware that clinical data exchange is different in both contexts. However, we believe that none of those differences are relevant.

According to Zakaria's et al. [37], the best-fit research model that can be used in order to understand the value of EMR would be through the evaluation of the three categories of service science (i.e. organizational, human/people, and technical/technological challenges). Regardless of the patients' role, the challenges to the introduction of EHR turn out to be the same. Also the benefits attend for doctor and patient are similar. Therefore, this paper tries to understand if a service science approach might facilitate the introduction (or increasing the development) of EHR. In order to analyse these concepts, it is used a case study "Kaiser Permanente". We have chosen this case for two main reasons. First of all, KP represents an important case for the EHR usage with an integrated patient health record portal, clinical transaction records, workflow, and account management. Secondly, we have had a particular access to the data (phenomenon), "an unusual access through friends" [38].

Moreover, we try to understand if and how service science can help diffusion of EHR in different countries. The literature review was enriched using practitioner references that include survey data from HIMMS Analytics (see Appendix). Data collection for the case study is conducted from archival data and publications drawing secondary data (2010–2013), architectural documentation, internal publications, and a review of KP Health Connect implementation documentation and the KP.org portal.

4   Case Study on Kaiser Permanente

Founded in 1945, Kaiser Permanente is a not-profit health care organization head-quartered in Oakland (California). With a vision of a "Real-time, Personalized Health Care", KP began offering online health services in 1996. Kaiser's business model is a closed network model of insurance, hospitals, pharmacies and health professionals (Table 2). The deployment of KP's EHR, *KP HealthConnect* ™, began in 2004 and cost about $4B to complete. It serves 9.6 million members in nine states. Nationwide, KP employs approximately 177,445 technical, administrative, and clerical staff 17,791 physicians 49,778 nurses and 14,000 physicians representing all specialties. KP is now building new hospitals without medical record storage areas.

Table 2. Kaiser Permanente 2014 - Online vs. on facilities based services (Source: KP Annual Report 2014)

Facilities:	
38 hospitals 608 medical offices and other facilities (659 total)	
Financials:	
$56.4B operating revenue	
$2.2B operating income	
$3.1B net income	
Facilities based services	**Online services (kp.org)**
98,000 babies delivered	*4.89 M members on My Health Manager*
224,943 inpatient surgeries	*37.4 M lab test results viewed*
40.2 M doctor office visits	*20 M secure emails sent*
1 M mammograms	*4.1 M appointments requests*
1.7 M colon cancer screenings	*17.5 M prescription filled*
74 M prescription filled	*1.3 M Mobile App download*
Benefits	
95 % reduction in dictation costs	
$1.4 M cost reduction on printed forms	
54 % reduction of archival storage space.	
2 day test results to patients	
57 % reduced medication errors	
12 % outpatient lab utilization	
4000+ Ongoing research / 1300+ Articles published	

The blended modalities of care between online services (kp.org) and facilities based services have enriched the services provided by this national provider. KP has reported benefits of its EHR implementation in form of cost reduction, reduced medication errors, and improved service to patients, members and research. The Web site's health information and related tools are free and available to the public. However, sign-on is required for members to access secure portions of the site, such as appointment scheduling or ordering prescription refills. My Health Manager, KP's personal health records (PHR), was fully deployed in 2007 and is linked to the EHR with 4.89 million registered members.

5   Discussion

5.1   EHR Value Co-creation in the Lens of Service Science

The key to service science is a focus on all aspect of the service as a system of interacting parts that include people (organizational), technology, and business. The review of the adoption maturity and challenges in this study helps focus the paper on the obstacles observed in the implementation of EHR.

The review in Sect. 2 reflects concepts of organizational dynamics (People) in the introduction of health services based on the use of EHR. Among the obstacles reported are in the need for structural changes at organizational level and the lack of time and the human resources required for patient care and practitioner's acceptance of the new tool sometimes shown related to their age. The required changes to interactions with patients that have now become actors in the treatment decision making process are complicated by the need to change practice style. This eventually raises systemic concerns about impacts on medical education and training and about the effects of health IT tools introduction on clinical care. On the other hand, focusing on the technology usability of intuitive system, with little training requirement is seen as critical to integrating clinical processes and encouraging adoption. The use of portals provides transparent patient access to health information and uses a system of engineering controls, such as encryption, electronic identification and control registers, in order to ensure privacy and the security of personal medical information.

The role of government through regulatory changes in the US helped promote the construction of user-friendly systems. Significant legislation on the architectural foundations with technical controls for encryption, access, patient privacy and data accuracy, through standards of semantic interoperability. Other obstacles to implementations were seen in the form of overambitious objectives of the project and some critical delays encouraging the UK authorities to phase the introduction into a federated approach to diffusion. State governmental influence is also reported through matched investments made for information technologies in healthcare in the countries of NE, state governments as opposed to the Italian government's lack of funding support causing non-uniform implementation strategies. And finally, while the US EMR introductions receive extensive Federal legislation support, Canada's central government focuses on strategies and expectations of improvements in efficiency and quality of care, leaving the governance of EMR programs and adoption policies at the provincial level.

5.2   Case Organizational Alignment

Kaiser Permanente's experience in EHR implementation was not without complexity. The delivery of healthcare involves many organizational units including hospitals, physicians' private practices, pharmacies, laboratories, etc. whilst none of these uniquely represent the boundary within within which value is truly created. Changes in work processes, organizational structures, and attitudes are required in the realizing the value from electronic health records implementations. A large portion of the costs incurred in deploying the KP system was attributable to training and workflow re-design of involved practitioners. The workflow is now standardized however, individual physicians still have considerable freedom in when and how they do things, such as reviewing available lab results and completing their charts. This freedom positively affects healthcare professionals EMR continuance behaviour. A study performed at the early stages of the implementation at KP indicated that a transient climate of conflict was associated with adoption of the system. Leadership, culture, and professional ideals played complex roles, each facilitating and hindering implementation at various points. Nevertheless, challenges in implementing an electronic health record range from selecting and testing an EHR system [13] to shifting in roles and responsibilities of the care provider. Clinicians participated in the decision-making process and collaborated with hundreds of stakeholders and IT experts worked to build the system requirements during the time span of the project; working groups were formed to address practices, standards, and modalities of care, then translated them into features in the system. This collaborative approach is a known critical factor in the success of EHR adoption.

5.3 Case Technology Enabled Capabilities

For the stakeholders at KP, the successful implementation of an EMR is likely with an intuitive system, with little training requirement, integrating clinical processes but allowing flexibility where clinicians are involved in selection and in modification in alignment with their department needs and the change capabilities of their team. KP developed standards of semantic interoperability for the disambiguation of data. The pervasiveness of the interoperability concept is necessary for data quality and error reduction [4]. To that effect HL7 specifies the structure and semantics of "clinical documents" for the purpose of quality data exchange.

In other EHR implemented in US, it is possible to note that EHR distracts the patient to doctor encounter, due to the extended time spent on the computer screen, especially in fixed computers setup. KP has deployed mobile computer carts that allow doctors to maintain their patient contact. Physicians and nurses are encouraged to use the system in front of the patient that can check this process.

5.4 Value Co-creation Through a Public Portal

In healthcare, value is co-created with patient participation. Potentially through patient's contribution to data diaries that could be useful in the treatment of the case at hand and a reference for other similar cases. The interactions between provider and patient are in the centre of Healthcare value co-creation, where the contribution from either side of the service chain is essential to the positive outcome of healthcare.

As an extension to the EMR system, KP accredits the web based EHR system for its patient facing access; a portal (Fig. 2) through which patients can enrol in the service online, complete surveys, review their lab tests and receive recommendations from their primary care physicians for continuity of care [10]. Powered by a secure patient-provider messaging available through a member Web site that also provides personal health records (4.89 million users); and an electronic inter-provider messaging (20 + million secure emails) about care that is automatically incorporated into patients' records. The importance of the process changes required yielding efficiencies for the healthcare team, with a reduction in number of clinic visits resulting in *"effectiveness of care"* benefits to the patient. Members, who are also KP's health Insurance Plan subscribers, can use KP provided tools to manage their health benefits, including estimating the cost of treatments and viewing medication formularies. KP members and the public may view health and drug encyclopaedia, take a health assessment, get information about popular health topics, and use health calculators (1.3 million users downloaded KP app). With a bilingual interface this online personal health record includes a patient health record with comprehensive documentation across care settings —inpatient and outpatient, clinical decision support, and complete, real-time connectivity to lab, pharmacy, radiology, and other ancillary systems. Blending traditional office visits with this modality of care has proven effective for this nationwide provider. The decrease in office visits in favour of scheduled telephone visits and secure e-mail messaging created operational efficiencies by offering non-traditional, patient-centered ways of providing care.

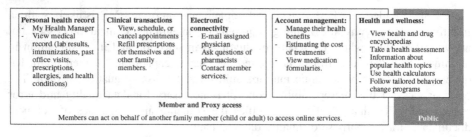

Fig. 2. Representation by the author from information in Silvestre et al. 2009 [10]

6   Conclusion

EHRs have existed for more than a decade. With the advent of EHR, e-health has an opportunity to become more widely available for providers and health care managers to broaden its potential use beyond individual patient care. Thus, the digitized healthcare IT ecosystem is comprised of many entities, all of which interact with the patient, including pharmacies, clinicians, insurance, laboratories, etc. These entities need to be connected to a secure IT infrastructure that provides technical and semantic interoperability and guarantees trust across healthcare environments. As healthcare data is stored, accessed and transferred in the healthcare ecosystem, it is necessary to track its provenance. The interaction between doctor and patient co-creates value not so much for knowledge supporting patient diagnosis (which could also be negative) than overall for Government research use. In fact, Government entities are holding a series of data that help patients to better understand the effectiveness of government expenditure and of cures. Moreover, the presence of a public portal as in the case of some implementations in Europe and NA encourages citizens to participate in the decision system and the data enrichment.

KP offers insight into practices used to improve the introduction of EHR. Looking through the lens of service science, the value realization from the EHR was dependent on a collaborative organizational dynamic, a purpose-built technical infrastructure and data rich source for research. Organizational alignment including the changes required to fully exploit the new system in the interaction among care practitioners and between care provider and their patients. Technology enabled capabilities powered by service oriented architecture ensured a platform for quality in data essential for the quality of health care. Kaiser's public portal accumulates patient data in an online record. This health-IT ecosystem offers secure member access to their information, an option for proxy access for family members and a public portal for community health management as in the case of Kaiser Permanente's implementation. Patients could contribute to their own wellbeing and health maintenance with a direct and secure interaction with their physician and care records. This new evolution of consumer-centric "defined-contribution" health-care reform is in giving patients access to their records assuming more responsibility for selecting and managing their own health-care benefits. In a look at the future, a vision of consumers in control of their information through Consumer Health Informatics is paving the way for fully transparent health records. These building blocks would facilitate the use of applications in a patient-centered medical home, patient decision aids and personal health management tools, and patient self-serve kiosks.

The vision for a Health IT ecosystem, projects the ability to use the atomic data (raw clinical data that is detached from patient information) as both analysis of aggregated data matched with local data at the point of care through targeted clinical decision support. The use of atomic data would assist practitioners in diagnosis, fuel big data analytics tools for clinical research and evidence-based data for policy governance of general public health. EHR implementations present considerable benefits, but not without significant challenges. Challenges persist on the ability to deploy a universal system where independent care providers could contribute and share patient records. Such challenges could be concerned with technical, adoption, security, and privacy concerns. At the moment our description is based on an instrumental study, used to understand more of what is obvious to the observer, using archival documents and data for a descriptive analysis. We are aware that the path is at the beginning that cultural differences are many between states more between continents but we think it would be interesting to study with qualitative research implementing the use of EHR through a public portal of this kind.

Appendix

See Tables 3 and 4.

Table 3. HIMSS Analytics EMR Adoption Model

Stage	Description
7	The hospital is paperless in delivering and managing patient care (discrete data, document and medical images). Data warehousing is being used to analyze patterns of clinical data to improve quality of care and patient safety and care delivery efficiency. Clinical information can be readily shared via standardized electronic transactions (i.e. CCD) with all entities that are authorized to treat the patient, or a health information exchange
6	Full physician documentation with structured templates and discrete data. Closed loop medication administration with bar coded unit dose medications environment is fully implemented. The Electronic medication administration record (eMAR) and bar coding or other auto identification technology (e.g. RFID) integrated with CPOE and pharmacy.
5	A full complement of radiology PACS systems provides medical images to physicians via an intranet and displaces all film-based images.
4	Computerized Practitioner Order Entry (CPOE) for use by any clinician licensed to create orders - a second level of clinical decision support capabilities related to evidence based medicine protocols.
3	Nursing/clinical documentation (e.g. vital signs, flow sheets, nursing notes, etc.) is implemented and integrated with the CDR for at least one inpatient service in the hospital.
2	Major ancillary clinical systems feed data to a clinical data repository (CDR) that provides physician access for reviewing all orders and results.
1	All three major ancillary clinical systems are installed (i.e., pharmacy, laboratory, and radiology).
0	The organization has not installed all of the three key ancillary department systems (laboratory, pharmacy, and radiology).

Table 4. EMR adoption in US Ambulatory EMR (outpatient & provider care)

Stage	Description	N = 34,115
7	HIE capable, sharing of data between the EMR and community based EHR, business and clinical intelligence	7.40%
6	Advanced clinical decision support, proactive care management, structured messaging	9.17%
5	Personal health record, online tethered patient portal	7.93%
4	CPOE, Use of structured data for accessibility in EMR and internal and external sharing of data	0.99%
3	Electronic messaging, computers have replaced the paper chart, clinical documentation and clinical decision support	12.03%
2	Beginning of a CDR with orders and results, computers may be at point-of-care, access to results from outside facilities	26.68%
1	Desktop access to clinical information, unstructured data, multiple data sources, intra-office/informal messaging	33.98%
0	Paper chart based	3.82%

References

1. Jha, A.K., Desroches, C.M., Campbell, E.G., Donelan, K., Rao, S.R., Ferris, T.G., Shields, A., Rosenbaum, S., Blumenthal, D.: Use of electronic health records in U.S. hospitals. N. Engl. J. Med. **360**(16), 1628–1638 (2009)
2. Panir, J.H.: Role of ICTs in the health sector in developing countries: a critical review of literature. J. Health Inf. Dev. Countries **5**(1), 197–208 (2011)
3. Cohen, B.C.: Press and Foreign Policy. Princeton University Press, NJ (2015)
4. Bonomi, S., Zardini, A., Rossignoli, C., Dameri, P.R.: E-Health and value Co-creation: The case of electronic medical record in an Italian academic integrated hospital. In: Nóvoa, H., Drăgoicea, M. (eds.) IESS 2015. LNBIP, vol. 201, pp. 166–175. Springer, Heidelberg (2015)
5. Spohrer, J., Maglio, P.P.: Toward a science of service systems - value and symbols. In: Maglio, P.P., Kielszewski, C.A., Spohrer, J.C. (eds.) Handbook of Service Science, pp. 157–193. Springer, Heidelberg (2010)
6. Maglio, P.P., Spohrer, J.: Fundamentals of service science. J. Acad. Mark. Sci. **36**(1), 18–20 (2008)
7. Spohrer, J., Kwan, S.K.: Service science, management, engineering, and design (SSMED): An emerging discipline - outline and references. Int. J. Inf. Syst. Serv. Sect. **1**(3), 1–31 (2009)
8. Dragoicea, M., Borangiu, T.: A service science knowledge environment in the cloud. In: Borangiu, T., Thomas, A., Trentesaux, D. (eds.) Service Orientation in Holonic and Multi Agent. SCI, vol. 472, pp. 229–246. Springer, Heidelberg (2013)
9. Vargo, S.L., Maglio, P.P., Akaka, M.A.: On value and value co-creation: A service systems and service logic perspective. Eur. Manag. J. **26**(3), 145–152 (2008)
10. Silvestre, A., Sue, V.M., Allen, J.Y.: If you build it, will they come? the kaiser permanente model of online health care. Health Aff. **28**(2), 334–344 (2009)
11. Hersh, W.R.: The electronic medical record: Promises and problems. J. Am. Soc. Inform. Sci. **46**(10), 772–776 (1995)
12. Health Level Seven International. Introduction to Health Level Seven (2013). https://www.hl7.org/permalink/?HL7OrgAndProcessPresentation
13. Hayrinen, K.: Definition, structure, content, use and impacts of electronic health records: A review of the research literature. Int. J. Med. Inform. **77**(3), 291–304 (2008)
14. Bates, D.W., Gawande, A.A.: Improving safety with information technology. N. Engl. J. Med. **348**(25), 2526–2534 (2003)
15. Garde, S., Knaup, P., Hovenga, E., Heard, S.: Towards semantic interoperability for electronic health records. Methods Inf. Med. **46**, 332–343 (2007)
16. Sittig, D.F., Singh, H.: Electronic health records and national patient-safety goals. N. Engl. J. Med. **367**(19), 1854–1860 (2012)
17. Buntin, M.B., Burke, M.F., Hoaglin, M.C., Blumenthal, D.: The benefits of health information technology: a review of the recent literature shows predominantly positive. Results Health Aff. **30**(3), 464–471 (2011)
18. Penoyer, D.A., Cortelyou-Ward, K.H., Noblin, A.M., Bullard, T., Talbert, S., Wilson, J., Schafhauser, B., Briscoe, J.G.: Use of electronic health record documentation by healthcare workers in an acute care hospital system. J. Healthc. Manag. **59**(2), 130–144 (2014)
19. Porter, M.E.: What is value in health care? N. Engl. J. Med. **363**(26), 2477–2481 (2010)
20. Øvreitveit, J., Scott, T., Rundall, T.G., Shortell, S.M., Brommels, M.: Improving quality through effective implementation of information technology in healthcare. Int. J. Qual. Health Care **19**(5), 259–266 (2007)

21. Richards, R.J., Prybutok, V.R., Ryan, S.D.: Electronic medical records: tools for competitive advantage. Int. J. Qual. Serv. Sci. **4**(2), 120–136 (2012)
22. Hikmet, N., Banerjee, S., Burns, M.B.: State of content: healthcare executive's role in information technology adoption. J. Serv. Sci. Manage. **5**(2), 124–131 (2012)
23. Rossignoli, C., Zardini, A., Benetollo, P.: The process of digitalization in radiology as a lever for organizational change: the case of the Academic Integrated Hospital of Verona. In: Phillips-Wren, G, Carlsson S., Respicio, A., Brezillon, P. (eds.) DSS 2.0-Supporting Decision Making With New Technologies, vol. 261, pp. 24–35 (2014)
24. McGinn, C.A., Grenier, S., Duplantie, J., Shaw, N., Sicotte, C., Mathieu, L., Leduc, Y., Legare, F., Gagnon, M.P.: Comparison of user groups' perspectives of barriers and facilitators to implementing electronic health records: a systematic review. BMC Med. **9**(1), 1–15 (2011)
25. Kierkegaard, P.: eHealth in Denmark: A Case Study. J. Med. Syst. **37**(6), 1–10 (2013)
26. Häyrinen, K., Saranto, K.: The core data elements of electronic health record in Finland. Stud. Health Technol. Inform. **116**, 131–136 (2005)
27. Doupi, P., Renko, E., Geist, S., Heywood, J., Dumortier, J.: Country Brief: Sweden. European commissions (2010)
28. Del Bufalo, P.: Il risparmio si fa investendo. (Saving is done by investments) Il Sole 24 Ore (2012). http://www.consorzioarsenal.it/c/document_library/get_file
29. Pelzang, R.: Time to learn: understanding patient-cantered care. Br. J. Nurs. **19**(14), 912–917 (2010)
30. Bonomi, S.: The electronic health record: a comparison of some European countries. In: Ricciardi, F., Harfouche, A. (eds.) Information and Communication Technologies in Organizations and Society. LNISO, vol. 15, pp. 35–50. Springer, Heidelberg (2016)
31. Cresswell, K.: Implementing and adopting electronic health record systems. How actor-network theory can support evaluation. Br. J. Clin. Gov. **16**(4), 320–336 (2011)
32. Katehakis, D., Halkiotis, S., Kouroubali, A.: Materialization of regional health information networks in greece: electronic health record barriers and enablers. J. Healthc. Eng. **2**(3), 389–404 (2011)
33. Maglogiannis, I.: Towards the adoption of open source and open access electronic health record systems. J. Healthc. Eng. **3**(1), 141–162 (2012)
34. de la Torre, I., Gonzales, S., Lopez-Coronado M.: Analysis of the EHR systems in Spanish primary public health system: the lack of interoperability. J. Med. Syst. **36**(5), 3273–3281 (2012)
35. Halas, G., Singer, A., Styles, C., Katz, A.: New conceptual model of EMR implementation in interprofessional academic family medicine clinics. Can. Fam. Physician J. **61**(5), 232–239 (2015)
36. Boonstra, A., Versluis, A., Vos, J.F.J.: Implementing electronic health records in hospitals: a systematic literature review. BMC Health Serv. Res. **14**(3), 14–37 (2014)
37. Zakaria, N., Affendi, M., Yusof, S., Zakaria, N.: Managing ICT in healthcare organization: culture, challenges, and issues of technology adoption and implementation. In: Zakaria N., Affendi, S. (eds.) Managing ICT in Healthcare Organization: Culture, Challenges, and Issues of Technology Adoption and Implementation, pp. 153–168. IGI Global (2010)
38. Eisenhardt, K.M., Graebner, M.E.: Theory building from cases: opportunities and challenges. Acad. Manag. J. **50**(1), 25–32 (2007)

Health Care Co-production: Co-creation of Value in Flexible Boundary Spheres

Maddalena Sorrentino[1](✉), Marco De Marco[2], and Cecilia Rossignoli[3]

[1] Department of Economics, Management and Quantitative Methods,
Università degli Studi di Milano, Milan, Italy
maddalena.sorrentino@unimi.it
[2] Nettuno University, Rome, Italy
marco.demarco@uninettunouniversity.net
[3] Università degli Studi di Verona, Verona, Italy
cecilia.rossignoli@univr.it

Abstract. Mounting pressure on governments to understand how well they can promote the health of their population is forcing national health systems to reconfigure their service delivery processes. The latest piece in the organisational puzzle is co-production: a concept that co-opts patients and informal caregivers in the self-management, realization and delivery of specific health care processes. Service management principles, especially those of value creation and co-production, acknowledge the need to engage the user and their personal network in a joint production effort. The paper supports this timely claim using the Outpatient Parenteral Antibiotic Therapy (or OPAT) illustrative case study to show how the concept of customer value-in-exchange and value-in-use applied to the successful health care co-production practice necessarily casts the patients and their informal caregivers as co-creators of value. From the theoretical perspective, the study shows how the provider sphere is not a closed dimension that limits itself to offering a value proposition. The study underlines the need for management to pay greater attention to the informal caregivers, given that these actors need to be orchestrated and that their role is set to become even more pivotal.

Keywords: Value · Co-creation · Service-dominant logic · Co-production · Public sector organizations · Healthcare · Home therapy · Informal caregivers

1 Introduction

Public management research is reaching agreement that the time is ripe to take a public service-dominant approach to both the discourse and the practice of innovation in the delivery of citizen services, ditching the transactional approach that has predominated up to now [1]. This is the thinking from which the paper takes its cue to make the central argument that service science and public management share many unharvested contact points, setting aside the differences between public and private organizations that prevent the transfer of *tout court* business practices to the public sector [2]. A particularly insightful work by Grönroos and Voima mines precisely the value creation concept to extract the

© Springer International Publishing Switzerland 2016
T. Borangiu et al. (Eds.): IESS 2016, LNBIP 247, pp. 649–659, 2016.
DOI: 10.1007/978-3-319-32689-4_49

opportunities offered by a 'cross-cutting phenomenon' [3] such as co-production in the context of a public service delivery [4].

Co-production is when a public service organization (PSO) expands its in-house production boundaries to jointly produce services with external entities, partnering with other public organizations, third sector, service users [5]. Co-production is a logical step taken by many kinds of public services [6], particularly in the health care sector which most OECD countries rate high priority [7, 8]. In many countries co-production is the flagbearer of an authentic paradigm shift especially to treat long-term conditions [8]. This means that the service must satisfy "the needs of current providers and recipients to engage in mutual value co-creation without decreasing the quality of future value co-creation" [9: 1209] - and encourage "ongoing and patient-tailored care" [10: 1450], taking into account that this personalisation requires "suppliers to have a complex strategic vision of customer's value in use" [11: 927].

Despite the scholars' valuable efforts, the challenge posed by the multi-dimensional nature of co-production within complex public service systems recently brought the research to a standstill as the sum of the parts is not adding up to a consummate whole. Most service management research has barely glanced at social and public services [9], which is surprising given the discipline's long intellectual history in the concepts of co-production, value-in-exchange and value-in-use. Academia has written much about the potential of the co-delivery of healthcare services, e.g., peer support groups, nurse-family partnerships [12: 39]. Nevertheless, this body of research seems to only skim the surface, going no further than the initial goal to optimise health outcomes. What does it mean – in terms of value creation - to embrace co-production integrating the provider's resources with those of the user instead of the mere "add-in" of new tasks to the PSO's organizational system? Which service provision phases generate true value for the service recipients?

These are tough questions to answer and the first logical step on this research path is to draw a timely, more complete picture by integrating the different views. The purpose of this qualitative paper is to build upon recent developments in the public management and service literatures to better understand health care co-production efforts. To usefully contribute to the ongoing debate on the OECD-wide shift towards the so-called New Public Governance (NPG) [13], the paper extends the Gronroos and Voima framework [4], highlighting how the informal caregivers involved in the home production of health care work alongside the PSO to create potential value for the patient-user.

To organize our discussion, the paper is split into six sections. After the introduction Sect. 2 discusses public services, co-production and value formation, from the managerial and the service science perspectives. Section 3 illustrates the chosen research method of a 'most-likely' case design, using a number of international studies as the empirical base. Section 4 analyses the provider, joint and customer spheres of the value-creation processes as applied to the Outpatient Parenteral Antibiotic Therapy (or OPAT). Section 5 discusses the findings. Section 6 sets out the implications and conclusions.

2   Public Services, Co-production and Value Formation

The theoretical roots of co-production are embedded in various traditions [3]. In the public management literature, Osborne and colleagues [1, 14] were among the first to notice that the growing fragmentation of society and citizen needs [1: 424] makes it paramount for PSOs to regain their service orientation and to take a public-service-dominant approach.

Recognising the inter-organisational dimension of public service delivery, the authors also seek to push past what has been defined as a "current short-term, transactional and product-oriented focus" [15]. Osborne and colleagues support their reasoning by pointing to the fundamentals of service theory and offer a conceptual model (called SERVICE framework) which incorporates co-production as an "inalienable element".

The SERVICE framework – like the concept of "service system" developed eight years earlier by Maglio and Spohrer [16] - assumes that the PSO can house diverse "configurations of people, technologies and additional resources" [17]. In the presence of multiple variables, the value that the providers and receivers create together (co-creating and re-creating) can vary considerably from one situation to the next. In addition, SERVICE emphasizes the need for the public providers to focus on external value creation and not just internal efficiency [1: 424]. Health care is highly cited as an example to show how the decision to put the patient at the centre (service user) of the clinical decision-making and service delivery effort not only raises patient service experience quality, but also the clinical outcomes [14]. Equally valid examples of how the PSOs "offer a service promise of what is to be delivered" can be found in diverse sectors: from social work to education, from community development to refuse collection (ibidem).

Exploring the nature of value creation in public services from the managerial perspective led Bovaird and Loeffler [12: 40] to propose a reworking of the value chain analysis of Porter [18]. The authors make a distinction between 'primary' and 'support' activities in the PSO production processes, where the former are performed sequentially in order to make the service available, and the latter sustain the appropriate performance of the primary activities. The new model offers an original approach on at least two counts. First, all the activities performed by the PSO are seen to be potentially co-produced by users and their community. Second, the value chain of a PSO is embedded within a wider "value system" consisting of both its 'upstream' supply chain of activities and its "downstream" customer value chain. For example, when the health care users use telecare systems or self-administer their drugs, these customer value chains can generate further value added for other citizens, such as informal caregivers, i.e., the family members and friends who provide care [19], and; for other users who can use the example to learn how to make better use of the service; for other individuals indirectly affected. In other words, any link in the co-production value chain can generate additional value and that it is entwined with the user value. However, the users are not motivated to co-produce merely by self-interest, but also because they are convinced it is an opportunity to "increase other elements of value", including social inclusion and/or community cohesion [12: 43-44].

The service literature treats the concept of co-production as being subordinate to that of value creation [20]. The latter takes place in the usage/consumption stage; the former may take place within the production process which precedes the usage stage (ibidem, p. 98).

Recent work by Grönroos and Voima [4] has conceptually unbundled the value creation processes in the services sector, identifying three separate spheres: the *provider sphere*, the only value facilitator (in which the supplier delivers the resources and organizational capabilities to be used by users-consumers to self-create value); the *joint sphere* (which sees supplier and customer get together to co-produce the service and co-create value); and the *customer sphere* (in which the customer is an independent value creator). Informed by a customer-grounded view, the authors focus on the inherent dynamicity of the size of the value spheres: for example, when the PSO invites the customer to join as a co-producer at different points of the production process, the service user crosses the boundary into the provider sphere [4: 141]. Conversely, the PSO can set up a call centre to encourage dialogue with users. In such situations, the provider and the customer spheres move closer to thus increase the potential value for the customer.

Grönroos and Voima observe that the dyadic interaction in the joint sphere can generate positive, negative or neutral impacts on the value creation process, which is influenced by the many satellites that orbit the sphere of the provider's jurisdiction but over which it has no sway [4]. The health care services delivered to chronically ill patients are a clear example of such an ecosystem. In fact, Sharma and colleagues [21: 23] claim that people with long-term conditions (LTC) are likely to have many contacts with various clinicians and health professionals in other services as they face different LTC-related choices and challenges over many years. The care setting of the chronically ill depends increasingly on informal caregivers who behave like formal care providers and medical personnel [7, 19].

In a nutshell, the value creation and co-creation processes occur in 'different spatial and temporal settings' [4] which emphasize the patient's experiences and logic. By interacting with the PSO and third parties, the customers co-create value [22]. Therefore, to fully grasp how the value creation processes unfold it is essential to analyse the shift in its real-life conditions, a factor that the next sections explore in more depth.

3   Research Approach

The present work aggregates a number of recent peer-reviewed studies of a widely adopted co-production clinical practice called Outpatient Parental Antibiotic Therapy (OPAT), which enables eligible patients to leave the clinical setting to administer their antibiotic treatment at home and participate in the care process. OPAT has been chosen as an illustrative example of a value-generating process for health care patient-customers because it can deliver the same therapeutic success as hospitalization; enable financial savings; and improve the patient's quality of life [23, 24].

Methodologically, the exploratory nature of this study leads us to address our research questions by means of a 'most-likely' case design, i.e., based on cases that are judged ex-ante to fit the theory [25]. The empirical base is made up of a number of international qualitative and quantitative studies developed in the healthcare field, some of which stem from comprehensive literature reviews. As exemplars of co-production applied to the clinical practice in question, such studies are ideally suited to a critical examination of the outcomes from the value perspective developed by Grönroos and Voima [4].

The authors believe that the research approach chosen can help clarify two key aspects of the OPAT in terms of how the scholars address this co-production clinical practice, and its connection with the empirical world, and have applied a triangulation approach to analyse and interpret the studies cited here.

4 Value Creation Processes: The Example of OPAT

OPAT is composed of five key service areas: multidisciplinary team setting; patient selection; antimicrobial management and drug delivery; monitoring of the patient during home therapy; outcome monitoring and clinical governance [26]. OPAT begins with the hospitalised patient's request to continue their final phase of antibiotic treatment at home. The patient has to satisfy specific eligibility criteria (average seriousness and absence of antibiotic-adverse reactions above all). This requires a multidisciplinary health care team to assess their clinical conditions and a physician and a social worker to ascertain the adequacy of the patient's home environment and that one or more care-givers are on hand to provide 24/7 monitoring throughout the treatment cycle. The transition from nursed patient to self-managed patient takes around 4/5 days. It starts with the OPAT-eligible patient receiving their first intravenous antibiotic therapy (IAT) in hospital alongside a targeted training course, when the nurse gives them the information and training needed to self-manage the complete OPAT cycle at home. The patient is not discharged until they have passed the OPAT-self-management course and the requisite drugs have been obtained from the hospital pharmacy.

The next step is for the nurse to schedule the haematological tests and blood chemistries and the clinical and physiotherapy check-ups scripted during the intensive hospital-administered IAT. The physician then sets the patient's Day Hospital check-up appointment to dovetail with the end of their home treatment course; this is the phase when the patient risks being readmitted to hospital if they show no improvement.

The goal of OPAT is to devise a course of reliable treatment that enables the lay person to administer intravenous medications with low-risk complications [27]. About 25 % of patients are estimated to suffer OPAT-related adverse events, mainly antibiotic reactions, intravenous access complications, or hospital readmission. The patients undergo regular follow-ups, including clinical and laboratory monitoring, to minimize complications [27].

Recognized internationally as a safe and effective way to manage selected patients [28], the risks related to patient/carer-administered OPAT are still a matter for concern. Many interrelated issues stop the mainstream from embarking on co-production, including the fact that the co-producing users rarely have the level of technical experience needed to deal with complications, that their behaviour is considered more unpredictable and less understood than that of more passive users [12: 47], and that the research has yet to fully enquire into the nature and quality of how the formal providers and informal caregivers interact [19]. A further checkpoint on the road to home-based

OPAT is the unwillingness of the public managers and health care professionals to relinquish the high ground [12, 29].

4.1 Provider Sphere

Generally speaking, the value-generating potential of the provider sphere is later turned into real value (-in-use) by the customers [4]. In the case of OPAT, the public hospital is the producer of the resources needed by the user to create value but, above all, is the enabler of a service, what is also termed a "value facilitator" (ibidem). For example, the hospital's multidisciplinary care team will not agree to a course of home care before first ascertaining the feasibility of this option from several viewpoints, not least the compatibility of the effort required and the psycho-physical conditions of the patient; personal skills and resources; the patient's home setting and type of facilities installed; and the presence or absence of informal caregivers. The latter "are asked to play an active role as member of the patient care team in managing care and carrying out medical interventions" [19: 141].

Not all patients are likely to engage in the different activities [30]. On the one hand, the hospital must build capability to identify motivated customers with the requisites to participate in service innovation [22]. On the other, it must invest in getting the stake-holders (OPAT service, primary care team, patient, informal caregivers) to reach mutual agreement on formulating a definitive care program. One of the key points in choosing a home treatment regimen is to keep the plan as simple as possible [27]. It also requires a dedicated administrative structure, supported ideally by an information system.

Moreover, the hospital needs to [31] ensure that all the interdisciplinary team members continue their professional development. A core aspect of ongoing education is keeping apprised of developments in antimicrobial stewardship and infection prevention and control as they relate to OPAT practice, which applies to everyone on the team, especially the non-medical prescribers.

In short, the shift to home therapy calls for: (a) redesigning the service processes; (b) rewiring the process interdependencies to chime with the activities redistributed among the extended cast of hospital and external stakeholders, and (c) bringing on board new actors without upsetting the continuity of care [29, 32, 33].

4.2 Joint Sphere

OPAT shows clearly that "organizational and client co-production are *interdependent*; the task cannot actually be performed without some contribution from both parties" (emphasis in the original) [34: 180]. The joint sphere creates a stream of continuous communication between the hospital and the "downstream care providers" [35]. To get the highest benefit from the co-producing relationship, the provider must make an effort to learn about the patient and their personal and collective situation, which, in turn, affects the value creation potential of both the joint sphere and the customer sphere [4].

Vice versa, the active customer may also venture across the frontier of the provider sphere to reshape the boundaries of the joint sphere and set the scene for a greater *platform* of *interaction* (or engagement [36]), thus enabling the organisation to sow the seeds of more joint value co-creation opportunities. The intensity of interactions is shaped by a continuum of cognitive, emotional and/or behavioural engagement (ibidem). When the value (-in-use) is created mainly in the customer sphere (e.g., at home) without direct interactions, the hospital is reduced to mostly or exclusively a value facilitator, providing *potential* value to service users [4].

As the "interactions between formal providers and informal caregivers may profoundly affect providers, caregivers and patients" [19: 141] so the provider's inter-action - their engagement with customer interactions - has a positive, negative or no influence at all on the customer's value creation. In fact it can even lead to the destruction of value. Examples of this are when the effective quality of the outcomes is far from that recommended by the clinical protocols, when adverse events arise, or the patient has to be readmitted to hospital. The organization thus misses opportunities to create value, such as when healthcare professionals neglect informal caregivers' needs or concerns [19], when a misalignment forms, or when the provider and the receiver spheres fail to reciprocate either partly or in full. To the contrary, successful practices construct an integrated circle of clinicians who constantly assess and engage patients: "When the pieces fall into place, patients receive timely appointments, understand their plan of care, and take the initiative for preventive measures, which is especially important for those with chronic illnesses" [37: s89].

4.3 Customer Sphere

Value creation in the customer sphere, or experiential sphere, is sole or independent, meaning that the customer creates self-value without tapping into the provider's processes. The customer interacts solely with the PSO-delivered resources, using other physical, virtual, and/or mental resources wholly unrelated to the provider [4]. Because the individual and the collective dimensions contain multiple temporal, spatial, physical, and social customer sub-dimensions, independent value creation is context-specific.

Given that the patient is the one to accrue the most benefits from home therapy [29], what the patient actually does when they create or co-create value depends on their personal characteristics and medical conditions. The decision of which one of the five practice styles of value co-creation elaborated by [30] - i.e., Team management, Insular controlling, Partnering, Pragmatic adapting, and Passive compliance – to opt for also is tied to the effective abilities of the patient to become involved in the process.

Tasks or points of the production process that substitute or supplement professional staff affect both the customer sphere and the joint sphere, such as in the case of admin-istering the antibiotic or controlling specific parameters during treatment. In other cases, inputs from the user and/or informal caregivers can help the staff to achieve their care goals, e.g., with regular visits to a physiotherapist or with healthier eating habits. "Downstream care providers" [35] interact with patient's resources in a social value creation process [4].

5   Discussion

Individual service in health care does not have the capacity to produce the same overall value for patients as the entire sequence of activities does. Shuttling the patient around a complex, fragmented system fails to increase patient value. To the contrary, the practice must be organized in tailored facilities taking account of the person's medical conditions. A combination of co-creation and co-delivery of care [6: 1108] is a determining factor in the quality of the patient's life and their ability to lead a normal existence.

The first source of customer value of home therapy is increased patient choice thanks to the provision of alternative models of appropriate care. Additional sources of value include: more rapid return to normality (work, education); greater comfort and privacy; nutritional and psychological benefits; reduced risk of hospital associated infection [26]. Interestingly, "normalization of illness" is how Bertocchi et al. [32][1] depict the first source of value.

The OPAT model describes "an equal collaboration between service users and providers in a way that uses the patient's experience … in designing and delivery of services" [21]. The studies analysed inform that one type of interaction is particularly significant in the co-production of potential value process, that between the formal and the informal caregivers.

In particular, the efficacious implementation of OPAT primarily depends on seamless communication between the hospital and the "downstream care providers" [35] to coordinate the tasks, which include the scheduling of appointments or arranging patient transportation. Again, training programmes held at the hospital or via web-based applications and the exchange of information on the patient's conditions [38] are another factor (e.g., when the outcomes of the therapy need to be monitored and reviewed during and after the treatment). Interaction between clinicians and informal caregivers is expected to enable effective knowledge transfer and shared decision making. In the words of Frow and colleagues [36: 473], this latter requires not only *cognitive* engagement – the acknowledgement and provision of own resources to the lead actor and/or its offering, but also engagement at the *behavioural* level (i.e., it impacts individual behaviour) and the *emotional* level (such as when the person "is committed and willing to invest and expend discretionary effort in engaging with the lead actor and its offering"). As the main resource integrator, the hospital draws on the contribution of the informal caregivers and ends up influencing the customer's value creation process.

When patients and families get involved in co-producing of care, the value of what they bring from their own daily experiences [39] is particularly evident in the customer sphere. Here informal carers are asked to contribute on a day to day basis, which means they must be mentally and emotionally prepared to get involved; curious enough to want to learn more; have the mindset to turn challenges into opportunities for improvement; have the ability to listen to everyone, learning and enacting what is relevant; and be ready to participate at a highly personal level [39: i90].

---

[1]   Special recognition for this reference given to Chiara Guglielmetti (University of Milano).

6   Implications and Conclusions

This paper has explored the potential of co-creation and co-production of value in healthcare, using the customer value perspective to analyse the OPAT practice. Using the model developed by Gronroos and Voima [4] as our springboard, the study argues, first, that a successful co-creation of value assumes the fullest integration of PSO and patient tasks, and, second, that the true value for the service recipients is indirectly generated by the interaction between the formal and informal caregivers. The active engagement of the latter is therefore a determining factor also outside the customer sphere, given that it enables the hospital to deploy the resources needed to produce the service and to allow its use by the receivers.

From the theoretical perspective, the study shows how the provider sphere is not a closed dimension that limits itself to offering a value proposition. Rather, it is an open place in which the resources produced autonomously by the provider - *in combination with* the resources of the informal caregivers – make customer value creation possible. However, further studies are needed to explore the logics of the interaction platforms where the various categories of caregivers converse and shape the potential value.

The study underlines the need for management to pay greater attention to the informal caregivers, given that these actors need to be orchestrated and that their role is set to become even more pivotal [7]. In a nutshell, expanding the focus to incorporate organizational coordination and ongoing feedback is essential to create an offering of authentic sustainable value for the patient - from the cognitive, emotional and behavioural standpoint – and for the home caregivers.

References

1. Osborne, S.P., et al.: The service framework: a public-service-dominant approach to sustainable public services. Br. J. Manag. **26**(3), 424–438 (2015)
2. Boyne, G.A.: Public and private management: what's the difference? J. Manag. Stud. **39**(1), 97–122 (2002)
3. Brandsen, T., Pestoff, V., Verschuere, B.: Co-production as a maturing concept, in New Public Governance, the Third Sector and Co-Production. In: Pestoff, V., Brandsen, T., Verschuere, B. (eds). Routledge, New York, pp. 1–9 (2012)
4. Grönroos, C., Voima, P.: Critical service logic: making sense of value creation and co-creation. J. Acad. Mark. Sci. **41**(2), 133–150 (2013)
5. Thomas, J.C.: Citizen, customer, partner: rethinking the place of the public in public management. Public Adm. Rev. **73**(6), 786–796 (2013)
6. Pestoff, V.: Co-production and third sector social services in europe: some concepts and evidence. Voluntas **23**(4), 1102–1118 (2012)
7. OECD: Health at a Glance 2015, OECD, Paris (2015)
8. Lega, F., Marsilio, M., Villa, S.: An evaluation framework for measuring supply chain performance in the public healthcare sector: evidence from the Italian NHS. Prod. Plan. Control **24**(10–11), 931–947 (2013)
9. Anderson, L., et al.: Transformative service research: An agenda for the future. J. Bus. Res. **66**(8), 1203–1210 (2013)

10. Temmink, D., et al.: Innovations in the nursing care of the chronically ill: a literature review from an international perspective. J. Adv. Nurs. **31**(6), 1449–1458 (2000)
11. Pires, G.D., Dean, A., Rehman, M.: Using service logic to redefine exchange in terms of customer and supplier participation. J. Bus. Res. **68**(5), 925–932 (2015)
12. Bovaird, T., Loeffler, E.: From engagement to co-production. How users and communities contribute to public services. In: New Public Governance, the Third Sector and Co-Production, Pestoff, V., Brandsen, T., Verschuere, B. (eds). Routledge: Abingdon, pp. 35–60 (2012)
13. Osborne, S.P. (ed.): Public Governance and Public Services Delivery. Routledge, Abingdon (2010)
14. Radnor, Z., et al.: Operationalizing co-production in public services delivery: the contribution of service blueprinting. Public Manag. Rev. **16**(3), 402–423 (2014)
15. Wright, G.H., Taylor, A.: Strategic partnerships and relationship marketing in healthcare. Public Manag. Rev. **7**(2), 203–224 (2005)
16. Maglio, P.P., Spohrer, J.: J.: Fundamentals of service science. J. Acad. Mark. Sci. **36**(1), 18–20 (2008)
17. Trischler, J., Scott, D.R.: Designing Public Services: The usefulness of three service design methods for identifying user experiences. Public Manag. Rev. **18**, 718–739 (2015)
18. Porter, M.E.: Competitive Advantage. Free Press, New York (1985)
19. Weinberg, D.B., et al.: Coordination between formal providers and informal caregivers. Health Care Manag. Rev. **32**(2), 140–149 (2007)
20. Etgar, M.: A descriptive model of the consumer co-production process. J. Acad. Mark. Sci. **36**(1), 97–108 (2008)
21. Sharma, S., et al.: Perceptions and experiences of co-delivery model for self-management training for clinicians working with patients with long-term conditions at three healthcare economies in UK. World Hosp. Health Serv. **47**(2), 22–24 (2011)
22. Sharma, S., Conduit, J., Hill, S.R.: Organisational capabilities for customer participation in health care service innovation. Australas. Mark. J. **22**(3), 179–188 (2014)
23. Esposito, S., et al.: Outpatient parenteral antibiotic therapy in the elderly: an Italian observational multicenter study. J. Chemother. **21**(2), 193–198 (2009)
24. Seaton, R.A., Barr, D.A.: Outpatient parenteral antibiotic therapy: Principles and practice. Eur. J. Intern. Med. **24**(7), 617–623 (2013)
25. Welch, C., Rumyantseva, M., Hewerdine, L.J.: Using case research to reconstruct concepts: a methodology and illustration. Organ. Res. Methods **19**(1), 111–130 (2016)
26. Chapman, A.L., et al.: Good practice recommendations for outpatient parenteral antimicrobial therapy (OPAT) in adults in the UK: a consensus statement. J. Antimicrob. Chemother. **67**(5), 1053–1062 (2012)
27. Halilovic, J., Christensen, C.L., Nguyen, H.H.: Managing an outpatient parenteral antibiotic therapy team. Ther. Clin. Risk Manag. **10**, 459–465 (2014)
28. Subedi, S., et al.: Supervised self-administration of outpatient parenteral antibiotic therapy. Int. J. Infect. Dis. **30**, 161–165 (2015)
29. Sorrentino, M., et al.: Health Care Services and the Coproduction Puzzle: Filling in the Blanks. Administration & Society, 1–26 (2015)
30. McColl-Kennedy, J.R., et al.: Health care customer value cocreation practice styles. J. Serv. Res. **15**(4), 370–389 (2012)
31. Gilchrist, M., Seaton, R.A.: Outpatient parenteral antimicrobial therapy and antimicrobial stewardship. J. Antimicrob. Chemother. **70**(4), 965–970 (2015)
32. Bertocchi, S., et al.: Diversi regimi terapeutici nel trattamento di bambini affetti da malattia emorragica congenita. Psicologia della salute **13**(3), 65–90 (2010)

33. Gilardi, S., et al.: Promuovere l'engagement dei pazienti con malattie croniche: un percorso di ricerca collaborativa (Promoting engagement in chronic illness patients: a collaborative research pathway). Psicologia della salute **17**(3), 58–79 (2014)
34. Alford, J., O'Flynn, J.: Rethinking Public Service Delivery. Palgrave Macmillan, Basingstoke (2012)
35. Gittell, J.H., Weiss, L.: Coordination networks within and across organizations: a multi-level framework. J. Manag. Stud. **41**(1), 127–153 (2004)
36. Frow, P., et al.: Managing co-creation design: a strategic approach to innovation. Br. J. Manag. **26**(3), 463–483 (2015)
37. Klein, D.B., Laugesen, M.J., Liu, N.: The Patient-Centered Medical Home: A Future Standard for American Health Care? Public Adm. Rev. **73**(s1), S82–S92 (2013)
38. Zardini, A., Rossignoli, C., Campedelli, B.: The impact of the implementation of the electronic medical record in an italian university hospital. In: Rossignoli, C., Gatti, M., Agrifoglio, R. (eds.) Organizational Innovation and Change, pp. 63–73. Springer, Heidelberg (2016)
39. Sabadosa, K.A., Batalden, P.B.: The interdependent roles of patients, families and professionals in cystic fibrosis. BMJ Qual. Saf. **23**(S1), i90–i94 (2014)

Work-Related Stress in Health Care Services: A Quantitative Study in Italy

Luisa Varriale[✉], Paola Briganti, Gloria Guillot, and Maria Ferrara

University of Naples Parthenope, Via Generale Parisi, n. 13, 80133 Naples, Italy
{luisa.varriale,paola.briganti,gloria.guillot,
maria.ferrara}@uniparthenope.it

Abstract. The measurement of work-related stress (WRS) for health providers is a crucial but cumbersome task. In this study a "WRS identity card" (WRS-ID) is proposed to self-monitor WRS risk in one organization, with an emphasis on health professionals and administrative employees at hospital. The method is based on a standard questionnaire purposely designed and validated by INAIL, the National Authorities for Prevention and Protection of Health at Workplace, which provides input data for a statistical inference analysis. The procedure is illustrated on a representative dataset from medical organization to discriminate between WRS levels between different departments. More specifically, thanks to over 3000 questionnaires anonymously administered by authors in hospital departments in one of the most relevant health care organization in the Southern Italy, it has been outlined how innovative and effective tools to monitor WRS are crucial, especially due to the specific health care workers' psycho-physical conditions. Theoretical and managerial implications have been provided.

Keywords: Work-related stress risk · WRS identity card · Health providers · Hospital

1 Introduction

In the last decades the deep changes occurred in the health care system in the overall world, and mostly in the European Union (EU) have contributed to a broad social, economic and political debate still ongoing. Since the Nineties, the European health care sector has been significantly changed, also affected by social and economic phenomena, such as the increasing technological innovation, the rise in demand for health care services, the progressive aging of the population, and the worsening of the general economic and financial conditions in essential public services, which require the application of efficiency and efficacy principles in managing and allocating the scarce financial resources [1, 2].

In this scenario the health care system in Europe started paying an increasing attention to issues completely neglected in the past, such as the adoption of effective policies for managing health care personnel with reference to exposure to professional risks and to the phenomenon of work-related stress (WRS) and burnout [3–5].

© Springer International Publishing Switzerland 2016
T. Borangiu et al. (Eds.): IESS 2016, LNBIP 247, pp. 660–673, 2016.
DOI: 10.1007/978-3-319-32689-4_50

Work-related stress represents a critical phenomenon in health care organizations, where unpredictable situations and emotional/physical load concern the workers and produce devastating effects, especially because of the specific context deeply changed and with high levels of uncertainty. Indeed, the daily pressure on health care professionals (i.e. medical, health care sector and administrative) is considerable and can significantly impair the level of performance, thus fueling the phenomenon of stress. Therefore, it is desirable to identify and quantify the level of stress for each employee and undertake the most effective actions to avoid exceeding certain thresholds by analyzing the main causes, models and management tools to keep work-related stress under control [6–8]. A methodology universally accepted is still missing and much desirable.

In this paper, we propose the application of a "WRS identity card" (WRS-ID) as an effective tool to measure and self-evaluate the stress levels in "Health Care Service providers". We start from the method developed on the basis of the procedures developed in the "INAIL manual" by INAIL organization (i.e. Italian National Work Insurance Institute) to measure WRS at workplace in any economic sector [9–11]. More specifically, the methodology adopted consists of collecting data through survey and analyze the results via statistical inference.

This study provides a first report that represents one preliminary outline aimed primarily at describing the main steps and the effectiveness of the WRS-ID proposed, in fact the research is still ongoing. The paper is structured as below: in the Sect. 2.

WRC phenomenon is conceptually described considering the main theoretical and regulatory frameworks with specific emphasis on the Italian context by identifying the causes, major events, evaluation methods, as well as tools for preventing and managing the same phenomenon. The Sect. 3 describes the methodology adopted in each step from data collection to measure WRS levels. In the Sect. 4 results are analyzed and discussed to examine a practical examples on a real numerical dataset from health care organizations in Italy. Finally, the Sect. 5 points out final considerations, future research trends and recommendations.

2   Regulatory and Theoretical Framework on Work-Related Stress and Technology Implications

In the early Nineties, the EU has promoted numerous health and safety provisions contained in different Directives to be implemented in individual Member States. In Italy the current legal framework is represented by the Legislative Decree no. 122/2010, and Legislative Decree no. 81/2008, which restricts any "employer", regardless of the economic sector, to engage in a risk assessment to preserve safety and well-being of the workforce, also against WRS. In particular, the Legislative Decree no. 81/2008 introduced the positive and holistic definition of well-being as a "state of complete physical, mental and social, not just the absence of disease or infirmity" (Article 2, paragraph 1, letter o). The practical tools to help all the organizations in respecting this diktat was elaborated by INAIL [9–11].

Health care professionals are continuously exposed to physical and psychological risks at workplace. Since Fifties and later Nineties of last century, Italian law underlined the significance for firms and employees in any economic sector to prevent and manage risks for workers' safety and health. The Italian Legislative Decree 626/1994 transposed the European Directives about safety, through the formal introduction of figures responsible for preventing risks at workplace (Managers of the Prevention and Protection - RSPP), underlining the active role of workers in protecting themselves. Subsequently the Law 39/2002 modified the Legislative Decree 626/1994 imposing to all public organizations and, hence, to health care public hospitals, the regular evaluation of "all risks to the health and safety of workers", in order to invite all the organizations to carefully consider the threats of a psychological equilibrium of employees. The Italian Legislative Decree 81/2008 makes it even more explicit reminder to the psychological aspects, naming in art. 2 (paragraph 1, letter "o") the definition of "health" proposed by the World Health Organization (WHO) as a "state of complete physical, mental and social wellbeing, not just the absence of disease or infirmity", and forcing companies to apply appropriate risk assessment work-related stress programs.

Stress of health care workers can be analyzed in relation to structural working conditions especially dangerous factors for the physical safety of employees, such as: musculoskeletal damage incurred during invasive medical diagnostics activities, such as gastroscopy, colonoscopy, and, in general, endoscopy; risks during surgical procedures in operating rooms, in particular, by infectious agents, anesthetic gases, radiations, latex allergies, infections with hepatitis B virus and HIV; dangers for hepatitis B, C and HIV contaminations in the clinical pathology laboratories [12–17]. Also, stress can be investigated considering neurological, endocrinological and psychological reactions, that characterize the human being.

Both interpretative lenses of the phenomenon can be framed within the framework proposed by the Theory of Organizational Acting and the Method of Organizational Congruencies, which consider the stress as a complex issue, just partially submitted to cognitive assessments, related to organizational decisions within structures with specific constraints, rather than a primarily psychological event, clearly revealed and with delineated borders, serially and rationally dependent by particular organizational factors and subjective characteristics [14, 18–20]. Therefore, there are internal stresses and/or environmental conditions that activate an alarm reaction, a step of resistance or biological adaptation by the body and a step of exhaustion, with neuroendocrine alterations, such as changes in hormonal level or biochemical area. Completed the process to restore homeostasis, in case of persistence of this disequilibrium, individuals develop adaptation diseases, such as: colitis, hypertension, diabetes, differentiated or not systemic autoimmunity disorders, psychosomatic diseases (asthma, allergies, dermatitis, etc.), carcinomas [20, 21]. In add, Selye [21] argues that patients subjected to surgical removal of the hypothalamus or general anesthesia experience such forms of stress, because this phenomenon is characterized by complex processes, not serial, and it is connected to the energy that nature requires for living. This is so far from the definition of psychological stress as nervous emotional tension, because it implies a broader set of factors involved and an existing, but not primary role of cognitive assessments as endogenous components. If you embrace this wider definition of stress, you may be able to prevent and manage specific stressful events, potentially dangerous, as some chemical and physical stimuli. Selye [21] has not proposed specific operational solutions, but common sense and the search of a living and working environment in line with the rules of the nature, as an antidote to contain negative stress or distress (negative form of stress, not leading to adaptation and rebalancing, opposed to eustress, positive form of stress and psychoneuroendocrine adaptation). Therefore, this extended interpretation of the phenomenon can contribute to find appropriate solutions in terms of preventing safety at workplace, through the specific research of greater congruence between production goals and workers' wellbeing [20].

However, since the end of the last century national rules and regulations to comply with the European Directives about the protection of workers' health have taken a reductionist approach to stress, regarded as mental and physical disorder, with attention focused on guidelines designed to analyze organizational factors as determinants of these phenomena [14, 21].

According to this advanced perspective, since Nineties, they have been developed interesting tools for evaluating psychosocial and stress risks at work: Job Content Questionnaire (JCQ) [23]; Occupational Stress Indicator (OSI) [24, 25]; Effort-Reward Imbalance (ERI) Model [26, 27]; Organizational Checkup System (OCS) [28, 29]; Objective Stress Factors Analysis (OSFA) Method [30]; Multidimensional Organizational Health Questionnaire (MOHQ) [31]; Testing of risk assessment work-related stress in the perspective of organizational wellness (Q-BO) [32, 33]; Maugeri Stress Index Questionnaire (MSIQ) [34]; Work Organisation Assessment Questionnaire (WOAQ) [35, 36]; M_DOQ10 Majer D'Amato Organizational Questionnaire 10 [37]. Some of these tools, mainly OCS, follow the traditional mold of the Maslach Bornout Inventory (MBI) [38–40].

The most common and spread tool used for evaluating and preventing WRS is JCQ, that identifies labor demand, social support and freedom of decision as organizational factors source of potential stress [23].

In the Italian context, three different types of logical approaches can be adopted to read the variegated landscape of tools for risk assessment and WRS [34]: in fact, there are evaluation models based on objective, subjective or mixed parameters for risk of occupational stress (OSFA) [30, 41, 42]; models based on subjective indicators tests rely on individual perceptions of stakeholders, such as JCQ [23] and ERI Model [23, 24, 43, 44]; mixed assessments finally integrate objective and subjective criteria [45].

The Legislative Decree 81/2008 was inspired by the prevailing trend due to the models of integrated study of workforce stress and proposed specific steps and evaluation tools, through a qualitative and quantitative case study analysis.

According to an international perspective, WRS phenomenon has been investigated [46–48] considering high levels of psychological distress which is pervasive in working population, in terms of mental disorders, also because of high-skilled jobs, increasing adoption of communication and information technology, and, consequently, higher demands and threats to the workers' mental health [49].

Most researchers developed three concepts to predict distress for workers exposed to psychosocial risks at work: the job demand-control theory [50], the organizational justice construct and equity theory [51], and the effort-reward imbalance model [52].

Indeed, scholars have outlined that some dimensions, such as high job demands (workload, work pressure) or low social support at workplace, represent predictive factors for stress related disorders of employees [46].

For instance, in the Netherlands and in the U.K., respectively, 79 % and 40 % of occupational physicians registered work-related common mental disorders [53]; in the U.S.A. high psychological distress disorders affect almost 10 % of employees [54]. Hence, work as a relevant aspect in the quality of life, also may negatively affect workers' health, generating distress disorders, significantly influencing workers' performance [55].

Academic studies and statistics on WRS are necessary to develop adequate primary preventing national initiatives, like the Management Standards developed by Health and Safety Executive Committee in U.K. and Italy to help work organization to reduce WRS risks, also through the adoption of temporary or permanent job rotation and psychological support [46, 56].

In addition, in the last decades in the health care context further significant changes occurred due to the adoption of innovative technologies, such as collecting medical information and data programs, sophisticated diagnosis instruments, electronic patient records (EPRs), billing and scheduling methods, laboratory result reporting, diagnostic instrument systems (e.g., in radiology and cardiology), e-care systems, intelligent emergency management system, pervasive healthcare data access, and ubiquitous mobile telemedicine [57–63]. Hence, health care organizations tend to manage patients and workers adopting innovative applications, such as Digital Smart Cards and so forth, but also new instruments are required to guarantee safety and healthy working conditions for all the health care professional providers.

In this study, starting from a brief review of the literature on WRS issue and technology impact on health care system, and following the INAIL manual procedure for assessing WRS at workplace, we aim to suggest a potential application, WRS-ID, to monitor, prevent, evaluate and manage work-related stress risks for health care workers.

2.1 INAIL Manual

The specific methodology, followed by employers in assessing WRS risk, is provided by the Permanent Advisory Commission for Safety and Health, created by the Ministry of Labor and Social Affairs, and consists in an appraisal process articulated in two phases: the preliminary assessment and in-depth evaluation.

The preliminary assessment explicitly concerns the detection of indicators objectively verifiable and numerically quantifiable, while the "in-dept" step is much more complex and it is possible only thanks to the assessment of subjective perceptions of those workers exposed to WRS risk. The second step can be carried out through the administration of questionnaires developed and collected according to INAIL manual [9: 53-55]. The questionnaires convey the subjective perceptions of workers about six dimensions of "Management Standards", related to the context and content of the work [9: 28], that is (1) demand (workload, work organization, work environment); (2) control (autonomy on the process of carrying out their work); (3) support (encouragement provided by supervisors and peers); (4) relationships (conflicts and tolerance of unacceptable behavior); (5) role (clarity on the position held in the organization); (6) changes (as they are managed and communicated in the organization).

The Management Standards are examples of ideal conditions or desirable states that organizations subject to WRS should attempt to reach and maintain, in particular those service providers most exposed to WRS like hospitals. In this study we endorse the questionnaire from the INAIL Manual. Apart from it, the WRS-ID proposed here does not use the evaluation system by INAIL but relies on general regression methods and it should be applied to the entire organization (not just to exposed workers).

3 Methodology: Data Collection and Analysis

The first element of our WRS-ID is the INAIL questionnaire, which comprises 35 questions (items), each of which requires an answer that maps a feeling of the interviewee (based on the late 6 months of time-lapse) onto the discrete quantitative 5 Likert scale [64] from very dissatisfied to very satisfied. For instance, some items concern employees' feeling at workplace in terms of expectations, level of autonomy, work duties (e.g. I am clear what is expected of me at work; I can decide when to take a break; Different groups at work require things that are hard to combine; I have unachievable deadlines) instead others regard the availability of helping colleagues and getting help by colleagues and so forth (e.g. If work gets difficult, my colleagues will help me; I give supportive feedback at work as I do; It's clear what my duties and responsibilities are).

The responses collectively gathered allow measuring in quantitative terms the WRS level of each individual (automatically given freely by INAIL according to a proprietary and validated algorithm), which represents a single statistical data point, and one organization, which represents a dataset of data points. Such information is very valuable and represents the fundamentals for: identifying either critical areas of a workplace or differences between subgroups/areas of the same organization; comparing stress levels to national averages tracked by INAIL for statistical purposes and against the model of Management Standard. In this paper the attention is mainly paid to the first aspect. In fact, because the management (general, administrative and medical managers), as required by the law, has to administer the INAIL questionnaire, there is a relevant opportunity to gather precious data to monitor trends in work-related stress risks in the different departments in the hospital. Over 3000 questionnaires during two years 2012-2013 were anonymously collected by the authors in departments from one of the most relevant hospital in the Southern Italy. A subset has been examined in Sect. 4 to illustrate how the WRS-ID can work. After the encoding of the questionnaires and the extrapolation of the related information, the dataset subdivided by Departments was processed by a statistical approach based on inferential "Hypothesis Testing" using the computerized package MINITAB 16© (other equivalent software can be used, e.g. SPSS©, SAS©, etc.), delivering a set of 35 plots per each department as output (e.g. Figures 1 and 2). The output can be equivalently expressed in tabular form. Statistical inference [65] is the process by which the characteristics of a population are deduced based on partial information from a random sample analyzed [66]. Statistical inference includes a very large class of heterogeneous approaches and tools, the most famous and effective is the "Test Hypothesis", which aims at testing a statistical hypothesis on the difference between an observation and estimated characteristics of the reference population.

4   Results and Discussion

We suggest a WRS-ID tool able to highlight the situations in medical service providers that are potentially more relevant by the viewpoint of the WRS risk. The WRS-ID developed consists, as already evidenced, in one instrument that can provide a picture of stress levels, more specifically of stress risks, for health care providers in departments outlining their criticisms. An illustrative example is examined, where five departments of a given (undisclosed) health care provider are compared against one reference distribution obtained by pooling all the available observations (over one thousand observations). In practice, for each of the 35 individual items (questions), the average judgments of each department were estimated and significant deviations "between departments" and against the "grand mean" level were observed to infer the propensity for WRS risk in each single department. For convenience, the total sample is referred to as "Group 99". The processing of questionnaires data has provided a WRS identification card for each department, rendering either consistency or discrepancy with the reference averages for the hospital for each 35 items. These indications have self-explanatory relevance for management purposes to prevent and reduce the WRS level. Regarding Department#1, that includes "Vascular surgery, Anesthesiologists, Maxillofacial, Surgery 1 and 2, Surgery Room, Thoracic Surgery, Top Management Department" with critical area concerning the Intensive Care Unit (ICU) post-surgery, as shown in Fig. 1, the 35 plots can represent the WRS-ID chart, where each plot compares the values of mean and standard deviation of Department #1 vs. values of Group 99. The statistical significance of any observed deviations are usually performed quantitatively by inferential statistical tests such as the t-value or the P-value (with a cut-off level of 5 %) which were both provided by MINITAB in the analysis of variance (ANOVA table). A significant difference is defined as a deviation (either positive or negative) between the average value of the department and the one of the reference Group 99 that yields a P-value < 0.05. While the ANOVA tables of significance are not provided here, the graphic information in Fig. 1 is eloquent and more intuitive to detect whether the average value of the Department #1 in certain areas is outside (significant) or inside (not significant) by confidence intervals (95 %) compared to the reference population Group 99 plotted aside.

The present approach is different from the standard INAIL approach, because the average values for a single department in this research work was checked against the intrinsic baseline offered by the average values computed for the same hospital (Group 99), as opposed to extrinsic baselines used in usual Management Standards (e.g. the INAIL procedure [9]), based on national averages or other reference statistics. In this regard, the proposed method can be helpful for the organization to self-evaluate and improve the WRS risk against the intrinsic baseline, by monitoring the phenomenon and removing/addressing stress causes.

In Fig. 1, the plots where Department # 1 departs significantly, either positively (+) (15 items) or negatively (−)(8 items), from Group 99 corresponds to 23 items against 35 total items. Of course, negative deviations (−) should be more worrying for the management as they support and implement sources of greater WRS risk and prompt for corrective actions to reduce dissatisfaction.

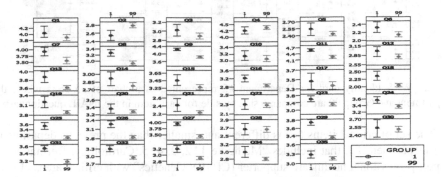

Fig. 1. WRS-ID card for Department #1 represented as a chart of 35 plots where the Department and Group 99 are compared side by side for each item.

From such self-evaluation, Department #1 exhibits criticisms of relational nature, whereas there is a likely absence of conflicts associated to performing tasks. Significant negative deviations were recorded for item 14 ("There is friction or anger between colleagues") and 34 ("Relationships at work are strained"), which clearly denotes relational conflicts that are otherwise masked by positively nuanced items 7, 8, 23, 24, 26, 27, 31, 33. These relational conflicts tend to emerge only in presence of questions that are negatively phrased with explicit reference to the presence of friction, while they are overlooked by the interviewees when questions are phrased in (positive) terms of support and collaboration with colleagues and boss. This may trace back to conflicts due to the presence of marked differences in personality or discipline in association with reduced decision-making freedom, e.g. in taking work breaks, as highlighted by item 2 ("I can decide when to take a break ") and 16 ("I am unable to take sufficient breaks"). This is reasonable conclusion outlines that harmony and cohesion from a technical-scientific standpoint exist between different workers, as it is supported by the positive items previously mentioned.

The following items do not seem to be source of stress and relationship conflicts in Department #1: unachievable deadlines (item 5), work overload (item 9), lack of clarity of tasks and responsibilities (item 11), partial ambiguity for the objectives of the unit (item 13), reduced decision-making autonomy on the content and the technical process of carrying out the work (item 19 and 15), pressures at work over the contractual working hours (item 18). The intensity of the possible relationship conflicts would misrepresent, however, the actual level of work-related stress, as pointed out by item 21 ("I am subject to bullying at work") and 34 ("Relationships at work are strained").

The situation is very different for each department. For instance, with reference to the WRS-ID card chart for Department #2, as shown in Fig. 2.

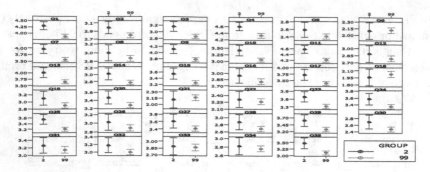

Fig. 2. WRS Identity card for Department #2 represented as a chart of 35 plots where the Department and Group 99 are compared side by side for each item in the INAIL questionnaire.

The set of critical items (−) is different and smaller than the previous department. The Department #2, that includes "Medicine 1, 2, 3, 4, 5, Cardiology, Dermatology, Expert professional healthcare supporter (CPSE), Genetics" with critical areas "Laboratory analysis and Blood Bank", turns out to be less exposed to WRS risk for the presence of several significant positive deviations, suggesting a situation better than the overall hospital on average, in areas such as: the clarity of the content and the process of carrying out the tasks (i.e. items 1, 4, 11, 13, 17); the degree of autonomy of the tasks (i.e. items 10, 15, 25); the structure of flexible working time (i.e. items 2, 30), the relationships among peers and supervisors (i.e. items 7, 23, 24, 29, 35). However, friction problems are highlighted here too but they are likely associated to rhythm and speed of work (i.e. work fast - item 20), as well as complexity (i.e. combining together conflicting requests - items 3, 14) and work intensity (i.e. item 9).

In general, the number of different stressors in each department needs to be properly related to organizational factors, as well as with the urgent or non-urgent nature of the activities, which both translate on the amount of the pressure being placed upon workers.

The approach can be extended to all five departments, addressing criticisms and WRS sources in each case. The other three departments concern: Administrative Department (D3), General Medicine Department (D4), and Emergency Department (D5), each one with specific areas. However, per se this is not the goal of this paper, which aims at ratifying the existence of critical WRS situations in hospitals and providing a methodology to monitor the phenomenon. The summary of the results in terms of the three possible statistical outcomes (i.e. significant positive or negative deviations and reference-like response "o") can provide the details of the statistical evaluation item by item and the total quotas of the three outcomes. A comparative plot is provided in Fig. 3, which presents the overall WRS-ID card chart of the organization and displays the three quotas for each department. It allows for a clearer visual comparison between the 5 subgroups, revealing immediately the departments with higher WRS risk, characterized by a large number of items with "strong" negative deviations (−) from the mean of the hospital.

An analysis of the patterns in Fig. 3 reveals that Department #1 is more critical, with about 23 highlighted deviations and 8 are strongly negative, pointing out that conflict between colleagues is the most serious problem to deal with. The Department #2 instead has 19 significantly deviating items with 4 strongly negative, confirming a lower risk of stress for the staff working in this department, who clearly understand tasks and has the ability/environment to handle the workload. Also, it is interesting to observe that the results from the Department #3 are sui generis, as this primarily deals with administrative tasks. Quit surprisingly this department highlights 2 critical items as reported, which is seemingly paradoxical for a workforce dealing with tasks characterized by "bureaucracy", harbinger of clarity, predictability, repetitiveness, high formalization and regulation (personnel in this department include office staff, protocol officers, general direction, health management, administrative management, legal department, technical department, accounting office, etc.). This is a relevant information suggesting an organizational problem which should be addressed to improve in the direction of WRS. In particular, the two recorded negative deviations referred to the lack in content and clarity of communication, together with the counter intuitiveness of task conduction, which resulted in "frustration and high pressure" on workers, due to overwork and under-representation of ethical and moral values at workplace. In contrast, the Department #4 instead exhibited the presence of a reasonable level of decision-making autonomy in the organization of the pace of work and constructive cooperation in the working groups. But at the same time conflict between colleagues exist. The Department # 5 presents criticisms with respect to the autonomy in managing breaks and working time and it is critical for job autonomy, stretched atmosphere, lack of respect and mutual overbearing and oppressive attitudes towards colleagues.

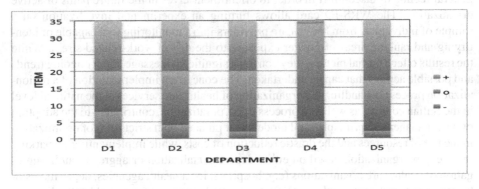

Fig. 3. Pictorial representation of comparison between Departments, highlighting quotas for positive deviations (+), negative deviations (−), an reference-like (o) items in the INAIL questionnaire.

5   Limitations, Future Perspectives and Concluding Remarks

This research is performed to build a picture of the state of WRS health care in the investigated hospital. This is a preliminary investigation to highlight the areas of the Departments that likely manifested situations of WRS for workers, to be weighed against different factors that impact this very critical and delicate matter.

The picture that emerges from the survey analysis encourages further research to develop appropriate and effective tools to prevent and resolve/reduce the causes of WRS phenomenon. It is, therefore, desirable and necessary in the light of this preliminary analysis, to think of appropriate initiatives for preventing and resolving criticisms. Following a comparative approach, most critical operational units, such as Department #1, need to be addressed first to prevent the escalation in the intensity of highlighted relational conflicts, and consequent degeneration of the organizational environment. Group meetings with quarterly basis were therefore recommended by the research team to promote recognition and awareness of the importance of managing emotions, learning strategies and cognitive behavioral techniques of psycho-relational management. This could allow monitoring the results of education and training paths, in addition to control the level of conflict over time. At the same time, Department #2 can be considered as an operational reference to develop as best practices on WRS regarding the organizational design of tasks and duties, leading to optimal management of relational dynamics among workers. For instance, in the Department #3 it would be appropriate to implement plans on overloading (overworked) by rationalizing the allocation of tasks and deadlines and programming training courses to align employees around common ethical values and moral principles, related to the welfare of individuals and the organization. Again, in the Department #4, it is desirable the reorganization of information flows, through processes of awareness and training aimed at the current managers of the system.

It is appropriate to point out that before promoting and making a radical restructuring of the work, it is necessary to fully understand the dynamics that led to this situation of general feeling of discomfort in order to orient themselves in the future paths of active organization. The WRS-ID card allows turning an experimental investigation on a sample of individuals from health care providers into a monitoring tool capable of identifying and ranking areas of greater exposure to the risk of work-related stress. While the results offer a partial picture, they convey a significant message about ongoing trends and possible actions that can be undertaken. The concurrent implementation of a regionalization process in handling the organization of health care services at the national level in the Italian context, as well as a process of corporatization, contributed to the adoption of new management principles and models that pursued both strict rules of optimization in the use of resources and the drastic reduction of costs, while implementing embarking in a deep reorganization based on either departmentalization or aggregation/disaggregation of health care organizations (e.g. hospitals, local health agencies, departments or health care departments, and so on), fostering the formation of regional health districts. In this context, the WRS-ID card could represent a very effective route for self-evaluation and stress management.

References

1. Tiraboschi, M., Fantini, L.: Il testo unico della salute e sicurezza sul lavoro dopo il correttivo (d.lgs. 106/2009), Milano, Giuffrè (2009)
2. NIOSH (National Istitute for Occupational Safety and Health): The changing organization of work and the safety and health of working people, Cincinnati, NIOSH, Report No. 2002_116 (2002)
3. Gottardi, D.: Lo stress lavoro-correlato: il recepimento dell'Accordo quadro europeo. Guida al lavoro **26**, 20 (2008)

4. Barling, J., Kelloway, E.K., Frone, M.R. (eds.): Handbook of work stress. California. Sage Publications, Thousand Oaks (2004)
5. Beehr, T.A., Newman, J.E.: Job stress, employee health, and organizational effectiveness: A facet analysis, model and literature review. Pers. Psychol. 31, 665–669 (1978)
6. Venturi, D.: Il decreto legislativo n. 81 del 2008. Uno sguardo di insieme, Bollettino Speciale Adapt, n. 5/2008, 8 (2008)
7. Bossche, S., van den Houtman, I.L.D.: Work stress interventions and their effectiveness: a review. Report for stress impact, Hoofddop: TNO Work and Employment (2004)
8. Collins, A.: Promoting well-being in the workplace: A tailored approach to stress management. Bowling Green State University, Bowl-ing Green, KY (2004)
9. INAIL: Valutazione e Gestione Del Rischio Da Stress Lavoro-Correlato, ISBN 978-88-7484-197-4 (free access available at 10. www.inail.it) (2011)
10. Gallo, M.: Stress lavoro-correlato: le linee guida Inail sulla valutazione e gestione del rischio, Guida al lavoro, 23 (2011)
11. Gallo, M.: Stress – Le nuove linee guida Inail sulla valutazione del rischio. Ambiente Sicurezza 11, 18 (2011)
12. Maciel, D.P., Millen, R.A.M., Xavier, C.A., Morrone, L.C., Silva-Júnior, J.S.: Musculoeskeletal disorder related to the work of doctors who perform medical invasive evaluation. Work 41, 1860–1863 (2012)
13. Abdelwahab, S., Rewisha, E., Hashem, M., Sobhy, M., Galal, I., Allam, W.R., Mikhail, N., Galal, G., El-Tabbakh, M., El-Kamary, S.S., Waked, I., Strickland, G.T.: Risk factors for hepatitis C virus infection among Egyptian health care workers in a national leaver diseases referral centre. Trans. Royal Soc. Trop. Med. Hyg. 106, 98–103 (2012)
14. Maggi, B., Rulli, G. (eds.): Lavoro organizzato e salute in un laboratorio di analisi cliniche. TAO Digital Library, Bologna (2010)
15. van den Berg-Dijkmeijera, M.L., Frings-Dresen, M.H.W., Sluiter, J.K.: Risks and health effects in operating room personnel. Work 39, 331–344 (2011)
16. Gutowski, C., Maa, J., Soo Hoo, K., Bozic, K., Philip, R.: Lee institute of health policy studies: Health technology assessment at the university of california-san francisco. J. Healthc. Manage. 56(1), 15–30 (2011)
17. Mele, A., Ippolito, G., Craxì, A.: Risk Management of HBsAg or anti-HCV positive healthcare workers in hospital. Digest Liver Dis. J. 33, 795–802 (2001)
18. Maggi, B., Rulli, G. (eds.): Decreto Legislativo 81/2008. Quale prevenzione nei luoghi di lavoro? (2011). http://amsacta.cib.unibo.it
19. Maggi, B., Rulli, G. (eds.): La prévention sur les lieux de travail et l'évaluation du stress en France et en Italie. TAO Digital Library, Bologna (2011)
20. Rulli, G.: Le stress au travail: évaluation du risque et prévention. TAO Digital Library, Bologna (2010)
21. Selye, H.: Stress in health and disease. Butterworths, Boston (1976)
22. Rulli, G.: Il 'caso' mobbing come occasione di riflessione biomedica sul disagio nel lavoro e sulla sua prevenzione. Quaderni di Diritto del Lavoro e Relazioni Industriali 29, 29–38 (2006)
23. Karasek, R.A.: Job demands, job decision latitude, and mental strain: Implications for job redesign. Adm. Sci. Q. 24, 285–308 (1979)
24. Cooper, C.L., Sloan, S.J., Williams, S.: The Occupational Stress Indicator. NFER Nelson, Windsor (1988)
25. Cooper, C.L., Sloan, S.J., Williams, S.: OSI, Occupational Stress Indicator. O.S. Organizzazioni Speciali, Firenze (2002)
26. Siegrist, J.: Adverse health effects of high-effort/low-reward conditions. J. Occup. Health Psychol. 1, 27–41 (1996)

27. Siegrist, J.: Adverse health effects of effort-reward imbalance at work: theory, empirical support and implications for prevention. In: Cooper, C.L. (ed.) Theories of Organizational Stress, pp. 190–204. Oxford University Press, Oxford (1998)
28. Leiter, M.P., Maslach, C.: Burnout and health. In: Baum, A., Revenson, T., Singer, J. (eds.) Handbook of health psychology, pp. 415–426. Lawrence Erlbaum, Hillsdale, NJ (2000)
29. Leiter, P.L., Maslach, C.: OCS Organizational Checkup System, Come prevenire il burnout e costruire l'impegno. O.S. Organizzazioni Speciali, Firenze (2005)
30. Argentero, P.: Una proposta di approccio obiettivo alla valutazione del rischio stress: il metodo Objective Stress Factors Analysis (OSFA). Risorsa Uomo 16(2), 185–200 (2011)
31. Avallone, F., Paplomatas, A.: Salute Organizzativa. Cortina Editore, Milano (2005)
32. De Carlo, N.A., Falco, A., Capozza, D.: Test di valutazione del rischio stress lavoro-correlato nella prospettiva del benessere organizzativo Q-BO). Franco Angeli, Milano (2008)
33. De Carlo, N.A., Falco, A., Sarto, F., Vianello, L, Marcuzzo, G., Dal Corso, L., Girardi, D., Magosso, D., Bartolucci, G.B.: The assessment of workrelated stress risk through the integration of objective and subjective measures: a contribution to the validation of the V.I.S method. In: Proceedings of 8th International Scientific Conference of International Occupational Hygiene Association, September 28–October 2, 2010, pp. 139–140, Rome (2010)
34. Giorgi, I., Baiardi, P., Tringali, S., Candura, S.M., Gardinali, F., Grignani, E., Bertolotti, G., Imbriani, M.: Il Maugeri Stress Index questionnaire per la valutazione dello stress lavoro correlato. Giornale Italiano di Medicina del Lavoro ed Ergonomia - Supplemento B Psicologia 33(3), 78–84 (2011)
35. Magnavita, N., Mammi, F., Roccia, K., Vincenti, F.: WOA: un questionario per la valutazione dell'organizzazione del lavoro. Traduzione e validazione della versione italiana. Giornale Italiano di Medicina del Lavoro ed Ergonomia 29, 663–665 (2007)
36. Griffiths, A., Cox, T., Karanika, M., Khan, S., Tomàs, J.-M.: Work design and management in the manufacturing sector: Development and validation of the Work Organisation Assessment Questionnaire. Occup. Environ. Med. 63, 669–675 (2006)
37. D'Amato, A., Majer, V.: M_DOQ10 Majer D'Amato Organizational Questionnaire 10. O.S. Organizzazioni Speciali, Firenze (2005)
38. Maslach, C., Jackson, S.E.: The measurement of experienced burnout. J. Occup. Behav. 2, 99–113 (1981)
39. Maslach, C., Jackson, S.E.: MBI: Maslach Burnout Inventory manual (research edition) (2nd ed, 1st ed. 1981), Consulting Psychologists Press: Palo Alto, CA (1986)
40. Maslach, C., Jackson, S.E., Leiter, M.P.: Maslach Burnout Inventory manual, 3rd edn. Consulting Psychologists Press, Palo Alto, CA (1996)
41. Argentero, P., Bruni, A., Fiabane, E., Scafa, F., Candura, S.M.: La valutazione del rischio stress negli operatori sanitari: inquadramento del problema ed esperienze applicative. Giornale Italiano di Medicina del Lavoro ed Ergonomia 32, 326–331 (2010)
42. Argentero, P., Candura, S.M.: La valutazione obiettiva dei fattori di rischio stress lavoro-correlati: prime esperienze applicative del metodo OSFA (Objective Stress Factors Analysis). Giornale Italiano di Medicina del Lavoro ed Ergonomia 31, 221–226 (2009)
43. Conway, P.M.: Gli strumenti per la valutazione soggettiva del rischio stress lavoro-correlato. Giornale Italiano di Medicina del Lavoro ed Ergonomia 31, 197–209 (2009)
44. Magnavita, N.: Due strumenti per la sorveglianza sanitaria dello stress da lavoro: il Job Content Questionnaire di Karasek e l'Effort Reward (2007)
45. Zoni, S., Lucchini, R., Alessio, L.: L'integrazione di indicatori oggettivi e soggettivi per la valutazione dei fattori di rischio stress-correlati nel settore sanitario [Integration of subjective and objective methods for stress related risks evaluation in the health care sector]. Giornale Italiano di Medicina del Lavoro ed Ergonomia 32, 332–336 (2010)

46. Nieuwenhuijsen, K., Bruinvels, D., Frings-Dresen, M.: Psychosocial work environment and stress-related disorders, a systematic review. Occup. Med. (Lond.) **60**(4), 277–286 (2010)
47. Stansfeld, S., Candy, B.: Psychosocial work environment and mental health–a meta-analytic review. Scand. J. Work Environ. Health **32**(6), 443–462 (2006)
48. Sembajwe, G., Wahrendorf, M., Siegrist, J., Sitta, R., Zins, M., Goldberg, M., Berkman, L.: Effects of job strain on fatigue: cross-sectional and prospective views of the job content questionnaire and effort-reward imbalance in the GAZEL cohort. Occup. Environ. Med. **69**(6), 377–384 (2012)
49. European Agency on Safety and Health at work: Expert Forecast on Emerging Psychosocial Risks Related to occupational Safety and Health. Eur. Communities, Luxembourg (2007)
50. Karasek Jr, R.A.: Job demands, job decision latitude, and mental strain: implications for job design. Adm. Sci. Q. **24**, 285–308 (1979)
51. Moorman, R.H.: Relationship between organizational justice and organizational citizenship behaviors: do fairness perception influence employee citizenship? J. Appl. Psychol. **76**, 845–855 (1991)
52. Siegrist, J., Siegrist, K., Weber, I.: Sociological concepts in the etiology of chronic disease: the case of ischemic heart disease. Soc. Sci. Med. **22**(2), 247–253 (1986)
53. Netherlands Center for occupational Diseases: Occupational Diseases in Figures, The Netherlands, Amsterdam (2009)
54. Carder, M., Turner, S., McNamee, R.: Work-related mental ill-health and 'stress' in the UK (2002-05). Occup. Med. (Lond.) **59**, 539–544 (2009)
55. Fink, G.: Encyclopedia of Stress, p. 723. Academic Press, San Diego (CA) (2000)
56. Kerr, R., McHugh, M., McCrory, M.: HSE Management Standards and stress-related work outcomes. Occup. Med. (Lond.) **59**, 574–579 (2009)
57. Dick, R.S., Steen, E.B., Detmer, D.E. (eds.): The Computer-Based Patient Record: An Essential Technology for Health Care. National Academies Press, Washington (1997)
58. Casalino, L., Gillies, R.R., Shortell, S.M., Schmittdiel, J.A., Bodenheimer, T., Robinson, J.C., Wang, M.C.: External incentives, information technology, and organized processes to improve health care quality for patients with chronic diseases. JAMA **289**(4), 434–441 (2003)
59. Jha, A.K., Doolan, D., Grandt, D., Scott, T., Bates, D.W.: The use of health information technology in seven nations. Int. J. Med. Inf. **77**(12), 848–854 (2008)
60. Denman, J., Yair, B.: Process for using smart card technology in patient prescriptions, medical/dental/DME services processing and healthcare management. U.S. Patent Application No. 10/819,882 (2008)
61. Yusof, M.M., Kuljis, J., Papazafeiropoulou, A., Stergioulas, L.K.: An evaluation framework for Health Information Systems: human, organization and technology-fit factors (HOT-fit). Int. J. Med. Inf. **77**(6), 386–398 (2008)
62. Shortliffe, E.H., Cimino, J.J.: Biomedical informatics: computer applications in health care and biomedicine. Springer Science & Business Media (2013)
63. Dünnebeil, S., Sunyaev, A., Blohm, I., Leimeister, J.M., Krcmar, H.: Determinants of physicians' technology acceptance for e-health in ambulatory care. Int. J. Med. Inf. **81**(11), 746–760 (2012)
64. Likert, R.: Technique for the measure of attitudes Arch. Psycho. **22**(140), 1–55 (1932)
65. Box, G.E.P., Norman, R.D.: Empirical Model-Building and Response Surfaces, p. 424. Wiley, New York (1987)
66. Fisher, R.A.: The fiducial argument in statistical inference. Annals of Eugenics, New York (1935)

New Technologies for Sustainable Health Care

Mauro Romanelli[✉]

University of Naples Parthenope, Via G. Parisi, 13, 80132 Naples, Italy
mauro.romanelli@uniparthenope.it

Abstract. Health care organizations and systems seem to benefit for the adoption and implementation of innovation driven by new technologies for seeking legitimacy and building trust with patients as to proceed towards a sustainable development. New technologies lead to develop health care as a process innovation-driven and patient-centered by improving quality and efficiency of health care services. Policies tend to help for diffusion and dissemination of innovation as to support the implementation of new technologies in health care service delivery. Sustainable health care organizations tend to develop or follow innovation by new technologies conforming to policies driving the diffusion of innovation for continuous improvement within health care delivery and systems.

Keywords: Sustainability · Legitimacy · Trust · Innovation · e-health care

1 Introduction

New technologies offer health care organizations and systems opportunities for proceeding towards a sustainable development as credible institutions working for wealth of people as to improve health and generate wider social value [1, 2]. Internet technologies are redesigning the relationship between health care institutions and patients leading the citizen as health-consumer to actively behave and act about their own health [3], driving health care from being institution-centric to becoming more and more patient-centric systems [4, 5]. Today, health care systems are facing some challenges related to the average life expectancy and the aging of population, the advances in informatics and medicine that require to build a sustainable development model [6]. E-health bridging medical informatics, Internet technologies and business relate to a new way of thinking for improving health care [3]. In health care technological innovation implies to be successfully implemented and supported in terms of diffusion or dissemination of innovation [7, 8].

The aim of this paper is to elucidate that e-health as innovation technology-driven helps health care systems and organizations seeking legitimacy for building trust with patients to proceed towards a sustainable development. Public policies as legitimate sources help support the adoption, the diffusion and dissemination of innovation within healthcare organizations driving or following the innovation. The study relies on the review and analysis of literature about the advent of new technologies and the role of e-health policies to sustain the innovation technology-driven in health care.

© Springer International Publishing Switzerland 2016
T. Borangiu et al. (Eds.): IESS 2016, LNBIP 247, pp. 674–682, 2016.
DOI: 10.1007/978-3-319-32689-4_51

2 Towards Sustainable Health Care Systems

Health care systems as complex social and political institutions are valued by people because of contribution for well-being of society as to improve health and generate wide social value. The State as a provider, funder, manager or regulator of health care services should play a central role for managing processes through which to establish the meaning and value contribution of the health system for society [1]. In the twenty-first century, health care systems are facing challenges related to development and aging of population, the average life expectancy, the advances in medicine and in human-computer interaction and informatics for better survival leading to develop a sustainable health care system [6]. Thereby, health as economic and social driving force in modern economies calls for policy innovation building for a network governance involving a broad range of actors and strengthening the role of citizens in health care [9]. Health and social protection systems should bridge social sustainability, co-responsibility and quality of life as the guiding principles for a new welfare system able to face and solve similar social, economic and political problems [10]. Sustainable health care implies that benefits produced are sufficiently valued by users and stakeholders to ensure resource able to support long-term activities and further benefits. Sustainable health services and care rely on organizational system with long-term ability to mobilize and allocate sufficient and appropriate human, financial and technological resources for activities meeting needs and demands of public health or the individuals [11]. Sustainable health care systems relying on the organizational awareness to contribute for continuous improvement [12] require to promote interventions on individual, organizational, community action and system level to achieve health promotion outcomes [13]. Promoting the sustainability of health care organizations relies on involving community for building a wide support to increase their credibility [14] by institutionalizing health programs in the organizational and community system for maintenance and continuation of health benefits [15].

3 Health Care Organizations and Systems Seeking Legitimacy for Building Trust

Health care systems and organizations are seeking legitimacy as credible institutions in order to restore trust with public and successfully proceed towards a sustainable development. Organizations seeking longevity within communities tend to consider trust as a necessary investment in order to emphasize their trustworthiness [16]. Trust influences performance and functioning of health care institutions leading to develop legitimacy for managing complexity of health systems [1].

3.1 Seeking Legitimacy

Health care organizations as complex systems acting in ways not always predictable tend to achieve greater legitimacy conforming to standards and expectations of the key stakeholders. Organizations tend to enhance credibility of their actions pursuing active or passive support in order to survive in front of complex and uncertain challenges and environments in terms of ongoing pressures for health care institutional reform and the emergence of new organizational governance structures [1, 17, 19]. Health care organizations tend to improve their survival chance and work actively to influence the normative assessments and feedback they receive from their multiple audiences [20]. Innovations that enhance legitimacy are desirable under conditions of uncertainty where the relationship between ends and means is no always clear. Regulatory programs lead organizations to comply with policies of government agencies and adopt formalized organizational practices as rationalized myths as a quest for legitimacy rather than for substantial organizational changes [21].

3.2 Building Public Trust

Trust facilitates cooperation and production of health care leading health systems to build wider social value by improving health [1, 2]. Trust helps reduce complexity being generally associated with a high quality of communication and interaction and providing a context increasing the likelihood that doctors and patients will tend to work cooperatively [16]. Today, health care organizations have to better define their own duties and obligations to build a patient-centred ethic [22] promoting trustworthiness to achieve the ends of medicine and medical ethics [23]. Health systems based on trust facilitate collective action and contribute to build social and economic value in society [1]. Responsive health care institutions tend to develop interaction and communication, providing information and involving greatly the patient to support trust-based relationships. Trust enhances exchange information and communicative interaction between health system and community encouraging a participatory process that tends to generate trust [24]. Public trust as trust placed by a group or person in a societal institution or system influenced by experiences of people in contact with representatives of institutions and by media images is expected to provide an information for measuring the performance of the health care system. Health care systems influence public trust providing good quality care and guaranteeing how healthcare providers protect the rights of patients too [25]. Changes in the institutional character of health care and cultural differences between countries tend to influence public trust as a multidimensional concept that relates also to health care institutions and system in terms of the worries of consumers about they will treated if necessary: patient focus, information and communication of providers, policies and quality of health care relate to health care as a system [26, 27]. Trust-based relationships can be built through institutions designing public policies at micro and macro levels patient centred care for improving quality of healthcare provision and enhancing public trust to restore lost trust [28, 29].

4 New Technologies for Innovation in Health Care

Internet technologies are redesigning the relationship between health care institutions and patients leading the citizen to assume a responsive orientation about their healthcare [4], driving the health care from institution-centric to patient-centric or consumer-centric systems in which patients can actively behave and act about their own health [5]. Successful implementation of technological innovation as organizational development and strategic change seems to rely on involving adequately the user and planning [30]. Innovation processes develop in dissemination, adoption, implementation and continuation as influenced by the socio-political context, the organization; the user or adopting person; complexity and relative advantage of the innovation [7]. While diffusion relates as passive spread, dissemination refers to active efforts to adopt. While implementation relates to mainstream an innovation, the sustainability refers to make innovation as routine until obsolescence [31]. In health care dissemination of innovation is more slow than its successful implementation. Diffusion of innovation depends on how organizations find sound innovation, support innovators and invest in early adopters making their activity observable trust and enable reinvention [8]. Thereby, service innovations seem to drive the adoption of e-health record even without financial incentives for the implementation [32].

4.1 E-Health Care Bridging Social and Technological Innovation

E-health care is related to technical development bridging medical informatics, Internet technologies, public health and business to deliver or enhance health services and information and focus on wider design about global health care improvement driven by technology [3].

Developing e-health implies to introduce and adopt information and communication technologies (ICTs) tools to improve quality and efficiency of healthcare increasing healthcare services accessibility and effectiveness of medical interventions as to support the interaction between patients and health-service providers. High levels of health information technology implementation tend to be positively associated to quality patient care and safety improvement and strategies that enhance patient satisfaction [33].

ICTs help health care organizations to acquire intangible gains looking beyond financial results to more qualitative impacts including patient and provider perceptions [34]. ICTs help quality of health care by reducing medication mistakes and developing innovation of care delivery driving increasingly pro active health consumers in their healthcare. E-health systems are evolving towards user-centricity by driving patients to control own their healthcare information, ensuring transparency and access to health records, fostering federation and integration of healthcare information between different providers and actors [35]. New Internet technologies have facilitated consumer education, disease management, clinical decision support, physician-consumer communication, administrative efficiency leading health care organizations to become fully aware of their role in the support of the e-health revolution putting people first, focusing on service and interactivity, offering appropriate training for physicians and support staff [36]. Technology helps improve health care as a process to support health professionals in their work and lifelong learning and assist citizens for reliable health information, disregarding organizational boundaries and functioning of the health systems [37].

The adoption of information technologies permits to innovate or re-engineer the healthcare sector and promote the economic sustainability, quality and cost efficiency of healthcare services that facilitate the interoperability among authorized healthcare professionals and promote collaborative, multidisciplinary and cross organizational health care delivery processes [38].

Internet technologies help improve the relationship physician-patient as to enhance communication, the access to health information, helping patients to make informed health care choices; a shared decision-making; collaborative teamwork approach; efficient use of clinical time [39]. Internet as source of health information seeking and channel of communication between citizens and doctors helps to supplement ordinary health services than replace them [40]. Internet technologies permit to design e-health interventions to develop an interactive communication and involve the users in health care promotion as to make e-health communication adapting to specific interests and orientation of different users [41].

E-health as a technological tool for patients achieving self management permits to tailor service to the specific needs and capabilities of patients and doctors coherently with empowerment components for patients and medical professionals in terms of ability to communicate own needs and using different channels, education and health literacy in terms of acquisition of relevant knowledge and transferring knowledge to patient, information about personal health situation, self-care, decision-making and contact with fellow patients [42]. Thereby, health care providers should incorporate patient's perspectives into medical decision making as to understand patient needs and offer patients education on the efficacy and safety of managing and sharing electronic health records and ensure the security of personal information in the health information exchange activities [43].

The implementation of e-health initiatives is uncertain and problematic as to fail. Initiatives coherent with existing organizational goals, staff skill sets and positive impact on patient-professional interactions and relationships between professional groups permit to understand the successful implementation and normalization of technologies into healthcare systems [44].

4.2 The Role of E-Health Policies to Support the Diffusion of Innovation in Health Care

E-health policies as a set of statements, directives, regulations, laws and judicial interpretation tend to direct and manage the life cycle of e-health [45]. The deployment of e-health application should require policies to support services innovation in health care because of overlap and interdependence between strategic, organizational, technological and professional dimensions [37].

E-health policies tend to facilitate the development of e-health programs enabling integration of e-health projects into regular services; implementing e-health successfully; guiding the process of evaluation and research for positive evidence of e-health adoption; transfer of information and provision of care between different jurisdictions; addressing the digital divide for diffusion of e-health [46]. For example, in the last decade European Union policies tend to help for the introduction and diffusion of new technologies within health care services and systems designing guidelines in order to exploit new technologies to improve health care service delivery and quality [47], by developing e-health tools and methodologies to increase sustainability and efficiency of health systems by spreading and introducing innovation, as to enhance patient/citizen-centric care empowering citizens by encouraging organizational changes [48] for building sustainable health care systems promoting the 'good health' and preventing diseases by sharing competencies and innovation technology-driven [49].

Policy makers should monitor continuous developments of health information technology, spur the development of new information tools and disseminate widely all promising technologies [50]. Furthermore, policies should be focused on aiding health care organizations to gain greater benefits from adoption and management of electronic health records [51]. In most countries the implementation of health information technology is crossing the beginning stages. Even if significant investments permit to gain benefits of health information technology for citizens the search for health information exchanges between countries is necessary for continuous progress [52]. E-health initiatives and policies should be planned to integrate local and regional health care organizations, to empower consumers in using information technologies and support the relationship between patients and health providers [53]. Policies should permit to overcome social, ethical and legal barriers that obstacle information technology implementation in health care providing incentives for certification and standardization of data [54]. The full potential of e-health seems to be far from meeting e-health objectives because of e-health strategies and policies not connected to health care delivery reality [55]. There are no clear strategies advancing to address best practices guidelines for effective development of applications. There is an emerging distance between what is postulated and empirically demonstrated about benefits of technologies for health care in helping storing, managing and transmission of data, clinical decision support and facilitating care from a distance [56].

5   Discussion and Conclusion

Sustaining the innovation driven by new technologies helps provision of health care services at low costs and responsive to needs of citizens-patients leading health care organization to improve communication with patients and restore trust with citizens proceeding towards a sustainable development of health care. Policies provide a context for health care organizations introducing technological and information system innovation in daily workings seeking legitimacy as credible and trustworthy institutions, working for wealth and quality of life of citizens and patients. Thereby, different responses to need to reconcile legitimacy and trust for achieving sustainability can emerge within health care systems driving or following innovation driven by other successful organizations and complying with guidelines of public policies.

The main contribution of this study is to identify a path leading health care organizations towards sustainable development by introducing, driving or following innovation offered by new technologies. Health care organizations embracing new technologies and medical informatics to improve efficacy, effectiveness and quality of cure and care tend to select a different path for proceeding towards a sustainable development along a *continuum* between seeking legitimacy and building trust with patients by driving the adoption and implementation of technological innovation or conforming to guidelines drawn by policies.

Policies that support the diffusion of technology contribute to enhance the legitimacy of health care organizations driving or following the innovation technology-driven. E-health policies tend to support for diffusion and dissemination of innovation in health care but do not exclude that best practices and successful technological innovation can emerge and address the investments driving the necessary organizational and operational arrangements meeting the approval of patients and satisfying ethical and quality standards for health care. Health care organizations following innovation technology-driven and drawn by other successful organizations tend to conform to policies that support diffusion of innovation and permit to ensure compliance by seeking legitimacy. Policies sustaining dissemination of innovation help health care organizations to build trust-based relationships with patients and design organizational arrangements for managing innovation in services and processes. Health care organizations driving technological innovation in services and relying on building public trust with patient need policies and interventions that support the adoption and the successful implementation of innovation for continuous improvement of processes leading towards a sustainable development of e-health care.

Future research perspectives require to further investigate how e-health care as opportunity is interpreted within Italian Regional care system relying on autonomous and decentralized local health care systems that emphasize different services innovation technology-driven.

References

1. Gilson, L.: Trust and the development of health care as a social institution. Soc. Sci. Med. **56**, 1453–1468 (2003)
2. Gilson, L.: Trust in health care: theoretical perspectives and research needs. J. Health Organ. Manag. **20**, 259–373 (2006)
3. Eysenbach, G.: What is e-health? J. Med. Internet Res. **3**(2), e20 (2001)
4. Eysenbach, G., Diepgen, T.L.: The Role of e-health and consumer health informatics for evidence-based patient choice in the 21st century. Clin. Dermatol. **19**, 11–17 (2001)
5. Demiris, G.: The diffusion of virtual communities in health care: concepts and challenges. Patient Educ. Couns. **62**, 178–188 (2006)
6. Haux, R., Ammenwerth, E., Herzog, W., Knaup, P.: Health care in the information society. A prognosis of the year 2013. Int. J. Med. Inform. **66**, 3–21 (2002)
7. Fleuren, M., Wiefferink, K., Paulussen, T.: Determinants of innovation within health care organizations. Int. J. Qual. Health Care **16**, 107–123 (2004)
8. Berwick, D.M.: Disseminating innovations in health care. JAMA **289**, 1969–1975 (2003)
9. Kickbusch, I.: Innovation in health policy: responding to the health society. Gac. Sanit. **21**, 338–342 (2007)
10. Garcès, J., Ròdenas, F., Sanjosè, V.: Towards a new welfare state: the social sustainability principle and health care strategies. Health Policy **65**, 201–215 (2003)
11. Olsen, I.T.: Sustainability of health care: a framework for analysis. Health Policy Plann. **13**, 287–295 (1998)
12. Radnor, Z.: Implementing lean in health care: making the link between the approach, readiness and sustainability. Int. J. Eng. Manag. **2**, 1–12 (2011)
13. Swerissen, H., Crisp, B.R.: The sustainability of health promotion interventions for different levels of social organization. Health Promot. Int. **19**, 123–130 (2004)

14. Brinkerhoff, D.K., Goldsmith, A.A.: Promoting the sustainability of development institutions: a framework for strategy. World Dev. **29**, 369–383 (1992)
15. Gruen, R.L., Elliott, J.H., Nolan, M.L., Lawton, P.D., Parkhill, A., McLaren, C.J., Lavis, J.N.: Sustainability science: an integrated approach for health-programme planning. Public Health **372**, 1579–1589 (2008)
16. Mechanic, D.: Changing medical organization and the erosion of trust. Milbank Q. **74**, 171–189 (1996)
17. Plsek, P.: Complexity and the adoption of innovation in health care. Accelerating Quality Improvement in Health Care: Strategies to Accelerate the Diffusion of Evidence-Based Innovations. Washington (2003)
18. Suchmann, M.C.: Managing legitimacy, strategic and institutional approaches. Acad. Manag. Rev. **20**, 571–610 (1995)
19. Yang, C.W., Fang, S.C., Huang, W.M.: Isomorphic pressures, institutional strategies, and knowledge creation in the health care sector. Health Care Manag. Rev. **32**, 263–270 (2007)
20. Ruef, M., Scott, W.R.: A multidimensional model of organizational legitimacy: hospital survival in changing institutional environments. Adm. Sci. Q. **43**, 877–904 (1998)
21. DiMaggio, P.J., Powell, W.W.: The iron cage revisited. Institutional isomorphism and collective rationality in organizational fields. Am. Sociol. Rev. **48**, 147–160 (1983)
22. Gray, B.H.: Trust and trustworthy care in the managed care era. Health Aff. **16**, 34–49 (1997)
23. Goold, S.D.: Trust and the ethics of health care institutions. Hastings Cent. Rep. **31**, 26–33 (2001)
24. Thiede, M.: Information and access to health care: is there a role for trust? Soc. Sci. Med. **61**, 1452–1462 (2005)
25. van der Schee, E., Groenewegen, P.G., Friele, R.D.: Public trust in health care: a performance indicator? J. Health Organ. Manag. **20**, 468–476 (2006)
26. van der Schee, E., Braun, B., Calnan, M., Schnee, M., Groenewegen, P.P.: Public trust in health care: a comparison of Germany, The Netherlands, and England and Wales. Health Policy **81**, 56–67 (2007)
27. Straten, G.F., Friele, R.D., Groenewegen, P.P.: Public trust in Dutch health care. Soc. Sci. Med. **55**, 227–234 (2002)
28. Abelson, J., Miller, F.A., Giacomini, M.: What does it mean to trust a health system? a qualitative study of Canadian health care values. Health Policy **91**, 63–70 (2009)
29. Calnan, M.W., Sanford, E.: Public trust in health care: the system or the doctor? Qual. Saf. Health Care **13**(2), 92–97 (2004)
30. Berg, M.: Implementing information systems in health care organizations: myths and challenges. Int. J. Med. Inform. **64**, 143–156 (2001)
31. Greenhalgh, T., Robert, G., MacFarlane, F., Bate, P., Kyriakidou, O.: Diffusion of innovations in service organizations: systematic review and recommendations. Milbank Q. **82**, 581–629 (2004)
32. Bhuyan, S.S., Xhu, H., Chandak, A., Kim, J., Stimpson, J.P.: Do service innovations influence the adoption of electronic health records in long-term care organizations? Results from the U.S. National Survey of Residential Care Facilities. Int. J. Med. Inform. **83**, 975–982 (2014)
33. Restuccia, J.D., Cohen, A.B., Horwitt, J.N., Shwartz, M.: Hospital implementation of health information technology and quality of care: are they related? BMC Med. Inform. Decis. Mak. **12**, 1–11 (2012)
34. Oecd: Improving Health Sector Efficiency. The Role of Information and Communication Technologies (2010). http://www.oecd-ilibrary.org/content/book/9789264084612-en
35. Deng, M., De Cock, D., Preneel, B.: Towards a cross-context identity management framework in e-health. Online Inf. Rev. **33**, 422–442 (2009)

36. Ball, M.J., Lillis, J.: E-health: transforming the physician/patient relationship. Int. J. Med. Inform. **61**, 1–10 (2001)
37. Moen, A., Hacki, W.O., Hofdijk, J., Van Gemert-Pijnen, L., Ammenwerth, E., Nykänen, P., Hoerbst, A.: eHealth in Europe– status and challenge. EJBI **8**(1), 2 (2012)
38. Serbanati, L.D., Ricci, F.L., Mercurio, G., Vasilateanu, A.: Steps towards a digital health eco system. J. Biomed. Inform. **44**, 621–636 (2011)
39. Wald, H.S., Dube, C.E., Anthony, D.C.: Untangling the Web– The impact of Internet use on health care and the physician-patient relationship. Patient Educ. Couns. **68**, 218–224 (2007)
40. Andreassen, H.K., Bujnowska-Fedak, M.M., Chronaki, C.E., Dumitru, R.C., Pudule, I., Santana, S., Voss, H., Wynn, R.: European citizens' use of E-health services: a study of seven countries. BMC Public Health **7**, 1–7 (2007)
41. Kreps, G.L., Neuhauser, L.: New directions in eHealth communication: opportunities and challenges. Patient Educ. Couns. **78**, 329–336 (2010)
42. Alpay, L., van der Boog, P., Dumaij, A.: An empowerment-based approach to developing innovative e-health tools for self-management. Health Inform. J. **17**, 247–255 (2011)
43. Qiao, Y., Asan, O., Montague, E.: Factors associated with patient trust in electronic health records used in primary care setting. Health Policy Technol. **4**, 357–363 (2015)
44. Murray, E., Burns, J., May, C., Finch, T., O'Donnell, C., Wallace, P., Mair, F.: Why is it difficult to implement e-health initiatives? A qualitative study. Implement. Sci. **6**, 1–11 (2011)
45. Scott, R.E., Chowdhury, M.F., Varghese, S.: Telehealth policy: looking for global complementarity. J. Telemed. Telecare **8**, 55–57 (2002)
46. Khoja, S., Durrani, H., Nayani, P., Fahim, A.: Scope of policy issues in e-Health: results from a structured literature review. J. Med Internet Res. **14**(1), e34 (2012)
47. Domenichiello, M.: State of the art in adoption of e-Health services in Italy in the context of European Union E-Government strategies. Procedia Econ. Finan. **23**, 1110–1118 (2015)
48. European Commission. eHealth Action Plan 2012-2020– Innovative healthcare for the 21st century. COM(2012) 736 final, 6.12.2012. Bruxels
49. European Commission. Proposal for a Regulation of the European Parliament and of the Council on establishing a Health for Growth Programme, the third multi-annual programme of EU action in the field of health for the period 2014–2020, Brussels; (2011)
50. Buntin, M.B., Burke, M.F., Hoaglin, M.C., Blumenthal, D.: The benefits of health information technology: a review of the recent literature shows predominantly positive results. Health Aff. **30**, 464–471 (2011)
51. Ben-Assuli, O.: Electronic health record, adoption, quality of care. legal and privacy issues and their implementation in emergency departments. Health Policy **119**, 287–297 (2015)
52. Jha, A.K., Doolan, D., Grandt, D., Scott, T., Bates, D.W.: The use of health information technology in seven nations. Int. J. Med. Inform. **27**, 848–854 (2008)
53. Harrison, J.P., Lee, A.: The role of e-Health in the changing health care environment. CNE Objectives Eval. Form **24**, 283–288 (2006)
54. Anderson, J.C.: Social, ethical and legal barriers to e-Health. Int. J. Med. Inform. **76**, 480–483 (2007)
55. Mars, M., Scott, R.E.: Global e-Health policy: a work in progress. Policies Potential **29**, 239–245 (2010)
56. Black, A.D., Car, J., Pagliari, C., Anandan, C., Cresswell, K., Bokun, T., McKinstry, B., Procter, R., Majeed, A., Sheikh, A.: The impact of eHealth on the quality and safety of health care: a systematic overview. PLOS Med. **8**, 1–16 (2011)

Interoperability of Medical Data Through e-Health Service in Romania

Elena Madalina Rac-Albu[1], Vlad Ciobanu[2], Marius Rac-Albu[1], and Nirvana Popescu[2(✉)]

[1] University of Medicine and Pharmacy "Carol Davila",
Bd. Eroii Sanitari 8, Bucharest, Romania
racalbu@gmail.com
[2] University POLITEHNICA of Bucharest,
Splaiul Independenei 313, Bucharest, Romania
{vlad.ciobanu,nirvana.popescu}@cs.pub.ro

Abstract. In the first part, the paper describes the Romanian e-Health service, the modalities of its operation in terms of patients medical data usage. The usage of medical data is very important, both administrative or medical point of view. Medically they have the ability to increase the efficiency of decision-making for all health care providers, both in the private and in the public area. It presents how a medical document model can be used nationwide and internationally and how it can facilitate the interoperability of medical data. In order to do that, a medical questionnaire is proposed (a model presentation of health data in a systematic and uniform way) that generates prerequisites standardization documents which represents in fact the patient's medical history and disease description. Once the questionnaire has been defined (which varies depending on existing medical specialties), the corresponding XML schema is generated that makes computer-computer interaction available.

Keywords: e-Health services · Medical data interoperability · Information system · EHR · HL7

1 Introduction

Interoperability for health related software environments consists of the ability of the information systems and heterogeneous applications to communicate and exchange data accurately, efficiently and consistently in order to allow further information processing [1].

The existence of interoperability brings many benefits to medical system, such as:

1. *Removing duplicate records within the system* - all presented data are accessed by all doctors of a patient, and upgrades are completed at each visit, having the opportunity to be consulted retroactive; so that it is impossible to appear different information (sometimes contradictory) about the same patient

© Springer International Publishing Switzerland 2016
T. Borangiu et al. (Eds.): IESS 2016, LNBIP 247, pp. 683–692, 2016.
DOI: 10.1007/978-3-319-32689-4_52

2. *Increasing the efficiency of medical and administrative staff* - medical staff can take medical decisions more quickly and accurately when they access patient's history, but the more important thing is that they can take vital decisions (saving lives) for patients who are unable to provide information about their health status (accidents, coma, etc.)
3. *Elimination of redundant data in the system* avoiding the storage of the same data in multiple contexts
4. *Streamlining the delivery of medical services*
5. *Avoiding to a very large extent of errors*

Interoperability of health information systems is only possible through the definition of standard messages, which must be adopted by all manufacturers of this type of technology to make effective functioning of these systems [2].

Among the various standards used, it should be highlighted through their characteristics HL7 (Health Level Seven) and DICOM (Digital Imaging and Communication in Medicine).

Electronic data exchange protocol - HL7 version 2.x is the standard used to transmit clinical and administrative information between health heterogeneous applications that rely on messaging. HL7 messages are XML documents (Extensible Markup Language) which can be validated against the XML schemas derived from the conceptual model, which is suitable for the transport of data between heterogeneous systems, allowing the separation of encoding structured information and content formatting [3].

In any hospital, information is managed by a generic application called HIS (Hospital Information System). Using this application, all the activities taking place in that hospital can be monitored and controlled. The application has such different interfaces that enable communication with all existing subsystems such as heart imaging (Radiology Information System), finance, human resources, pharmacy, etc. To connect with the "outside world" a web-based application is used. This allows reading and writing information in the hospital database. HL7 enables communication between different software applications existing in hospital, each being developed by various companies.

For better communication between the hospital and other medical institutions, HL7 standard can be used to carry data traffic. It is sufficient for the information systems of these institutions having a HL7 compliant interface. HL7 is the standard used to exchange information about patients, doctors, resources and documents between hospitals. There are also data synchronization protocols that provide persistence of data between applications. By using the HL7 standard, this data exchange can be carried out independently of existing software solutions and operating systems on the devices target. What is important is that the information is contained in the HL7 message.

HL7 provides the ability to access information / medical records and processing them independently, regardless of the software solution chosen by each institution. Thus, no matter who is the supplier for a particular software application, as long as it is in accordance with standard specifications and does not limit in any way the existing options to acquire other systems (they do not necessarily have to be developed by the same company).

2 Interoperability Models of Public Health System Services

2.1 Interoperability of Medical Data in Romania in the Present Days

The medical records in Romania are currently performed and managed by SIUI (Unique Integrated Information System) [4], whose main purpose is to aggregate, store medical data of insured patient while allowing web management. The system is administrated by the National Unique Fund of Health Insurance, part of CNAS (National Health Insurance Agency). Access to the system is given to CNAS and County Health Insurance Agencies. Physicians and health care providers entered into this system all consultations, diseases and treatments of their insured patients with settlement purposes.

SIUI process transactions of social insurance as payer of health services; SIUI is also able to perform authentication issues, management requests and reimbursements. In addition, there are centralized data about statistics, records and transactional data of healthcare providers (e.g.: hospitals, pharmacies and practitioners, as well as day clinics and outpatient clinics).

The current implementation of SIUI is structured into three modules: the Health Card, ePrescription and EHR (Electronic Health Record).

By using the Health Card component, each patient that is insured in CNAS is granted with an access card which acts as a key for accessing patient data. Therefore the system is in fact an authorization mechanism that assures patient data privacy by disabling the medical personnel access to the patient file without patient approval and ensures fraud detection and prevention in the Romanian medical system. Another important part of SIUI is the Electronic Prescription component (ePrescription), which increases the quality of health care by controlling drug prescription and also monitors the drug consumption in Romania.

From the EHR point of view, the system has not yet been launched and is still under implementation and testing. In the near future, once released, the EHR component is supposed to be the most important step in ensuring interoperability in the medical field by implementing interfaces and communications protocols standardized in the central component of the EHR system.

2.2 EHR (Electronic Health Record)

Electronic health records keep track of any diagnostic or therapeutic measure in a standardized manner. By reducing or avoiding redundancy in medical records, EHR facilitates the presentation of medical concepts in an optimized way, unambiguous, preserving the original context.

Electronic Health Record reflects the chronology of events and supports different views of the data according to user (doctor or insured).

Electronic health records provides:

- a patient's clinical data consolidation covering its entire lifetime;
- a medium for delivering accurate, complete and timely information through a permanent online system;
- a private and secure ensuring access to EHR data made available through the health card infrastructure;
- a scalable solution and extensible which will allow continued growth, extensive clinical information stored;
- an interoperability with other systems using open standards; a health using open standards, such as HL7;
- an information interoperability among many service providers, both nationally and internationally;
- an online access for doctors to the content of previous episodes of care;
- a support for the introduction of information;
- an accessibility and availability of patient information;
- a reduction in time spent on administrative activities.

EHR should interconnect multiple health registries, including chronic diseases registries, where they exist, on a standard computer interface. For healthcare providers in the public domain interoperability can be made directly within EHR, but in the private sector things are more complicated - the health computer systems of the private sector must be prepared to exchange medical information necessary treating patients in the two systems in an interleaved mode.

The current phase in Romania is the data entry process, where GP (General Practice) doctors are required to enter patient information, the most difficult and expensive part of the project which involves a large volume of work from GPs.

On the other hand, another issue consists of the current implementation of information systems inside hospitals, which require further developments so they can communicate effectively with EHR (meaning reading data from it, and the subsequent charging of medical data obtained through modification of the patients health respectively).

Although in Romania the system is not fully functional, one can find such an integration in Italy, within the Lombardia region. Here another approach has been developed by using a middleware solution that ensures the safe transfer of patient data between heterogeneous data sources within healthcare organizations and healthcare professionals following international health standards [5].

The middleware integration that enables electronic documents to be exchanged or shared when needed is based on Java Composite Application Platform Suite (JCAPS http://ers.sun.com/javacaps/development). JCAPS was used to implement the HL7 standard. Lombardia Informatica has provided middleware solution based on JCAPS all medical organizations (private practices, private hospitals, clinics, etc.) wishing to connect to the Regional Health System. JCAPS, based on Service Oriented Architecture (SOA) provides the integration of different applications via HL7 messages, creating integration adapters to be used in non-native HL7 applications and the management server integration services [5].

There are two types of applications to be integrated: HL7 interface with native applications and native applications without an HL7 interface. In both cases adapters are used as environmental technology integration: in the first case, technological adapter interfere with the content of the message, while in the second case, AC (technological adapter) provides HL7 messages from non-native HL7. JCAPS is essentially a hub that aims to manage and integrate all HL7 messages exchanged between different hospital departments [5].

2.3 Interoperability Schema Model for Romania

In Romania, implementing an interoperable environment at the national level involves direct integration with CNAS, which is the binding element of all medical services.

The Electronic Health Record file is the key to interoperability and it is fully managed by CNAS. That is why it is very important for EHR to apply measures for data protection and consistency, regardless of where or when the treatment is performed. User authentication is performed optimally by using Health Card implemented in the composition of SIUI eCard. Cases of card usage and information to be stored in the system will be established during the development process of EHR.

By centralizing documents from different EHR systems, an integrated perspective on the data is provided while securing access to users based on their rights in the context of patient records. In order to increase the security context, the authenticity of information is assured by signing it electronically with a digital signature. EHR enables efficient data collection through authorized persons through various environments online data input (keyboard and import using web services).

Other countries have already made several efforts in developing and Electronic Health Record, with a higher or lower success rate. For example, Canada has started implementing the system in the early 2003 and had the target of covering 50 % of the whole population by 2010. In the 2009 report, they admitted that the goal will not be reached by the end of 2010 even if the budget allocated over seeded 2 billion $ [6].

A successful case study can be found in Denmark, where a national strategic plan has been developed that allows physicians to obtain patient summaries throughout the country using a national Internet-based portal. The technical achievements and the organizational considerations that have led to a leading edge national program for electronic health records are described in [7].

After studying and analyzing interoperable systems in other countries such as Iceland and Norway [8], some innovations and improvements can be proposed, that will make life easier for care and health of patients while lowering costs. Thus an interoperability scheme is defined to be used at nation level that has the following advantages (Fig. 1):

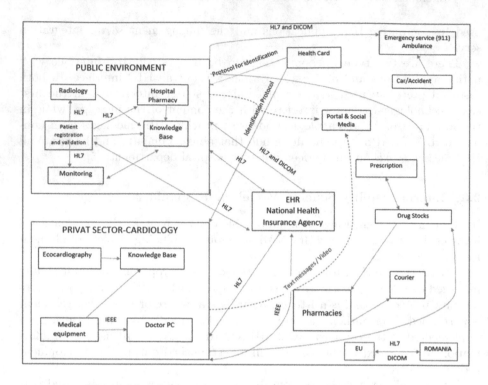

Fig. 1. Model for medical data interoperability in Romania

1. Reduces the data transfer between private clinics and / or hospitals
2. Benefits of increased failover mechanisms
3. Follows standardized communication protocols - the same ontology with other medical entities in the EU
4. Assures data safety by using the classification of the Health Card
5. Increases the trust in the medical decision making process by using a portal or social media service for doctors
6. Helps the drug prescription by providing live information of the pharmacies stocks therefore eliminating the situation in which a drug that is not available is prescribed.
7. Integrates the information from heterogeneous sources such as MRI scans, ultrasounds, etc. from both public and private medical units.
8. Allows real-time information sharing such as medical data, photos or videos between the all participants to the medical process: ambulances, emergency units, hospitals, thus increasing the quality of the medical act and allows fast decision making.
9. Supports new types of data sources, such as intelligent vehicles that automatically alert the emergency services in case of an accident as presented in the new 2016 standard.

3   Interoperability Model of Medical Data in Private Healthcare Services

Finding a pattern in private e-Health services requires a standardize model for medical data storage and presentation. Thus, a necessary step is the creation of a common questionnaire in order to be used by all the service providers in the same sector (e.g. cardiology - branch "Arrhythmology / Heart rhythm disorder"). By following the flow of the questionnaire, the relevant data allows further offline processing in order to facilitate the diagnosis and can be used for future faster pathology detection.

Heart rhythm disorders play an important role in cardiac pathology. Understanding underlying mechanisms of arrhythmias is a topic of ongoing research that has experienced an important development in the recent years.

Correct identification of the type of arrhythmia is important for taking a correct therapeutic decision, of vital importance for patient, many of these heart rhythm disorders being a potentially life threatening for patients.

In the proposed questionnaire (Fig. 2), supraventricular rhythm disorders are targeted, as presented in the ACC / AHA / ESC guidelines for the management of patients with supraventricular arrhythmias [9].

Based on the questionnaire, an XML schema can be developed that standardizes the targeted medical information, thus allowing computer-computer world-wide communications.

This model should be adapted for every medical field and by following the same pattern, which will make interoperability of medical data easy to accomplish.

4   XML Schemas

XML schemas allows the standardization of XML files, by describing the exhaustive internal structure of the documents, rules of completion and dependencies. An XML schema has been designed for the questionnaire shown in Fig. 2 and contains the following data types:

– *PersonalData* - complex type that should have at least the following children: Name, Surname, Date of Birth, Gender, City, Phone, Email address
– *Symptomatic* containing:
  – *Palpitations* - complex type that has three simple types as children: Rhythm, Type and NumberOfEpisodes, all enumerations
  – *HeartRate* - simple enumeration
  – *Syncope* - can be missing, a simple enumeration
  – *Fatigue* - simple enumeration using the POMS scale [10]
  – *ChestPain* - can be missing and consists of several enumeration-like children
  – *Dyspnea* - a simple enumeration
– *Debut* and *End* - simple enumerations

A.   The patient's personal data (*Name, Surname , Date of Birth, Gender , City, Phone, Email address*)
B.   Symptoms
    a.   Asymptomatic
    b.   Symptomatic
        1.   Palpitations
            a.   If YES
                i.   With fast / slow rhythm
                ii.   Regular
                iii.   Number of episodes
                    • Daily
                    • Several times per week
                    • A few weeks
                    • Monthly
                    • A few months
        2.   Heart rate
            i.   < 60 / min
            ii.   60 – 80 / min
            iii.   > 80 / min
        3.   Patient had syncope (loss of consciousness)
            a.   If Yes
                i.   When?
                    • At the beginning of arrhythmia
                    • At the end of arrhythmia
        4.   Fatigue (quantification using the scale Profile of Mood States (POMS))
        5.   Chest Pain
            a.   If YES
                i.   Location: Precordial, Retrosternal, Epigastrium, Back, Left Arm, Other
                ii.   Irradiation: Neck, Jaw, Shoulder (left or right), Back, Arms (left or right), Others
                iii.   Duration: Seconds, Minutes, Hours, Days
                iv.   Appears on: Stress, Rest, Cold, Night, Emotions, After meals, Other
                v.   Relief with: Nitroglycerin, Anti-inflammatory, Pain relievers, Rest, Other
                vi.   Amend breathing: Yes, No
                vii.   Amend position: Yes, No
                viii.   Number of seizures/episodes: Daily, Weekly, Monthly, Yearly, Other
        6.   Dyspnea (breathlessness)
            a.   If YES
                i.   At Effort
                ii.   Paroxysmal nocturnal (occurs in the first half of night)
                iii.   With orthopnea (not tolerate lying)
C.   Debut
    a.   Sudden
    b.   Gradually
D.   End
    a.   Sudden
    b.   Gradually
    c.   Vagal maneuvers
E.   Rhythm
    a.   Fast (> 80 – 100 heart beats / min)
    b.   Slow (<60 heart beats/min)
    c.   Regular
    d.   Irregular
F.   Arrhythmia duration: Seconds, Minutes, Hours, Days, Weeks, Months, Years
G.   Possible triggers: Physically/Mentally Stress, Drugs (specify which one), Nicotine, Alcohol, Coffee, Period

Fig. 2. The proposed questionnaire

- *Rhythm* - simple type
- *Duration* - enumeration
- *PossibleTriggers* - string

Figure 3 shows the logical diagram for the XML generation. In this case, the main blocks are used for the principal values as Personal Data, Palpitations, Syncope, Fatigue, Chest pain, Dyspnea, Arrhythmia duration, Possible triggers etc. These blocks are detailed in Fig. 3. The XML schema is used for the data interchange between systems.

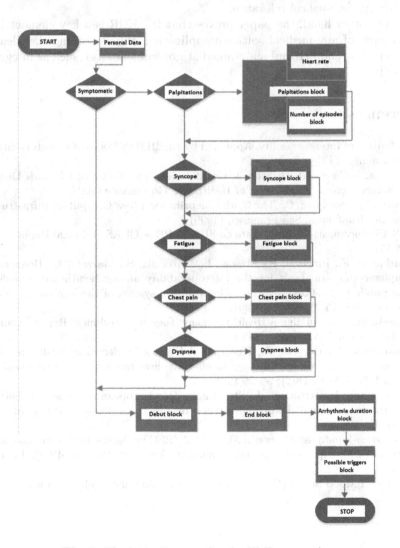

Fig. 3. The logic diagram for the XML generation

5   Conclusions

This paper is the starting point for the achieving the interoperability for medical software systems for both public and private services in Romania. Although the case study was made with cardiology aspects in mind, it can be easily extended for any other medical field.

This paper emphasizes also the importance of the strong cooperation that is necessary between doctors and IT specialists in order to assure the consistency and standardization of medical information stored in software systems, but, more importantly, the medical relevance.

On the other hand, the paper proves that the EHR is a key element in the development of any medical software application, thus enforcing the idea that EHR should be adopted and maintained at government level, such as integrating it into SIUI.

References

1. Definition of Interoperability, Approved by the HIMSS Board of Directors. https://www.himss.org
2. Chheda, N.C.: Standardization & Certification: The Truth Just Sounds Different. Technical Report, Application of Healthcare Governance (2007)
3. Foster, I., Kesselman, C.: The Grid: Blueprint for a New Computing Infrastructure. Morgan Kaufmann, San Francisco (1999)
4. CNAS: Specificatii de interfatare cu SIUI + PE + CEAS. Tehnical Report, CNAS (2015)
5. Barbarito, F., Pinciroli, F., Mason, J., Marceglia, S., Mazzola, L., Bonacina, S.: Implementing standards for the interoperability among healthcare providers in the public regionalized healthcare information system of the lombardy region. J. Biomed. Inf. **45**(4), 736–745 (2012)
6. MacAdam, M.: Building a Healthy Legacy Together. Technical Report, Canadian Policy Research Networks (2009)
7. Kushniruk, A., Borycki, E., Kuo, M.: Advances in electronic health records in denmark: from national strategy to effective healthcare system implementation. Acta Inform Med. **18**(2), 96–99 (2010)
8. Stroetmann, K., Artmann, J., Stroetmann, V.: European countries on their journey towards national eHealth infrastructures. Technical Report, eHealth Strategies (2011)
9. Blomstrm-Lundqvist, C., et al.: ACC/AHA/ESC guidelines for the management of patients with supraventicular arrythmias. J. Am. Coll. Cardiol. **42**(8), 1439–1531 (2003)
10. Profile of Mood States (POMS). http://www.brianmac.co.uk/poms.htm

Implementing the Patient Clinical Observation Sheet as a Service in Hospitals

Florin Anton[✉] and Silvia Anton

Department of Automatic Control and Applied Informatics,
University Politehnica of Bucharest, Bucharest, Romania
{Florin.Anton,Silvia.Anton}@cimr.pub.ro

Abstract. Currently in many countries in Europe there is a lack of medical staff in hospitals, and mostly physicians, also the physicians employed are overwhelmed by different activities and by a high number of patients. In many cases due to the lack of time the physicians are helped by other medical staff to fill the observations in the observation sheet. Many times some observations are recorded badly or omitted. This paper offers a solution to this problem, by proposing an electronic patient clinical observation sheet which will store the physician observations in audio files. This can bring noticeable improvements regarding the time spent by the physician to write on the observation sheet the evolution of the patient and the recommended medication. The observations are recorded in audio files converted in text using cloud services. The text files are added to the observation sheet, allowing the physician to use the time efficiently.

Keywords: Patient clinical observation sheet · Cloud computing · Mobile computing · Medical record confidentiality

1 Introduction

The clinical observation sheet represents a very important tool in the physician hands, which can be used in order to see how the prescribed medication influences the evolution of the patient in the hospital. The structure and the content of the observation sheet vary from hospital to hospital and sometimes vary also inside the same hospital for different specializations, and it is modified in order to offer better information regarding the healing process [1, 2]. Even if the structure of the observation sheet differs one thing remains in the structure of this document, and this is (among others) the section reserved for physician observations. By consulting the literature we can see that in [1] the purpose of the study was to create a newly devised child observation sheet (COS-5) as a scoring sheet, based on the Childhood Autism Rating Scale (CARS), for use in the developmental evaluation of 5-year-old children, especially focusing on children with suffering from autism, and to check its validity. In [2] the purpose was to describe and analyze the infrastructure and function of OUs (Observation Units) within self sustained children's hospitals and to verify and analyze characteristics between hospitals which are using or not OUs.

© Springer International Publishing Switzerland 2016
T. Borangiu et al. (Eds.): IESS 2016, LNBIP 247, pp. 693–702, 2016.
DOI: 10.1007/978-3-319-32689-4_53

The physician should analyze the medical record and the observation sheet, but many times other experts are requested to present their opinions in order to help the recovery of the patient. If the observation sheet is kept only on paper, in hard copy, this process will be cumbered. One solution for this problem is the electronic medical record/observation sheet, this approach was proposed and implemented in many hospitals. By using an electronic medical record /observation sheet will allow a much easier retrieval of data [3, 4], analysis [5, 6], and a big improvement from the point of view of efficiency of the medical process [7]. Even if the electronic medical record /observation sheet brings new major advantages, there are unfortunately some question marks related to privacy [8].

The discussion in literature [3] focuses on how to retrieve encrypted private medical records which are gathered from remote (not trusted) cloud servers in the case of special situations like medical accidents or disputes. In [4] is presented the problem of ambiguous medical queries, and is proposed a new semantic-based approach to achieve the diversity-aware retrieval of EMRs (Electronic Medical Records), in this case both the relevance and novelty are considered in order to rank the EMR. Using the ontologies in the medical domain, the authors extracted the potential semantics (concepts and relations linking them) from a query and use these semantics in order to model multiple query aspects.

In [6] a study regarding data analysis revealed that a set of items representing the examination template can be selected when the analysis considers not only exact matches but also similarities in terminology.

The privacy of EMR was discussed in a considerably large number of papers in literature, and is a problem which is still debated; research in [9] presents the results of a literature review regarding the privacy and security of electronic health record (EHR) systems. One of the problems is how to publish data from EHR, [10] presents a survey of methods proposed for making available publicly structured patient data, but the privacy to be preserved in the same time. The problem of sharing and accessing EHR data without loosing privacy was also discussed in [11].

Research in [12] is trying to preserve privacy by proposing a general framework to allow the accurate application of statistical disclosure control (SDC) methods to non-numerical clinical data, having the focus on the preservation of *semantics*. SDC methods have been used in order to mask sensitive attributes but in the same time preserving, the utility of data which is not related to a certain patient (anonymous data). Many of these methods are focused on continuous-scale numerical data.

In [13] is proposed a set of rules for good practice in order to ensure the protection of privacy in the usage of medical records, in [14] an open platform for personal health record applications with platform-level privacy protection is presented.

On the evolution scale, the next step for storing and processing medical data is cloud computing, this technology is used because solve multiple problems: storing, accessing, and processing medical data, but in the same time offers security services. This problem is discussed and validated in a number of papers in the literature, for example paper [15] presents a method of sharing personal health records in cloud in a secured way, in [16] is presented an implementation of a cloud-based electronic medical record.

Integrating technologies in cloud and processing medical data using cloud infrastructures has been discussed in [17–21], while data privacy in cloud for medical records has been analyzed in [22].

This paper presents an electronic system which uses cloud services in order to aid in the process of adding information and the diagnostic of the physician to the patient observation sheet.

2 The Architecture of the System

The system which we will describe further, is a system designed to acquire, process and retrieve the physician observations from and to the patient clinical observation sheet.

The system was created in order to help the physician in his daily work during the patient visits when he needs to fill his observations in the observation sheet. The approach is to use a recording device, and the most frequent recording device found in almost everyone pocket is nowadays the mobile phone (smart phone), to record the physician observations and to transform the recorded voice in a text file which later will be added to the observation sheet in electronic format but also in hard copy next to the bed of the patient.

The architecture of the system, presented in Fig. 1, is composed by the following elements:

- A mobile phone (smart phone) which has as a operating system iOS or Android

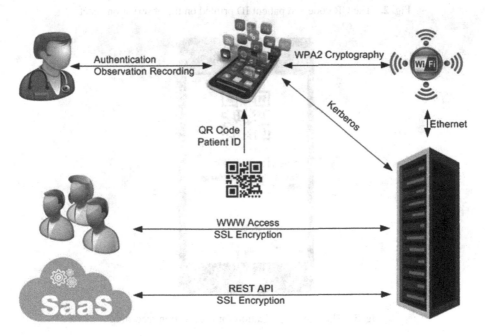

Fig. 1. The architecture of the system

- A server placed in the hospital, which offers connectivity services with a cloud voice processing system
- A speech to text SaaS (Software as a Service) cloud service offered by Vocapia

During the visiting program the physician will start on his mobile phone an application ("Visit Tour"), when the application starts it will connect on the local server allowing the physician to authenticate using a username and a password, the authentication process is based on the Kerberos protocol. The connection to the server is local using only the Wi-Fi Hot Spots in the hospital, in this way a connection from outside is not allowed and, because the authentication is based on Kerberos, the authentication data resides on the server, and the phone application does not allow to store de authentication data on the phone increasing in this way the security of the system.

After the authentication process completes the physician can start his visits to the patients. The observation sheet of each patient has a QR code and an identification code printed (Fig. 2).

The QR code (Quick Response Code) stores the same information (patient code) and also the patient name, and can be used to identify the patient using the phone.

PATIENT CODE:
162438992

Fig. 2. The QR code and patient ID printed on the observation sheet

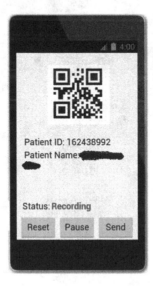

Fig. 3. The phone application for observation recording

After the physician has evaluated the patient he will scan the QR code or type the code in the application and, in order to record his observations, he will press record on the application and he can start to speak on the phone microphone. If the physician wishes, at any time, he will be able to restart or place in pause the recording (the pause is the default behaviour if the application is placed in background, for example if the phone is ringing or another application is used). When the recording ends, the physician will press the send button (Fig. 3) in order to send the recording to the server, and then he can go to the next patient.

The result of the recording is an mp3 file which, along with the identification number of the patient, is sent to the local server which stores the recording in an archive (a database) along with other information like the author of the recording. The role of the local server is not only to store the recording but also the server will generate a service request to the SaaS cloud system by sending the mp3 file, the file is tagged with the ID of the patient in order to assure the consistency of data.

The SaaS Speech to Text service returns in maximum 3 min the text obtained after processing the mp3 file. The resulting text is placed in an xml file which tags each word with the timestamp from the audio file, this feature allows a fast review and proof reading if it is the case (this action can be done by the physician or by other authorized users using a web application). The Speech to Text cloud service is able to process 24 h of recordings per day and can be accessed using REST API (Representational State Transfer Application Program Interface).

3 The Phone Application

On the smart phone is installed an application which is called "Visit Tour", the application is build in C ++ using the Appmethod Development Environment from Embarcadero.

Appmethod was selected in order to develop the application due to its features: it can help to rapidly develop and deploy an application; the most important advantage is that the user can build the same application for iOS and Android without making any change of the application code.

The phone application implements the following functions:

- Allows remote authentication using Kerberos
- Receives the patient ID by direct input from the phone virtual keyboard or by scanning the QR code in order to identify the patient
- Allows recording of physician observations in mp3 format and sends the file to the local server, tagged with the patient ID, for further processing

The application does not allow storing the credentials used for authentication or any information about the patient; moreover the mp3 file is deleted after the server confirms the receipt of the mp3 file.

Even if the application was carefully written in order to avoid security risks, this is not a 100 % safe system due to the fact that resides on a mobile phone which can be compromised if is not properly used (the system should be updated, an antivirus application should be installed, applications from unknown sources should not be installed, etc.).

4   The Local Server

The local server offers the following services:

1. Authentication service for the users (physicians) who are using smart phones in order to add observations in audio format to the patient observation sheet. In order to authenticate the system uses the well known Kerberos protocol [23–25].
2. The local server accepts the mp3 files sent by the mobile application and places them in a database which includes also other patient data, the file is stored without alteration; after receiving the file, the server contact the SaaS service for converting the audio file in text. The audio file can be later used as proof in cases of malpractice investigations. When the file is sent to the SaaS service, it doesn't need to be encrypted because the patient personal information is not contained in it.
3. The local server needs to connect to the SaaS service in cloud (this is done using SSL Encryption) in order to request the conversion of the mp3 file in text, this is done by using REST API, the same service receives the xml file (which represents the text conversion) from the SaaS service when the data is ready and places this file into the same database where the mp3 file is stored.
4. Another service offered by the local server is a web application which allows viewing/editing the patient observation sheet, based on the privileges associated with each user. The application offers an interface which integrates forms for displaying the observation sheet, a text editor for the transcript and an mp3 player. The application can be accessed using a regular SSL Encrypted connection using any web browser (and this can be done only from the hospital). The physician who has made the observations, or other authorized user can edit the speech to text xml file, any change in the file is tracked, the system being able to keep the history of changes, and stores this history in the database. This editing feature is very useful because the speech to text system is not 100 % error free, some words being converted wrongly and needs to be corrected.

The web application is using the timestamps from the xml file, each word from the transcript being tagged with a timestamp; this allows a fast editing/correction of the transcript. In such way the editor of the transcript is able to correct the wrong converted words easily by double clicking on the wrong word. The integrated player will jump on the file at the point when the word is pronounced, the editor will hear the word, and then he will be able to correct in the transcript.

The services offered by the local server are implemented using four distinct applications (agents). The database system is implemented using IBM DB2 Express-C for testing purposes. IBM DB2 Express-C was selected between other database products because of the native support for pureXML, XML files being stored in pages in the database offering a superior performance. Also DB2 Express-C is free to use, because of that this database solution comes with some limitations regarding the hardware resources which can be used (only 2 processor cores and 2 GB of RAM). The advantage of this solution is that it can be easily upgraded to a commercial edition which can use more resources and also has support like DB2 Express or other variant, also commercial variants have the possibility to use add-ons like High Availability and Disaster Recovery.

The relation between services which are offered by the system and the messages exchanged between these services can be seen in Fig. 4.

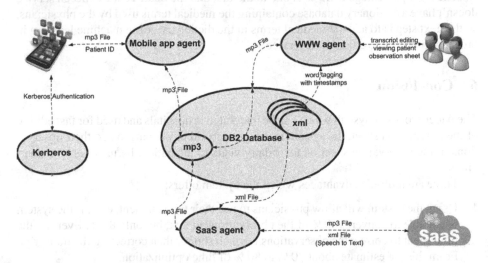

Fig. 4. The phone application for observation recording

5   Experimental Results

The designed system allows the physician to record the observations (in Romanian) in an mp3 file, then extracts from this file the transcript using a Speech to Text SaaS service, and then, later, the physician can review and correct the transcript if needed.

Three sets of tests have been conducted:

1. For the first test the audio file was processed without any modification, the file contained background sound: noise and other voices. After processing the file the percentage of the correctly recognized words has been 56 %.
2. In the second test a filter was applied in order to remove or diminish the background sound, this filter was implemented in the mobile application. In this case a significant improvement has been observed in the quality of the result, the recognition level was 72 %, (an improvement of 16 %).
3. Inspecting the results from the second test we found that some of the errors are generated due to the inflexions of the voice of the physician and also due to the other voices (of the personnel near the physician: colleagues or resident students). In the third test we asked the physician to speak using a constant voice the other personnel

reduced the talking during the recording. In these conditions the recognition level grew up to 85 %.

For the first test we used 12 mp3 files, for the second test 10, and for the third test 16 files. Even if the total improvement was of 29 % (the difference of results obtained from the first and the last test) for recognizing the words correctly, a level of 85 % means that the physician must spend an important amount of time to correct the transcript.

The error percentage of 15 % is due to the fact that the SaaS Text to Speech service doesn't have a dictionary database containing the medical terms used by the physicians, so the next step is to add the medical terms in the dictionary or use machine learning in order to improve the conversion service.

6 Conclusion

The paper propose a system which can be integrated in hospitals and used for fast editing of the observation sheet; the system is designed to aid physicians to add their observations in the observation sheet on their daily visits to the patient by using only a smart phone.

There are multiple advantages which the system offers:

1. Using the system will allow physicians to use their time efficient, even if the system is not able to convert 100 % of the observations in text, but only 85 %. Even so, the time spent to correct the observations is much shorter than correcting the transcript. From this we estimate about 70 % to 80 % of time optimization.
2. The system can be used for investigating malpractice cases, and is protected from tampering, being designed not to erase or alter the original information, but only to add more information. As we mentioned before, when a change in done at the level of transcript, the original information is also stored in the database, in this way the system allows you to track the changes and the users which executed them. Another advantage is that the audio file is kept unaltered in the database.
3. In situations when another medical opinion is needed, the system can be used to export or visualize all the information about the condition of the patient and the history of treatment, allowing a fast decision in urgent cases.
4. An increased quality of the medical services offered to the patient due to the fact that the physicians can now to focus on the diagnostic and medication and not on writing observations, the observations which the physician reads from the observation sheet are now reflecting exactly what the physician recorder last time, and lastly because the medical personnel is much focussed knowing that their actions and decisions are now recorded.
5. The system offers a high level of security because almost all connections are made in the local network, encryption is used (WPA2 and SSL), and no personal information is sent in internet (using the SaaS connection). The connection of the mobile phone in the Wi-Fi local hospital network is using WPA2 encryption level, the authentication uses Kerberos which keeps the credentials on the server and not at the client. After the authentication has been completed, the phone application

connects to the local server using an SSL connection. The mp3 file is not encrypted, because contains only observations about the condition of the patient and the treatment, no other personal information is recorded. The ID of the patient is sent to the server and then further in internet, but the ID is only a number used on the local server to link the mp3 file to the patient, and has no signification outside the local server. The connection between the local server and the SaaS service is encrypted using SSL, a protocol which is also used for the connection between the local server and the web application.

One problem that we see regarding the security is the Kerberos protocol which uses DES cipher (Data Encryption Standard) which now is considered as a weak cipher. In the next version of the application AES will be used (Advanced Encryption Standard) with 256 bit keys which is considered acceptable from the point of data confidentiality.

Another security problem is related to the smart phone usage, which if is not properly used as we mentioned before can be compromised, this issue can be solved by using correct security settings on the phone, and by training the users about basic security rules.

Further developments will include:

- a new mobile application which will be able to run on multiple types of devices like tablets and smart watches;
- a new encryption method (AES) which will be used by the Kerberos authentication protocol;
- a machine learning algorithm, "learn by example" which will be used to increase the percentage of recognized words from the audio record of the physician observations.

In the current stage the system can be used as a useful tool in the hands of the physicians, and can be extended to allow implementations in any hospital.

References

1. Fujimotoa, K., Nagai, T., Okazaki, S., Kawajiri, M., Tomiw, K.: Development and verification of child observation sheet for 5-year-old children. Brain Dev. **36**(2), 107–115 (2014)
2. Shanley, L.A., Hronek, C., Hall, M., Alpern, E.R., Fieldston, E.S., Hain, P.D., Shah, S.S., Macy, M.L.: Structure and function of observation units in children's hospitals: a mixed-methods study. Acad. Pediatr. **15**(5), 518–525 (2015)
3. Wang, H., Wu, Q., Qin, B., Domingo-Ferrer, J.: FRR: Fair remote retrieval of outsourced private medical records in electronic health networks. J. Biomed. Inform. **50**, 226–233 (2014)
4. Li, J., Liu, C., Liu, B., Mao, R., Wang, Y., Chen, S., Yang, J.J., Pan, H., Wang, Q.: Diversity-aware retrieval of medical records. Comput. Ind. **69**, 81–91 (2015)
5. Chauhan, R., Kumar, A.: Cloud computing for improved healthcare: techniques, potential and challenges. In: E-Health and Bioengineering Conference (EHB), pp. 1–4 (2013)
6. Rosenbeck Gřeg, K., Chen, R., Randorff Hřjen, A., Elberg, P.: Content analysis of physical examination templates in electronic health records using SNOMED CT. Int. J. Med. Inform. **83**(10), 736–749 (2014)
7. Carter, J.T.: Electronic medical records and quality improvement. Neurosurg. Clin. North Am. **26**(2), 245–251 (2015)

8. Stan, O., Sauciuc, D., Miclea, L.: Medical informatics system for Romanian healthcare system. In: E-Health and Bioengineering Conference (EHB), pp. 1–4 (2011)
9. Fernández-Alemán, J.L., Señor, I.C., Oliver Lozoya, P.Á., Toval, A.: Security and privacy in electronic health records: a systematic literature review. J. Biomed. Inform. **46**(3), 541–562 (2013)
10. Gkoulalas-Divanis, A., Loukides, G., Sun, J.: Publishing data from electronic health records while preserving privacy: a survey of algorithms. J. Biomed. Inform. **50**, 4–19 (2014)
11. Perera, G., Holbrook, A., Thabane, L., Foster, G., Willison, D.J.: Views on health information sharing and privacy from primary care practices using electronic medical records. Int. J. Med. Inform. **80**(2), 94–101 (2011)
12. Martínez, S., Sánchez, D., Valls, A.: A semantic framework to protect the privacy of electronic health records with non-numerical attributes. J. Biomed. Inform. **46**(2), 294–303 (2013)
13. Riou, C., Fresson, J., Serre, J.L., Avillach, P., Leneveut, L., Quantin, C.: Guide to good practices to ensure privacy protection in secondary use of medical records. Rev. Epidemiol. Sante Publique **62**(3), 207–214 (2014)
14. Van Gorp, P., Comuzzi, M., Jahnen, A., Kaymak, U., Middleton, B.: An open platform for personal health record apps with platform-level privacy protection. Comput. Biol. Med. **51**, 14–23 (2014)
15. Liu, J., Huang, X., Liu, J.K.: Secure sharing of personal health records in cloud computing: ciphertext-policy attribute-based signcryption. Future Gener. Comput. Syst. **52**, 67–76 (2015)
16. Haskew, J., Rř, G., Saito, K., Turner, K., Odhiambo, G., Wamae, A., Sharif, S., Sugishita, T.: Implementation of a cloud-based electronic medical record for maternal and child health in rural Kenya. Int. J. Med. Inform. **84**(5), 349–354 (2015)
17. Hsieh, P.J.: Healthcare professionals' use of health clouds: integrating technology acceptance and status quo bias perspectives. Int. J. Med. Inform. **84**(7), 512–523 (2015)
18. Dhivya, P., Roobini, S., Sindhuja, A.: Symptoms based treatment based on personal health record using cloud computing. Procedia Comput. Sci. **47**, 22–29 (2015)
19. Lin, W., Dou, W., Zhou, Z., Liu, C.: A cloud-based framework for Home-diagnosis service over big medical data. J. Syst. Softw. **102**, 192–206 (2015)
20. Zhuang, Y., Jiang, N., Wu, Z., Li, Q., Chiu, D.K.W., Hu, H.: Efficient and robust large medical image retrieval in mobile cloud computing environment. Inf. Sci. **263**, 60–86 (2014)
21. Arka, Hossain: I., Chellappan, K.: Collaborative Compressed I-cloud Medical Image Storage with Decompress Viewer. Procedia Comput. Sci. **42**, 114–121 (2014)
22. Yang, J.J., Li, J.Q., Niu, Y.: A hybrid solution for privacy preserving medical data sharing in the cloud environment. Future Gener. Comput. Syst. **43–44**, 74–86 (2015)
23. Todd, C., Johnson Jr., N. L.: Chapter 3 – Kerberos Server Authentication. In: Hack Proofing Windows 2000 Server, pp. 63–104, (2001)
24. De Clercq, J., Grillenmeier, G.: 6 – Kerberos. In: Microsoft Windows Security Fundamentals, pp. 303–408, (2007)
25. Russell, D.: High-level security architectures and the Kerberos system. Comput. Netw. ISDN Syst. **19**(3–5), 201–214 (1990)

Service and IT-Oriented Learning and Education Systems

Innovation for Sustainable Development by Educating the Local Community. The Case of an Italian Project of Food Waste Prevention

Sabrina Bonomi[1(✉)], Sara Moggi[2], and Francesca Ricciardi[2]

[1] eCampus University, Novedrate, Italy
sabrina.bonomi@uniecampus.it
[2] University of Verona, Verona, Italy
{sara.moggi,francesca.ricciardi}@univr.it

Abstract. Service oriented perspectives represent an opportunity of innovation and an answer to current challenges for social welfare, sustainable development and everyday life. The prevention of food waste requires new networked and collaborating competences, in the light of the increasing inefficiencies of modern economic growth models and the improvement of new paradigms for sustainable development. This research presents the case of a project that, while addressing food waste at the level of several organizations throughout the supply chain, implemented a recovering process to reduce food impairment. The project (R.e.b.u.s.) applies the efficiency system originally developed for school and university canteens to other food donors. In order to support this project, a far-reaching educational program for sustainable development was started in schools, universities and through public events. By educating the local community and enhancing processes that drive a change in behaviour, this initiative proved essential for the successful prevention of food waste.

Keywords: Value co-creation · Sustainability education · Italy · Sustainable development · Food waste

1 Introduction

The increasing attention on sustainable development contrasts with the inefficiencies of modern economic growth models, driving the development of new paradigms of services to improve the quality of life and cost efficiency.

Several studies have examined inefficiency in resource use, in particular considering the for-profit point of view and analysing tools and managerial approaches for a more sustainable production. Despite the wide literature on these issues, little is known about food waste prevention, related strategies, instruments and levers to gain an effective implementation. The main streams of research consider measures to prevent food waste by leveraging consumer's behaviour, production and supply chain management.

Our study enlarges the literature on food waste prevention by studying education for sustainable development (ESD) as a valuable way to address this problem. A well-designed educational initiative, in fact, allows strengthening and integrating the

© Springer International Publishing Switzerland 2016
T. Borangiu et al. (Eds.): IESS 2016, LNBIP 247, pp. 705–716, 2016.
DOI: 10.1007/978-3-319-32689-4_54

competences of the parties that may be involved for value co-creation. The service science approach suggests taking advantage of the network of stakeholders in order to build a shared vision on the expected performance of a given service, and to design a new service system based on stakeholders' cooperation [1, 2]. The literature on service science often refers to educational services as particularly suitable to address this challenge [1].

Education can be seen as a very stimulating issue for service science studies and projects [3]. For this reason, in this paper we ask whether education can be a useful way to build a new perspective in order to create a more efficient eco-system for the food value chain. To this aim, we present the R.e.b.u.s. project, and focus on its educational initiatives, which are aimed to increase the awareness on food waste in the local community, starting in childhood. The core of R.e.b.u.s. activities, indeed, is to identify food waste in the area of Verona (Northern Italy) and to implement the process to reduce food waste through a network of several coordinated actors. Through the efficiency system developed by a non-profit organisation (NPO) supervising the project, and enabled by ICT, the food, instead of being wasted, can be shared with people affected by food poverty. The project was developed thanks to the network created by this supervising organization. With the aim to prevent food waste, R.e.b.u.s. is also promotes a far-reaching educational programme aimed to increase the awareness on waste. This programme embraces several initiatives involving local authorities and the local education system, engaging a wide number of subjects like teachers, students and managers. Our analysis of this case of ESD contributes to the literature by highlighting the role of service science to address food waste prevention and environmental sustainability, and provides insights to support similar initiatives.

The remainder of this study is structured as follows. In the next section, a brief overview of the European Union's recommendations, Italian legislation and local authorities' initiatives are described and then commented in the light of the service science approach. The methodology section lists the main steps carried out during this path of research, underlining the main features of the data collection phase and data analysis. The case study description concerns the origins, aims and peculiarities of the R.e.b.u.s. project, paying particular attention to the numerous educational aspects of the initiative. Finally, the conclusions of this research are presented.

2   Food Waste and Education for Sustainable Development

The studies on sustainable development strongly highlight the importance to satisfy both our, and the future generation's, needs [4]. As environmental, social and economic implications, the unsustainable use of resources and waste generation [5] enhance the priority of waste management from the final disposal of waste to actions that can prevent waste production [6].

The production of food waste impacts society from the agricultural to the manufacturing processes and from the household to the supply chain. Although food waste concerns are linked with a wide range of political, social and economic structures, the individual consumer demand has a power that, over time, can influence these structures, driving the change to a more sustainable production, consumption and disposal [7]. In light of this, consumers are identified as subjects to educate regarding sustainable practices in order to prevent the surplus of food and food waste. By definition [8], "food losses or waste are the masses of food lost or wasted in the part of food chains leading to edible products going to human consumption".

As presented by the Papargyropoulou et al.'s model [4], it is important to gather our efforts on food waste reduction, considering the waste hierarchy framework that presents levels in which the food, because of its nutritional properties, still has an economic and social value [9]. Moving from this model, our study adds a new item on the prevention dimension (Table 1), depicting how prevention of food waste can be promoted and made more efficient through a far-reaching program on education, involving the local community, non-profit organizations, elementary schools, higher education and local authorities.

Table 1. The food waste hierarchy, adapted from Papargyropoulou et al. [4].

Area of intervention	Actions
Prevention	Avoid surplus food generation throughout food production and consumption; Prevent avoidable food waste generation throughout the food supply chain and education
Re-use	Re-use food for human consumption through redistribution networks and food banks
Recycle	Recycle food waste into animal feed or via composting
Recovery	Treat unavoidable food waste and recover energy
Disposal	Dispose unavoidable food waste into engineered landfills with landfill gas utilization systems in place.

Because the first step is to recognise the individual behaviour as part of a collective change, education aims to increase the awareness of the citizens' actions. As underlined by Redman and Redman [10], education plays a pivotal role in creating long-term changes [11, 12]. In this sense, the Education for Sustainable Development (ESD) can provide helpful tools to foster the change involving all the educational levels into a process of behaviour change. UNESCO declares that ESD "should be of a quality that provides the values, knowledge, skills, and competencies for sustainable living and participation in society" [13]. Under this perspective, it also becomes crucial to recognise the importance of ESD since childhood, considering children as young citizens [14] and educating them about sustainable citizenship regarding everyday life, including food consumption [15]. Furthermore, the introduction of sustainable development dimensions into the higher education programmes and projects would encourage the holistic handling of sustainable development issues; promote the development of ethical behaviours; motivate people to play their role in preserving natural resources, in the way they consume goods; foster building among participants on sustainability courses and projects; create awareness on sustainable development [16, 17]; and help managers of tomorrow to be more sensitive to sustainability issues [18].

3   The Analysis of the Legislative Context

The European Union (EU) has promoted several dispositions on food waste in all life stages [19] through an integrated product policy [20], resource efficiency initiative [21] and bio-economy support [22]. In particular the EU [21] explained its concerns on unsustainable European consumption—in which the food and drink value chain causes 17 % of greenhouse gas emissions and uses 28 % of the material resources—referring to the importance of a common effort for food waste reduction. In the milestones for 2020, the EU declared "incentives to healthier and more sustainable food production and consumption will be widespread and will have driven a 20 % reduction in the food chain's resource inputs. Disposal of edible food waste should have been halved in the EU". Furthermore, the EU stated "action to reduce food waste is the introduction of targeted awareness-raising, information campaigns and education programmes" [23].

The Italian government, through the Law n.155/2003, named the Law of the Good Samaritan, considers non-profit organisations that collect and distribute food to the poor as equal to the final consumer, based on the individual responsibility of the organisations that spontaneously decide to involve themselves in this activity. Before this law, these charities had to provide guarantees for the food donated (preservation of the food, transport, storage and use of the food) even after the delivery to the non-profit organisations. This imposition discouraged potential donors. On one hand, non-profit organisations have to manage the health and security of the food donated, from the harvesting to the delivery to the consumer, by deploying technical procedures and adequate equipment. On the other hand, donors have to be formally recognised as food business operators and be subjected to the national legislation on food safety, granting that the food donated is perfectly edible.

The economic and financial crisis has increased the number of people affected by poverty and social distress. The Veneto region dedicated the Law 11/2011 to tackling these problems through the redistribution of the surplus food. The aim of this law is to pursue specific actions: (1) to increase the quality of life of individuals and families in hardship situations; (2) to raise a nutritional culture; (3) to establish partnership networks between food companies, catering services and NPOs that redistribute still-edible food to people affected by food poverty; and (4) to develop IT systems to ease the food waste reduction and food redistribution between donors and non-profit beneficiaries. The Regulation n. 196/2012 formalised the constitution of a working group aimed at identifying local needs and strategies for food redistribution.

This group was composed of delegates from several NPOs involved in the management of food waste, such as the Italian Red Cross and Caritas. In light of the Regional Law, this group has worked on two fronts in order (1) to ensure and implement the amount of food for beneficiaries and (2) to rationalise and monitor the process of collection and (re) distribution of food in order to avoid an unequal distribution or production of waste. The regional working group was responsible for implementing the three phases of the programme: to develop a digital platform to coordinate donors and beneficiaries; to define common criterions of access to the programme; and to coordinate social marketing events, working inclusion and educational programmes.

Finally, regarding the local context of Verona, thanks to the evidences presented by R.e.b.u.s., local authorities have decided to reward the large retail (e.g., supermarkets) and catering (e.g., canteens) organisations that have a virtuous behaviour in the social, local context. If these organisations contribute to the prevention of food waste, redistributing food and meals produced, local authorities have approved a reduction (up to 80 %) on the payment of the local tax on the production of solid waste (TIA: Tariffa d'Igiene Ambientale). Through these organisations, all unsold products and undistributed, and edible, meals will be donated to non-profit organisations, helping disadvantaged populations in the local community.

4   The Lens of Service Science

The service science approach suggests leveraging the network of stakeholders in order to build a shared view on the expected performance of a certain service, and to consistently design a new service system and a roadmap for innovating services based on stakeholders' cooperation. Organizational inertia and resistance to change are taken into account to make the strategic choices between radical or incremental service innovations and periodically adjust the program [1, 2]. Looking through the lens of service science, the value realization from the R.e.b.u.s. project was dependent on a collaborative organizational dynamic, a purpose-built technical infrastructure and a data rich source for research and for the educational program. According to Lusch et al. [24], one of the primary reasons why people engage in co-production is for pure enjoyment—the psychic (experiential) benefits, coming from activities like education or learning a new skill. Looking at the cooperation among local authorities, enterprises and NPOs, coordinated by an association of social promotion that has the role of service integration, facilitated through an ICT tool, that involves numerous citizens (for example as consumers, beneficiaries or voluntaries), education can be a useful service to build a new perspective in order to create an eco-system more efficient in solving problems of food waste.

5   Methodology

The analysis on this case study was carried out by a participant observer directly involved in the project, who collected data from numerous sources, such as surveys, semi-structured interviews with the key-informants in the educational project and internal and external documentation.

The researchers employed the case study methodology to a particular initiative. This methodology helps researchers to understand a unique context and a complex phenomenon set within its real-world context [25]. The analysis of this case study was carried out longitudinally from 2008 to 2014 through a participant observation research conducted by one of the authors who was directly involved in the project, and by other two researchers involved as non-participant observers and interviewers. Participant observation constitutes a research strategy that "simultaneously combines document analysis, interviewing of respondents and informants, direct participation and observation, and introspection" [26]. In this sense, in our study, a wide range of sources were available directly from the field of research, such as internal documents regarding the strategic decisions, the long and short plans on the use of resources and the reports provided to the several stakeholders involved in the project.

The data collection is further enriched by a number of semi-structured interviews and surveys with the key-informants involved in the project, such as teachers, managers and beneficiaries. The analysis of the numerous data collected was based on an interpretative approach [27] in the labelling phase on the educational aims of the R.e.b.u.s. project.

6   Case Study Analysis: R.E.B.U.S. and the Innovative Process

6.1   Origins of the Project and Current Scenario

The main idea for the R.e.b.u.s. project came from a group of people who observed a negative educational impact from the amount of food wasted inside the canteens of Verona's schools. Looking into the process, these people discovered that the local government spent public funds in three ways: buying food for school canteens, for garbage disposal and buying food, through charities, for poor people.

Consequently, it was created a partnership among the local government, companies that supply meals and manage waste, and non-profit organisations feeding people affected by food poverty in order to reuse the surplus of meals and to give it to the poor people. After doing an environmental analysis, it was shaped the process of food waste reduction, guaranteeing the hygienic and fiscal standards level. In light of the increasing complexity of the process and the number of subjects involved, a NPO, an association of social promotion, was introduced to supervise the entire process and to promote public meetings to discuss the results of this good practice, share knowledge on food waste reductions and educate citizens on their consumption behaviour.

Formally, the so-called R.e.b.u.s. project (it is an acronym that means Recupero Eccedenze Beni Utilizzabili Solidalmente, *eng. trad.* Re-use of goods in surplus, usable for charities) was started up at the end of 2008. Thanks to the local authorities' support and the local network created among public organisations, companies, and NPOs, it is possible to re-use unsold and/or unused goods that have a reduced market value, but that still have an intrinsic value, so can be perfectly used. Moreover, the donors involved could request a reduction on their taxes paid on solid waste. The goods transfer, consisting of mainly food, came from companies' donations to NPOs involved in the social assistance for people in marginal and uncomfortable situations. Regarding the educational aspects of the project, the programme called 'R.e.b.u.s. Informs' was started up in 2010. This specific programme considered several topics, such as waste reduction, correct nutrition, respect for the environment, subsidiarity and was addressed to children, students and citizens. Nowadays, the project is fully operational in the Verona area. Additionally, the supervisor supports other local networks in northern Italy, such as Vicenza, Padua, Rovigo, Bergamo and Mantua.

Focusing on the Verona area, in 2014, about 1,430 tons worth of food was reused, which is an increase of about 32 % compared with 2013; the economic value of the recovered food is about 1,800,000 euro. The companies involved in the project as donors of their surplus food, are fruit and vegetable markets; farms; the companies that manage the scholastic, academic and hospital canteens; pharmacies; supermarkets; organisations of agricultural producers; and some occasional donors. The public organisations involved are the local government of Verona, the Province of Verona, the local health authority, the prefecture and an important role is also played by the municipal organisation responsible for waste logistic management. There are more than 70 NPOs involved, assisting over 60,000 people in situations of marginality or disadvantage. Thanks to the R.e.b.u.s. project, charities involved can save funds otherwise spent buying food, receiving about 80 % of their meals from donors and, in some cases, 100 %. The money saved through the project helps feed more subjects and develops additional social actions. Furthermore, with all of the vegetables and fruits as part of the food donations, the people attending the charities' canteens also receive highly nutritious, balanced meals.

6.2   Peculiarities of R.E.B.U.S

For non-profit organisations, the distribution of food to people in disadvantaged situations is a usual practice [28, 29]. For example there is a similar project in Ferrara city; network isn't alike neither supervised by a local NPO but rather by an external consultant: it has been recovered 555 t in 10 years. It is true that Ferrara is smaller that Verona, but results are very smaller. There are also other projects, based on different logic (charity) but made by well-structured organizations; they miss the involvement of Public Administration so results are proportionally minor (295 t in 2012, but in 28 Italian cities). In Brescia's city, instead, there is a cooperative organization that works in very similar way to Verona's case and similar is also its result (300 t in 2012) [30].

On the other hand, R.e.b.u.s. gives the possibility to the participants of the inclusion in a process that contrasts the opportunistic behaviours, guarantees administrative and fiscal fulfilments, transparency and legality, prosecutes nutritional education, environmental and health prevention, achieving economic, social and environmental sustainability, thanks to a win-win logic [30, 31], and a value co-creation. R.e.b.u.s. is derived from the co-design of a shared strategy of service science that aims both to solve problems and to answer the requests coming from the local community. Service science is defined as the study of the configurations of people, technology and the connections of internal and external services of sharing information (e.g., language, laws, measures and methods) to create systematic service innovation. Procedures, processes and norms are standardised, shared in all network members through ICT tools, which eases the replication of the model and its diffusion [2].

The aim of R.e.b.u.s. is twofold: on one hand, it tries to prevent food from ending up in landfills through the solidary re-use of food; on the other hand, it promotes a lifestyle careful to rationally use natural resources for sustainable development and increases subsidiarity for the local community [32], improving citizens', especially children's, education. The educational initiatives cover several topics: to observe and avoid the supply chain waste, to reduce domestic waste, to correct nutritional habits, improve public health and to respect the environment by waste prevention (art.3, Law Decree n.22/1997)—and not only through recycling, recovery and disposal—as sustainable development requires [33]. In particular, R.e.b.u.s. Informs focuses on 'food security', that means the possibility to guarantee to everybody "the physical, social and economic access to sufficient, safe and nutritious food that meets their needs and preferences, so as to enable him to lead an active and healthy life" [34]. For both these objectives, the project demonstrates the importance of education for sustainable development at the local community level [10–12]. Indeed, food waste education drives consumer behaviour and becomes pivotal in fostering change through targeted educational programmes and shared information. With the aim to create virtuous circles in surplus management, these programmes show citizens and enterprises a number of best practices on waste reduction, recovery, reuse and recycling. Educating citizens to play their role in society permits the use of the unsold or unutilized products till the end of their life cycle, thus reducing the presence of recyclable materials into landfills, CO_2 emissions, methane and greenhouse gases [4].

6.3   Issues on Education for Food Waste Prevention

The key to service science is a focus on all aspect of the service as a system of interacting parts that include people, technology, and business. The review of the existing situation and challenges in this study helps focus the paper on the obstacles and the inter-organizational dynamics observed in the implementation of food waste prevention. The need for cultural changes, in the entire community but also in relationships among different organizations and at intra-organizational levels, could be performed creating a stakeholders' network correlated to educational services.

Because R.e.b.u.s. involves several subjects, several organisations (public, profit and NPOs) and also private subjects (e.g. aided by associations, voluntaries, employees, citizens, and teachers), the educational programme R.e.b.u.s. Informs has manifold applications. Analysing the project's different stakeholders, different kinds of people to involve in the project's educational program were found. The educational activities can be summarised in three main frames:

1. tutorial: educational and training courses and activities, based on Regulation CE n. 1234/2007 e, Executive Regulation UE n. 534/2011 and on specific procedures, such as sanitary, fiscal, corporate and social responsibility to support donors and beneficiaries in their specific tasks on the reuse of surplus, improving their efficiency and their inter- and intra-organisational relationships; it started in 2009 when the supervisor association opened a specific office for the project. The tutorial programme has been expounded every year in three different steps. First, general aspects of R.e.b.u.s. are discussed during a meeting at the beginning of the year. In this meeting, the non-profit organisations involved as beneficiaries to the project review standard procedures, define future developments and exchange best practices. Second, employees and volunteers of new organisations included into the project are trained in the field, i.e., 'learning by doing'. Finally, ad hoc training is usually organised to answer specific requests or educational needs.
2. Education: lessons within focused programmes for students of primary and secondary schools and for undergraduate students. The educational project in the schools aims to increase teacher and student awareness of the R.e.b.u.s. project and other related issues through the use of slide, video, debate and group game. Topics considered during the

lessons are, for example, the importance of correct nutrition, the human solidarity, the food waste reduction, and environmental aspects. The program was presented in 35 classrooms in 2014. During these occasions, children demonstrated their learning ability and increased awareness on topics discussed by presenting final results, papers, drawings, compositions or posters. The teachers involved completed a survey about the experience. This survey included 38 questions about the material prepared and presented by the children, the aim of the laboratory, the expectations and the achievements of the educational course, the methods employed, the change of behaviour and the objectives reached after the end of the educational programme. In addition to schools, the educational programme was developed through several other channels, such as universities, or the 'European week for waste reduction', promoted by UE and Unesco; regarding this last, more than 20 groups of children participated for 2014 Verona's edition.

3. Informational: public conferences and open debates aimed at sensitising and educating citizens on food waste and sustainable development. Sharing good practices stimulates people to change their behaviour and to join the project. The sharing of knowledge increases the network of organisations involved in the project (e.g., participants suggested new potential donors, or connections with other projects, such as 'urban vegetable gardens', from which the recovery and re-use of surplus fresh vegetables is possible). The programme is usually developed by public debates open to citizens and organised in partnership with institutions like universities or local authorities. The topics discussed are varied, such as the role of civil economy and its social consequences, food, waste and recovery. To spread knowledge about R.e.b.u.s., the project was also presented in scientific conferences in the European context. Data collected through surveys on the people involved in the project underlined the increasing awareness of participants regarding food waste reduction. In scholar canteens, for example, a combined effort with the municipal ecological sector, called 'Red miles', measured food waste before and after courses and found an average reduction of 20 % of refuses.

The data analysis also demonstrated that, from the beginning of the tutorial, 2009, and the educational programmes on food waste reduction, 2011, the project has seen a

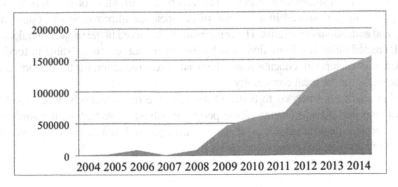

Fig. 1. The trend of recovery from 2004 to 2014

high increase in food reuse (Fig. 1). The data on recovery, in particular, show a huge increase between 2010 and 2011, after the introduction of "R.e.b.u.s. Informs".

7   Conclusions

According to Papargyropoulou et al.'s model [4], it is necessary to consider the actions involved in food waste reductions, placing such actions at the top of the food waste hierarchy. The food, even if it is reduced or lost its commercial value, often maintains its nutritional properties and still has an economic and social value. Moving from this model, our study considers education as an additional tool to enhance food waste prevention, demonstrating this through the study of the R.e.b.u.s. case. Our study also reveals how this program can be an effective tool for change people's behavior, about food waste prevention and sustainable development in general. In effect, as our findings show, the effectiveness of the project is also based on the development of "R.e.b.u.s. Informs", an ESD initiative designed to improve the awareness of consumer behaviour [35] and increase the knowledge of food waste reduction by creating several educational paths through school classes, tutorial courses and meetings for the entire local community. The educational service system is a good engine for the project and, consequently, for the food waste reduction.

Beneficiaries, donors, public administrations and citizens as operant resources become the primal source of innovation, organizational knowledge, and value. The role of the supervisor is a servant-supervisor who is there to support the organizations involved in the project; it uses Information Technology (IT) in order to facilitate the service-integration function, both within the organization and across the entire value-creation network including the user, enables the ability of all entities in the value- creation network to collaborate [24]. In R.e.b.u.s. case, IT accelerates the relationships among all the organizations involved and between organizations and individuals. All can share, increase and disseminate knowledge about arguments proposed in the educational program. We could observe the implementation of a collaborative service process based on co-creation of value between educational service providers, consumers [36] and food donors.

The educational programs can foster service innovation to achieve more satisfying results in a collaborative and interactive environment. The co-creation of value can be increased by software and the coordinator's relationships permit to access to more resources and information that stimulate to improve humans behaviour; all information is shared and all organizations are assisted in a process of competence improvement through internal training and educational programs. The organizations involved in the project, thanks to their network created through information tools by the supervisor, co-create value in food waste reduction, mutual support, education and the waste taxes reduction for the donors, creating social progress for the local community.

Further studies are needed to better understand the relationship between food waste reduction and the lifestyle change of the people involved; nevertheless, the study on the R.e.b.u.s. project demonstrates that, if people are educated and actively involved in the sustainability change, this change is possible.

References

1. Vargo, S.L., Lusch, R.F.: Service-dominant logic: continuing the evolution. J. Acad. Mark. Sci. **36**(1), 1–10 (2008)
2. Maglio, P.P., Spohrer, J.: Fundamentals of service science. J. Acad. Mark. Sci. **36**(1), 18–20 (2008)
3. Cantino, V., Devalle, A., Gandini, S., Ricciardi, F., Zerbetto, A.: Business school innovation through a service science approach: organizational and performance measurement issues. In: Nóvoa, H., Drăgoicea, M. (eds.) IESS 2015. LNBIP, vol. 201, pp. 278–288. Springer, Heidelberg (2015)
4. WCED: Our common future. World Commission on Environment and Development. Oxford University Press, Oxford, New York (1987)
5. Stern, N.: Stern Review: The Economics of Climate Change. HM Treasury, London (2006)
6. Papargyropoulou, E., Lozano, R., Steinberger, J.K., Wright, N., bin Ujang, Z.: The food waste hierarchy as a framework for the management of food surplus and food waste. J. Cleaner Prod. **76**, 106–115 (2014)
7. Heller, M.C., Keoleian, G.A.: Assessing the sustainability of the US food system: a life cycle perspective. Agric. Syst. **76**(3), 1007–1041 (2003)
8. Gustavsson, J., Cederberg, C., Sonesson, U., Van Otterdijk, R., Meybeck, A.: Global food losses and food waste. Food and Agriculture Organization of United Nations, Rome (2011)
9. European Parliament Council: Directive 2008/1/EC of the European Parliament and of the Council of 15 January Concerning Integrated Pollution Prevention and Control, Brussels (2008)
10. Redman, E., Redman, A.: Transforming sustainable food and waste behaviours by realigning domains of knowledge in our education system. J. Cleaner Prod. **64**, 147–157 (2014)
11. Kelder, S.H., Perry, C.L., Klepp, K.I., Lytle, L.L.: Longitudinal tracking of adolescent smoking, physical activity, and food choice behaviours. Am. J. Public Health **84**(7), 1121–1126 (1994)
12. Pooley, J.A., O'Connor, M.: Environmental education and attitudes: emotions and beliefs are what is needed. Environ. Behav. **32**(5), 711–723 (2000)
13. UNESCO: The Bonn declaration. http://www.desd.org/ESD2009_BonnDeclaration080409.pdf
14. Eriksen, K.G.: Why education for sustainability development needs early childhood education, the case of Norway. J. Teach. Educ. Sustain. **15**(1), 107–120 (2013)
15. Gadotti, M.: What we need to learn to save the planet. J. Educ. Sustain. Dev. **2**(1), 21–30 (2008)
16. Leal Filho, W.: About the role of universities and their contribution to sustainable development. High. Educ. Policy **24**(4), 427–438 (2011)
17. Leal Filho, W.: Teaching sustainable development at university level: current trends and future needs. J. Baltic Sea Educ. **9**(4), 273–284 (2010)
18. Cortese, A.D.: The critical role of higher education in creating a sustainable future. Planning High. Educ. **31**(3), 15–22 (2003)
19. Mirabella, N., Castellani, V., Sala, S.: Current options for the valorisation of food manufacturing waste: a review. J. Cleaner Prod. **65**, 28–41 (2014)
20. European Commission: Communication from the Commission to the Council and The European Parliament, Directive 2003/1/EC of 18 June, Integrated Product Policy. Building on Environmental Life-Cycle Thinking, Brussels (2003)

21. European Commission: Communication from the Commission to the Council, the European Parliament, the European Economic and Social Committee and the Committee of the Regions, Directive 2011/1/EC of 20 September, Roadmap to Resource Efficient, Brussels (2011)

22. European Commission: Communication from the Commission to the Council, the European Parliament, the European Economic and Social Committee and the Committee of the regions, Directive 2012/1/EC of 13 February, Innovating for Sustainable Growth. A Bio economy for Europe, Brussels (2012)

23. European Commission: Policies to encourage sustainable consumption, Technical report 061, European Communities (2010)

24. Lusch, R.F., Vargo, S.L., Wessels, G.: Toward a conceptual foundation for service science: contributions from service-dominant logic. IBM Syst. J. **47**(1), 5–14 (2008)

25. Yin, R.K.: Validity and generalization in future case study evaluations. Evaluation **19**(3), 321–332 (2013)

26. Denzin, N.K.: The Research Act: A Theoretical Introduction to Sociological Methods. McGraw-Hill, New York (1978)

27. Crotty, M.: The Foundations of Social Research, Meaning and Perspective in the Research Process. Sage, London (1998)

28. Bremner, R.H.: Giving: Charity and Philanthropy in History. Transaction Publishers, New Jersey (1996)

29. Poppendieck, J.: Sweet Charity? Emergency Food and the End of Entitlement. Penguin, London (1999)

30. Elkington, J.: Towards the suitable corporation: win-win-win business strategies for sustainable development. Calif. Manage. Rev. **36**(2), 90–100 (1994)

31. Adams, W.M., Aveling, R., Brockington, D., Dickson, B., Elliott, J., Hutton, J., Roe, D., Vira, B., Wolmer, W.: Biodiversity conservation and the eradication of poverty. Science **306**(5699), 1146–1149 (2004)

32. Porta, P.L.: Subsidiarity and new welfare. In: Bruni, L., Zamagni, S. (eds.) Handbook on the Economics of Philanthropy, Reciprocity and Social Enterprise, pp. 354–362. Edward Elgar, Cheltenham (2013)

33. Bonomi, S., Ricci, M., Tommasi, M.: The relationships between different organizational units for the development of an integrated strategy to reduce food waste and waste management. In: Proceedings of SUM Second Symposium on Urban Mining, paper 034 CISA Publisher (2014)

34. FAO: The State of Food Insecurity in the World. FAO, Rome (2001). http://www.fao.org/docrep/003/y1500e/y1500e00.htm

35. Pavlova, M.: Technology and Vocational Education for Sustainable Development: Empowering Individuals for the Future. Springer, Berlin (2008)

36. Dragoicea, M., Borangiu, T.: A service science knowledge environment in the cloud. In: Borangiu, T., Thomas, A., Trentesaux, D. (eds.) Service Orientation in Holonic and Multi agent, SCI, vol. 472, pp. 229–246. Springer, Heidelberg (2013)

The Assessment of Performance of Educational Services: The Case of Portuguese Secondary Schools

Maria C.A.S. Portela[1] and Ana S. Camanho[2(✉)]

[1] Católica Porto Business School, Porto, Portugal
csilva@porto.ucp.pt
[2] Faculdade de Engenharia da Universidade do Porto, Porto, Portugal
acamanho@fe.up.pt

Abstract. This paper describes the assessment of performance of educational services recurring to benchmarking. We adopted two perspectives for the evaluation of secondary schools, aligned with the objectives of different stakeholders. In the society perspective schools are viewed as promoting students achievement (ideally including not only academic results but also interpersonal capacities) given the students characteristics in terms of academic abilities and socio-economic backgrounds. In the educational authorities perspective schools are viewed as transforming a set of resources (including students with given characteristics in terms of academic abilities and socio-economic backgrounds and also school resources, such as teachers) into students achievement. The relative performance assessment was carried out using Data Envelopment Analysis models, followed by an exploratory analysis of contextual indicators that potentially affect schools' performance, in order to understand their impact on the educational process.

Keywords: Educational services · Secondary schools · Data Envelopment Analysis · Benchmarking

1 Introduction

This paper describes a formative performance assessment of Portuguese secondary schools. These are an essential component of the educational service continuum. Secondary education determines students' access to university, and thus influences to a large extent students' future career prospects. As a member of the European Union, Portugal is committed to the goal defined in 2000 by the Lisbon Council of "making Europe the most dynamic and knowledge based economy in the world". However, according to the OECD indicators [1], Portugal is the country with the lowest average number of years of the adult population in the educational system, one of the lowest performance of pupils in the mathematics and problem solving PISA tests (Program for International Student Assessment), and with below average performance in several other education indicators. In addition, OECD reports show that Portuguese schools have a high between-school variance in the PISA mathematics test, meaning that the schools attended by pupils matter in their attainment. It is therefore important to

© Springer International Publishing Switzerland 2016
T. Borangiu et al. (Eds.): IESS 2016, LNBIP 247, pp. 717–731, 2016.
DOI: 10.1007/978-3-319-32689-4_55

investigate differences between schools and to provide tools for the self and external evaluation of schools, so that they can improve the quality of their educational practices.

In the majority of the European countries, the evaluation of schools is at the heart of the educational system as a means to guarantee the quality of education. For example, in the UK the Department for Education publishes School performance Tables, whereas in France, the Ministry of Education publishes three indicators of school performance. In Portugal, there is legislation since 2002 that establishes the self-evaluation of schools compulsory and also contemplates their external evaluation.

This paper intends to put forth a framework based on which schools can be evaluated on a comparative basis. The main contribution of our approach consists on the development of a quantitative and contextualized analysis of educational services' performance using a benchmarking technique. This approach allows considering interactions between students, teachers, resources availability and family context in the educational value co-creation process. This process is explored from two stakeholders' perspectives: a society perspective and an educational authorities' perspective.

The quantitative methodology used to compare schools and calculate their relative efficiency is Data Envelopment Analysis (DEA).

2   Performance Evaluation in Education

Much has been written on schools evaluation as can be seen, for example, in the literature review of [2] that outlines a number of conclusions from previous studies regarding the variables affecting the educational achievement, or [3] that reviews frontier efficiency measurement techniques in education. After some decades of research, the literature reached a finding that is undisputed: schools can make a difference [4].

"Education is a service that transforms fixed quantities of inputs (that is, individuals) into individuals with different qualities" [2]. This definition of education is thorough since it outlines a number of characteristics of the production process that takes place in schools. Namely, schools provide a service that has the usual characteristics of services like intangibility and heterogeneity, which hamper standardization, and the educational service is carried out on the actual pupil, who is at the same time an input and an output of the production process. These characteristics make the evaluation of schools a particularly difficult task. [5] described some other characteristics of the education process that should be carefully taken into account in the assessments of school efficiency: (i) the time dimension of the education process, as many components of this process are only revealed a few years after the students completed the education process at school; (ii) the cumulative nature of the education process, which makes it difficult to assign the students achievements to a given school, since they are influenced by previous years of education; and (iii) the importance of elements exogenous to the school, which also determine the success of the education process for each pupil. The uniqueness of the educational production process implies that a "significant effort must be made to filter out what is really provided by each school" [5, p. 133] so that it is possible to measure correctly school efficiency and value-added.

Regarding the methodology, [5] concluded that DEA is an attractive methodology to be applied in a context as peculiar as educational services, and [3] showed that DEA has dominated educational assessment studies.

The choice of variables to be used in an educational assessment depends on the level of analysis (pupils, schools, and groups of schools). We will concentrate in this paper on the variables used in school efficiency studies, which is the focus of the empirical analysis.

The studies that use the school as the level of analysis have reached a generalized consensus about the variables that should be used in the assessments. On the input side, three groups of variables are usually considered: (i) those reflecting characteristics of pupils (like prior attainment, social-economic characteristics, etc.), (ii) those reflecting characteristics of the school (like number of teaching and non-teaching staff, expenditure per pupil, size of school, or class size), and (iii) those reflecting characteristics of teachers (like their salary, experience, or level of education). Outputs are in general related to results of students in standardized test scores, aggregated at the school level in various forms like the median [6], the mean [7, 8], or the proportion of pupils achieving more than a certain grade [9]. Other relevant outputs also related to pupils' achievement are the number of approvals or success rates [7, 10, 11], attendance rate [9, 12], number of graduates [10], and percentage of students who do not drop out from school [12]. For recent reviews on educational studies see [13, 14].

The generalized use of standardized test scores is related with the availability of these variables and the non-availability of others reflecting equally important outcomes of schooling, such as pupils' attitudes, the type of employment they get when leaving school, the preparation they are offered at school for future jobs, or the quality of their daily lives whilst at school [15]. In spite of the general agreement that pupils academic outcomes tell just a part of the story that goes on in schools, it is true that these are the only objectively measurable outcomes of schools. Empirical evidence is, however, "inconclusive about the strength of the link between test scores and subsequent achievement outside the school" [2, p. 1154]. We believe that the use of test scores is especially problematic during compulsory or basic education. Pupils that decide to follow on secondary education in general wish to continue education at universities and for that purpose achieving good academic results is perceived as a main objective. As mentioned in [2, p. 1154] "a more persuasive argument for the use of test scores relates to continuation in schooling".

3 Variables and Data

Secondary education in Portugal happens for a period of 3 years, so we collected data on this three-year period rather than on a single year. We considered in the assessment pupils that attended general courses and technological courses in secondary education.

Schools have many stakeholders, each with a different perspective of school performance. We believe it is important to define carefully the perspective since some variables may be important from one perspective but unimportant from others. In this paper we adopt two perspectives for the assessment of school performance. We called the first society perspective, which intends to be a perspective of external accountability to the society, i.e., if parents could choose the best school to foster the academic development of their children, which school would be considered the best? In this perspective schools are viewed as promoting students achievement (ideally including not only academic results but also interpersonal capacities) given the students characteristics in terms of academic abilities and socio-economic backgrounds. The second was called educational authorities perspective, where school resources, other than pupil related, are also accounted for in the performance evaluation. In this perspective schools are viewed as transforming a set of resources (including students with given characteristics in terms of academic abilities and socio-economic backgrounds and also school resources, such as teachers) into students achievement. From this perspective schools with less resources are required less in terms of achievement than schools with more resources.

There are in the literature previous distinctions between types of assessments that can be used for schools. For example [16] distinguish between the assessment of efficiency and effectiveness in schools. According to these authors, effectiveness corresponds to an assessment that uses school outcomes, like test scores, whereas efficiency corresponds to an assessment based on outputs rather than outcomes, like FTE students. Another classification can be found in [17], who considers that the distinction between efficiency and effectiveness lies on the consideration or not of expenditures and school resources. For this author efficiency is value for money (where school resources including expenditures are considered), and effectiveness (where these school resources are not accounted for) is value added. Our two perspectives can be considered comparable to the value added and value for money perspectives of [17], although under our educational authorities' perspective school resources do not need to be necessarily expenditure related.

Table 1 summarizes the input and output variables used in the DEA model for the society perspective. The input variables reflect school resources (student related variables and socio-economic context) and the outputs reflect student academic achievements.

The student related input intends to reflect the students' academic potential, which is associated with the average prior attainment of the cohort under study. This variable in measured by the average scores obtained by students on a number of subjects attended in the first trimester of the 10th year of secondary education. Note that we used a selection of subjects from general courses and technological courses, where scores vary between 0 and 20. Ideally this variable should be defined by the average scores in the national exams taken at the end of the previous educational cycle (basic education), but this variable was not available at the time of this study.

In order to reflect the socio-economic context of the school, we used two variables: the average number of years of education of parents of the cohort of students under analysis, and the percentage of students that are not subsidized by the state. The first variable intends to reflect the cultural background of pupils. We assume that parents with higher academic degrees can foster in their children motivation towards studying, leading to better academic achievements. The second variable intends to reflect the economic context where the school is located, which is known to have an impact on performance [2]. Schools in a deprived economic context will have more students applying for grants and subsidies than schools in wealthy areas. Note that we used a

Table 1. Inputs and outputs for society perspective assessment.

Inputs	Outputs
Student related variables	Average scores on exit on national exams
Average scores on entry	% students entering public higher education
Socio-economic variables	% students completing secondary education in 3 years
Avg number of years in school for the parents	% students not abandoning secondary education
% secondary students not subsidized by state	

measure of economic advantage rather than economic disadvantage so that the input is positively related to the outputs.

The outputs reflect the students' academic achievements at the end of secondary education and were measured by the following variables: Scores on national exams at the end of secondary education, Percentage of students entering public universities, Percentage of students that successfully completed secondary education in three years, Percentage of students that did not abandon secondary education.

Considering the educational authorities perspective, the list of inputs in Table 1 was extended so as to consider indicators relating to internal resources. These were represented by the variable expenditure on teacher salaries per pupil. This variable reflects the major running cost of schools. Teacher salaries are a function of the number of teachers and their position in the career. In relation to the number of teachers, schools with more staff can either have small class sizes or, in alternative, some teachers may be allocated to the promotion of extracurricular activities/projects, which are expected to have a positive impact on learning. In relation to the position in the career, that is also reflected in the teacher salaries, high positions indicate that teachers have good qualifications or experience.

As a result the input and output variables of the DEA model representing the education authorities' perspective are similar to those in Table 1, but added of the input 'Teacher salaries per pupil'.

22 schools, 12 public and 10 private were analysed in this study. The descriptive statistics for the input and output variables are reported in Table 2.

4 Model Specification

4.1 Data Envelopment Analysis Model

The DEA model used in this study is an output oriented model with constant returns to scale. Since all the variables used are ratio type variables with upper bounds on the percentage variables (100 %), we imposed restrictions on targets to guarantee that they are not higher than the upper limit, as described in [18]. The model used in this paper is identical to the one used by [19] for assessing school efficiency.

Table 2. Descriptive statistics of data.

Inputs and output variables	Average	St. Dev.	Min	Max
Average scores on entry	10.7	0.94	9.1	13.9
Average years in school for parents	10.9	1.47	9.4	15.5
% of secondary students not subsidized	86.7	12.1	50.8	100
Teacher salaries per pupil	2775.2	833.4	784.4	4074.6
Average scores on exit	11.1	1.02	9.5	13.5
% students entering universities	44.4	16.6	24.8	75.9
% students completing education in 3 years	38.5	11.5	21.9	58.8
% students that did not abandon school	89.5	9	62.9	100

We consider an input vector $\mathbf{x} = (x_1, \ldots, x_m) \in R_+^m$ used to produce an output vector $\mathbf{y} = (y_1, \ldots, y_s) \in R_+^s$ in a technology involving n production units, schools in our case. For each school $_o$ under assessment the following DEA model was used:

$$\max\{\beta_o | \sum_{j=1}^n \lambda_j y_{rj} \geq \beta_o y_{ro}, r = 1, \ldots, s, \sum_{j=1}^n \lambda_j x_{ij} \leq x_{io}, i = 1, \ldots, m$$

$$\sum_{j=1}^n \lambda_j y_{rj} \leq 100, r = 1, \ldots, s, \lambda_j \geq 0\}$$

(1)

In model (1) β_0 and λ_j are the decision variables, corresponding to the efficiency score of the school under assessment and the intensity variables that identify its peers, respectively. This was the first stage model where the radial expansion of outputs was sough to be maximised. We also run a second stage model to assure Pareto-efficiency [20].

4.2   Single Weights Model

One of the advantages of DEA is that the DMUs are given complete freedom in assigning weights to input and output variables. This reinforces certainty about inefficiencies, but may raise doubts about efficiencies, since some units might appear efficient just because they used a certain combination of weights that implied, for example, neglecting most inputs and/or outputs. In order to shed light on the performance of those units identified with 100 % efficiency in the free weights model, we assessed all the schools in the sample in relation to the same weighting scheme. This weighting scheme was not defined a priori. It was determined by a DEA model developed in this paper for the purpose of assessing all DMUs with a common set of weights. The schools that are able to maintain their efficiency status under this restrictive assumption confirm their benchmark status. The idea of using a common set of weights in a DEA analysis was first explored by [21] and also applied in [22]. However, the approaches proposed by these authors used the weights identified by the free-weights DEA model, despite the problem of multiple optimal solutions [23], or implied solving a number of DEA models with restrictions on the weights. We tried to simplify the procedure of finding a common set of weights by adapting the model of [24] to assess all DMUs with a unique set of weights. The model of [24] has the advantage of assessing all units with a single LP model, instead of requiring a specific LP model for each DMU. The model we used is shown in (2), and corresponds to the multiplier output oriented formulation.

$$
\min \begin{cases} \sum_{k=1}^{n} g_k = \sum_{k=1}^{n} \sum_{i=1}^{m} v_{ik} x_{ik}| - \sum_{r=1}^{s} u_{rk} y_{rj} + \sum_{i=1}^{m} v_{ik} x_{ij} \geq 0, j = 1, \ldots, n, k = 1, \ldots, n \\ \sum_{r=1}^{s} u_{rk} y_{rk} = 1, k = 1, \ldots, n, \qquad\qquad\qquad (b) \\ v_{ik} = v_i, i = 1, \ldots, m, u_{rk} = u_r, r = 1, \ldots, s, \qquad (a) \\ u_r, v_i \geq 0, r = 1, \ldots, s, i = 1, \ldots, m \end{cases} \Bigg\} \ (2)
$$

In model (2) the decision variables are the weights v_{ik} assigned to input $i(i = 1, \ldots, m)$ and the weights u_{rk} assigned to output $r(r = 1, \ldots, s)$ for the DMUs $k\,(k = 1, \ldots, n)$ under assessment. Without the restrictions (2a) this model is equal to the model proposed in [24] and returns for every unit $k = 1, \ldots, n$ the same efficiency score as that obtained using (1), which is given by g_k. Imposing constraints (2a) all units are assessed with the same weights v_i and u_r assigned to each input $i(i = 1, \ldots, m)$ and output $r(r = 1, \ldots, s)$. Model (2) simplifies to the formulation shown in (3) by replacing the normalizing constraints (2b), which are defined for every DMU $k\,(k = 1, \ldots, n)$ individually, by a single normalizing constraint applicable to the sum of the output from all DMUs analysed. This change in the normalization constraint is essential to ensure the feasibility of the optimization model.

$$
\min\{ \sum_{j=1}^{n} g_j = \sum_{i=1}^{m} v_i(\sum_{j=1}^{n} x_{ij})| - \sum_{r=1}^{s} u_r y_{rj} + \sum_{i=1}^{m} v_i x_{ij} \geq 0, j = 1, \ldots, n
$$

$$
\sum_{r=1}^{s} u_r(\sum_{j=1}^{n} y_{rj}) = n, u_r, v_i \geq 0, r = 1, \ldots, s, i = 1, \ldots, m\}
$$

(3)

Model (3) has the particularity of using aggregate inputs and aggregate outputs in the assessment. Therefore, the objective function value provides an aggregate efficiency score for the educational services provided by the set of schools analysed. The efficiency of each school (DMU) can be computed as the ratio of the weighted sum of inputs and the weighted sum of outputs for each school, using the common weights obtained at the optimal solution of model (3). The issue of aggregation is closely linked with the issue of common weights or common prices (since weights are shadow prices or opportunity costs that are in general unknown to the researcher). [25] addressed this issue and used a model that is very similar to model (3) except that it is a cost efficiency model rather than a technical efficiency model.

5 Analysis of Results

5.1 DEA Model

Our small sample of schools results in limited discrimination of the DEA scores, that must be interpreted with caution. The results reported intend to show the potentialities of the framework proposed and the type of results/conclusions that can be obtained. The DEA results produced for both the authorities and society perspectives revealed that 14 out of the 22 schools analysed are efficient under both perspectives. Two schools (26 and 37 are inefficient only under the society perspective, with scores 92.9 % and 80.1 %). Six schools are inefficient under both perspectives, with the average efficiency of the authorities' perspective equal to 94.3 % and average efficiency of the society perspective equal to 93.3 %.

We can conclude that the efficiency scores are quite high for both perspectives. This finding is, in our opinion, a result of two factors: (i) the small number of schools analyzed, and the corresponding small discriminant power of DEA models given the number of inputs and outputs we used; and (ii) the fact that the schools used in this study are schools that are already engaged in external evaluations and are in general concerned with quality improvements and efficiency issues. It should also be noted that the efficiency scores are relative, meaning that the high average efficiency of the schools analyzed should be interpreted as a sign of homogeneity in terms of efficiency, and cannot be extrapolated to a conclusion that Portuguese schools are very efficient.

In terms of the comparison between the society and authorities' perspective, we note that the efficiency scores for the authorities' perspective can only be greater or equal to the scores for the society perspective. When the scores differ, it is an indication that the school achieves the academic results with limited resources available in terms of teacher salaries per pupil. The greatest difference between the efficiency scores of the two perspectives was observed in schools 37 and 26, which are inefficient only in the authorities perspective. These schools have an average salary per pupil of 1887 and 2195 thousand Euros, respectively, values that are clearly below average (2775.2 thousand Euros), which can be due to a combination of effects like unexperienced teachers in the beginning of their careers, or a small number of teachers. Therefore, some of the inefficiencies detected in terms of the ability to generate good academic achievements can be explained by the lack of teacher related resources, such that these schools should not be penalized in the authorities' perspective assessment.

One way to differentiate between the efficient schools is to count the number of times each school appears in the reference set of other schools. Following this criterion, there are 3 schools that stand up as benchmark schools: school 33, school 45 and school 47 under both the educational authorities' perspective and the society perspective. When considering each perspective alone, we can add to this set school 17 for the authorities' perspective, and school 13 for the society perspective.

To illustrate what a school can learn from the DEA assessment, take for example one of the worst performing schools under the educational authorities perspective: school 40. The targets and peers for this school are shown in Table 3.

The comparison between input and output levels of inefficient school 40 with its peers can be illustrated using radar graphs (in Fig. 1), where the strengths and

Table 3. Targets and peers of school 40 in educational authorities' assessment.

Input and output variables	Observed	Target	School 47 ($\lambda = 0.828$).	School 33 ($\lambda = 0.090$)	School 17 ($\lambda = 0.021$)
Average scores on entry	10.3	10.3	11.0	11.4	10.2
Average years in school for parents	82.1	82.1	87.9	91.2	50.8
% of secondary students not subsidized	10.3	9.6	10.0	12.5	9.9
Teacher salaries per pupil	2790.9	2790.9	2247.0	3834.5	3902.8
Average scores on exit	36.4	67.8	72.4	75.9	45.4
% students entering universities	45.0	50.5	54.0	58.3	26.1
% students completing education in 3 years	80.8	90.8	97.6	90.5	80.1
% students that did not abandon school	9.5	10.7	11.3	13.0	9.5

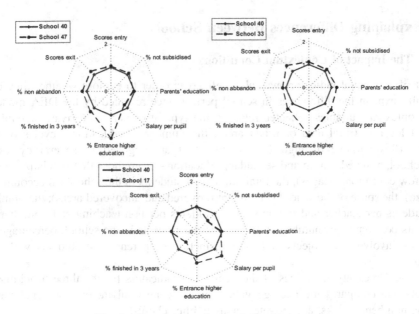

Fig. 1. Comparison of school 40 with its peers.

weaknesses of the unit assessed become clear. The values in these radars are normalized by the observed input and output levels of school 40 to make comparisons easier.

Figure 1 shows that the main weakness of school 40 is the percentage of pupils that this school places on higher education, especially when compared with schools 47 and 33. In addition, the mean scores on exit are well below the level of school 33. Note that the use of school 17 as a peer of school 40 is not very relevant, as the lambda value is quite low. Clearly the strength of school 17 is the fact that it has more disadvantaged students than most schools in the sample (it has the minimum value in the sample for the percentage of students not subsidized by the state) and even so manages to place a high percentage of its pupils in higher education.

5.2   Single Weights Model

Using the single weights model, our set of benchmarks, corresponding to the schools achieving a 100 % efficiency score in both the society and educational authorities perspectives, only comprises one public school (school 33, located in an urban area) and two private schools with association contracts (schools 45 and 13, located in peripheries of urban areas). These benchmarks are the same under the educational authorities and the society perspective as a weight of zero was placed on the input 'teacher salaries'. These 3 benchmark schools are large, with a total number of students exceeding 1500.

6   Explaining Differences Between Schools

6.1   The Impact of Contextual Conditions

A list of contextual indicators was also defined in order to explore whether they can partially explain the differences in school performance revealed by the DEA models. The contextual variables collected relate to the type of ownership (private or public), school location (rural area or urban area), the number of educational cycles of the school (this variable distinguishes schools that are engaged in several cycles – pre-school, basic education and secondary education – from those that specialized only on a few educational stages), the total number of students in the school (to account for its size), the space of the school per student (covered and uncovered areas), the number of students per teacher and the number of students per non-teaching staff, number of students per computer, number of extracurricular projects in the school, percentage of students involved in projects and the satisfaction of parents and students with the school.

Table 4 presents the values of the contextual indicators for the three benchmarks schools and compares the average values of the contextual factors for benchmarks versus non-benchmarks, and private versus public schools.

The analysis of benchmark schools revealed that the public benchmark (school 33) is different from the private benchmarks (schools 45 and 13) in terms of the contextual conditions. The contextual conditions of the public school are less favourable than

Table 4. Descriptive statistics of contextual data.

Variables	Benchmarks			Averages			
	U33	U45	U13	Bench	Nonbench	Public	Private
Total number of students	1950	1791	1512	1751	1397	1398	1515
Covered area per student (m2)	3	5	7	8	8	4	12
Uncovered area per student (m2)	8	31	38	26	22	12	38
No. students per teacher	8	12	15	12	10	9	13
No. students per non-teaching staff	36	31	20	29	27	29	24
No. students per computer	13	10	13	12	22	22.8	16.7
No. projects in the school	4	25	32	20	13	12	17
% students involved in projects	3 %	39 %	54 %	32 %	32 %	28 %	37 %
Students satisfaction with school	60	65	68	65	62	60	65
Parents satisfaction with school	56	72	73	67	66	63	71

those of the private benchmark schools in terms of the uncovered space available per student (8 m^2 in the public school, against 31 m^2 and 38 m^2 per student for the private schools). The number of projects and percentage of students involved in projects were also smaller in the public school. However, this information must be interpreted with caution, as most projects of this school are integrated in the curricular subjects, and involve all students attending classes (and therefore were not classified as extra-curricular). Parents' and students' satisfaction with the school is also lower for the public benchmark than for the private benchmarks.

The diversity in the profile of the benchmark schools in terms of the contextual factors suggests that these factors cannot explain the differences in efficiency between schools. Average values for the contextual variables observed are basically the same for the benchmark and non-benchmark schools. This is an indication that what makes schools different is associated with intangible or qualitative factors such as school management, organization or leadership.

In relation to the comparison between public and private schools in terms of the contextual variables, we found that in general private schools have better contextual conditions that public schools in all dimensions analysed except for the number of students per teacher. t-tests were run to analyse differences between private and public schools. Differences for the covered and uncovered area, and students per teacher are statistically significant (95 % confidence).

A result of interest from the comparison of private and public schools is the significant difference for the variable teachers per student. This confirms that public schools have an excessive number of teachers when compared to private schools. This is a result of the centralized recruitment of teachers in public schools, under the state responsibility, that leads to significant inefficiencies. Our models could not identify these inefficiencies in spite of considering the variable teacher salaries per pupil. This may have been a result of using a large set of input and output variables with a small number of schools. Clearly this would be an issue worth investigating further if a larger sample of schools was available.

6.2   Factors that Make a School Effective

An evaluation of schools based solely on quantitative variables, as in the analysis above, can only indicate where best practices may exist. It is important to complement this analysis with visits to schools, to explore the actual practices and processes at the schools which cannot be revealed by quantitative methods.

Our visits included all the benchmarks and also a few other schools. These visits had a double objective: first to validate the results obtained from the quantitative models, i.e. to assess whether the schools identified as benchmarks by our models can be in fact considered so, and second, to identify the practices at the benchmark schools that are worth disseminating through all the schools under analysis.

Regarding the first objective, the visits to the three benchmark schools (13, 33 and 45) corroborated the quantitative analysis that identified these schools as benchmarks. Although the benchmark schools had different features, they all had a set of common traces that justifies their classification as benchmarks.

Previous research has identified a list of qualitative factors that can make some schools more effective than others. Such listings can be found for example in [4] or [26] and include aspects such as professional leadership, learning environment, concentration on teaching and learning, high expectations, positive reinforcement, monitoring progress or home-school partnership. Guided by these previous studies we identified the following factors that differentiated our benchmark secondary schools:

- Good resources and infrastructures. All benchmark schools had good resources, including computer rooms, well equipped laboratories, working space for teachers, a library with multimedia and a reasonable number of books, and spaces allocated to the parent's association and to the psychologic assistance department.
- Motivated and stable body of teachers. The schools had experienced teachers, although one school had a significant number of young teachers. All schools considered the stability of teachers very important. The working environment amongst teachers and between teachers and students was good and friendly.
- A well-defined and inclusive school mission. A big emphasis was placed in the development of human and social characteristics of students as well as preparing them to achieve good results in national exams. All schools provided extra classes at the end of the academic year aiming at preparing students for national exams. In addition, throughout the year the school ensured the curricular goals of all subjects were achieved and provided tutorial classes for students needing extra help.
- Effective control. Students are controlled in terms of class attendance, in terms of results (students with bad results are identified and measures taken to try to improve their academic performance), in terms of evaluation (the schools seek a uniform behaviors from all teachers regarding student evaluation), and in terms of discipline (anti-social behaviors are strictly forbidden, and civil work is used as compensation for eventual damages caused).
- Self-evaluation and rigorous use of student performance data. All schools performed statistical analysis of students' results, although the sophistication of the

self-evaluation procedures varied among schools. All benchmark schools mentioned that they have already implemented or are going to start using procedures for evaluating teachers. One of the schools had a procedure for evaluating non-teaching staff and teachers with managerial positions.

- High number of extra-curricular activities with a reasonable involvement of teachers and students. All benchmark schools listed a number of extra-curricular activities available for students. In most cases these extra-curricular activities were organized in clubs, such as dance, school journal, radio station, theater and chess.
- Involvement of students' parents. In all cases the parents associations was pro-active in the school, with a room for meeting and organizing their activities.
- Leadership well adapted to the school context. The managerial styles of school management were different in the three benchmark schools visited. However, a few common traces of directors from these schools were their availability (there was always someone in the direction to whom people could address) and a good capacity to obtain extra funds from the community (city councils and firms).

7 Conclusions

This paper assessed a small sample of Portuguese secondary schools using DEA. Schools were assessed from two perspectives - a society perspective and an educational authorities' perspective - that imply a different specification of the input set used to evaluate schools. A CRS model with additional constraints on targets was used because all variables were ratios and most of them had an upper limit of 100 %. The model allowed schools to freely choose the weights assigned to each of the factors considered in the assessment, but in order to improve the discrimination of the efficiency results and to identify best performing schools we also applied a model with common weights for all schools.

The results showed that the relative efficiency of the schools analyzed is quite high, meaning that the performance of these schools is homogenous. Nevertheless, the comparison between benchmark and inefficient schools pointed directions for performance improvement.

A major limitation of this study related to the use of a small sample of schools, which means that the analysis reported serves mainly to illustrate the potential of the method employed. There are also limitations associated with missing data. Although this limitation was overcome in the DEA analysis, it prevented the use of more sophisticated techniques to analyze *a posteriori* the drivers of efficiency.

Some visits to benchmark and worst performing schools were conducted as a way to try to identify best practices. This qualitative analysis of schools proved important to reinforce our belief that schools identified as benchmarks could indeed be considered so. These visits also enabled the identification of a set of common characteristics shared by the benchmarks, which can contribute to improved school effectiveness.

References

1. Organisation for Economic Co-operation and Development. Education at a glance, OECD indicators 2005 - executive summary. Technical report, OECD publishing (2005)
2. Hanushek, E.: The economics of schooling: production and efficiency in public schools. J. Econ. Lit. **XXIV**, 1141–1177 (1986)
3. Worthington, A.C.: An empirical survey of frontier efficiency measurement techniques in education. Educ. Econ. **9**(3), 245–268 (2001)
4. MacBeath, J., Mortimore, P.: Improving School Effectiveness. Open University Press, Philadelphia (2001)
5. Mancebón, M., Bandrés, E.: Efficiency evaluation in secondary schools: the key role of model specification and of ex post analysis of results. Educ. Econ. **7**(2), 131–152 (1999)
6. Bessent, A., Bessent, W.: Determining the comparative efficiency of schools through data envelopment analysis. Educ. Adm. Q. **16**(2), 57–75 (1980)
7. Muñiz, M.A.: Separating managerial inefficiency and external conditions in data envelopment analysis. Eur. J. Oper. Res. **143**, 625–643 (2002)
8. Mizala, A., Romaguera, P., Farren, D.: The technical efficiency of schools in Chile. Appl. Econ. **34**, 1533–1552 (2002)
9. Bradley, S., Johnes, G., Millington, J.: The effect of competition on the efficiency of secondary schools in England. Eur. J. Oper. Res. **135**, 545–568 (2001)
10. Kirjavainen, T., Loikkanen, H.A.: Efficiency differences of Finnish senior secondary schools: an application of DEA and Tobit analysis. Econ. Educ. Rev. **17**(4), 377–394 (1998)
11. Oliveira, M.A., Santos, C.: Assessing school efficiency in Portugal using FDH and bootstrapping. Appl. Econ. **37**, 957–968 (2005)
12. Arnold, V., Bardhan, I., Cooper, W., Kumbhakar, S.: New uses and statistical regressions for efficiency evaluation and estimation - with an illustrative application to public secondary schools in Texas. Ann. Oper. Res. **66**, 255–277 (1996)
13. Johnes, J.: Operational research in education. Eur. J. Oper. Res. **243**(3), 683–696 (2015)
14. De Witte, K., López-Torres, L.: Efficiency in education: a review of literature and a way forward. J. Oper. Res. Soc. (2016). doi:10.1057/jors.2015.92
15. Gray, J.: A competitive edge: examination results and the probable limits of secondary school effectiveness. Educ. Rev. **33**(1), 25–35 (1981)
16. Banker, R.D., Janakiraman, S., Natarajan, R.: Analysis of trends in technical and allocative efficiency: an application to Texas public school districts. Eur. J. Oper. Res. **154**(2), 477–491 (2004)
17. Mayston, D.: Measuring and managing educational performance. J. Oper. Res. Soc. **54**, 679–691 (2003)
18. Cooper, W.W., Seiford, L.M., Tone, K.: Data Envelopment Analysis: A Comprehensive Text with Models, Applications, References and DEA-Solver Software. Kluwer Academic Publishers, Boston (2000)
19. Ray, S.C.: Resource-use efficiency in public schools: a study of connecticut data. Manage. Sci. **37**(12), 1620–1628 (1991)
20. Charnes, A., Cooper, W.W., Rhodes, E.: Measuring the efficiency of decision making units. Eur. J. Oper. Res. **2**, 429–444 (1978)
21. Roll, Y., Cook, W.D., Golany, B.: Controlling factor weights in data envelopment analysis. IIE Trans. **23**(1), 2–9 (1991)
22. Cook, W.D., Kazakov, A., Roll, Y., Seiford, L.M.: A data envelopment approach to measuring efficiency: case analysis of highway maintenance patrols. J. Socio-econ. **20**(1), 83–103 (1991)

23. Cooper, W., Ruiz, J., Sirvent, I.: Choosing weights from alternative optimal solutions of dual multiplier models in DEA. Eur. J. Oper. Res. **180**, 443–458 (2007)
24. Post, T., Spronk, J.: Performance benchmarking using interactive data envelopment analysis. Eur. J. Oper. Res. **115**, 472–487 (1999)
25. Kuosmanen, T., Cherchye, L., Sipilainen, T.: The law of one price in data envelopment analysis: Restricting weight flexibility across firms. Eur. J. Oper. Res. **170**, 735–757 (2006)
26. Sammons, P., Hillman, J., Mortimore, P.: Key characteristics of effective schools; a review of school effectiveness research. Report by the Institute of Education (University of London) for the Office of Standards in Education (1995)

Examining Cloud Computing Adoption Intention in Higher Education: Exploratory Study

Gheorghe Militaru[✉], Anca Alexandra Purcărea, Olivia Doina Negoiță, and Andrei Niculescu

Department of Management, Faculty of Entrepreneurship,
Business Engineering and Management, University Politehnica of Bucharest,
Splaiul Independentei 313, 060042 Bucharest, Romania
{gheorghe.militaru,anca.purcarea}@upb.ro,
negoita.olivia@gmail.com, andrei@niculescu.com

Abstract. The purpose of this study was to examining the factors that lead to cloud computing adoption in a higher education setting. This cross-sectional empirical research is based on the Technology Acceptance Model (TAM) framework. Data was collected by surveying 96 students from University Politehnica of Bucharest, Romania. The factors that affect cloud computing adoption in higher education were identified and tested using LISREL software. The findings suggested that factors identified can be successfully integrated in our conceptual model. Perceived value and usefulness have a strong positive influence on intentions to use cloud computing in higher education, but student's attitude towards technology had no significant effects on dependent variable. Perceived risk has significant negative effects on students' intentions to use cloud computing. The findings are expected to enhance the understanding of cloud computing adoption for students and faculty members. The implication of these findings for faculty members and students are discussed.

Keywords: Cloud computing · Higher education · Virtualization · TAM model

1 Introduction

Universities must become more flexible in order to attract the best and brightest students in a highly competitive market. The quality of teaching depends on the capacity of university to attract and retain the best talent. With rising student expectations of employability and intense competition, universities need to invest in infrastructure and teaching process. On the other hand, teaching and learning costs are increasing rapidly. A solution to cost reduction is cloud computing adoption in which dynamically scalable and often virtualized resources are provided as a service over the internet to students and faculty members [1].

A large number of organizations are expected to rely on the cloud for more than half of their IT services by 2020 [2]. They are turning on external suppliers of infrastructure, software and services. Users pay for the service as an operating expense without incurring any significant initial capital expenditure. Universities cannot stay away from these

© Springer International Publishing Switzerland 2016
T. Borangiu et al. (Eds.): IESS 2016, LNBIP 247, pp. 732–741, 2016.
DOI: 10.1007/978-3-319-32689-4_56

changes because they can reduce their investment in IT infrastructure and improve accessibility of students anytime and anywhere.

Cloud computing is a pool of computing resources that are accessible over the internet and dynamically configured to optimize resource utilization [1]. Thus, cloud computing is a cluster of service solutions based on computing resources, such as databases services, virtual servers, service workflows or configurations of distributed computing systems [3]. Virtualization enables application consolidation on the same physical hardware infrastructure. Virtualization is the technology that hides the physical characteristics of a computing platform from the users by its emulating.

Many universities increasingly discover that their substantial capital investments in information technology are often underutilization. Some studies found that desktop computers have an average capacity utilization of less than 5 % [4]. A variety of factors may influence the adoption of Cloud computing solutions. Many universities are concerned about such issues as data security, reliability, reduced implementation and maintenance of IT infrastructure, develop a flexible and scalable infrastructure, storage and software application that are configurable based user requirements [5]. Nonetheless, the issue of how to identify significant factors influencing cloud computing adoption takes on considerable importance. Although many studies have investigated the potential of cloud computing and development trends in terms of the adoption of cloud computing in business environment, few studies have investigate in depth this issue in higher education context.

Despite the existence of several studies about cloud computing, it is not clear how it can improve the teaching and learning processes in higher education institutions to determine its adoption. Consequently, the aim of this study is to explore the relationships between various factors on students' intentions to use cloud computing. This study attempts to extend the scope of research by incorporating technical, affective and behavioral factors in our investigation. However, there is little research that explicitly links between students' attitude towards technology, internet self-efficacy and students' intentions to use cloud computing.

Next follows a literature review and hypotheses development. Then a section is dedicated to test our model and hypotheses on data collected from respondents. Next, we present our research methodology, which is followed by our empirical analysis results. The paper concludes with a discussion of our findings, the theoretical and practical contributions of our work, and future research directions.

2   Theory and Hypothesis Development

In this section, we present our theoretical setting and the construction of a model that present a set of factors relevant to understanding the intention to use of cloud computing in higher education institutions. The factors and conditions enabling cloud computing adoption can be identified using the predictive power of various frameworks based on the theory of planned behaviour. Previous studies examined the opportunities and risks associate with cloud computing acceptance in business.

Cloud computing represents a convergence of IT efficiency and organization agility. Thus, students can use computational tools through resources that are shared, dynamically scalable, rapidly provided, and virtualized. Resources such as CPU, memory, network, and bandwidth can be flexibly allocated on demand according to the workload intensity [6]. Cloud computing involves making computing, data storage, and software services available via the Internet [7]. Generally, cloud services can be divided into three categories: Software as a Service (SaaS), Platform as a Service (PaaS), and Infrastructure as a Service (IaaS).

SaaS enables users to access a software application as a service through the web (e.g., Google Apps, Google Mail, Google Docs, CRM, Facebook, and Twitter). The user pays for the serviced based on the use of application, university focus on core its activities integrating learning services in the cloud. PaaS provides a development platform in the network cloud and allows users to customize, deploy and test their new applications (e.g., Microsoft's Azure Service Platform, Google App Engine, and Amazon's Relational Database Services). IaaS uses virtualization extensively for processing, storage, network as a service on a pay-as-you-use basis whereby storage and compute capabilities are offered as a service (e.g., Amazon's S3, Education ERP, EC2 computing platform). Cloud providers supply users with requisite infrastructure to support their teaching and learning processes, including the hardware, operating system, storage, servers, and networking equipment in an on-demand service [8].

The technology acceptance model (**TAM**) was developed for predicting individual behaviour. We examined cloud computing acceptance from the perspective of students' perceptions. According to the expectation-value theory individual attitudes toward a specific behaviour depend on beliefs and evaluations of behaviour outcomes (e.g., perceived usefulness and perceived ease of use) [9]. These consequences were proposed in [10] a study about the Unified Theory of Acceptance and Use of Technology (UTAUT) model. The most recent TAM 3 developed in [10] is based on the initial TAM after refinements and is presented in Fig. 1.

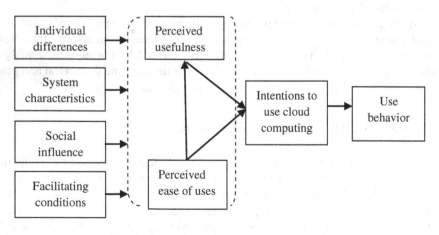

Fig. 1. Technology Acceptance Model 3 [10]

The attitude toward cloud computing services is one individual factor included for assessing individual evaluation and intention to use these services in higher education institutions. Perceived usefulness is the degree to which a person believes that using cloud computing solution would enhance his or her learning performance. This construct is used to capture the value of the cloud computing utility in accomplishing activities specific teaching, learning and research processes. Perceived usefulness influences directly the user's intention to adopt this solution in an education system [9]. Thus, we hypothesise that:

H1: *Perceived usefulness will have a positive effect on student intention to use cloud computing services in higher education.*

Perceived ease of use is defined as the degree to which an individual can use the cloud computing services to accomplish his tasks specific teaching, learning and research processes. Universities can use cloud computing technology and its virtualisation capability to build many virtual parallel computing environments which supports various multidisciplinary programs and various research programs. The virtualization of computer resources enables savings on hardware, software, and maintenance costs leads to a lowering of operational costs and improving the quality of educational services. Increased student access to professional and research tools, for example, access to Virtual Computing Lab, can multiply the working capacity of the physical server. This dimension influences directly the individual's intention to accept cloud computing solution in his university. Consequently, we hypothesise that:

H2: *Perceived ease of use will have a positive effect on student intention to use cloud computing services in higher education.*

Behavioural intentions differ in terms of duration, intensity and frequency. The critical predictor of behaviour is intention. Attitude toward using cloud computing directly influence one's behavioural intention to use this solution in high education institutions [9]. For education, higher congruence between a student's or teacher's work style and the activities supported by cloud computing services results in greater perceived usefulness. The integration of existing learning tools with cloud computing services in a flexible way can support the student-cantered learning activities (e.g., by collaboration, interaction, and monitoring of student progress). Based on literature review, we expect that the perceived ease of use is positively related to perceived usefulness. Consequently, we formulate the hypothesis that:

H3: *Perceived ease of use is positively related to student perceptions of the usefulness of the cloud computing use.*

Cloud computing services can be accessed in several access media such as desktops, laptops, smart phones and tablets. Thus, students can use computing resources from their terminal devices anywhere and anytime without knowing the physical location to those computing resources. Applications and storage spaces hosted on central server can be accessed by using various computers, and students can access them using a standardized interface. Virtualization can create learning environments more cost effectively.

Moreover, student attitudes about mobility are hypothesized to influence perceived ease of use because a technology that is more compatible with learning or teaching activities is more likely to be recognized as easy to use [9]. The following hypothesis is proposed:

H4: *Students' attitude towards technology is positively related to perceptions regarding usefulness (H4a) and ease of use of the cloud computing use (H4b).*

Risk perceived of cloud computing is an essential driver of cloud adoption in higher education institutions. It denotes the levels of performance, reliability, security, privacy, trust, and service availability. Reliability refers to a person's perception of a system's reliability and responsiveness during normal operations [9]. Cloud reliability refers to hardware and software facilities offered by cloud providers, connectivity and user's digital skills. Bandwidth, security, privacy, reliability risks and connectivity to the cloud is a concern for all users. Cloud provider distributes the computing resources in several locations, but in case of bugs, the cloud provider can redirect the end user request to other physical locations where a back-up of computing resources can be found [11]. The adoption of cloud computing is negatively associated with perceived risk. Perceived risk can hinder the adoption of cloud computing in higher education [12]. Consequently, we formulate the hypothesis that:

H5: *Risk perceived is negatively related to perceptions regarding usefulness (H5a) and ease of use of the cloud computing in higher education (H5b).*

Cloud computing ads value with small capital expenses because cloud providers have the ability to add capacity quickly and easily, and with no capital. Technical IT capabilities are important facilitators of the cloud adopted and interoperability and portability are required to migrate to cloud computing. In this case, cloud computing offers advantages, such as collaboration, analytics, and application development [13]. Cloud provider enables universities to focus on their core teaching, learning, and research processes because they can free up resources, which can be used in other areas that create value [14]. How a university uses its capabilities to successfully meet student's needs and offer high teaching quality is the key for its future. A centralized cloud at the level of higher education institution may improve operational efficiency, security, scalability, interoperability and students' performance [11]. For example, lower operational and capital expenses can be achieved by reducing the software licensing and software. Consequently, we hypothesise that:

H6: *Perceived value is positively related to perceived usefulness of cloud computing used in higher education institutions.*

Students may differ substantially in their skills, especially in their internet experiences and capabilities. Internet self-efficacy refers to one's belief in his or her capability to accomplish online tasks or assignments, including understanding of internet software and hardware [15]. Online learning environments are designed to promote personalization and adaptability to the students' needs. Liang and Wu [16] indicated that higher internet self-efficacy led to higher motivations for web-based learning and show preference for cloud computing. Cloud providers will enable students' access to expansive software from anyplace and anytime. Therefore, it is hypothesized:

H7: *Internet self-efficacy will have a positive effect on perceived ease of uses of cloud computing in higher education institutions.*

To reduce the variance caused by other factors, we controlled for the age and gender of respondents. The conceptual framework is shown in Fig. 2. Relationships among the constructs were empirically tested as follows.

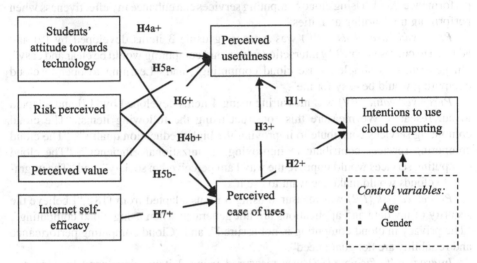

Fig. 2. Conceptual framework

3 Method

3.1 Research Context

To test the conceptual model and hypotheses, we conducted a survey using a paper-based questionnaire and some interviews with faculty members at University Politehnica of Bucharest (UPB). This university is the largest and the oldest technical university in Romania. As for research, a survey instrument was created using a combination of existing and newly development measures. This study used cross-sectional survey data. The use of technological information in education and professional training are elements that define the university profile. The proposed model will be empirically examined using the Structural Equation Model (SEM) to analyze data collected by a survey. The data for this study were collected using a questionnaire consisted of seven constructs that was administrated to the students from UPB. The sample consists of engineering students aged between 20 and 26 years old. The sample also represents a higher number of females (54 or 56 %) compared to males (42 or 44 %). The majority of respondents who participated in the survey have good digital skills.

3.2 Measures

Most of the variables involved in this study were measured with items using a seven-point Likert scale with anchors ranging from strongly disagree to strongly agree. To measure the dependent variable – *intentions to use cloud computing (IUC)*, respondents were asked to present their opinions about the following statements [9]: "Using cloud computing is pleasant for me", "I like to use the cloud computing services", and "I find using cloud computing services enjoyable".

Perceived usefulness (PU) was measuring using 2 items developed by [9] and adapted to our research: "Using cloud computing services improves my academic performance", and "Using cloud computing services can enhance my effectiveness when performing my learning activities".

Perceived ease of use (PE) was measuring using 3 items developed by [9] and adapted to our research: "My interaction with cloud computing would be clear and easy", "In general, it is simple to use cloud computing", and "Learning to operate cloud computing would be easy for me".

Perceived value (PV) was measuring using 4 items developed by [17] and adapted to our research. We measure this construct using the following items: "The cloud computing services contribute to improving the higher education quality". "The cloud computing services contribute to improving organizational efficiency", "The cloud computing services would improve the way I am perceived in society", and "The migration to clouds would make me want to use it".

Perceived risk (PR) was measured using 3 items adapted from [18]: "I believe the security of my data and applications are not generated when using cloud computing", "The privacy in cloud computing is not assured", and "Cloud computing performance and reliability are not guaranteed".

Internet self-efficacy (ISE) was measured using 2 items developed by [15] and adapted for this study: "The extent to which students feel confident with the internet hardware and software" and "The extent to which students can gather data through internet".

Students' attitude towards technology (SAT) was measured using 2 items: "I believe that technology enhances my learning experience", and "I believe that technology gives me the opportunity to acquire new knowledge and increase my satisfaction".

Control Variables: Following previous studies, we controlled for student age and gender. *Gender (G)*, as dummy variable, was included to control for the specific impact on the engineering student preferences for cloud computing. As the distribution of student age differed from normality, we employed its logarithmical terms. Thus, *student age (SA)* was represented as the log of the number of years.

4 Analyses and Results

The data were subjected to factor analysis in order to validate the instruments. A principal components factor analysis was employed to identify constructs and to isolate a small number of factors for our prediction. All factors have eigenvalues equal to or greater than 1.00 [19].

The conceptual model was tested for reliability and validity. For each latent variable we calculate the composite reliability and average variance explained (AVE). Convergent validity is established by analyzing the average variance extract (AVE), whose value should exceed 0.5 and composite reliabilities 0.6. Convergent validity is strong because all latent variables have high loading score, higher than 0.7 [19].

A correlation matrix between latent variables with descriptive statistics (mean and standard deviation) for the final constructs is shown in Table 1. We found that there were very low correlations between variables.

Table 1. Descriptive and correlation matrix (N = 96)

Construct	Mean	S.D.	1	2	3	4	5	6	7	8
IVC (1)	5.21	1.53	–							
PU (2)	4.69	0.87	.356	–						
PE (3)	5.87	1.16	.243	.283	–					
PV (4)	5.43	1.63	.379	.152	.277	–				
PR (5)	4.36	1.41	.275	.352	.124	.281	–			
ISE (6)	3.64	0.98	.176	.271	.238	.262	.326	–		
SAT (7)	3.87	1.07	.453	.311	.341	.178	.166	.376	–	
G (8)	0.44	0.13	.337	.166	.218	.226	.322	.271	.351	–
SA (9)	3.18	1.3	.132	.171	.128	.155	.331	.221	.127	.341

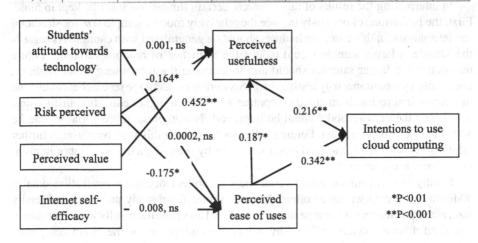

Fig. 3. Data analysis results

The results of the structural model test (LISREL) are presented in Fig. 3. Of the 9 paths examined, we found 6 are significant. Broadly speaking, most of the hypotheses are supported, except H4a + , H4b + , and H7 + . The path coefficient of perceived usefulness to students' intention to use cloud computing ($\beta = 0.216$) is significant at $p < 0.001$. Also, the path coefficient of perceived ease of uses to students' intention to use cloud computing ($\beta = 0.342$) is significant at p < 0.001. The path coefficient of perceived ease of use to perceived usefulness ($\beta = 0.187$) is significant at p < 0.01. However, the paths from students' attitude towards technology to perceived usefulness or from students' attitude towards technology to perceived ease of uses or from internet self-efficacy to perceived ease of uses are not significant ($\beta = 0.001$, $\beta = 0.008$, $\beta = 0.0002$, ns).

The path coefficient of risk perceived to perceived usefulness ($\beta = -0.164$) is significant but negatively at p < 0.01. Also, the path coefficient of risk perceived to perceived ease of uses ($\beta = -0.175$) is significant but negatively at p < 0.01. Finally, the path coefficient of perceived value to perceived usefulness ($\beta = 0.452$) is significant at p < 0.001.

5   Conclusions

This study investigates the influence of students' attitude towards technology, perceived risk, perceived value, interest self-efficacy, perceived usefulness, and perceived ease of uses on students' intentions to use cloud computing in higher education institutions. However, some factors (students' attitude towards technology and interest self-efficacy) no support hypotheses related. We found that students' intentions to use cloud computing was negatively influenced of risk perceived. This study contributes to the existing literature by providing empirical support for the cloud computing adoption in higher education institutions.

In interpreting the results of this research, certain limitations must be kept in mind. First, the limitations of our study include the relatively modest sample size for structural model analysis. In this case, our findings should be generalized with caution. As regards the sample, a larger sample would reduce the influence of random variation. Future research using larger samples should aim to examine the robustness of our findings, preferably by simultaneously testing them. Second, we encourage researchers to engage in longitudinal research on cloud computing adoption in higher education institutions. Third, any theoretical model could be improved. Nonetheless, more variables can be added to our research model. Future studies look to refine this variable through further pilot testing with academics and practitioners, or by selecting a different set of items to represent this construct.

Finally, we encourage future researchers to collect objective innovation data in addition to the data we have collected, for example, about study programs, university size, academic leadership or type of university, and compare the results with our finding. We need a better understanding why universities adopt or not the cloud computing services to improve teaching and learning processes.

References

1. Shawish, A., Salama, M.: Cloud computing - paradigms and technologies. In: Xhafa, F., Bessis, N. (eds.) Inter-cooperative Collective Intelligence: Techniques and Applications. Studies in Computational Intelligence, vol. 495, pp. 39–67. Springer, Heidelberg (2014)

2. Garrison, G., Wakefield, R.L., Kim, S.: The effects of IT capabilities and delivery model on cloud computing success and from performance for cloud supported processes and operations. Int. J. Inf. Manage. **35**, 377–393 (2015)
3. Goscinski, A., Brock, M.: Toward dynamic and attribute based publication, discovery and selection for cloud computing. Future Gener. Comput. Syst. (2010). doi:10.1016/j.future.2010.03.009
4. Marston, S., Li, Z., Bandyopadhyay, S., Zhang, J., Ghelsari, A.: Cloud computing – the business perspective. Decis. Support Syst. **51**, 176–189 (2011)
5. Garrison, G., Kim, S., Wakefield, R.: Factors leading to the successful deployment of cloud computing. Commun. ACM **55**(9), 62–68 (2012)
6. Vouk, M.: Cloud computing – issues, research and implementations. J. Comput. Inf. Technol. **16**, 235–246 (2008)
7. Wu, W.W.: Mining significant factors affecting the adoption of SaaS using the rough set approach. J. Syst. Softw. **84**, 435–441 (2011)
8. Wang, W., Rashid, A., Chuang, H.M.: Toward the trend of cloud computing. J. Electron. Commer. Res. **12**(4), 238–242 (2011)
9. Davis, F.D., Bagozzi, R.P., Wasshaw, P.R.: User acceptance of computer technology: a comparison of two theoretical models. Manage. Sci. **35**(8), 982–1003 (1989)
10. Venkatesh, V., Bala, H.: Technology Acceptance Model 3 and a research agenda on interventions. Decis. Sci. **39**(20), 273–315 (2008)
11. Sasikala, S., Prema, S.: Massive centralized cloud computing (MCCC) exploration in higher education. Adv. Comput. Sci. Technol. **3**(2), 111–118 (2010)
12. Alotaibi, M.B.: Exploring users' attitudes and intentions toward the adoption of cloud computing in Saudi Arabia: an empirical investigation. J. Comput. Sci. **10**(11), 2315–2325 (2014)
13. McAfee, A.: What every CEO needs to know about the cloud. Harvard Bus. Rev. **89**, 125–132 (2011)
14. Levina, N., Ross, J.W.: From the vendor's perspective: exploring the value proposition in information technology outsourcing. J. Manage. Inf. **27**(3), 331–364 (2003)
15. Eastin, M.S., LaRose, R.: Internet self-efficacy and the psychology of the digital divide (2000). http://jcmc.indiana.edu/vol6/issue1/eastin.html
16. Liang, J.C., Wu, S.H.: Nurses' motivations for web-based learning and the role of internet self-efficacy. Innovations Educ. Teach. Int. **47**(1), 25–37 (2010)
17. Sweeney, J.C., Souter, G.N.: Consumer perceived value: the development of a multiple item scale. J. Retail. **77**, 203–220 (2001)
18. Benlian, A., Hess, T.: Opportunities and risks of software-as-a-service: findings from a survey of IT executives. Decis. Support Syst. **52**(1), 232–246 (2011)
19. Hair, J., Black, B., Anderson, R., Tatham, R.: Multivariate Data Analysis, 6th edn. Prentice-Hall, Upper Saddle River (2006)

Service Science Textbooks: Opportunities of an Interdisciplinary Approach

Johannes Kunze von Bischhoffshausen[✉], Peter Hottum, and Ronny Schüritz

Karlsruhe Institute of Technology, Englerstr. 11, 76131 Karlsruhe, Germany
{johannes.kunze,peter.hottum,ronny.schueritz}@kit.edu

Abstract. With the rise of service science, management and engineering as an independent and interdisciplinary research school, several courses and entire study programs emerged in several universities around the world. Several textbooks address teaching service science from the perspective of a specific discipline such as marketing, operations management or computer science. Therefore, so far teaching service science requires the preparation and combination of lecture material from different textbooks and other teaching material, since there was a lack of interdisciplinary and integrated textbooks for teaching service science. This paper reviews existing service textbooks for motivating the need for an integrated service science textbook. Furthermore, the outline of a new forthcoming interdisciplinary service science textbook is presented. This textbook integrates several disciplines, such as business and economics, quantitative sciences, and computer science. The textbook therefore provides an interdisciplinary map of the world of service science that conquers the challenges to explain service systems to students and practitioners. This enables lecturers to organize their courses along a comprehensive and integrated course concept which has been the result of teaching service science at universities for several years.

Keywords: Service science · Service systems · Teaching · Textbook

1 Introduction

Service Science, also "Service Science, Management, and Engineering" (SSME) is inherently interdisciplinary, integrating multiple disciplines from economics, marketing, computer science, etc. [1]. Most textbooks dealing with services are dominated by a certain discipline (marketing, operations, computer science). This requires the use multiple textbooks and other teaching material for university courses dealing with service systems, which can be very cost-intensive and inconvenient for both, students and lecturers. This short paper therefore presents the outline of a forthcoming textbook on service systems, integrating content from multiple disciplines in order to create a holistic teaching concept for service science and service systems.

The structure of this paper is as follows: Sect. 2 summarizes the origin of service science and its implications for teaching, Sect. 3 reviews existing service textbooks from service marketing, service operations, and computer science. Section 4 subsequently

© Springer International Publishing Switzerland 2016
T. Borangiu et al. (Eds.): IESS 2016, LNBIP 247, pp. 742–749, 2016.
DOI: 10.1007/978-3-319-32689-4_57

presents the outline of the new interdisciplinary service textbook. Section 5 concludes this paper and discusses its implications for teaching.

2   Service Science and Service Systems

As Service Science is an interdisciplinary research school, originated i.a. in the domains of "economics, operations research, industrial engineering, management of information systems, multi-agent systems, or the science of complex systems" [1], it is based on multiple traditions and research fields in academia. Service Science raises the claim to integrate methods from those originated disciplines and apply them to diverse service industries, scientific research as well as teaching concepts following this idea should be interdisciplinary as well. To address these requirements, this paper and the presented analysis is rooted in different disciplines.

Service Science as a research discipline was initially fostered by IBM and the Cambridge University's Institute for Manufacturing in the 2000s [2]. It is based on the work of Vargo and Lusch, who set the foundation of a 'service-dominant logic' (SD logic), where "value is defined by and co-created with the consumer rather than embedded in output" [3]. Instead of a goods-centered dominant logic, where goods are the "primary unit of exchange" [3], with their perspective the exchange "to acquire the benefits of specialized competences (knowledge and skills), or services" [3] is the essential part of a service-centered dominant logic and a huge shift in examining economical collaboration. Based on this SD logic the exchange of competencies and information between several partners raises more attention in research as well as education. Hereby, especially the activities of the customer, who was mainly a consumer in the goods-dominant logic (GD logic), and the different interactions with the provider become more important as all involved parties may provide competencies and information. Textbooks that educate service students as well as practitioners have to address this shift in provider-customer interaction and common creation of value.

Originally, Service Science is the shortened term for "Service Science, Management, and Engineering" (SSME) [1]. The term points out the targeted interdisciplinary dialogue between different disciplines from science, management and engineering with one main goal: examine the service provision within a systemic view.

The service provider, the provider's network and the customer(s) are seen as parts of a system, so called service system, which collaborates to achieve a certain value. This is realized by the application "of competences [...] through deeds, processes and performance for the benefit of another entity or the entity itself" [3]. Based on [4] this implies two different aspects. On the one hand, it focuses the importance of information, knowledge and competencies as operant resources for the application and the common exploitation of the service(s). On the other hand, it emphasizes the understanding of value creation through the application of a service.

Both aspects, the importance of those service-specific aspects as well as the understanding of value creation, are essential for textbooks on Service Science, that address students and practitioners. As managing value co-creation within service systems is not meant to optimize the inputs of a party at the expense of another party, ways to address potentially contradictory targets have to be discussed in according textbooks.

3   State-of-the-Art in Service Textbooks

Originated from several research disciplines, textbooks related to service science have been published. This review focuses on traditional textbooks only, although more and more teaching material is published in other formats such as online courses. In the following, a comprehensive selection of these textbooks is reviewed and discussed: Firstly, textbooks that have been written by scholars from the services marketing community; second, textbooks that are related to service operations; and lastly, textbooks that are related to computer science disciplines have been taken into account for a short review (Table 1). The traditional service disciplines service marketing and service operations are the primary focus of this review, supplemented by a selection of IT textbooks. Only academic textbooks, which are intended to be used as a course textbook at universities, have been considered in the review of service marketing and service operations textbooks.

Table 1. Overview of reviewed service textbooks

Textbook	Discipline	Focus
Zeithaml, Bitner, Gremler [5]	Marketing	GAP model
Lovelock, Wirtz [7]	Marketing	7 P's
Fisk, Grove, John [8]	Marketing	Theater model and IT
Grönroos [9]	Marketing	Nordic school's services marketing view
Fitzsimmons, Fitzimmons, Bordoloi [10]	Operations	Designing a service enterprise, service operations, quantitative methods
Johnston, Clark [11]	Operations	Service operations, customer-supplier relationships, delivery, performance management
Daskin [12]	Operations	Quantitative methods, mostly from operations research
Orand, Villarreal [13]	IT	IT Service Management
Krafzig, Banke, Slama [14]	IT	Web Services, SOA

3.1   Marketing Textbooks

The first reviewed textbook is *Services Marketing – Integrating Customer Focus Across the Firm* by Zeithaml et al. [5]. This widely adopted[1] service marketing textbook uses the service quality GAP model [6] as the basic conceptual framework to structure the book. Therefore, twelve out of sixteen chapters are related to the four initial gaps of the model [6]. After an introduction into fundamental concepts of service marketing, such as service conceptualizations and consumer behavior, two chapters (Part 2) deal with addressing the market research gap through performing market research and building

---

[1] This service textbook has by far the highest international amazon ranking (in December 2015).

customer relationships. The following three chapters (Part 3) address the service design gap, including chapters on service innovation and design, customer-defined service standards and physical evidence and the servicescape. Five chapters (Part 4) are concerned with delivering and performing service. Those chapters detail the roles of employees and customers, electronic service delivery, capacity management and service recovery. Two chapters (Part 5) are then related to the perception gap and how to manage service promises, including marketing communications and pricing in a service context. The last chapter (Part 6) breaks down the financial impact of service quality.

The second reviewed service marketing textbook is *Services Marketing – People, Technology, Strategy* by Lovelock and Wirtz [7]. It is a marketing textbook structured according to the seven P's of service marketing. The first part of the book is concerned with service definitions and basic concepts such as consumer behavior and service competition. The second part of the book details the application of the classical four marketing P's to services. This part includes chapters on developing service products, distributing services, service pricing and promoting services. The third part is about managing the customer interface, including designing and managing service processes, capacity management, crafting the service environment and managing people. The last part is about implementing profitable service strategies through managing relationships, service recovery, improving service quality and productivity, and striving for service leadership.

The third reviewed service marketing textbook is *Services Marketing – An Interactive Approach* by R.P. Fisk, S.J. Grove and J. John focusing on managing service experience [8]. The obligatory foundations part on understanding service marketing, frameworks for managing customer experience and the influence of the information age on services. The second part focuses on creating the interactive service experience, including planning and producing the service performance, designing the service setting, leveraging the people factor, and managing the customer mix. The third part is about making service promises through service pricing and service promotion. The fourth part deals with delivering service experience and ensuring its success. This part includes customer loyalty and service quality, service recovery and researching service success and failure. The last part details management issues specific to services, such as developing a marketing strategy, dealing with fluctuating demand and globalization.

The last reviewed service textbook originated in the marketing domain is *Service Management and Marketing – Customer Management in Service Competition* by C. Grönroos. This service marketing textbook is mostly based on research from the Nordic school of marketing. Seventeen chapters present concepts such as service quality, service productivity, service culture, and internal marketing [9].

Service marketing textbooks inherently take a front-office perspective and focus on customer management. At least to a certain extend, every service marketing textbook also deals with service operations in topics such as empowerment, service recovery, and managing capacity and demand. In addition to this, with a focus on teaching service science, dedicated service management and operations textbook provide more details on the back-office perspective.

3.2   Management and Operations Textbooks

The first reviewed example for a textbook bridging the gap between service marketing and service operations is *Service Management: Operations, Strategy, Information Technology* by J.A. Fitzsimmons and M.J. Fitzsimmons [10]. In four parts, different topics on service management are presented. The first part introduces the nature of service and its implications for service operations. Part two details how to design a service enterprise. Part three covers the classical service operations topics, such as managing capacity and demand, managing waiting lines, and supplier management. Part four subsequently presents corresponding quantitative methods and models which are applied in service operations.

The second reviewed service operations textbook is *Service Operations Management - Improving Service Delivery* by Johnston and Clark [11]. After an introduction into service operations and definitions of services in the first part, the second part deals with managing customer and supplier relationships. Part three focuses on service delivery and how to design and manage service processes, how to manage people in service businesses, how to utilize resources and leverage technology. Part four is dedicated to performance management and how to measure performance and drive operational improvement. Part five deals with the strategic change of service organizations, including service culture and handling organizational complexity.

The last reviewed service operations textbook is *Service Science* by Daskin [12]. This textbook is very much focused on quantitative methods, in particular methods from mathematical optimization. Consequently, topics such as workforce scheduling, resource allocation planning, location problems, and vehicle routing are presented.

While service operations textbooks are already very much concerned with implementing and delivering services, the question of which technology is relevant in a service context is left open in the reviewed service marketing, as well as service operations textbooks.

3.3   Computer Science Textbooks

There is a number of computer science textbooks which are related to service science. They can be classified into two major streams: IT service management and literature on services as a programming paradigm for loosely coupled computation entities with well defined interfaces. Because of this huge amount of textbooks, only one representative of each category is reviewed.

An example for an IT service management textbook is *Foundations of IT Service Management with ITIL* by Orand and Villarreal [13]. This textbook covers the entire ITIL service lifecycle, including IT service strategy, IT service design, IT service transition, IT service operation, and IT continual service improvement. The proposed best practices and frameworks are mostly only applicable to IT service management.

An example for a textbooks dealing with services as a programming paradigm is *Enterprise SOA - Service-Oriented Architecture Best Practices* by Krafzig et al. [14]. This textbook describes how companies can leverage technologies such as web services for organizing and integrating their IT systems.

4 An Interdisciplinary Service System Textbook

This short paper presents the outline of a forthcoming textbook (blinded for review) integrating several disciplines related to service science, such as business and economics, quantitative sciences, and computer science. The textbook consists of ten chapters: Foundations, Electronic Services, Service Innovation, Service Design, Service Semantics, Service Analytics, Service Optimization, Service Co-creation, Service Markets, and Service Research.

The first chapter (Foundations) describes the growing importance of services due to several reasons. It provides several service definitions and makes use of the IOT concept from service operations to explore the nature of services. Furthermore, services are contrasted with goods with regards to their marketing and management implications.

The second chapter is dedicated to electronic services with regards to two paradigms: the automation of services with ICT and service as programming paradigms. Furthermore, a classification of service systems with regards to their role of information technology, service architectures, strategies, and business models is presented. In addition, various service types and paradigms that exist are detailed and set into context: electronic services, web services, service-oriented architectures, cloud services, and internet of services.

The third chapter (Service Innovation) introduces basic definitions and types of innovation. Furthermore, particular challenges and opportunities of innovation in services firms are faced with are presented. Methods which can be applied in the context of service innovation are presented. Lastly, servitization and different types of product-service-systems which are important for manufacturers to innovate their service business are introduced.

The fourth chapter (Service Design) introduces service design as a human-centric approach for creating and improving services. The chapter explores the relationship between service innovation and service design and explores the role of service design within the last decades. Furthermore, key characteristics of service design are explored. A typical service design process is detailed, and specific core methods of service design, such as stakeholder maps, personas, customer journey maps, and blueprints are discussed.

The fifth chapter (Service Semantics) deals with enriching the description of cloud services with semantic knowledge. Therefore, the limitations of describing cloud services with natural language are explained. The chapter details how cloud services are programmatically accessed by means of Web APIs. Linked USDL and semantic technologies are introduced as a means to describe cloud services. Furthermore, graph patterns for describing REST services and search algorithms making use of semantic service descriptions are introduced.

The sixth chapter (Service Analytics) deals with capturing, processing, and analyzing the data generated from the execution of a service system to improve, extend, and personalize a service to create value for providers and customers. Therefore, the concept of service analytics and its various related tasks are detailed. Furthermore, data mining methods such as classification, prediction, and association rules and their application to service systems are explored. Lastly, a real-world scenario how analytics can support the execution of IT services is presented.

The seventh chapter (Service Optimization) introduces the application of mathematical optimization for planning problems in a service context. After a short introduction into the basic concepts of mathematical optimization, a number of planning problems are detailed. Furthermore, OPL models for solving these problems using IBM's ILOG CPLEX are discussed.

The eighth chapter (Service Co-creation) describes the relationship between co-creation of value in service systems, service encounters, service quality, and service productivity. In addition, the nature of relationships in a service co-creation context and concepts and methods to manage customer relationships are introduced.

Finally, the concept of customer participation, different customer roles and how to manage customer participation is detailed.

The ninth chapter (Service Markets) studies the economic and business components of services. This chapter starts with an introduction into the application of basic microeconomic systems in a service context. Furthermore, business and pricing models in service markets are introduced. Key challenges in addressing economic questions with an implicit understanding of their core assumptions are explored in a service context. Lastly, multi-agent systems as a methodological framework for addressing economic questions in service systems are introduced.

The tenth chapter (service research) presents two examples of research streams in service science: service network analysis and service level engineering. The first stream includes describing service networks and detail how service networks can be reconstructed using the web as a large-scale database. The second stream highlights the importance of service level objectives and presents a methodology for determining customer-optimal service level objectives.

5   Conclusion

This paper reviewed existing service textbooks and and discussed their shortcomings with regards to teaching service science. While a number of textbooks exist for established and isolated fields such as service marketing, there has been no integrated and interdisciplinary source, which can be utilized as a text for teaching service science. This paper presented the outline of such a new textbook, integrating content from several disciplines such as economics, business, IT, operations research, and math. This enables lecturers to supplement their lecture material with a corresponding textbook or build an entire course based on the provided and class-proven teaching material.

References

1. Spohrer, J., Maglio, P.P., Bailey, J., Gruhl, D.: Steps toward a science of service systems. Comput. (Long. Beach. Calif). **40**, 71–77 (2007)
2. Spohrer, J.C., Gregory, M., Ren, G.: The Cambridge-IBM SSME white paper revisited. In: Maglio, P.P., Kieliszewski, C.A., Spohrer, J.C. (eds.) Handbook of Service Science, pp. 677–706. Springer, Heidelberg (2010)
3. Vargo, S.L., Lusch, R.F.: Evolving to a new dominant logic for marketing. J. Mark. **68**, 1–17 (2004)
4. Hottum, P., Schaff, M., Müller-Gorchs, M., Howahl, F., Görlitz, R.: Capturing and measuring quality and productivity in healthcare service systems. In: Proceedings of the 21st International RESER Conference, pp. 1–11 (2011)
5. Zeithaml, V.A., Bitner, M.J., Gremler, D.D.: Services Marketing: Integrating Customer Focus Across the Firm. McGraw-Hill Irwin, New York (2006)
6. Zeithaml, V.A., Berry, L.L., Parasuraman, A.: Communication and control process in the delivery of service quality. J. Mark. **52**, 35–48 (1988)
7. Lovelock, C.H., Wirtz, J.: Services marketing: people, technology, strategy. Pearson Education International, Upper Saddle River (2004)
8. Fisk, R.P.: Services Marketing - An Interactive Approach. Cengage Learning (2013)
9. Grönroos, C.: Service Management and Marketing. Customer Management in Service Competition. John Wiley and Sons, Hoboken (2007)
10. Fitzsimmons, J.A., Fitzsimmons, M.J.: Service Management: Operations, Strategy, and Information Technology. McGraw-Hill/Irwin, New York (2006)
11. Johnston, R., Clark, G.: Service Operations Management: Improving Service Delivery. Pearson Education, Boston (2005)
12. Daskin, M.S.: Service Science. Wiley, Hoboken (2011)
13. Orand, B., Villarreal, J.: Foundations of IT Service Management: With ITIL. CreateSpace Independent Publishing Platform (2011)
14. Krafzig, D., Banke, K., Slama, D.: Enterprise SOA: Service-Oriented Architecture Best Practices (2004)

Research and Education in Service Science Management and Engineering: The Case of the Italian Service Management Forum

Sergio Cavalieri[1(✉)], Mario Rapaccini[2], Giuditta Pezzotta[1],
and Nicola Saccani[3]

[1] CELS, Department of Management, Information and Production Engineering,
Università degli Studi di Bergamo,
Dalmine, BG, Italy
{sergio.cavalieri,giuditta.pezzotta}@unibg.it
[2] IBIS LAB - Department of Industrial Engineering,
Università di Firenze, Florence, Italy
mario.rapaccini@unifi.it
[3] RISE Laboratory, Department of Industrial and Mechanical Engineering,
Università degli Studi di Brescia, Brescia, Italy
nicola.saccani@unibs.it

Abstract. The paper describes an initiative carried out on the Italian territory, the ASAP Service Management Forum, as an exemplary practice contributing to spreading the service management culture across firms as well as cross-fertilizing good practices and the development of joint academia-practitioners's research and education initiative. Within the ASAP Service Management Forum community, in particular, an extensive study has been carried out about the competence needed for service management roles and the professional lifelong training activities carried out at company level. Moreover, an analysis of the educational activities carried out at the M.Sc. or post-master level in Italy and abroad has been carried out. The results of these studies show that despite the growing interest and development of activities and educational activities in the field there is still a largely untapped potential in this area.

Keywords: Servitization · Education · Courses · ASAP service management forum · Community

1 Introduction

Servitization has been defined as "market packages or 'bundles' of customer-focused combinations of goods, services, support, self-service and knowledge" in the seminal paper by [1], and more recently as "the innovation of an organisation's capabilities and processes to better create mutual value through a shift from selling product to selling Product-Service-systems." [2].

Besides the benefits that a manufacturing company can achieve from servitization pointed out by the scientific literature [3], this transformation implies several challenges [4]. If not thoroughly addressed, such challenges may lead to the so-called

© Springer International Publishing Switzerland 2016
T. Borangiu et al. (Eds.): IESS 2016, LNBIP 247, pp. 750–760, 2016.
DOI: 10.1007/978-3-319-32689-4_58

"servitization paradox" [5] and an increased service offering can even reduce the chances of survival of a firm [6].

In such a context, servitizing manufacturers should emphasize the diffusion of a service culture within the firm, and the development of a service orientation among its employees. As identified by [7] one of the main challenges in service oriented research is to develop and maintain a service culture. They identified five main topic areas to enhance the service culture:

1. Recruiting, training, and rewarding associates for a sustained service culture
2. Developing a service mind-set in product-focused organizations
3. Creating a learning service organization by harnessing employee and customer knowledge
4. Keeping a service focus as an organization grows, matures, and changes
5. Globalizing a service organization's culture across different countries

To support the dissemination of the service culture, it results fundamental to look at current higher education and lifelong training offerings in order to direct them to match the emerging demand for service-oriented education [8] and to increase the collaborations between the Academia and manufacturing companies in research, education and transfer projects.

Manufacturing firm top management have often little knowledge about services and are ill-equipped to face the heterogeneity of the problems related to the servitization of their business [8]. To facilitate and accelerate the servitization process in the manufacturing companies it is first of all necessary to carry out executive training in order to provide a direct channel to those who may already have the power to introduce changes in the manufacturing companies [9].

However, the development of training and education offering is still inadequate as the service economy continues to grow [10]. In fact, even if university education is a prime outlet of knowledge for students during [8] and allows having people already trained in service, service-oriented courses both in business and in engineering schools are still lacking, in particular in the Italian case - object of this study.

To overcome the above mentioned gaps, the ASAP Service Management Forum (ASAP-SMF), an Italian industry-academia initiative, has been established with the purpose of promoting the service culture and excellence in service management and engineering (Fig. 1).

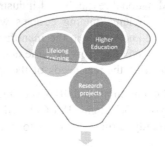

Service-oriented culture

Fig. 1. ASAP service management forum ingredients for increasing a service-oriented culture

In this sense, the ASAP-SMF operates today as a community where scholars and practitioners of several leading manufacturing companies, consulting firms and service providers, collaborate in developing both training and education about service management and service-oriented research projects and share findings in the servitization and product-service management fields (see Fig. 1).

2   The ASAP Service Management Forum: A Community Model

The ASAP Service Management Forum is a scientific and cultural initiative that originated as a follow-up of a two year research project funded by the Italian Ministry of Research, named "ASAP - After Sales Advanced Planning - new logistics and organizational models for the integrated management of after-sales service". Five Italian Universities carried out in the period 2002-2004 an extensive and thorough survey on the current state of the art of the Italian after sales market focusing in particular on four main industries: automotive/motorbike, consumer electronics, domestic appliances and micro-informatics.

Given the high pressure from industry, consultancy, software vendors and academia, involved in this research initiative, to proceed on investigating, an Industry-Academia Service Management Forum was established in 2005.

The Mission of the ASAP-SMF is to promote service culture and excellence in service management. It operates today as a community where scholars and practitioners of several leading manufacturing companies, consulting firms and service providers, collaborate in developing research projects, share findings and educate students and employees in the servitization and product-service management and engineering fields.

More specifically:

- It aims at eliciting industry "best practices" within service activities, by working in close partnership with a wide range of actors playing in the Italian panorama: from small-medium enterprises to large companies.
- It provides knowledge, competencies, services, fellowship and peer-to-peer connections in the field of product-service systems, supporting managers and executives within their decision, organizational and operative processes.
- It promotes and catalyses companies' involvement in research projects within the umbrella of European and national research and industrial programs.
- It co-designs and delivers lifelong training courses with companies in order to improve the service-oriented knowledge in the manufacturing context.
- It supports Universities in creating service oriented courses at graduate and post-graduate levels considering the real needs of the market.

In 2015 the Forum could count on around 40 associated companies, among which Electrolux, Cannon, IBM, ABB, DeLonghi, IVECO, IBM, a.o. The ASAP Service Management Forum is currently structured into four sections, each specifically industry-oriented:

- *Durable consumer goods*, inclusive of domestic appliances, consumer electronics, heating systems;
- *Automotive*, for private, industrial and commercial vehicles, and motorbikes;
- *Machinery*, spanning from tooling machines to power plant systems;
- *Digital Systems*, inclusive of server and networking systems, printers and copiers, and professional imaging systems.

The main activities carried out by the ASAP-SMF are:

- *Research*, including Industry and Cross-industries Surveys; R&D funded Projects; Editing of papers and books on Service Management
- *Networking and dissemination*, through Conferences on Service Management & Industry Workshops
- *Training and Education*, through company or multi-company projects and training and educational programs

The main topics on which the Forum operates are reported in Fig. 2.

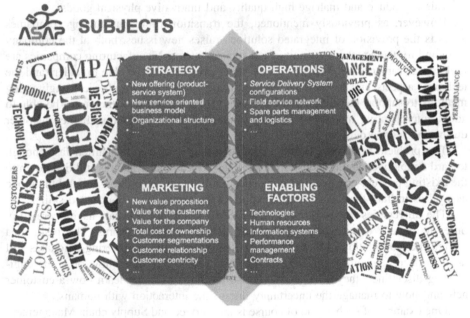

Fig. 2. Main topics with which the ASAP forum operates

The Forum also adopts a web-based tool to foster the discussion about service management through its website, and the social networks (a Twitter account and a closed group on LinkedIn), where feedbacks from the managers are collected.

Moreover, it carries out *Focus Groups*, based on roundtables involving interested companies on a specific topic preceded and followed by research and benchmarking activities concerning the same companies, which are designed and discussed in the roundtables.

Focus Groups have been or are being carried out so far on the topics:

- Industrial and light commercial vehicles service network management and service offering
- Full service contracts and Business Process Outsourcing
- Installed Base information management
- The Servitization of car manufacturers
- Customer centricity
- ICT and digitalization of service processes

The next sections will provide more details about the education and training activities carried out within the umbrella of the Forum.

3   The Educational Activities at the Master Level

In Italy, the education of engineers is mainly oriented towards the technical requirements since, in the general understating, those professional figures have to be educated to design, produce and manage high quality and innovative physical goods.

However, as previously mentioned, the transition of manufacturing companies towards the provision of integrated solutions raises new issues, both at the company level and for the country's economic and social systems. Manufacturing companies are looking for career briefs with new skills; these profiles must be able to understand the technical aspects and the new technology issues, and to adopt classical engineering methods to support the design and execution of a product. Also, they must be able to adopt interpretative models to properly understand and interact with the customer during the service delivery process.

The problem is that the world's educational system has not shifted fast enough toward a rapidly changing industry [11] and the educational system is still tied down to the existing product-oriented discipline silos. Only in few institutions around the globe as well as in Italy there has been an explicit will towards service-oriented skills.

The universities involved in the ASAP-SMF in the last 10 years have operated in order to include service oriented courses in engineering programs. The main idea behind the introduction of these courses is that even if the engineering graduates still need to deeply acquire technical expertise and technology know-how on some engineering disciplines, they also need to get softer skills [12] and learn how a customer acts and how to manage the uncertainty due to the interaction with humans.

One example of such a kind of course is the Service and Supply chain Management course developed at the University of Bergamo for students of the Master of Science in Management Engineering.

In particular, during the Service and Supply Chain Management course, the student acquires the necessary elements and concepts related to the service business both in pure service and in manufacturing industries. The course deals with service design and engineering, organization, management and performance measurement.

Table 1. Service and supply chain management course syllabus at Bergamo University

Title	Main contents
Introduction	Definition of service; the main characteristics of services (intangibility, inseparability, perishability, variability); the driving forces behind the growth of services; the servitization of manufacturing
Classification of services	A service portfolio management framework; Lovelock's matrixes; Product-Service offerings: classification dimensions
Service Engineering & Operations	Definitions; service engineering process models; Service Engineering & operations methods (service blueprinting, value & functional analysis, service QFD); Service Engineering tools: ServLab, service explorer
The Service Capacity	Capacity management in service, waiting time vs. customer satisfaction, queuing theory, determining the capacity level; yield management
Performance measurement of Services	An integrated performance measurement system; customer satisfaction and customer loyalty; the determinants of customer satisfaction; the gap model; the SERVQUAL model

At the end, the student has the basic knowledge and skills of a service manager and engineer and they should have assimilated an understanding of (Table 1):

- the main service characteristics and classification models
- service capacity management
- the main service engineering characteristics and methods

Another example is the Service Management course carried out at the University of Florence. The main aim of the course is to provide to students a general understanding of service business, of its distinctive characteristics and how these characteristics affect the way service should be managed. The syllabus is reported in the Table 2:

Table 2. Course syllabus of the Service Management course at the University of Florence

Title	Main contents
Fundamentals	Unified Services Theory Basics
	Services Fundamentals: Planning
	Services Fundamentals: Execution
	Understanding Non-Services (manufacturing)
Service Business Strategy	Identifying Strategic Opportunities
	Identifying Strategic Threats
Managing Service Processes	Cost Issues
	Human Resources Management
	Marketing in Services
	Production and Inventory Control
	Service blueprinting

(Continued)

Table 2. (*Continued*)

Title	Main contents
Service Quality and Value	Defining Service Quality
	Challenges in Delivering Service Quality
	Service Recovery
	Measuring Service Quality and Productivity
Servitization of manufacturing	Servitization of manufacturing

4   The Professional Lifelong Training

As said, servitization is quite challenging as it requires changes to operational practices [2], as well as the shift of people mindset [13].

As long as managers became aware that this transition can get hindered by significant competency gaps, they start claiming for professional training. This was observed in a number of times, as managers participating to workshops and focus groups continuously solicited the ASAP-SMF to provide answers to how service managers and service networks could be effectively trained.

Determining which competences should be developed in a servitizing environment became so relevant that the committee decided to dedicate one annual conference to the topic "Human resources: the key to compete in a service business".

We surveyed the internet and found information about +80 initiatives regarding professional training of service networks, mostly promoted by product manufacturers through the corporate training centres (e.g. company university or academy). We then purposively selected some leading firms in business and consumer markets. Initially we focused on the automotive industry, and visited the Fiat Training Academy in Turin, the BMW training center in Milan, and the Toyota Headquarter in Rome. We explored which courses were provided, to which professionals, to create which skills, how frequently, through which systems/practices, which resources were involved, what benefits/incentives people would expect from training. In detail:

- It came out that leading companies were actually reconsidering how they should train their direct or indirect field-force to provide superior quality services. Especially in situations in which there was a clear attempt to differentiate the company's offering through services, lifelong training of service professionals was considered a must-have.
- Firms just recruited managers with specific expertise, asking them to reorganize the way service networks were trained, and to create training centres.
- We found that firms were commonly introducing distance-learning platforms, to enable always-on access to on-line courses. Training programs were completely re-designed, and efforts were put in determining the kind and amount of training that professionals should receive initially to be qualified for certain roles, and lifelong to maintain the company qualification and receive professional certifications. The most structured program for initial qualification did span over three years.
- Generally, calls for new training were issued as new products were developed. In some cases, this was a major issue, since shorter innovation cycles were pushing for

higher training needs that were perceived as not sustainable. To this concern, managers placed great expectation on distance learning systems.

- Another interesting finding relates to the fact that most manufacturing firms had shaped the organizational models of their assistance centres, to decide which kind of skills should be trained for each role. This model included also non-technical roles such as operating managers, marketing and communication managers, administration staff whose responsibilities, activities and competences were clearly defined. Therefore, training catalogues also included non-technical courses such as business management, accounting, marketing, communication, quality and environmental management, and so on.
- We collected clear evidences that interest around soft skills was arising: approx. 50 % of the catalogues included this kind of courses, and we found manifold initiatives to assess and improve communication and relational skills, leadership and such skills in front-line people and directors. Conversely, we found that less than 10 % catalogues included language courses.

Three interviews to HR managers of Canon Europe, SKF, and Kyocera pointed out the necessity of balancing vertical skills (e.g. known-how about product and process technologies) with managerial and relational skills.

After claiming for interdisciplinary education as the base of T-shaped professionals in service management, we showed that, at that time, only four of the MBA programs offered by top business schools in U.S included elective courses on service design, engineering and management.

Very few universities renowned for research on service management, such as the Center for Excellence in Service at Maryland University, the Center for Service Research and Education at Lally School of Management, the Center for Service Leadership at Arizona State University have in place master degree courses on topics related to service science, management and engineering. An outlook to Italian universities showed that there was still paucity of education initiatives for service managers. In the following months we started a focus group whose aim was to determine: (a) a model to represent - in the most general way - organization and roles of service divisions in manufacturing firms; (b) the set of key competences for each role.

Again, supported by service managers from manufacturing and service firms (e.g. Samsung, Kyocera, Mediamarket, Brembo, Stream Global Services, Candy, Indesit Group, LG, Electrolux Professional, Canon, Whirpool) we firstly confronted manifold organizational charts. We then agreed on a common architecture and went through pointing out the responsibility of each role (e.g. service director, marketing, technical support, product specialist, operations manager), and the competences requested for covering them successfully.

We distinguished among propaedeutic competences (e.g. math, statistics, business languages), technical and managerial competences (e.g. business management and accounting, marketing, operations management, legal, maintenance engineering, project management, health & safety issues) and relational/soft skills and attitudes (problem solving, empathy and emotional intelligence, ability to collaborate, and so on).

This work was quite useful as, in the following months we designed a catalogue of training courses, and created a project framework for delivering short (1 or 2 days) courses to service professionals. In 2010 this project framework was funded by Fondimpresa, and we provided +600 h of classes on different topics, ranging from spare parts logistic management to CRM and servitization strategies.

5 In-House Professional Courses

ASAP-SMF has also developed specific training courses commissioned by companies operating within the Forum with the aim to update the knowledge and other pertinent information of the employees working in the service department or with a close relation to it.

In Table 3 below examples of courses developed and of the main approaches used to support the learning process are reported.

Table 3. Examples of executive courses carried out by the ASAP Service Management Forum

Course Title	Industry	Main course content	Leaning approach used
Service Engineering	Power and automation industry	Servitization	
		Service Engineering	Theoretical lecture
		Application in the Truck Industry	Case Study Method
		Case study	
		Workshop: developing a restaurant service	
Service Management	Bank	Definition of service and of the main characteristics	Theoretical lecture
		The classification of pure services	Case Study Method
		Service Engineering & Operations	
		Performance Measurement System	
		The Service Capacity	
		Workshop: developing a restaurant service	
After-sales management	Textile machinery and electronics industry	Definition of service and of the main characteristics	Theoretical lecture
		Servitization of Manufacturing	Case Study Method
		Service Engineering & Operations	
		Performance Measurement System	

(Continued)

Table 3. (*Continued*)

Course Title	Industry	Main course content	Leaning approach used
		Spare Parts Management	
		Workshop: developing a restaurant service	
Spare parts management	Household and professional appliances	Spare parts distribution and logistics network configuration	Theoretical lecture
		Spare parts demand characteristics and forecasting methods	Case Study Method
		Supply chain collaboration for spare parts management	
Service network management	Household and professional appliances	Service network structure and configuration	Theoretical lecture
		Outsourcing vs. insourcing	Case Study Method
		Repair shops process model	
		Repair shops performance analysis	

6 Conclusions

In order to successfully undertake the servitization transformation, manufacturers should emphasize the diffusion of a service culture within the firm, and the development of a service orientation among their employees. Executive training is required in order to provide a direct channel to those who may already have the power to introduce changes in the manufacturing companies. The paper describes an initiative carried out on the Italian territory, the ASAP Service Management Forum, as an exemplary practice that contributes in spreading the service management culture across firms as well as the cross-fertilization of good practices and the development of joint academia-practitioners research and education initiative. Within the ASAP Service Management Forum community, an extensive study has been carried out in particular about the competence needed for service management roles and the professional life-long training activities carried out at a company level. Moreover, an analysis of the educational activities carried out at the M.Sc. or post-master level in Italy and abroad has been performed. The results of these studies show that despite the growing interest and development of activities and educational activities in the field there is still a largely untapped potential in this area. The academic community should therefore cover a leading role in addressing and understanding the needs of the practitioners' community about service management and promote joint initiatives.

References

1. Vandermerwe, S., Rada, J.: Servitization of business: adding value by adding services. Eur. Manage. J. **6**(4), 314–324 (1998)
2. Baines, T., Lightfoot, H.W., Evans, S., Neely, A., Greenough, R., Peppard, J., Roy, R., Shehab, E., Braganza, A., Tiwari, A.: State-of-the-art in product-service systems. Proc. Inst. Mech. Eng. **221**(10), 1543–1552 (2007)
3. Neely, A.: Exploring the financial consequences of the servitization of manufacturing. Oper. Manage. Res. **1**, 103–118 (2008)
4. Alghisi, A., Saccani, N.: Internal and external alignment in the servitization journey–overcoming the challenges. Prod. Plann. Control **26**(14–15), 1219–1232 (2005)
5. Gebauer, H., Fleisch, E., Friedli, T.: Overcoming the service paradox in manufacturing companies. Eur. Manage. J. **23**(1), 14–26 (2005)
6. Benedettini, O., Neely, A., Swink, M.: Why do servitized firms fail? A risk-based explanation. Int. J. Oper. Prod. Manage. **35**(6), 946–979 (2015)
7. Ostrom, A.L., Bitner, M.J., Brown, S.W., Burkhard, K.A., Goul, M., Smith-Daniels, V., Rabinovich, E.: Moving forward and making a difference: research priorities for the science of service. J. Serv. Res. **13**(1), 4–36 (2010)
8. Bitner, M.J., Brown, S.W.: The evolution and discovery of services science in business schools. Commun. ACM **49**(7), 73–78 (2006)
9. Gummesson, E., Lusch, R., Vargo, S.: Transitioning from service management to service-dominant logic: Observations and recommendations. Int. J. Qual. Serv. Sci. **2**(1), 8–22 (2010)
10. Borangiu, T., Curaj, A., Dogar, A.: Fostering innovation in services through open education and advanced IT. In: International Joint Conference on Computational Cybernetics and Technical Informatics (2010)
11. Maglio, P.P., Srinivasan, S., Kreulen, J.T., Spohrer, J.C.: Service Systems, Service Scientists, SSME and Innovation. Commun. ACM **49**(7), 81–85 (2006)
12. Cunha, J.F., Patrício, L., Camanho, A., Fisk, R.: A master program in services engineering and management at the University of Porto. In: Hefley, B., Murphy, W. (eds.) Service Science, Management and Engineering Education for the 21st Century, pp. 181–190. Springer, Heidelberg (2006)
13. Oliva, R., Kallenberg, R.: Managing the transition from products to services. Int. J. Serv. Ind. Manage. **14**(2), 160–172 (2003)

Author Index

Printed in the United States
By Bookmasters